Estimation	*Result*
Bilirubin (P, S)	0·1–0·5 mg./100 ml.
Glutamic oxaloacetic transaminase (S)	10–110 μ moles/hour/100 ml. (Modified from King, 1958)
Glutamic pyruvic transaminase (S)	10–110 μ moles/hour/100 ml. (Modified from King, 1958)
Aldolase (S)	Under 2 years: up to 25 Bruns units/ml. Over 2 years: 5–15 Bruns units/ml. (Bruns, 1954)
Cholesterol (S)	Under 1 month: 80–160 mg./100 ml. Over 1 month: 100–220 mg./100 ml. (Carr and Drekter, 1956)
Protein-bound iodine (venous; S)	3·3–7·4 μg./100 ml. (Grossman and Grossman, 1955)
Iron (P, S)	27–153 μg./100 ml.
Iron-binding capacity (P, S)	168–500 μg./100 ml.

N.B.—Great variation from day to day

Lead (B)	Under 40 μg./100 ml.
Uric acid (P, S)	1–4 mg./100 ml.
Cortisol (venous; P)	7–14 μg./100 ml. (Sweat, 1955)
Amylase (S)	Newborn—none Appears at 2 months After 1 year: 60–180 Somogyi units/100 ml.

Normal findings in other body fluids are shown at the back of the book.

SICK CHILDREN

DONALD PATERSON'S
SICK
CHILDREN

DIAGNOSIS AND TREATMENT

by

REGINALD LIGHTWOOD

M.D.(Lond.), F.R.C.P.(Lond.), D.P.H.(Eng.)

Director, Pædiatric Unit, St. Mary's Hospital Medical School, University of London, and Physician-in-Charge, Children's Department, St. Mary's Hospital, London. Physician to The Hospital for Sick Children, Great Ormond Street, London. Pædiatrician to the Research Unit for Juvenile Rheumatism, Canadian Red Cross Memorial Hospital, Taplow. Senior Examiner in Medicine, University of London. Examiner for the Diploma of Child Health, Conjoint Board in England.

and

F. S. W. BRIMBLECOMBE

M.D.(Lond.), F.R.C.P.(Lond.), D.C.H.

Pædiatrician, Royal Devon and Exeter Hospital, Exeter City Hospital, Torbay Hospital and North Devon Infirmary; Consultant Pædiatrician, Exeter Clinical Area. Sometime Acting Assistant Director, Pædiatric Unit, St. Mary's Hospital Medical School, University of London.

EIGHTH EDITION

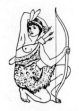

CASSELL · LONDON

CASSELL & COMPANY LTD

35 Red Lion Square · London WC1

and at

MELBOURNE · SYDNEY · TORONTO · CAPE TOWN
JOHANNESBURG · AUCKLAND

———

New material in this edition © Cassell & Co. Ltd. 1963

First published	-	-	1930
Seventh Edition	-	-	1956
Reprinted	-	-	1956
Reprinted	-	-	1957
Reprinted	-	-	1960
Eighth Edition	-	-	1963

Printed in Great Britain by The Chapel River Press Ltd., Andover, Hants.

PREFACE TO THE EIGHTH EDITION

WHEN, in 1948, Dr. Donald Paterson left the Westminster Hospital and The Hospital For Sick Children, Great Ormond Street, to return to Canada, his departure created a vacuum in British pædiatrics. He was not only the sole author of " Sick Children " and part-author of " Modern Methods of Feeding in Infancy and Childhood " (Constable & Co., Ltd.), but he had manifold activities besides. His foresight and tireless energy had enabled him to take the lead in founding the British Pædiatric Association and to bring out two editions of " Diseases of Children ", a major work published by Edward Arnold & Co. Indeed, it could be said that during most of the decade before his return to Canada, he came to dominate pædiatrics both in London and in the home counties. Yet it is not just for these achievements that his pupils and colleagues remember him, but rather for his happy knack of stimulating to further endeavour, encouraging despite every reverse.

Dr. Paterson, now in retirement in Vancouver, is still active in supporting health programmes for Canadian children. In England, he has not been forgotten by his old colleagues or by his former patients; a " Donald Paterson Essay Prize " is to be awarded biennially by the British Pædiatric Association to commemorate his work for the Association.

The preparation of the present edition has necessarily been our entire responsibility, and with the wide-ranging advances in pædiatrics the revision has had to be a radical one. The emphasis on diagnosis and treatment has been retained, and although we have concerned ourselves primarily with the common disorders, we have not hesitated to make brief mention of rare diseases, particularly those in which recent advances in knowledge have occurred. At the same time, we have endeavoured to strike a balance between physical and emotional disorders, as they present in childhood, and to describe the variations that occur in normal development. The final result does not purport to be a complete reference book; it is intended rather as a working manual for the medical student, the postgraduate undergoing pædiatric training, and the practising doctor at home or overseas.

Our task of revision could not have been achieved without the advice and help of colleagues. We owe a special debt of gratitude to Dr. Mildred Creak, Physician-in-charge of the Department of Psychiatry at The Hospital For Sick Children, London, who has written for this edition a new and most valuable chapter on the " Emotional Disorders of Childhood ". Professor Cicely Williams, who is an inspiration to all who are interested in the welfare of children in the emerging

v

countries, has again brought up to date her chapter on " Diseases of Children in the Tropics ", and Dr. J. P. M. Tizard, Reader in Child Health in the University of London, has kindly revised his chapters on " Disorders of the Nervous System " and " Mental Subnormality "; to both of them, we express our appreciation for giving so generously of their knowledge and skill.

Pædiatricians and colleagues in other disciplines in many parts of the world have sent us constructive suggestions for the improvement of the book, while overseas doctors, during their postgraduate studies in Britain, have helped us to understand the varying needs of children of different races living in different climates.   To these and many others who do not appear by name in the text we extend our grateful thanks.

R.L.

1963.   F.S.W.B.

EXTRACT FROM THE PREFACE TO THE
FIRST EDITION

In this Manual I have attempted to deal with the commoner diseases of childhood as completely as the limits of space allowed, keeping constantly in view the needs of the senior student and the general practitioner.   The reader, I hope, will find that the descriptions of symptoms, though concise, are adequate, nor have ætiology and pathology been neglected;   but, as the title suggests, the main stress has been laid on diagnosis and treatment as the surest way of making the book practical and helpful.

1930.   Donald Paterson.

ACKNOWLEDGEMENTS

OUR thanks are due to Dr. Barbara Clayton, Consultant Chemical Pathologist at The Hospital For Sick Children, Great Ormond Street, who has kindly revised the tables of normal values which appear on the end pages of this book; to Dr. J. M. Tanner, Reader in Growth and Development at the Institute of Child Health of the University of London, who has allowed us to reproduce the tables of normal heights and weights in Appendix 5; to Dr. P. J. N. Cox, Assistant Director of the Pædiatric Unit, St. Mary's Hospital, London, for helpful criticisms of Chapter 11; and to Mr. A. G. Allnutt, Chief Pharmacist at The Hospital For Sick Children, who has given us much assistance concerning the proper names and dosages of drugs.

We are indebted to Dr. Dorothy Taylor, lately Senior Medical Officer for Maternity and Child Welfare, Ministry of Health, for information on designated milks; and to Dr. Mary Paterson, London County Council Deputy Divisional Medical Officer, who advised on Appendix 7. Acknowledgements are gratefully given to Dr. J. L. Hamerton, Pædiatric Research Unit, Cytogenetic Section, Guy's Hospital Medical School, for the illustrations of karyotypes of human chromosomes in Fig. 58; to Sir Wilfred Sheldon, Professor A. A. Moncrieff, Dr. L. G. Blair, Dr. R. E. Bonham Carter, Dr. A. P. Norman, Sir Denis Browne and Mr. D. Waterston, and also to The Hospital For Sick Children for Figs. 4, 9, 10, 16, 17, 26, 28, 29, 42, 44, 46, 47, 48, 49, 50, 51, 54, 56, 61, 63, 64, 66, 76, 79, 83, and Plates V, VIII, IX, XII, XIV, and XVIII; to Dr. P. N. Cardew, Director of the Photographic Department, St. Mary's Hospital, for Figs. 8, 37, 38, 45, 52, 59 and Plate X; to Mr. Norman Capener and Mr. Geoffrey Blundell Jones, as well as to the Princess Elizabeth Orthopædic Hospital, Exeter, for Plates XIII, XV, XVI and XVII; to Mr. P. J. Fiske, A.I.B.P., A.R.P.S., Medical Photographer to the Special Unit for Juvenile Rheumatism, Canadian Red Cross Memorial Hospital, Taplow, for Figs. 30, 31, 34, 73 and Plate VI; to the Royal Devon & Exeter Hospital for Plates I, II and XI; to Messrs. Butterworth & Co. Ltd. for Fig. 6, for the diets on pp. 53-54 from "Pædiatrics for the Practitioner" edited by Gaisford and Lightwood, and for the children's diets on pp. 66-67 from the "British Encyclopædia of Medical Practice"; to the Editor of the *British Medical Journal* for the diet sheet on pp. 682-683; to the Editor of the *Lancet* for the Tables and diet on pp. 684-689; to the Editor of the *Archives of Diseases of Childhood* for Fig. 62; to the Editor of *Thorax* for Fig. 23; to the Year Book Publishers, Chicago, for the adaptions from "Inborn Errors of Metabolism", by Dr. David Hsia, used in Figs. 1-3; to Mr. Paul Bierstein for Fig. 89; to Dr. Ursula Shelley, Pædiatrician to the Royal Free Hospital, for Plate XXII;

vii

to the Perinatal Mortality Survey, The National Birthday Trust Fund, for Table XI; to Dr. E. D. Irvine, Medical Officer of Health for the City of Exeter, for Tables XXVI and XXVII; to Dr. E. M. M. Besterman for phonocardiograms recorded by him at the Canadian Red Cross Hospital; to the late Dr. Paul Wood for Plate IV; to Dr. W. W. Brigden for Plate VI; to Dr. J. F. Goodwin and Dr. R. E. Steiner for the angiocardiogram, Plate VII; to Dr. C. E. Stroud for Fig. 44; to Mr. Derek Martin, Assistant Curator at The Hospital For Sick Children, for advice on the illustrations; to Mr. I. W. J. Evans for technical help; and to Oxygenaire Ltd. for Fig. 5.

Our grateful thanks are due to Miss Edna Tilley of the Pædiatric Unit, St. Mary's Hospital, and to Miss Aileen Gubb, Miss E. Gwynn and Miss Elizabeth Preece for ever-willing secretarial help. The tolerance and courtesy of the printers and publishers have been unlimited, and they have earned our admiration and respect.

CONTENTS

ix

x

LIST OF PLATES

CHAPTER 1

History Taking and Clinical Examination

HISTORY TAKING

THE physician's task in eliciting an accurate history of the development
of an illness is usually as important as the subsequent physical examination of the patient, for often the diagnosis is suggested by the history
and is then confirmed by the examination.

In pædiatric practice the history of the illness has frequently to
be taken from a third person, usually the mother, and in assessing the
evidence the physician has to exercise considerable powers of judgement and experience before he can estimate, for example, the severity
of a pain *felt by that particular child as described by that particular mother.*
In organic disease the parent's attempted interpretation of the symptoms and accounts of the opinions of others are of little value, whereas
a factual report of symptoms is vital evidence. The mother, through
constant care of her child, is often a most reliable observer of small
temperamental and habit changes, and so reports of alterations of this
kind require close attention. Sometimes part of the reason, and
occasionally the whole reason, for the consultation is a secret fear of
disease, such as tuberculosis, on the part of the parents, rather than
any of the actually observed symptoms of illness. On the other hand,
where a nervous mother has good grounds for suspecting organic
disease, the presence of serious symptoms may be denied at the first
consultation and only admitted later, when a definite diagnosis has
already been made and explained to her.

Symptoms can often be suggested to a child by the parents. A
young girl may complain of the identical type of headache and
lassitude which she has heard so often described by her mother at
home. The whole circumstances of the home, the overcrowding, the
tenants underneath who dislike noise, the degree of stability of the
parents' marriage—all these reflect upon the child's reaction to
disease, be it organic or functional, and upon the description of the
child's symptoms as given by the mother. Where the doctor suspects
that a part or the whole of the patient's complaint is not organically
determined but is of emotional origin, he must be prepared, either
then or at a subsequent consultation, to set aside time in which the
mother may have the opportunity of confiding to him the underlying
problems that are disturbing the child and the whole family. On
such occasions it is the doctor's part to *listen* and to allow the mother

1

to give her account in her own way. Direct questioning should be reduced to the absolute minimum. However trivial the apparent reason for the consultation, the doctor has been consulted because a problem exists, and he has been paid the compliment of being asked to solve it.

DOCUMENTATION

Should the patient have been referred for consultation by another doctor, the physician should reply promptly with the report of his findings. Many hospitals justly acquire a bad reputation with general practitioners because of their delay in replying to letters, and it is clearly of the first importance to the patient that the liaison between practitioner and hospital should be very close. In the United Kingdom, at the present time, there is a danger of duplication of medical care. Welfare clinics or school clinics may make diagnoses and give treatment independently of the family doctor. It is of the greatest importance that doctors in each of these fields should make certain that this does not occur. On occasion the hospital pædiatric department, which should be aware of this danger, can, by sending copies of the findings and recommendations to both parties, resolve these difficulties.

In the general field of child care, there may be many people interested in the care of one child. Family doctor, medical officer of health, child psychiatrist, children's officer, health visitor and psychiatric social worker may, for example, all be concerned with one patient. It is vital that all such persons concerned with one child, or with one family, should be punctilious in their duty to consult with each other on questions of general management. Good manners, attention to detail and awareness of each other's problems will go far to avoid the friction and duplication of effort which will otherwise inevitably occur from time to time.

If a good history is to be obtained, it is important that both mother and child should be put as much at their ease as is possible at the start of the consultation. It is often helpful to interest the child in a toy or game before beginning to take the history, after which the mother can give her undivided attention to her account. Usually it is advisable that children with behaviour disorders be out of earshot while the mother recounts the symptoms. A nervous mother may often be put at her ease by the paying of a compliment on some aspect of the child's appearance or clothing.

Scheme of History Taking

The patient's name, address, date of birth, and father's occupation should be noted; if referred by another doctor, his name and address should be obtained, together with information as to the relationship of the person from whom the history is being taken.

Complaint. The reason for the consultation should be written in the original words of the person giving the history, e.g. " Very breathless on climbing one flight of stairs," *not* " Dyspnœa on exertion."

Present Illness. This is often the most important part of the whole consultation, and no trouble should be spared to obtain as accurate an account as possible. The mode of onset should be recorded in the fullest detail, and the appearance of additional symptoms should be carefully noted in the order in which they developed. Leading questions should be avoided as far as possible, but, if used a note should be included to that effect. Details of bodily functions, such as bowel movement, micturition, appetite, sleep, cough, and gain in weight, should be recorded as a routine.

PREVIOUS HISTORY

Birth History. The mother's health during pregnancy, the length of gestation, details of delivery, birth weight and neonatal state should be noted.

Infancy. The method of feeding, the age of weaning and ease with which it was carried out, and details of vitamin supplements to the diet should be recorded, together with details of all immunization procedures carried out.

Development. Sufficient details should be elicited at all times to provide a rough estimation of the rate of physical and mental development of the child. The age at which the first tooth erupts, of sitting up, crawling, standing, walking, talking, and the development of continence of urine and fæces, provide sufficient evidence in most cases; but where any possibility of special retardation of physical or mental growth is suspected, a much fuller enquiry will be required (*see* p. 20).

Past Illnesses. The details of all past illnesses, accidents and operations should be recorded, together with the dates at which they occurred. If hospital admission has been necessary, the address of the hospital and the date of admission should be noted.

Family History. The health of the other members of the family and people with whom the child is in close contact should be noted. Special enquiry should be made as to the child's contact with anyone known to be suffering from tuberculosis.

Particular problems require detailed enquiry along particular lines; for example, in cases of obesity or dwarfism the heights and weights of the parents are extremely important; in suspected mongolism the age of the mother at the time of the child's birth may be valuable (*see* p. 470), and in possible genetic disease an enquiry as to consanguinity in the parents is required.

SOCIAL HISTORY

The home circumstances, number of rooms and type of residence occupied, sleeping accommodation of the child, dampness or other defect of the house, availability of lavatory and washing facilities, and presence of a garden or accessible recreation ground or park should be noted.

EMOTIONAL DISORDERS

Throughout this book emphasis is laid upon the importance of emotional disorders in childhood (*see* particularly Chapter 18). No formal scheme of history taking can be adopted in such cases, for much depends upon the doctor's own ability to gain his patients' confidence and so permit them to confide in him concerning the underlying anxieties and disharmonies which may beset the child and the family. When such problems are being described, the patient or parent must never be hurried and each should be allowed to tell his story in his own way. The doctor will learn infinitely more by *listening* than by asking questions.

EXAMINATION

MUCH greater care is necessary in examining a child than an adult. The physician is helped by the adult's own description of his symptoms, but with a child he must very often depend on the observations of the mother or nurse, which may be either helpful or the reverse.

For a thorough examination, an infant or child should be quiet and happy, and the co-operation of the mother or nurse is necessary to keep him amused. The physician will be amply repaid for the expenditure of a few moments spent at the beginning, chatting with the parents and the child so that the latter becomes accustomed to the physician's voice and person and gains confidence. A consulting room brightly furnished with toys and objects of interest to children of various ages will remove much of the fright of a visit to the doctor. There is much to be said for avoiding the use of a white coat, which may have become associated in the child's mind with an immunizing injection in a welfare clinic or with a previous hospital admission. Infants and small children are happiest when seated on the mother's knee, and they often cry if forced to lie down. Palpation, percussion and auscultation of the chest should be performed with warm fingers and stethoscope. Very often a play of examining a doll before listening to the child's chest will reassure him. Above all, there must be no hurry or brusqueness if the examination is to be made without tears. Young practitioners need not be discouraged, despite early failures, for experience will lead to success.

No examination is complete unless it includes a careful inspection of the ears and throat, for which patience is required. To see the tympanic membranes the physician must use a good auriscope and a fresh battery. When the rest of the examination is done, the throat should be quickly and carefully examined under good illumination. This often requires a degree of skill only attained with practice. The urine should always be examined and, where appropriate, a recently passed stool should be inspected.

THE HEAD

The measurement of the skull circumference gives valuable information in infancy. A very small head suggests microcephaly; a head which is too large suggests the possibility of hydrocephalus. Details of the average measurements are given in Table XXXIII, p. 679.

The shape of the head is also important. As infantile rickets heals, the parietal bones, and sometimes the frontal eminences, become thickened or bossed, with shallow grooves between the bosses. When these grooves run like the arms of a cross between the frontal and parietal bones, the shape of the skull resembles a hot-cross-bun. In lesser degrees of rachitic bossing, the head is merely large and square. With this may be contrasted the more spherical enlargement of hydrocephalus and its overhanging forehead. Rachitic grooves may also be found along the occipital sutures, in the situation where craniotabes (eggshell crackling) occurs at an earlier stage of the disease. *Plagiocephaly* is the name given to cranial asymmetry; it is not a serious condition and is usually the result of foetal posture; congenital torticollis is frequently associated with it. *Brachycephaly*, in which the antero-posterior diameter of the skull is greatly reduced and the occiput flattened, is characteristic of mongolism. In *dolicho-cephaly* the antero-posterior diameter is disproportionately long, as in Morquio's disease (*see* Fig. 62).

THE FONTANELLES

With the notable exceptions of microcephaly and craniostenosis, the anterior fontanelle remains patent as a rule until after 12 months, and in most infants properly protected from rickets it is usually closed at about 15 months. Delay in its closure after 18 months is regarded as abnormal; it may be an indication of past rickets, or a sign of hydrocephalus, or perhaps mongolism, cretinism, or achondroplasia. The posterior fontanelle and the sagittal fontanelle are usually almost closed at the time of birth, except in hydrocephalus and mongolism when these two apertures, together with the sagittal suture, close more slowly (p. 472).

THE SCALP

Normally the infant has a little soft down at birth, but occasionally there is thick black hair; by 6 months there is a good growth of new hair. In cretinism, the hair is straight, scanty and dry. In mongolism, the hair is straight, but softer. The scalp should always be examined to exclude ringworm and patches of alopecia, scurf and impetigo. In newborn babies a swelling of the scalp often appears at the site of presentation; this is the *caput succedaneum* and is really an œdema of the subcutaneous tissues (p. 99). Occasionally a cephal-hæmatoma may form (p. 99).

THE EYES

The condition of the eyelids, conjunctivæ, lens and cornea should be noted. Is there *strabismus*? In suitable cases the lens, vitreous and fundus should be examined with an ophthalmoscope, the pupils being dilated with homatropine if necessary. The disc of the newborn baby is usually pale compared with that of a child or adult.

An infant should begin to follow light at 3–4 weeks old and should see objects clearly by 2 months old. If not attracted by a light or unable to focus by this age, the baby is probably blind or mentally defective, or both. *Blindness* may be due to congenital cataract, congenital optic atrophy, congenital cerebral agenesis or to acquired conditions such as retinoblastoma or retrolental fibroplasia (*see* p. 83). Congenital abnormalities include ptosis, coloboma of the iris, etc., albinism and abnormalities of the retina and optic nerve (*see* p. 522).

Ptosis of the eyelids may be unilateral or bilateral, and the congenital variety is often familial. Acquired ptosis may be due to a lesion of the third cranial nerve or the cervical sympathetic.

In mongolism, the epicanthic folds are prominent, the palpebral fissure is almond-shaped and slants upwards.

Nystagmus may be congenital and familial, or it may be caused by imperfect central vision, as in congenital cataract or degeneration of the macula. In a rare condition called *spasmus mutans* (head nodding), a peculiar wobbling type of nystagmus is seen.

Squinting is common. A slight degree of internal strabismus is often seen in the early weeks of life, and this will frequently disappear as the acuity of vision increases. Other cases of internal strabismus may be due to imbalance of the extrinsic muscles, sometimes associated with errors of refraction. Paralytic squint is likely to be a sign of brain disease, such as cerebral palsy, meningitis or neoplasm. Squint may be more apparent than real, due to the eyes being set close together. In such a case, the absence of a true squint can be shown by standing in front of the child and looking to see if the reflection of light, visible in the pupil, is equally placed on the two sides.

THE NOSE

Patency of the nasal airway should be checked, and the presence of nasal discharge noted. When nasal obstruction is present, it is often caused by enlarged adenoids, sinusitis or by allergic rhinitis. In the newborn period, choanal atresia, in which a septum is found across the posterior nares, may cause acute respiratory obstruction. Nasal blockage in older children gives rise to mouth-breathing and perhaps a pinched-in appearance of the nose.

Chronic rhinitis often causes cough, usually because a post-nasal discharge causes pharyngitis or bronchitis (often alluded to as sinobronchitis). A foreign body in the nose causes a brown or bloodstained discharge from one nostril. Mouth-breathing is often associated with malocclusion of the teeth, with or without under-development of the mandible (micrognathia).

THE EARS

Deafness may easily be overlooked in the first years of life. Delay in talking or apparent backwardness should always arouse suspicion, but occasionally minor degrees of deafness, and particularly deafness limited to the higher tones only, may pass undetected well into school life (*see* p. 235).

An examination of the drums should be a routine procedure and is of especial importance where there is a fever without apparent cause. Wax may obscure the examination and must then be removed. Dry wax may need initial softening with olive oil drops. Syringing of the ears should be reserved for older children only.

COMPLEXION AND FACE

A healthy child is pictured as pink-cheeked and fair-skinned, but this varies with his parentage. The newborn infant is usually rather red-complexioned, then within a week or two his face becomes relatively pale and remains so until he is at least 2 or 3 months old, when a little more colour begins to appear. Certain children, especially those with auburn hair, are always pale-faced, although not anæmic; and very dark-haired families often have sallow skins.

Extreme thinness of the face is a sign in *lipodystrophia progressiva*. In the extreme emaciation of the marasmic infant the sucking-pads protrude in the cheeks, the rest of the face being wasted.

THE MOUTH, LIPS AND GUMS

The lips are cracked and excoriated in congenital syphilis (*rhagades*), and dry and cracked in feverish conditions. *Herpes* may appear as small blisters or crusts. The mouth is carp-shaped, or turns down at the corners, in mongolism and is open widely, allowing the huge tongue to protrude, in cretinism. The lips are pale and almost colourless in extreme anæmia and may become cyanosed in heart disease or pneumonia.

In scurvy the gums may be swollen, red and hæmorrhagic; in ulcerative stomatitis they are swollen and ulcerated. Koplik spots appear at the end of the prodromal stage of measles; they consist of tiny grey lesions with a surrounding halo of erythema situated on the buccal mucosa opposite the premolar teeth.

THE THROAT

When examining a child's mouth and throat, it is best to wrap him in a blanket or shawl, or else he should sit on his mother's knee. She should take both his hands in one of hers and hold his head firmly against her by placing her other hand over his forehead. The tongue can be depressed with a teaspoon, and the mouth and throat inspected with a pocket torch. The number and condition of the teeth should be noted. A glance should be sufficient to detect ulceration or thrush. Depressing the tongue brings the tonsils into view, and the presence or absence of exudate or of tonsillitis can be noted.

THE GLANDS

By palpating at the angle of the jaw, enlarged tonsillar glands can be felt and the glands draining the adenoid region can be detected behind the sternomastoid. The glands in the axilla and inguinal region should be palpated as a routine, and a careful examination made of the abdomen. When the glands of one axilla are enlarged, look for an infective lesion of the upper limb. With inguinal adenitis, look at the skin of the leg and the anal region. Generalized adenitis occurs in glandular fever, leukæmia and certain neoplastic conditions.

THE NECK

Palpation of the sternomastoid in a young infant will often reveal a small hard lump, due to a hæmatoma in the sternomastoid. Generally this disappears completely within a few weeks although very occasionally torticollis follows. Torticollis may also be due to congenital shortening of the sternomastoid muscle, causing the head to be held to one side. In such cases the child should be so placed on its pillow as to press the head into the correct position; simple stretching of the muscle under the direction of a physiotherapist makes operation unnecessary in the great majority of patients. Head retraction is seen in meningitis or hydrocephalus, or there may be a stiffness of the neck only, as in meningism, poliomyelitis, spinal caries and cervical adenitis.

THE CHEST AND ITS SHAPE

The chest should be examined first by inspection. Beading of the lower costochondral junctions is found in active rickets. Backward subluxation of the sternum suggests scurvy. In *osteogenesis imperfecta* there is a marked tendency to fracture of the ribs. If the chest be examined posteriorly the shape of the spine can be seen. Kyphosis may be due to faulty posture, but, if the deformity is fixed, vertebral disease should be sought.   Scoliosis, with or without malformation of the vertebræ, may be of congenital origin or may be the result of poliomyelitis or rickets.   More commonly, however, it is due to faulty posture and general hypotonia of the muscles.   Pigeon-chest results from rickets, accentuated by some form of respiratory obstruction or other cause of dyspnœa; thus it is seen in congenital heart disease, chronic pulmonary disease and nasal obstruction.   In asthma the chest may be barrel-shaped.   Marked depression of the sternum may be familial in origin and is often associated with an abnormal anterior attachment of the diaphragmatic tendon.   In the most severe cases, where the heart's action is embarrassed or where the vital capacity is greatly reduced, the deformity can be corrected surgically.

THE LUNGS

The breath-sounds in children are harsh, and expiration can be heard almost as prolonged as inspiration.   In a crying or teething child who is salivating, sounds referred from the trachea are heard throughout the chest.   Frequently, a slight diminution of air-entry, or an occasional crepitation, may indicate considerable underlying disease, but, on the whole, slight changes are much less significant than they are in the adult.   Percussion should be light and not carried to any extent below the angle of the scapula, as the liver and kidneys may give rise to dullness which will mislead.

THE HEART

Percussion of the area of cardiac dullness does not give information as accurate as palpating the apex-beat and feeling for the general cardiac impulse under the præcordium.   On auscultation the basal sounds are best heard to the left of the sternum.   The presence of a thrill over the præcordium, suggesting congenital malformation, should be noted.   The presence of normal pulsation of the femoral arteries should be noted as a part of the routine examination to exclude the presence of coarctation of the aorta.

THE ABDOMEN

The abdomen of the infant is normally rounded, and this fullness persists sometimes into the third or fourth year; by the age of five the abdominal muscles are firmer and the abdomen flatter.   An unduly large abdomen may be due to rachitic " pot-belly," ascites, cœliac disease, fibrocystic disease, tuberculosis, renal or other tumours, a distended bladder or gross enlargement of the liver or spleen.   Wind-swallowing and Hirchsprung's disease should also be considered.   The condition of the navel should be noted, especially in the newborn.

On palpating the abdomen, the liver should be outlined.   Normally this extends one to two fingers' breadths below the costal margin.   In cœliac disease, frequently it cannot be palplated.   In cirrhosis it can be felt, firm and hard, and enlarged to a greater or lesser extent. Enlargement of the liver is found in infective hepatitis, cardiac failure, leukæmia, syphilis, von Gierke's disease, Gaucher's disease, neoplasms, and other systemic diseases. The spleen is normally not palpable. The causes of splenic enlargement are very numerous. It is usual to find that the spleen is palpable in almost all generalized systemic infections, such as septicæmia, glandular fever, miliary tuberculosis, brucellosis and enteric fever. Malaria and leishmaniasis are among the infections in tropical countries which make splenomegaly almost a routine finding. Infective hepatitis and portal obstruction occasionally cause splenic enlargement. Other causes include blood diseases such as leukæmia, Hodgkin's disease and thrombocytopenic purpura. Both liver and spleen may be low in position and easily palpated when the thorax is narrowed by a deep Harrison's sulcus and the abdominal wall is flabby. Deep palpation of the abdomen for enlarged kidneys or other masses should be carried out. The child should be examined in a good light, standing, if possible, to allow herniæ to be seen, and the presence or absence of the testicles in the scrotum should be ascertained by palpation. Rectal examination should always be done whenever an acute abdominal condition is present. Pain on defæcation or a history of blood on the stool is an indication for a careful inspection of the anal margin to exclude an anal fissure.

THE LEGS AND ARMS

The shape of the legs and arms should be noted. Knock-knee or bow-leg suggests rickets. Abnormal shortness of the arms and legs is present in achondroplasia. Congenital dislocation of the hip should be detected in early infancy; there is limitation of abduction of the affected hip, and, when this movement is attempted passively, a click may be heard or felt by the manipulator (Ortolani's sign). Limping may be seen in simple trauma of the foot, leg or hip, or in tuberculous disease and pseudo-coxalgia. Talipes equinovarus should be detected at birth and treatment instituted forthwith. Pain on movement of the limbs in an infant suggests scurvy.

THE NERVOUS SYSTEM

Examination of the nervous system requires much patience and the child's co-operation; crying and resistance can make this examination almost valueless. First, the patient should be watched in movement and at play, then the limbs should be handled, and the rest of the examination will follow.

The tendon reflexes are obtained by tapping the tendon while the joint is at rest at about the mid-point of its range of movement and *with the muscles relaxed.* Reinforcement can be used in a doubtful case. In chorea, the knee-jerks are sometimes prolonged (" sustained ") or they may be absent, especially in the so-called " limp type " of chorea. In athetosis, rigidity of the muscles makes the limbs stiff (*extrapyramidal rigidity*); deformities may be present. In lesions of the pyramidal tract the affected limbs are also stiff, but in this case it is due to *spasticity*. On first stretching spastic muscles, the spasm may suddenly increase (spastic stretch reflex) and then suddenly relax (clasp-knife spasticity). The tendon reflexes will be increased, clonus may be present and the plantar reflexes extensor. But remember that in patients under 12–18 months the plantar reflex may be equivocal and a quick upward movement is a normal response. Absence of tendon reflexes is found in peripheral nerve injuries, polyneuritis, poliomyelitis, myopathy and Friedreich's ataxia.

Hypotonia and *inco-ordination* should be noted. Often formal tests of co-ordination are impracticable; if so, then the child's movements should be noted when he handles toys, undresses and dresses, or moves about in play. Through such observation, the presence of a tumour of the posterior fossa may come to be suspected.

Testing of sensation is often neglected in young children, yet this is usually feasible. In congenital hemiplegia, under-development of the affected limbs may be associated with unsuspected sensory loss (*see* p. 442).

The optic fundi should always be examined and the presence of strabismus recorded.

CONCLUSION

IN CONCLUSION the student should bear in mind that a medical consultation should have a definite form. First, the history, in which the parent or child is allowed ample time to describe in detail the symptoms for which medical advice has been sought, supplemented by the minimum of direct questioning necessary to obtain a clear picture of all the relevant factors. Second, the examination, which, together with the history, enables the doctor to make a diagnosis or at least to plan further investigation.

Invariably there should follow, in some measure, an explanation to the parents of the probable cause of the symptoms and the likely outcome of the illness. It is a matter of clinical judgement and experience, and indeed of the whole art of medicine to decide how detailed in any particular instance this explanation should be, but it should never be omitted altogether. Finally, the form of any treatment or further investigation should be explained to the parents and arrangements made to put it into operation.

This chapter must end with a few words of comfort and exhortation to the young practitioner. More errors are made from the failure to take a careful history and carry out a thorough clinical examination than from any other cause. If this simple rule is remembered, the foundations upon which medical practice is conducted are firm and upon them clinical judgement can be built.

CHAPTER 2

Heredity, Genetics, and Normal Development

HEREDITY AND GENETICS

As a result of new knowledge and of new hazards, the study of human genetics is assuming ever-increasing importance in medicine. In pædiatrics the investigation of inherited disorders has become one of the growing points of research at the present time.

Expressed in its simplest terms, the nuclear structure of a human cell contains 23 pairs of chromosomes, one of each pair being derived originally from each of the parents. As each cell divides, the daughter cells retain this same chromosomal pattern. An exception to this occurs in the gametes—spermatozoa and ovum—in which only one set of 23 chromosomes, one from each original pair of chromosomes, is represented. These will join to make up the 23 pairs of chromosomes in the newly formed embryo.

Each chromosome is subdivided longitudinally into innumerable areas or loci which contain the particular gene substances that determine the inherited characteristics of the individual. The different genes are distributed in a constant order along the length of each particular chromosome. One pair of chromosomes only is associated with sex differences, the female chromosome of this pair being designated X and the male Y. The remaining 22 pairs of chromosomes are known as autosomes.

Throughout the countless processes of cell division the individual genes remain extremely stable in their action. Only as a very great exception does a gene alter in its characteristic effect on the individual, but once such a change in genetic qualities (mutation) has occurred that gene will retain the new characteristic in all subsequent cell divisions. Thus, as a result of different mutations, an individual gene may exist in the population in several different forms, each of which is known as an *allele* form. If an individual inherits from each parent the same allele form of a particular gene he is said to be *homozygous* for this particular gene. If, however, the two allele forms of the particular gene under review are different then he is said to be *heterozygous* in this respect.

Where a particular allele form gives rise to an obvious physical characteristic when present only in the *heterozygous* form, it is said

12

to be a *dominant* gene, but if the particular characteristic only appears in the individual when the gene is *homozygous* it is said to be *recessive*.

Certain genes exert their action by modifying cell metabolism, a number of these processes being now identifiable by biochemical techniques; in such instances an individual who is heterozygous for a particular characteristic, but who does not overtly show the condition due to its suppression by the normal gene, can now be detected by biochemical testing. Thus, in a recessively inherited condition, such as phenylketonuria, in which the disease only appears in individuals homozygous for the particular gene, those relatives who are apparently normal, but who are in fact carriers of the particular allele gene, can be identified by the administration of large quantities of phenylalanine. In these individuals such overloading uncovers their relative inability to metabolize this amino-acid and abnormal metabolic products appear in the urine.

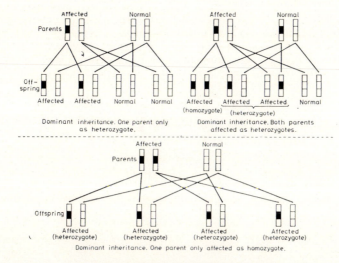

Fig. 1.   Mode of expression of dominant genes.

In Figs. 1-3[1] the manner in which dominant, recessive and sex-linked characteristics are transmitted is illustrated.

It will be noted that in *dominant inheritance*, where only one parent possesses the dominant allele gene, the chance is that half the siblings will be affected; if both parents are carriers then the chance is increased to three out of four. Should one parent be homozygous then all the siblings will be affected.

---

[1] Adapted from Hsia, D.Y-Y. (1959). " Inborn Errors of Metabolism." Chicago: The Year Book Publishers Inc.

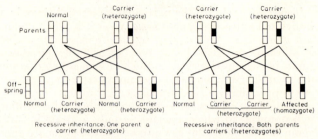

Fig. 2. Mode of expression of recessive genes.

In *recessively inherited conditions* the characteristics can only be manifest when both parents carry the particular allele form. In such circumstances the chances are that 1 in 4 of the siblings will show the abnormality and a further two will be heterozygotes. If only one parent is a heterozygote then none of the siblings will exhibit the characteristic, but the chance is that half of them will be heterozygotes. Where a particular allele form is uncommon, heterozygotes are likely to come from a common stock. Thus, in recessively inherited diseases, affected siblings are eight times more likely to originate from marriages between first cousins than from unions between previously unrelated parents.

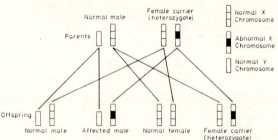

Fig. 3. Mode of expression of sex-linked genes.

In *sex-linked inherited diseases*, such as hæmophilia, in which the particular genetic characteristic is carried on the female or X chromosome, four different types of sibling can be produced: a normal female offspring who does not carry the gene, a normal male offspring, a female offspring who carries the particular gene but who like her mother does not exhibit the *trait*, and finally a male offspring who manifests the condition. Such a male can transmit the *trait* to his daughters, who will be carriers of the condition. If he should marry a female who carried the gene, then both male and female offspring of such a union may exhibit the *trait*; such circumstances have but rarely been encountered in human genetics.

TABLE I
DISORDERS TRANSMITTED BY DOMINANT INHERITANCE. A PROPORTION OF
THESE SHOW INCOMPLETE GENE PENETRANCE (*see* TEXT)

Skeleton
Achondroplasia.
Arachnodactyly.
Cleido-cranial dysostosis.
Cranio-facial dysostosis.
Enchondromata, multiple.
Marble-bone disease—one form
  (Albers-Schonberg).
Osteogenesis imperfecta.

Muscles
Dystrophia myotonica.
Myotonia congenita (Thomsen).

Central Nervous System
Epiloia.
Huntingdon's chorea.
Muscular dystrophy—some forms.
Neurofibromatosis (von Recklin-
  hausen).

Blood
Acholuric jaundice.
Porphyria acute—one form.
Sickle-celled anæmia (heterozygous
  form).
Thallassæmia minor.

Metabolic
Alkaptonuria—one form.
Hypercholesterolæmia (primary).
Pitressin-sensitive diabetes insipidus.
Renal glycosuria.

Cutaneous
Ectodermal dysplasia.
Ehlers-Danlos syndrome.
Epidermolysis bullosa.

Vascular
Lindau's disease.
Sturge-Weber syndrome.
Telangiectasia, multiple (Osler).

Eyes
Congenital cataract—one form.
Ptosis.
Retinitis pigmentosa—rare form.

Intestines
Peutz's syndrome.
Multiple polyposis of the colon.

TABLE II
DISORDERS TRANSMITTED BY RECESSIVE INHERITANCE. CERTAIN OF THESE
ARE DETECTABLE EVEN IN THE HETEROZYGOUS FORM (*see* TEXT)

Skeleton
Gargoylism.
Morquio's disease.

Muscles
Muscular dystrophy—some forms.

Central Nervous System
Amaurotic familial idiocy.
Deafness—some forms.
Laurence-Moon-Biedl syndrome.
Infantile progressive spinal atrophy
  (Werdnig-Hoffman).

Blood
Afibrinogenæmia.
Fanconi's anæmia.
Congenital methæmoglobinæmia.
Congenital porphyria.
Sickle-celled anæmia.
Thallassæmia major.

Metabolic
Albinism.
Alkaptonuria.

Cystinosis (Lignac-Fanconi).
Cystinuria.
Fructosuria.
Galactosæmia.
Glycogen storage disease.
Goitrous cretinism.
Hartnup disease.
Congenital hyperbilirubinæmia.
Hypophosphatasia.
Maple syrup disease.
Pentosuria.
Phenylketonuria.
Wilson's disease.

Cutaneous
Epidermolysis bullosa—most forms.
Ichthyosiform erythrodermia.

Eyes
Buphthalmos—one form.
Colour blindness.
Retinitis pigmentosa.

Miscellaneous
Mucoviscidosis (fibrocystic disease).

TABLE III

Disorders Transmitted by Sex-linked Inheritance

Skeleton
Multiple exostosis (diaphyseal aclasis).

Blood
Agammaglobulinæmia.
Christmas disease.
Hæmophilia.
Glucose-6-phosphate-dehydrogenase deficiency.

Muscles
Pseudo-hypertrophic muscular dystrophy.

Metabolic
Pitressin-insensitive diabetes insipidus.
Vitamin-resistant rickets.

Eyes
Partial colour blindness.

In addition to the inherited diseases included in these tables (which are those described in the text), there are a large number in which genetic influences play some part in the ætiology. Some depend upon more than one gene for their clinical expression (multifactorial origin), whilst others are greatly influenced by environmental factors, e.g. infantile pyloric stenosis, epilepsy, essential hypertension and diabetes mellitus, to mention only a few.

In theory, where an hereditary disorder is dependent on the effect of a single gene, the progeny of a particular mating should follow the clearly defined patterns described above. In practice, many inherited syndromes depend upon more than one particular gene for their clinical emergence. Moreover, environmental factors may also play a part in suppressing genetically determined characteristics. Thus, in many inherited disorders, the actual frequency of the abnormality is considerably less than would be expected in terms of pure dominant or recessive inheritance. Where environmental factors are active in suppressing hereditary disease, the term *incomplete gene penetrance* is used. Where more than one gene is required for the expression of a particular recessive *trait*, the condition may only become manifest when each and all of the mutant forms required are represented in both parents.

In general terms, therefore, studies of individual families may often fail to show a clear mode of inheritance of a particular abnormality. Dominant *traits* may apparently affect a first- and third-generation and miss the second-generation members of the family. In other cases, second-generation individuals may show only minor forms of the abnormality.

Certain disorders, such as sickle-celled anæmia, require the homozygous state for their complete expression but show a partial form of the disease among heterozygotes. Such conditions are therefore partly dominant and partly recessive.

Tables I–III provide a list of the more commonly inherited diseases, but it must be stressed that present knowledge is not sufficient in many instances to allow accurate predictions of actual frequencies of expression.

Normal and Abnormal Chromosomes in Man[1]

In 1956, Ford and Hamerton[2] and Tjio and Levan[2] showed that the chromosomes of the nucleus of the human cell numbered 46 instead of 48, as had been previously taught. Advances in technique now permit the differentiation and classification of the 23 different pairs of chromosomes and have shown that abnormal chromosomal patterns may be associated with specific clinical abnormalities.

Special techniques are used to display chromosomes, since they can be recognized as such only during cell division. These procedures involve the use of short-term cultures to provide actively dividing cells, the treatment of the cell culture with colchicine (which modifies cell mitosis at the phase most appropriate to reveal the chromosomes), and the use of hypotonic solutions to disperse the chromosomes immediately prior to fixation; finally, the chromosomes are displayed in single layer preparations. Camera lucida drawings and photographic prints at magnifications of 3,000 diameters provide records in which the 46 individual chromosomes are matched in pairs, according to their individual shape and size, and classified according to the internationally agreed Denver classification.[3] Cell cultures may be made from bone marrow, skin, or from circulating leucocytes from peripheral blood. The study of cytogenetics has produced a highly technical vocabulary and brief descriptions are now given of some of the terms employed.[4]

Chromosome.   One of a finite number of small bodies occurring in pairs into which the chromatin material of a cell nucleus resolves itself prior to cell division. *Homologous* chromosomes are the two members of one pair, one of maternal and one of paternal origin. At mitosis the longest human chromosome measures 8–10 μ and the smallest 1·2–1·5 μ. It is the unit structure bearing the carriers of hereditary traits, the genes.

Sex-chromosome.   The chromosomes concerned with the determination of the sex of the offspring. In the human, they comprise one pair of the total of 23 pairs of chromosomes in the cell nucleus. They differ from the remaining 22 pairs of chromosomes (autosomes) in that the female sex chromosome, designated X, is larger than the male sex chromosome, designated Y. In the remaining 22 pairs of autosomes, each member of an homologous pair of chromosomes is identical in shape and size in the normal individual. The somatic cell nuclei of females contain two X chromosomes (XX) while those of males contain one X and one Y chromosome (XY).

Autosome.   A non-sex chromosome (*see also* under sex-chromosome described above).

Karyotype.   The number, size and shape of the chromosomes of the cell nuclei which predominate in all the somatic cells of a particular individual and which thus identify his particular chromosomal pattern. The diagrammatic representation of the chromosome make-up of an individual is termed an idiogram.

[1] Penrose, L. S., Brown, A. C. (1961). "Recent Advances in Human Genetics." London: Churchill.
  Hamerton, J. L. (1962). "Chromosomes in Medicine." Little Club Clinics. London: Heinemann Medical Books.
[2] Ford, C. E., Hamerton, J. L. (1956). *Nature,* **178**, 1020.
  Tjio, J. H., Levan, A. (1956). *Hereditas (Lund)*, **42**, 1.
[3] Denver Report (1960). *Lancet*, 1, 1063.
[4] Sohval, A. R. (1961). *Amer. J. Med.*, **31**, 397.

Mitosis. The process of cell division in which the chromosomes participate, resulting in daughter cells which are qualitatively and quantitatively counterparts of the parent cell. The process is divided into several stages.

Meiosis. A specialized type of cell division which provides for the halving of the number of chromosomes of the somatic cell to the haploid number of the gamete cell (spermatozoa or ova). Fertilization subsequently restores the somatic or diploid number in the zygote (fertilized ovum). In the first stage of meiosis, the homologous pairs of chromosomes separate, one to each daughter cell, to give the reduction in the number of chromosomes; in the second stage a mitotic division takes place without further reduction in the chromosome number.

Non-disjunction. Abnormal chromosome behaviour during either meiosis or mitosis. Meiotic non-disjunction may be primary or secondary. In the primary variety, the two members of an individual pair of chromosomes may fail to separate during meiosis so that two different gamete cells are formed, one containing both members of the particular pair of chromosomes whilst the other receives none. Secondary meiotic non-disjunction refers to the types of gametes that will be produced by an individual who already has an abnormal karyotype and who at meiosis must inevitably develop abnormal gametes (second generation effect). Mitotic non-disjunction relates not to the formation of the gametes, but to the zygote; non-separation of a pair of chromosomes at the first mitotic cell division after fertilization will give rise to two kinds of cell of different chromosome pattern; these will be the forebears of two lines of cells which will co-exist within the one individual (mosaicism).

Monosomy and Trisomy. As a result of such chromosomal behaviour as meiotic non-disjunction, alternative gametes are produced which contain either both chromosomes of one homologous pair or no chromosome material of that pair. In the case of a female with non-disjunction of the normal sex chromosomes (XX), one gamete would contain both chromosomes (XX), whilst the other would contain none (O). If the first type of female gamete (XX) is fertilized by a normal male gamete bearing a single (X) chromosome, the resulting zygote will have the sex chromosome pattern (XXX) or trisomy X. If the alternative female gamete with no sex chromosome (O) is fertilized by a similar spermatozoon bearing the single female (X) chromosome, the resulting zygote will have a sex chromosome pattern (XO) or monosomy X, as in Turner's syndrome. By contrast, if a normal male gamete bearing the single chromosome (Y) is concerned, the resulting zygotes would be respectively (XXY) which is designated trisomy XY, as is found in Klinefelter's syndrome, or conversely (YO) which has yet to be detected clinically and is therefore probably incompatible with life. Similar examples of trisomy and monosomy also occur in relation to autosomes.

Translocation. A type of aberration in which fragmentation of a chromosome occurs, the broken-off portion becoming attached to another chromosome, often of a different pair. Once survival of a translocated chromosome is assured, the new characteristic will persist in subsequent mitoses and meioses. The best known example is the translocation of part of one of the chromosomes designated 21 in the Denver classification to one of the chromosomes of another pair, most commonly 15 or 22. This abnormality is found in a minority of mongol children, often those born to a young mother, or where other mongol children have been born in the same family. The translocation defect may also exist in one of the parents.

Deletion. A chromosomal aberration characterized by detachment and loss of a portion of a chromosome. The deleted portion fails to survive if it lacks a centromere.

Polysomy. An individual in whom one or more chromosomes are reduplicated and are found represented three or four times. This is usually the result of meiotic non-disjunction and may involve autosomes in addition to sex chromosomes.

Mosaicism. The presence of cell nuclei of different chromosomal patterns within the same individual. A minor degree of mosaicism, in which a small proportion of the cell nuclei have a different number of chromosomes than that present in the great majority of cell nuclei, is more common in man than was originally thought likely. Mosaicism may occur as a result of non-disjunction in the early mitoses of the zygote or from simple loss of a chromosome (deletion).

Nuclear Chromatin. Apart from the full investigation of the karyotype, information related to an individual's sex chromosome pattern may be obtained from the staining reaction of the sex chromtain of somatic cells. Barr and Bertram[1] have shown that the chromatin of the nuclei of cells from females, which contain the XX sex chromosomes, stain readily with basic dyes (chromatin positive), but that the nuclei of cells from males containing XY sex chromosomes fail to take up these stains (chromatin negative). The positive staining reaction depends upon the presence of two female sex chromosomes within the nucleus. Such examinations may be carried out directly on the leucocytes of peripheral blood or on cells obtained from buccal smears without recourse to cell cultures.

Such investigations are valuable, for example, in genetic males with Turner's syndrome (XO) who prove to be chromatin negative on examination, and in genetic females with Klinefelter's syndrome (XXY) from whom a chromatin positive reaction will be obtained.

CLINICAL APPLICATIONS

EXAMINATION of karyotypes (*see* Fig. 58, p. 473) is a relatively new tool in its application to clinical medicine.

Abnormalities of Autosomes

Knowledge of the association of specific abnormalities of the auto-somal pattern with particular clinical disorders is still far from complete, but a number have now been identified.

MONGOLISM (*see also* p. 472)

In the majority of mongol children, trisomy of 21 or 22 chromosome due to non-disjunction is frequently present and appears to be associated with the well-recognized tendency among mothers in the later years of child-bearing to have mongols. Due to this trisomy, such mongols have 47 chromosomes.

In a minority of mongols, there is a familial incidence. In this type, the chromosomal abnormality is one of translocation of part of chromosome 21 to chromosome 15 or 22, so that the total number of chromosomes remains at 46. Such a condition is inherited, and either or both parents may be found to have the translocation defect although they show no stigmata of mongolism. In this type the incidence of mongolism is unrelated to maternal age.

LEUKÆMIA (*see also* p. 347)

In a small proportion of patients with leukæmia, a morphological defect of chromosome 21 (the same chromosome usually found to be abnormal in mongolism) has been reported. The abnormality appears to be a translocation or deletion defect and bears some relationship to the chromosomal defects found in mongolism.

[1] Barr, M. L., Bertram, E. G. (1949). *Nature*, **163**, 676.

MENTAL DEFICIENCY WITH MULTIPLE ANOMALIES

Cases have been reported of mental retardation together with multiple anomalies in association with trisomy of certain autosomes. One group involves the chromosomes 17–18 in the Denver classification and another the chromosomes 13–15. Present methods do not permit a more precise identification of the chromosome involved.

Abnormalities of Sex Chromosomes

The relationship of non-disjunction of the sex chromosomes to Turner's syndrome (p. 163) and Klinefelter's syndrome (p. 165) has already been mentioned. Trisomy X (i.e. a sex chromosome distribution XXX) has been found in women in whom the only abnormality may be inferior intelligence.

More complex sex chromosomal abnormalities, with mosaicism due to meiotic non-disjunction and complicated by subsequent mitotic non-disjunction and deletion defects in the zygote, have also been found in patients with hypogonadism in both sexes.

NORMAL DEVELOPMENT

NORMAL growth can be described as a unified development of intelligence, emotional maturation, adaptation to society and increasing physical size and prowess. For the purposes of description these aspects of normal growth have to be considered separately, although they are closely dependent upon each other.

Intellectual Development

Intellectual development cannot be measured in absolute terms. Instead, comparative estimates are made of the age of attainment of particular skills so that a particular child can be assessed as of retarded, average, or above average ability compared with the mean for his age group. Whilst innate intelligence is considered to be genetically determined, performance can undoubtedly be modified by emotional difficulties, environment and physical defects and illnesses. For example, deprivation of maternal affection in the early years may cause the child to show regressive tendencies to a pattern of behaviour usually encountered at an earlier age. Similarly, lack of stimulus and of the normal experiences of childhood may result in apparent retardation of development. Physical defects, such as high tone deafness, may give rise to poor school performance and poor speech development.

The following table lists some of the " milestones " in accomplishment and the ages at which they are normally reached. There are, however, considerable individual variations, and lateness in one particular should not be taken as evidence of mental defect. The backward child is late in every respect, although not necessarily to the same degree, whilst perfectly normal children may be late in learning to walk or to talk or to control the bladder. Moreover, allowances must be made for prolonged illness, which may cause general retardation, and for physical handicap; for instance, a child with congenital dislocation of the hip will walk late, and one with congenital deafness will be late in learning to talk.

TABLE OF MILESTONES[1]

At birth. The activities of a newborn baby seem to be largely of a more or less simple reflex nature.[2] Some of these " automatisms," such as turning the head to one side when placed prone, crying when hungry, " rooting " for the breast, sucking, sneezing, and withdrawal of a limb from a painful stimulus, have obvious survival value to the infant. Other reflexes, such as the startle reflex (Moro), the palmar and plantar grasp, the walking and crawling reflexes, have no obvious purpose but may be of ontogenetic or phylogenetic significance. All this activity seems to be largely independent of functioning cerebral hemispheres—possibly the fixing of gaze on the mother, noticeable in most newborn babies when feeding, may be an exception.

The following are brief notes on behaviour after the newborn period:

At 1 month	The infant follows a bright light with the eyes. He smiles (normal range 4 to 6 weeks).
At 2 months	He coos and gurgles. He can lift his head when lying prone and turn his head to watch someone moving.
At 3 months	He recognizes his mother. He turns his head towards a sound. When held sitting, he holds his head up with only occasional wobbles. He watches his hands. He " talks " when spoken to.
At 5 months	He examines his hands and feet. He reaches out with both hands and can grasp objects. He recognizes his parents' voices. He laughs.
At 6 months	He can sit upright. He can reach out for an object with one hand, can put it into his mouth or change it from one hand to the other.
At 9 months	He can sit himself up from the lying position. He makes a definite effort to crawl. He can pick up an object between finger and thumb and release it deliberately. He can feed himself with a biscuit. He is

[1] Recommended for further reading:
Gesell, A., *et al.* (1940). " The First Five Years of Life." London: Methuen.
Illingworth, R. S. (1960). " The Development of the Infant and Young Child, Normal and Abnormal." Edinburgh: Livingstone.
[2] André-Thomas, Chesni, Y., Dargassies, S. (1960). " The Neurological Examination of the Infant." London: National Spastics Society.
Illingworth, R. S. (1962). " An Introduction to Developmental Assessment in the First Year." London: National Spastics Society.

tremendously interested in his environment, and continually handles all objects in his vicinity. He has begun to be frightened of strangers.

At 1 *year*   He can pull himself up to a standing position and walk holding on. He can say a few words. He can drink from a cup, unscrew the top off a bottle, and unwrap the paper covering from a sweet. He gives evidence that he experiences the emotions of rage, fear, joy, affection, jealousy, disappointment and anxiety. He has learned various tricks, such as waving goodbye, pat-a-cake, etc.

At 18 *months*   He walks unaided and can climb on to a chair. He can throw a ball and begins to build bricks. He can hold a cup securely with two hands and feeds himself untidily with a spoon. He can identify objects in a picture book. He has a vocabulary of about a dozen words. He obeys simple commands.

By 2 *years*   He can now run. He holds a cup in one hand and he can turn the pages of a book one by one. He can now say sentences of several words, and has a vocabulary of two to three hundred words. He wishes company and playfellows. He may know some of his colours. He will pull a stool over to an object which is too high to obtain from the ground. He has gained control over the bladder during the day, and very often at night. He has complete control over defæcation.

By 3 *years*   One has ceased to think of him as a baby. He can ride a tricycle, play by himself and scribble with a pencil. His language abilities have so developed that one ceases to think of his having a vocabulary. He knows his colours. He listens to stories. One can begin to reason with him. He can feed himself completely and help to dress and undress himself.

By 4 *years*   He can say nursery rhymes, knows his colours and the names of a large number of objects. He can count a little and knows several of his letters. He appreciates signs and knows which is the longer of two lines. He can make drawings of familiar objects and plays nicely with toys, showing much make-believe and fantasy in his play. He is now old enough to be reasoned with. He asks endless questions and likes showing off.

By the fifth year he knows his letters, and can count up to 10 or more.

By the sixth year he can read short words, and from then on his learning is largely determined by the interest his school can arouse in him. By the *seventh* or *eighth year* he can reason and form judgements, and can profit by his experience. His play is much less make-believe, and he likes school games.

By the ninth or tenth year he develops hobbies, is keen on games, and can reason for himself.

By the thirteenth year he can adapt himself in an intelligent manner to new situations as they arise in life, and he shows a considerable degree of intelligence, wisdom and general knowledge.

At puberty there is a tendency to emotional disturbances, but the mental powers forge ahead.

At the sixteenth year the development of the purely intellectual processes of the mind have attained completion.

MENTAL TESTS

A skilled psychologist can obtain a more accurate estimate of a child's intelligence by using standardized tests. Gesell's developmental tests are used to measure gross motor activity, manipulation, adaptive behaviour, language and play, and social reactions in the infant and young child. Modifications of Binet's intelligence tests are used to estimate intelligence in children from two to three years of age and upwards. Although these tests have been devised to minimize the effect of education and environment, they cannot be said to measure only innate intellectual capacity. The results are expressed in the form of mental age (MA) or intelligence quotient (IQ). The mental age is an estimate of the age at which the child's level of intelligence would be normal. The IQ is the mental age expressed as the percentage of the real age. Thus, if a child of eight years is found to have a MA of six years, his IQ is said to be 75. Children of average intelligence have IQs of between 90 and 110; the highly intelligent of 130 or more; the educationally subnormal 50 to 70; imbeciles 20 to 50; and idiots under 20. The IQ is useful in comparing the intelligence of groups of children of different ages, or of a single child when tests are repeated at intervals of months or years, but when applied to the results of a single test on one child may give a misleading and spurious idea of accuracy. The results of a single test are best expressed in the form of the approximate mental age, and any variability in different test performances should be stated. The results of intelligence testing are obviously influenced by the child's emotional state and physical health at the time of the test, but an experienced psychologist will take these factors into account. Special methods of testing must be used for physically handicapped children.

Emotional Development

Much has been written in recent years concerning the emotional development of children. The reader is referred particularly to the writings of such authors as Gesell, Winnicott and Illingworth[1] who have contributed so much to our knowledge of this subject. There is still a great deal more to be learnt.

In the first years of life, the continuing growth of the mother-child relationship and an undisturbed home background will promote a sense of security, in which an awareness of " belonging " and individual personality can develop. It is easy to see that failure to provide this loving maternal care and stable background may seriously imperil this vital aspect of development. Increasing awareness of this problem has, for example, brought about a much more liberal approach to the problem of visiting children in hospital. After the initial phase of complete dependence upon the mother, come the first immature expressions of independence characterized by minor rebellion against authority (negative stage). Subsequently, through ordinary daily life at home and at school, the child begins to come to terms with society, with a subconscious realization of the needs of others as well as his own.

Inevitably, behaviour difficulties arise at any or all of these stages of development and are to be expected in their minor forms as normal aspects of growing up. Presenting symptoms vary according to the age of the child. Thus the doctor, consulted over the problem of an infant who will not sleep or who cries persistently or who refuses to take his weaning diet, must think in terms of emotional as well as physical causes. In a slightly older age group, abdominal pain, failure to gain control of the bowels or bladder, and temper tantrums may have similar origins. In the investigation of the school child with such symptoms as habit spasms and tics, limb pains and headache, lassitude, a relapse into enuresis and anti-social behaviour, such as aggressiveness to other children, emotional as well as physical causations must be considered.

Stable personality in the parents and a good marriage relationship, including a normal desire for and acceptance of their children, provide the background against which a child is able to achieve satisfactory emotional maturity. Where the home background is bad or non-existent, it may be easy to appreciate the overt causes of persistent emotional disturbances in the child. Where the home background is superficially satisfactory, the family doctor or pædiatrician must be prepared to spend a considerable amount of time and patience in listening to the parent's description of the problems besetting the child and the family, before deciding whether he can help best by his own advice or whether he should obtain help from a psychiatrist.

The whole subject of emotionally determined illness is considered in detail in Chapter 18.

[1] Gesell, A., Amatruda, C. S. (1947). " Developmental Diagnosis." New York: Hoeber.
Gesell, A., Ilg, F. L. (1943). " Infant and Child in the Culture of Today." New York: Harper.
Winnicott, D. W. (1957). " The Child and the Family." London: Tavistock Publications.
Winnicott, D. W. (1957). " The Child and the Outside World." London: Tavistock Publications.
Illingworth, R. S. (1960). " The Development of the Infant and Young Child, Normal and Abnormal." Edinburgh: Livingstone.

Physical Growth[1]

The normal growth of a child is not a uniformly continuous process but contains three separate periods of accelerated growth. The first is a continuation of the rapid growth of the fœtus and lasts until the end of the first post-natal year. The second is a small increase in growth rate between 6 and 8 years of age (second dentition) and is called the mid-growth spurt. The third is the adolescent growth spurt associated with the development of puberty.

Whilst boys tend to remain both slightly taller and heavier than girls throughout childhood, there is little difference in growth rate until the onset of the adolescent growth spurt.

There is, however, considerable variation in the rate of growth of different tissues and body organs. The head is disproportionately large at birth and has attained about 95 per cent. of its total growth by the age of ten years. The growth of the lymphatic tissues is remarkable in that the total size of such organs as the thymus reach their peak in the age group 5–10 years and then gradually regress in size. In both sexes a transient increase in fat precedes the start of adolescent growth.

Puberal development is associated with the adolescent growth spurt. In girls the growth spurt takes place usually between the ages 11–14 years and the menarche occurs shortly after the peak of the growth spurt has been passed. In boys the growth spurt occurs a little later, usually in the age group 13–16 years, and is of greater magnitude than in girls. Towards its conclusion there develops a considerable increase in muscular strength coinciding with the completion of puberty development. In both sexes, if the growth spurt is delayed it tends to be of lesser magnitude and is associated with a later onset of puberty.

The development of the female type of pelvis occurs at the time of adolescent growth and is thought to be due to the influence of œstrogens on the pelvic cartilage. Similarly, the increased shoulder growth of boys occurs at adolescence stimulated by androgen secretion.

Although growth is taking place throughout the year, in the Northern hemisphere the maximum weight increase in children occurs in the months October to December, whilst most height is gained between April and June. In the Southern hemisphere the reverse happens. The reason for it is not known.

In the past 100 years there has been a significant increase in height and weight of children of comparable ages which is only partly due to improved nutrition. The nutritional effect was shown in Germany both in World War I and II when the relative increase in height and weight was temporarily reversed. The increase in rate of growth is associated with an increase in ultimate height which may be under separate genetic control. This acceleration of growth is associated

[1] Tanner, J. M. (1962). " Growth at Adolescence." Oxford: Blackwell Scientific Publications.

with an onset of both the adolescent growth spurt and puberty significantly earlier than in the past.

Ultimate height is mainly determined by hereditary factors as, indeed, is a constitutional tendency to obesity.

The bony epiphyses develop their centres of ossification in a constant sequence so that from observations on large numbers of children it is possible to determine a pattern of skeletal age correlated with chronological age (Appendix 5). Thus, an individual child can be assessed from the x-ray appearances of the epiphyses as having retarded, normal, or advanced bone age. Retarded bone age is observed particularly in patients with cretinism, and advanced bone age in children with precocious puberty.

For a description of such abnormalities of growth as *gigantism*, *dwarfism* and *infantilism*, *see* Chapter 11.

For normal growth, a well-balanced diet containing an adequate content of all the vitamins is essential. Children require especially an adequate supply of protein. A severe illness, particularly of a nutritional nature, may temporarily arrest growth. In such instances a transverse line of relatively denser calcification develops across the long bones which will persist even after normal growth has been resumed.

NORMAL WEIGHT GAIN

In Europe, the average weight of a newborn infant is about 7 lb. There is a loss during the first four days of anything up to half a pound, but this is quickly made up, and by the tenth to twelfth day the birth weight is regained. Thereafter, from 6 to 8 ounces a week are gained for the first five months, and about 4 ounces per week from five months to one year. At five months most infants have doubled their birth weight and at one year have trebled it. It is not uncommon for a 7-lb. infant to weigh 18 lb. at 6 months and 25 lb. at one year; this does not necessarily mean that the child is more healthy. Cutting teeth, a change of feed, or vaccination may all temporarily cause stationary weight. The most important guide to normal progress is a happy, contented, vigorous baby. Much unnecessary anxiety is seen in mothers who have been persuaded, either by their families or by other well-intentioned but misguided advisers, to believe that their child's weight gain is inadequate. Subsequent attempts at overfeeding may then cause a reaction in the child and produce a real feeding difficulty. A mother should be allowed flexibility in the care of the child and should be encouraged to enjoy and rear her baby as a healthy human being; she should not be bedevilled by feelings of guilt about her handling of her child as a result of over-zealous advice. Most infants are remarkably adaptable and will thrive on the most unexpected regimes. What an infant finds much harder to tolerate is a mother who has been made to feel guilty and over-anxious.

In *older children*, emaciation or wasting may be due to over-activity or to nervous fatigue, or to physical disorders, such as cœliac disease, rheumatism or tuberculosis. The constitutionally over-active child is extremely difficult to fatten and may be a problem in practice (*see* " Nervous Exhaustion," p. 383). In many instances, however, the parents may feel a misplaced anxiety concerning a child who, they consider, is underweight. Provided the child is active and enjoys life, the practitioner will often find that his problem is to reassure the parents rather than to treat the child (*see also* p. 384). Some children gain in the summer only and are stationary or gain very little in the winter, and vice versa. Others gain in the holidays but not in term.

Details of the normal ranges of height and weight gains are included in Appendix 5 (p. 672); there is also a simple formula which gives the approximately expected weight of boys and girls up to 11 years with only a small margin of error: age in years $+ 3 \times 5 =$ weight in pounds, e.g. 6 (years) $+ 3 = 9 \times 5 = 45$ lb.

Dentition

Good teeth sometimes run in families, and there are important hereditary factors which determine the size, character and positioning of the teeth. Rickets has been regarded as a cause of delayed dentition and of caries, but the situation is not so simple; both those dental features may occur in the absence of rickets, and rickets without either. Nevertheless, in the formation of good teeth diet is of outstanding importance—the prenatal diet for the first teeth, the diet in infancy for the permanent teeth. Any deficiency in the diet of the pregnant mother should be supplemented and the child should receive a cod-liver oil supplement from the earliest weeks and an adequate diet. Excess of carbohydrates, especially sugar, increases any liability to caries.

In the preservation of the teeth, good dental hygiene is important. The mouth should be cleaned twice a day, once after breakfast and again after the last meal of the day has been taken. A small brush with good bristles should be used to clean the gums and between the teeth to remove food debris. A meal should end with fibre-containing foods, such as an apple or nuts, rather than with flour or sugar-containing foods.

Fluoridation of water supplies to produce a fluorine content of 1 part per million has been shown to cause a striking reduction in the incidence of dental caries. Where the natural water supply contains this amount of fluorine there is only one-third of the dental caries that there is in areas in which the water contains less than 0·4 parts per million. If the natural content of fluorine is over 5 parts per million, then some discoloration of the dental enamel is found, but no other harmful effects have been noticed.

The nutrition of the jaws and their growth is encouraged by chewing; their shape can be affected by thumb sucking and mouth breathing, hence the importance of correcting chronic nasal obstruction.

FIRST SET OF TEETH OR PRIMARY DENTITION

Individual variations in the date of eruption of the teeth are considerable, although they are usually cut in the following order and at the following times:

1. Lower central incisors, 5 to 10 months.
2. Upper central and lateral incisors, 8 to 12 months.
3. Lower lateral incisors and lower and upper first molars, 12 to 14 months.
4. Lower and upper canines, 16 to 22 months.
5. Lower and upper second molars, 24 to 30 months.

SECOND SET OF TEETH OR PERMANENT DENTITION

1. First molars appear between the ages of				5	and	7	years	
2. Central incisors	,,	,,	,,	6½	,,	8	,,	
3. Lateral incisors	,,	,,	,,	7	,,	9	,,	
4. First bicuspids	,,	,,	,,	9	,,	11	,,	
5. Second bicuspids	,,	,,	,,	10	,,	12	,,	
6. Canines	,,	,,	,,	10	,,	12	,,	
7. Cuspids	,,	,,	,,	11	,,	14	,,	
8. Second molars	,,	,,	,,	11	,,	13	,,	
9. Third molars	,,	,,	,,	16	,,	21	,,	or later

SYMPTOMS OF TEETHING

Some doctors think that teething is responsible for nothing but the cutting of teeth, while others are ready to attribute many minor and some major symptoms to teething; the latter can be overdone.

It seems certain that some infants may experience local discomfort as the teeth are erupting, and they appear to obtain relief by rubbing the gum with a teething ring. Infants liable to eczema may have exacerbations as each tooth comes through; *lichen urticatus* and various other urticarial rashes also appear and disappear at this time.

Purgatives, grey powders and teething powders should be avoided. If the disturbance at night is severe, causing loss of sleep, aspirin is recommended.

Training in Micturition and Defæcation

The value placed on very early training in control of the bowels and bladder by the nannies of a past generation was almost certainly misplaced. Their assertion that from the age of one month old a child could be trained to urinate into a chamber pot is explained by the presence of the handling reflex, so familiar to many medical practitioners and mothers. When a baby's napkin is removed and the perineal or genital area handled, micturition will frequently occur; this reflex disappears well before the age of one year.

Routine potting should be commenced about the time that the child is able to sit on the chamber with only slight support, usually about the age of six months. At first this should be limited to once or twice a day, usually after breakfast and lunch, to gain control of the bowels.   Later on the child should be potted after every meal and at such other times as he indicates his needs, in order to start to gain control of micturition.   Success should always be a matter for congratulation and praise, and not too much should be made of failure in the early days.

There are wide variations in the times when children attain control; delay may be familial and it is well to enquire in appropriate cases at what age the parents attained it.   What is called " toilet training " is partly a misnomer for, in the early stages, it is the mother who trains herself to recognize the signs by which her young child indicates his needs.   Except for occasional lapses, many a child will have gained control of the bowels before the age of one year.   Bladder control is often accomplished during the day in the early part of the second year and by night a little later.   By $2\frac{1}{2}$ years the child should be able to ask during the day to be attended to, and this may be only on waking, after breakfast, at dinner, at tea, and at bedtime.   During the night, some children require to be lifted up at 10 p.m., but this should be discontinued as soon as possible.   Giving the last meal at 5 p.m. with no drinks afterwards is a very great help in getting some children to remain dry during the night.

The problem of constipation is considered on p. 189, but a word of warning must be given here to emphasize the harm that can be done to normal training habits should defæcation become painful due to the presence of hard bulky stools and the possible complication of an anal fissure.   In such circumstances the child may associate the pain with the presence of the chamber pot rather than with the act of defæcation itself.   He may then refuse to sit on the pot, and even the mere sight of it may produce screaming or temper tantrums.   In such circumstances the constipation must be overcome along the lines suggested on p. 190, and great patience and tact will be required to restore the child's confidence in normal training habits.

Clothing

The infant requires light warm clothing which should consist of a short-sleeved woollen vest, a garment of wool and fibre mixture and, in winter, a woollen jacket.   Socks may be required for the first three months in winter.   Cotton can be substituted for heavier materials in hot weather.   At 5 to 6 months the infant wants more freedom to move, and short dresses or knitted suits can be used.   A binder is not needed after the umbilicus is healed.

Infants born in the summer need not wear bonnets or caps out of doors, but those born during the winter require some protection until the hair has grown sufficiently.   All children require woollen caps or some form of head-covering during severe weather.

At the age of one year, when the infant begins to walk, it is best to provide him with shoes having firm, non-slipping soles and small heels.   The heel should be narrow enough to fit snugly, whereas the toe should be broad, allowing plenty of room. For children who show a tendency to flat-foot, from laxity of muscles or overweight, exercises should be prescribed to tone up the muscles. The presence of knock-knee and valgus ankles is also an indication for exercises to strengthen the foot and ankle. Leather lace-up shoes should be worn in which the heels may have to be wedged $\frac{1}{8}$ inch to $\frac{3}{16}$ inch on the inner side, tapering away to nothing on the outer side.

Sleep

THE NORMAL CHILD

Although there is a wide individual variation, the following table shows the average amount of sleep required by children at various ages:

Birth	20–24 hours
Six months	18 ,,
One year	14–16 ,,
Two years	12–14 ,,
Five ,,	10–12 ,,
Ten ,,	10–11 ,,
Sixteen ,,	9 ,,

For children up to the age of four or five it is well to continue a midday rest: during the toddler period this often comes before dinner, say from 11 a.m. to 1 p.m.; later on it is more convenient after dinner between 1.30 and 2.30 p.m.

ABNORMALITIES OF SLEEP

Infants require more sleep than children, children more than adults, yet the requirements of individuals vary widely at all ages. Some small children seem ready to drop off to sleep at any hour and under any circumstances. Other young children may be in the habit of waking at 3 or 4 a.m., after a few hours of sound sleep; they then seem to require no more sleep and will sing or play until their parents must also abandon sleep. The next day these children will show no signs of sleepiness. The handling of such a situation is difficult. Some children are better in *a separate room* and with a later bedtime. Firm handling may solve the problem. Restlessness during sleep is different. It may be caused by fatigue or excitement and results in further fatigue the next day. Children who become too excited or who are allowed to be on their legs too much sleep badly. Digestive disturbances, late supper and over-fatigue tend to produce night terrors and disturbed sleep. Nasal obstruction and, in infants, hunger pains and wind colic may produce broken sleep. Some infants waken each time water is passed and refuse to settle down again unless changed.   A cough or a fever will disturb sleep, and earache or teething pain is commonly the cause of screaming at night.   Insomnia and night screaming are sometimes found in children of over-anxious parents.   There is a use for a sedative or hypnotic, such as chloral hydrate, given for a limited period to re-establish a habit of sleeping (*see also* pp. 388–390).

Fresh Air, Sunshine and Exercise

Fresh air is invaluable and from the earliest weeks an infant should be put to sleep out of doors, both morning and afternoon.   A city child needs about 4–6 hours in the fresh air every day.   *Sunlight* is valuable because it helps the skin to synthesize vitamin D and thus prevent rickets, and it has a further asset in that it benefits children and adults in indirect ways, mainly psychological.   Artificial sunlight has lost its vogue, and it is not good practice to crowd children into a room for exposure to ultra-violet light because of the time wasted and the risk of infection; equal or more good accrues from a teaspoonful of cod-liver oil and a game in the open air.

During the summer months, whenever possible, the child should be stripped and, with the sun shining directly on the body, allowed to run and play.   This, combined with sea air, is of the utmost value to every normal child and especially to those who have been debilitated by illness.   Exposure to sunlight should be gradual, particularly after a long illness.

EXERCISE

Although many children have to suffer confinement and lack of fresh air, very few children, once they are able to walk, lack exercise. A very few, highly strung children are too active and take more exercise than is beneficial; fatigue and thinness may result.

Normal Variations of Development

In growth and development, as in most things, the normal shades into the pathological.   Members of some families develop early, others mature late.   The disparity between two boys of the same age, one an early, the other a late, developer, may be remarkable.   There is almost as much variation, too, in the menarche as there is in the menopause.   A mother giving a history of a very early or a very late menarche will sometimes have a daughter with a similar history. The result of comparing the rate of development of their own children either with the siblings or with their neighbour's children, without appreciating the striking variations in the range of normal develop-ment, often causes anxiety to parents.   Such comparisons may be made of physical growth, motor development or intellectual attain-ment.   The doctor must not dismiss these fears lightly.   Time taken to allow a parent fully to express her apprehensions, followed by a thorough examination of the child to exclude any genuine abnormality of development, coupled with a reasoned explanation of the variation between the children, will remove a source of anxiety which might otherwise lead to serious difficulties within the family.

Adoption of Children

Various legal enactments control the adoption of children[1]; generally speaking, the interests of the child are well protected but those of the adopting parents somewhat less so. There ought to be an obligation on the adoption societies and other agencies to provide the examining doctor with all the information available as to the likelihood of inheritable disease. At the present time, parents, rightly anxious to receive such necessary knowledge through their medical representatives, may be fobbed off with a general and meaningless statement such as " both the father and the mother are healthy stock. "

The doctor representing the adopting parents should start by making a careful physical examination, looking for deafness, visual defect, or other signs of organic disorder, such as spasticity, cerebral palsy, congenital heart disease and dislocation of the hips. He should also pay attention to the general appearance and alertness of the child. A Wassermann test should be done and the urine examined. Any unusual condition of the bones, lungs, etc., would indicate that an x-ray examination should be made. Then the doctor should do his best to obtain details of the family history of the child's parents, especially in relation to inheritable mental disease, alcoholism, suicide, nervous disorders, such as epilepsy, and other conditions, such as diabetes mellitus and allergy.

Not only is it essential that the child should be judged fit for adoption, but it is also necessary that the third party who arranges the adoption should ascertain details concerning the suitability of the prospective parents. Adoption societies have an excellent record in this respect, tending to reject persons approaching the end of the child-bearing age, those beyond it and those who show evidence of mental instability or who seek to adopt a child for unworthy motives. Societies are also best equipped to maintain anonymity between the natural and the adopting parents.

Private individuals acting as third parties may be less impartial in rejecting the claims of unsuitable persons who wish to adopt a child. Generally speaking, family doctors are well advised not to make themselves the third party in an adoption but to recommend childless couples, and others who seek their advice, to consult an adoption society. In particular, local adoptions where both sets of parents are known to each other and continue to live in the same area are to be deprecated strongly. It is unfortunate that at the present time only one-third of all adoptions in the United Kingdom are arranged through societies.

[1] *See* Appendix 7, p. 690.

CHAPTER 3

Breast-Feeding

THAT breast-feeding and breast-milk are admirably suited to the needs of the normal infant is a truism which needs no stressing; except under conditions of first-class hygiene, mortality and morbidity are greater among artificially-fed than among breast-fed infants. Some women can entirely, and the majority partially, breast-feed their children, but in England less than 50 per cent. suckle for more than three months.

By breast-feeding an infant, the mother saves the cost of the artificial food, as well as much work and worry, and she has the added advantage of aiding involution of the uterus. Breast-milk is virtually sterile, and there is a lower morbidity and mortality among breast-fed babies than among those artificially fed. The only disadvantage is that breast-feeding takes a considerable amount of the mother's time; she must be prepared to sacrifice herself in this respect.

Not every woman can wholly feed her baby, and it is essential for the doctor when advocating breast-feeding to study the individual mother. Some mothers will not make the attempt to breast-feed or will give it up altogether for inadequate reasons. It is the physician's duty to point out to the mother the advantages of breast-feeding and to emphasize the superiority of natural over artificial feeding.

The breast should be massaged daily from the sixth month. The nipples should be drawn forward and rolled gently between finger and thumb. A little lanolin can be used and a properly fitting brassiere is essential. Even retracted nipples can often be improved by these means. The late Dr. Waller[1] made important contributions to an understanding of lactation and how to overcome its difficulties. He advocated that colostrum should be expressed from the breasts daily in small quantities for six weeks before term, in order to prevent, after parturition, painful distension of the breasts caused by thick colostrum retained in the ducts and sinuses of the breast. The nipples should not be scrubbed or rubbed with spirit to " harden " them. When the newborn baby is first put to the breast, it should be allowed to suck for only 2 or 3 minutes so as to avoid bruising the nipples, which harden up after a few days to allow longer feeds.

In the first few days after delivery, before the milk comes in, colostrum is secreted by the breasts. Because it is richer in protein than milk it is rather thicker, but it is low in fat and sugar.

[1] Waller, H. (1939). " Clinical Studies in Lactation." London: Heinemann.

BREAST-MILK

It will be seen from Table IV that the fat content of breast-milk varies from 3 per cent. to 5 per cent. The globules, however, are extremely small in comparison with those in cows' milk and the emulsion therefore finer. This makes for easier digestion. The fat

TABLE IV

Showing Composition of Cows' and Human Milk and Variations which may occur in the Composition of Breast-milk

Components	Cows' Milk Per Cent.	Human Milk Per Cent.	Variations in Human Milk Per Cent.
Water	86–87	88·05	87·82–85·50
Fat	4·00	3·50	3·00– 5·00
Proteins	3·50	1·25	1·00– 2·25
Milk sugar	4·50	7·00	6·00– 7·00
Mineral salts	0·75	0·20	0·18– 0·25

content of the milk cannot be varied by giving a richer or poorer diet to the mother, provided she is adequately fed. Protein is $1\frac{1}{2}$ to 2 per cent., compared with $3\frac{1}{2}$ to 4 per cent. in cows' milk. The bulk of the protein is present as lactalbumin and lactglobulin, only a small proportion as casein. In cows' milk, on the other hand, the casein content is from four to five times as great as the albumin content. The curd formed in the stomach of the infant fed on breast-milk is fine. By diluting cows' milk, thus reducing the protein from 4 to 2 per cent., an attempt may be made to approximate cows' milk to breast-milk, but the proportion of insoluble casein in cows' milk cannot by this means be made to approximate to that of breast-milk; therefore attempts at " humanizing " milk by dilution can never be successful. The carbohydrate in breast-milk is lactose, the amount approximately 7 per cent., which gives breast-milk a much sweeter taste than cows' milk. The salts in breast-milk, mainly calcium and phosphates, are present in a smaller quantity than in cows' milk.

Breast-feeding

Breast-feeding is the ideal for the infant. At times, however, a mother is unable to supply her baby with enough breast-milk, perhaps because of social duties, or having to go out to work, or her physical condition. Sometimes, the longer the attempt is continued the more the infant deteriorates. Under such circumstances *complementary feeding*, that is giving cows' milk at the end of the breast-feed, can be adopted with great benefit. The individual mother must be studied, just as the individual child is studied in artificial feeding.

CONTRA-INDICATIONS TO BREAST-FEEDING

When the mother has open tuberculosis she should not attempt breast-feeding, as there is a risk of infecting the child. However, a syphilitic infant can be nursed by its own mother without risk of infection. In acute infections, such as typhoid fever or pneumonia, the mother will be too ill to breast-feed, but in mild infections as a rule there is no contra-indication. In heart disease, nephritis, anæmia and epilepsy, each case must be considered individually. Insanity in the mother may contra-indicate breast-feeding. The onset of menstruation during lactation should not be taken as an indication for weaning. The infant may require artificial food for 24 hours but should resume its breast-feeds thereafter. If the mother becomes pregnant while still feeding her baby, weaning should be carried out.

VARIATION IN QUANTITY AND QUALITY OF BREAST-MILK

(See Table IV)

The first feed in the morning is probably the largest in quantity. From that time the feeds get smaller and in the middle of the day are the smallest, remaining deficient until the evening when the amount again increases. The quantity of the milk seems to vary with the activity of the mother, but the composition appears to be constant for any particular woman. Worry or fatigue may reduce the flow of milk but this effect is, normally, only temporary.

LACTATION AND ITS ESTABLISHMENT

A normal baby can be put to the breast of a healthy mother 8 hours after birth; it could be even sooner. Feeding can then be at approximately four-hourly intervals, provided that the time of sucking is at first restricted to two or three minutes. This is because the epithelium of the nipples is delicate and easily damaged until it hardens after a few days. At first soreness or excoriations may result from the avid sucking of a strong baby. If the breasts become over-engorged it may be difficult for the infant to engage the nipple properly in its mouth. This difficulty should be met without delay by expression, using the hand or a breast pump. Excessive lactation sometimes occurs as a temporary condition soon after the coming in of the milk. This can be controlled by giving less fluid to the mother or by small doses of stilbœstrol.

COMPLEMENTARY FEEDS, AND WHEN THEY SHOULD BE STARTED

Once the flow of milk is established both breasts can be used for the feeds, the infant being kept at each for 7 or 8 minutes. Often, however, there is delay in the complete establishment of lactation, and during this time the infant cries constantly, swallows air, and may have loose stools, with the result that breast-feeding is often abandoned. The weight should be taken daily, and if the loss continues beyond the fourth day, small complementary feeds should be given after each breast-feed. This, however, should be merely a temporary measure, to be continued only until the flow of milk is fully established.

TIMES OF FEEDING

Flexibility is desirable in the times and frequency of feeding; the size of the infant, the supply of breast-milk and the length of time that the baby will remain contented between feeds must all be considered. If arbitrary feeding times are to be recommended, it is suggested that infants under 6 lb. require at least six feeds in 24 hours, those from 6 to 7 lb. require five or six feeds in 24 hours, and those over 8 lb. five feeds in 24 hours. For the average infant of 6 lb. and over it is customary to feed at 6, 10, 2, 6, and 10. Satisfactory results are also obtained by allowing the mother to follow a more flexible routine, permitting the infant's natural rhythm of feeding to determine the intervals and his appetite the amounts. This is called *self-demand feeding*. It has the advantage of being moulded by the instincts of mother and baby; denial of food to a hungry baby and attempts to feed him when not hungry can be emotionally upsetting to both.

DURATION OF FEEDINGS

The great bulk of the feed is obtained in the first five minutes, and 15 minutes ought to be sufficient time for the whole. Some babies will feed faster than this without harm. At the end of the feed the baby should be wrapped in its shawl and placed upright against the mother's shoulder to allow him to " break his wind." This should always be done after feeds because all sucklings swallow some air which should be allowed to be eructated, otherwise discomfort, vomiting, and sometimes colic, will ensue. It is also as well to hold the baby up to bring up wind before the feed and again half-way through it.

MATERNAL DIET IN PREGNANCY AND LACTATION

In order to supply the needs of the fœtus, the diet of the pregnant woman must contain plenty of protein and sufficient salts, and protective food factors. During lactation also she requires extra first-class protein, calcium, phosphorus, iron and vitamins. Protein is found mainly in meat, fish, cheese, milk and eggs. Milk, cheese and vegetables are the main sources of calcium and phosphorus. Iron and the other essential elements are contained in meat and vegetables. If her diet does not provide sufficient of any of these essentials it is necessary to give special supplements; in Great Britain pregnant and nursing mothers are usually given extra milk (protein, calcium, phosphorus), eggs (protein), iron salts, and vitamins.

Vitamin Supplements.—The widespread use of cod-liver oil and fruit juice as adjuvants in infant feeding has practically eradicated rickets and scurvy from England. Theoretically, if the mother's diet is ideal, there should be no need for these supplements to be given to a breast-fed infant. In Great Britain, however, supplements are almost always given, usually as orange juice concentrate and " welfare " cod-liver oil, or some equivalent preparation (*see* p. 65).

Failure to Breast-feed

This may be due to a defect in the infant or to a defect in the mother.

1. *Defect in the infant.* Anything which interferes with strong suction may cause a failure in lactation. Nasal obstruction due to rhinitis, also hare-lip, cleft palate, or micrognathos may cause difficulty in sucking. Sometimes the infant is premature or too weak from some other cause, e.g. congenital malformation of the heart, to suck properly. For these infants the milk may have to be expressed and the feed given with a spoon or bottle. In some infants the co-ordination between sucking, breathing and swallowing is poorly developed. Success in such cases depends on the skill with which the situation is handled.

2. *Defect in the mother* arises usually from one or more of the following conditions:—

(i) Worry or mental upset is a potent cause, and if she is over-worked and undernourished the supply of breast-milk may also be deficient.

(ii) Failure on the part of the mother, nurse and doctor to persevere in getting the infant to take the breast in the first fortnight after birth.

(iii) Cracked or sore nipples; infection of the breast.

(iv) Depressed nipples, or poorly-developed breasts.

METHODS OF INCREASING THE FLOW OF BREAST-MILK

Once lactation has been established, it is maintained by a conditioned reflex and the strong suction of the infant emptying the mother's breasts at regular intervals. An insufficient supply of breast-milk may be increased by:

1. Adequate rest.
2. Sufficient intake of fluid.
3. The calmness and confidence produced by good nursing and a careful doctor.
4. Making certain that the baby is emptying the breasts at each feed; otherwise expressing the residue.

UNDERFEEDING ON THE BREAST

Underfeeding may either prevent gain in weight or cause sleepless nights, or both. The infant may become constipated when the amount is only slightly deficient, but later the motions are small,

TABLE V

Average Chemical Composition of Cows' and Human Milk[1]

(Figures refer mainly to the middle period of lactation)

Constituent			Cow	Human	Remarks
Lactose			4·75 G. per 100 ml.	6·5 G. per 100 ml.	Rises in human milk for a fortnight after birth and then remains fairly constant throughout lactation.
Fat			3·75 G. per 100 ml.	3·6 G. per 100 ml.	Subject to wide variations in human milk and in milk of different breeds of cow.
Protein	Caseinogen ..		3·0 G. per 100 ml.	0·8 G. per 100 ml.	Total protein in human milk falls during the first month after birth from 1·7% to 1·2% after which it remains fairly constant till towards the end of lactation when it falls gradually to 0·9%.
	Lactalbumin ..		0·4 G. per 100 ml.	0·4 G. per 100 ml.	
	Lactoglobulin ..		Trace	(?)	
	Total		3·4 G. per 100 ml.	1·2 G. per 100 ml.	
Salts	Calcium	Soluble	0·03 G. per 100 ml.	0·016 G. per 100 ml.	Rises in human milk to reach a maximum at the end of 4 months and then slowly declines
		Insoluble	0·09 G. per 100 ml.	0·020 G. per 100 ml.	
		Total	0·12 G. per 100 ml.	0·036 G. per 100 ml.	
	Phosphorus	Soluble	0·038 G. per 100 ml.	0·014 G. per 100 ml.	Shows in human milk a rise and fall similar to that of calcium, but less marked.
		Insoluble	0·057 G. per 100 ml.	0·004 G. per 100 ml.	
		Total	0·095 G. per 100 ml.	0·018 G. per 100 ml.	
	Iron		0·027–0·14 mg. per 100 ml.	0·05–0·19 mg. per 100 ml.	
	Copper		0·012–0·02 mg. per 100 ml.	0·04–0·08 mg. per 100 ml.	
	Manganese		4–5γ per 100 ml.	(?)	
	Iodine		4–7γ per 100 ml.	4·3–4·6γ per 100 ml.	Depends on the iodine content of the diet.
	Total		0·7 G. per 100 ml.	0·2 G. per 100 ml.	

[1] Reproduced from Wilson, G. S. (1942). "The Pasteurization of Milk." London: Edward Arnold

Constituent		Cow	Human	Remarks
Vitamins	Carotene ..	5–75γ per 100 ml.	5–60γ per 100 ml.	Higher in cows' milk in summer than in winter depending on diet.
	A	20–130 i.u. per 100 ml.	160–270 i.u. per 100 ml.	
	Total A potency	28–280 i.u. per 100 ml.	200–500 i.u. per 100 ml.	
	B_1	15–25 i.u. per 100 ml.	1·6–4·4 i.u. per 100 ml.	Fairly constant in cows' milk. If present in human milk, not usually in free state.
	Riboflavin ..	0·1–0·3 mg. per 100 ml.		
	Nicotinic acid ..	0·5–1·4 mg. per 100 ml.	(?)	
	C	about 2 mg. per 100 ml.	about 3–5 mg. per 100 ml.	Fairly constant in cows' milk.
	D	Winter 0·3–1·7 i.u. per 100 ml. Summer 2·4–4·9 i.u. per 100 ml.	Usually less than in cows' milk	In cows' milk depends on amount of sunshine to which cows are exposed.
	E	Very small	(?)	

slightly greenish, and often frequent—so-called " hunger stools." Aerophagia is common and vomiting may occur. An unformed stool may be passed, with flatus, during or immediately after each feed with consequent loss of calories. On being put to the breast, a very hungry baby will gulp what little milk there is, swallowing air at the same time. When this air is returned, some of the milk may come up as well, thus a portion of the meagre supply of milk is lost, so that at the next feed the baby is even more hungry. It is this picture which has given rise to the expression " windy milk," but no such thing as " windy milk " exists; usually the quantity is insufficient. An infant who is underfed cries a great deal, especially before the feeds are due. He also cries after being fed, having colic from swallowed wind. This crying gives the impression that the baby has indigestion, so the parents think the breast-milk is too rich or that he is getting too much. Consequently water is often given before the feed to dilute the strength. If truly underfed, the infant's condition will be aggravated by such treatment.

TEST-FEEDS

The method of confirming that an infant is underfed is to measure the daily intake by doing test-feeds for 24 hours. To perform a test-feed the infant should be weighed in a shawl before and after the feeds; if a stool or urine has been passed he should not be changed until after the test. The increments in weight obtained at each feed are added together to give the total daily intake. If this intake is much below the baby's estimated requirements, underfeeding has been shown and appropriate advice should be given.

AMOUNT OF BREAST-MILK REQUIRED IN THE DAY

The amount of breast-milk required by a normal and healthy infant can be estimated. For the first four or five months the infant will need approximately 45 to 50 calories per pound of body-weight per day (100–110 calories per kilo). An average sample of breast-milk yields approximately 20 calories per fluid ounce (70 calories per 100 ml.). Thus, using the higher figure for the calculation, it is seen that a 10 lb. infant requires $10 \times 2\frac{1}{2} = 25$ oz. of breast-milk in the day. Since the yield of breast-milk varies at the different feeds, it is easy to see that one isolated test-feed is no criterion and that it must be the amount of breast-milk given during a particular day that is ascertained. Each infant is a law unto itself; some infants require much more food than others, and nervous, highly-strung infants especially require more food than placid infants who sleep much. In cold weather more food is required than in hot, sultry weather, and therefore the figure given above is only an average. It should be clearly understood, however, that the minimum of $2\frac{1}{2}$ oz. of breast-milk per pound of body-weight per day applies to the normal healthy infant. If an infant is underweight, calculation should be made on *expected weight*, not on actual weight. For example, an infant that fails to gain adequately and at six weeks weighs $7\frac{1}{2}$ lb. instead of the expected 9 lb. should received $9 \times 2\frac{1}{2}$ oz. per day.

COMPLEMENTARY FEEDS

When an infant is not gaining and test-feeds have shown that the flow of breast-milk is not sufficient, then *complementary feeds* should be given, i.e. additional food at the end of each breast-feed but not in place of a breast-feed. A sufficient quantity is given in the bottle immediately after the breast-feed to make up the deficit.

An example of this would be an infant weighing 10 lb. and fed four-hourly—that is, getting five feeds in the day—who is obtaining from its mother 15 oz. of milk only. This baby would only be getting an average of about 3 oz. at each of the five feeds, but an infant weighing 10 lb. ought to have $10 \times 2\frac{1}{2} = 25$ oz. in the day, which is an average of 5 oz. at each of the five feeds. Therefore, 2 oz. of a complementary feed should be offered to this child at the end of each breast-feed.

Rules for Complementary Feeding. 1. The infant should be left at the breast only long enough for the breast to be properly emptied, that is, if very little milk is present, for not more than three to six minutes. Sucking at the empty breast fills the infant with wind.

2. The complementary feed should be given after the breast-feed, and never before. This ensures that the breast is properly emptied.

3. Both breasts should be given at every feed, and each should be given first, alternately.

4. The complementary feed should not be made very sweet, or the infant will refuse the breast and prefer the complementary feed.

5. Where possible, all the breast-feeds should be test-feeds and the deficiency made up to an exact quantity. Probably the smallest feed is in the middle of the day and therefore the largest complementary feeds will be required then.

6. Action should be taken to increase the supply of breast-milk (*see* p. 37).

Overfeeding on the Breast

This fault comes less often to the notice of the doctor because nature tends to correct the error herself.

SYMPTOMS
1. At first the weekly gains will be excessive, the baby contented and without symptoms.
2. Then there are small vomits or regurgitations after feeds not usually produced by eructations of wind.
3. Sometimes there will be an increased number of stools which may become loose.

MANAGEMENT
1. Test-feeds should be made to ascertain the amount being taken.
2. The time at the breast should be shortened.
3. Three-hourly feeds should be changed to four-hourly ones.
4. A little water may be given before the breast-feed.

Weaning and the Commencement of Mixed Feeds

The process of weaning should be gradual so that the infant can get used to the new foods as the mother's milk flow slowly decreases. The age of weaning is an arbitrary choice. When an infant weighs 15 lb. it will be getting about 35 oz. of breast-milk from its mother, and it is seldom that the average woman can produce more than this without inconvenience. Before this point is reached, the infant should have been accustomed to small amounts of broth (*see* p. 42) and vegetable purée (2 teaspoonfuls); one of the homogenized vegetables may be used (such as Brand's, Heinz, Libby's or Nestlé's), or lightly boiled egg (1 teaspoonful) at the 2 p.m. feed, the quantities being gradually increased. These foods are often introduced between $4\frac{1}{2}$ and 5 months. The second stage, which comes at six months, is to give a cereal, first at 10 a.m. and later at 5 p.m. also. The most convenient cereal preparations are those which require no cooking, e.g. Farex, Farley's, or those quickly prepared, e.g. Cow and Gate Cereal Food. So far all the feeds are fluid; they should be given with a spoon from a cup. Before the incisor teeth come through the baby can start sucking and chewing a rusk or a bone. When the teeth appear, solid foods are gradually introduced.

In recent years the practice of introducing cereal foods at an earlier age in infancy, i.e. 2 to 3 months old, has become a fashion. The composition of milk, in which the carbohydrate is in the form of lactose, makes it probable that cereal feeding is unphysiological in the early months of life. Babies easily become fat and flabby with such feeding.

Between six and eight months, the breast-feeds given at 6 a.m. and 10 p.m. will be changed to milk (5 oz.) and water (2 oz.) with a heaped teaspoonful of white sugar, and the small breast-feeds given at 10 a.m. and 6 p.m. will be discontinued as the size of the cereal feeds is increased.

When breast-feeding is gradually cut down in this way, there is seldom discomfort for the mother, but if the breasts should become uncomfortable lactation can be stopped by giving stilbœstrol.

WEANING DIET FOR A HEALTHY BREAST-FED INFANT FROM FIVE TO EIGHT MONTHS OLD. (WEIGHT 14 TO 18 LB.)

Feeding Times. 6 a.m., 10 a.m., 2 p.m., 10 p.m.

6 a.m. Give both breasts, 7 minutes at each side.

10 a.m. 1. Boiled milk ....2 ounces.
Water ....1 ounce.
Sugar ....1 level teaspoonful.
or National full-cream dried milk ....2 measures.
Water ....3 ounces.
Sugar ....1 level teaspoonful.
To this add one to three heaped teaspoonfuls of a prepared cereal, such as Farex or Cow and Gate Cereal Food. Half a teaspoonful of the yolk of a lightly boiled egg can be given with this feed and gradually increased to two teaspoonfuls if well tolerated.
2. After this feed give a small breast-feed.

2 p.m. 1. Milk mixture as at 10 a.m.
Add to this 2 tablespoonfuls of bone and vegetable broth or thickened broth (*see* p. 54). One or two tablespoonfuls of Brand's, Libby's, Heinz or Nestlé's homogenized vegetables may be added.
2. Give the breast.

6 p.m. 1. Give a cereal feed as at 10 a.m., but omit egg.
2. Give a small breast-feed.

10 p.m. Give the breast only.

Fruit Juice.—Orange or tomato juice, two to three teaspoonfuls, diluted with water and sweetened with sugar, or a similar quantity of black-currant purée or rose-hip syrup, diluted with water, should be given daily at tea-time.

Cod-liver Oil.—If the feeds are made up with liquid cows' milk, the baby should have one teaspoonful of " welfare " cod-liver oil (containing 400 i.u. of vitamin D) or a corresponding amount of a suitable vitamin preparation. If dried milk is used, then the recommended amount of " welfare " cod-liver oil is 7–8 drops daily because the dried milks are fortified with calciferol.

CHAPTER 4

Artificial Feeding

Most infants can and should be fed at the breast, but since breast-milk will not always be available, the practitioner must make himself acquainted with the principles of artificial feeding. The importance of these principles is being more and more appreciated by the profession and the public, and no doctor is completely trained without knowledge of them. These principles should underlie the practice of infant nutrition and this practice can be made relatively simple by pruning it of unnecessary detail. Indeed, it is a subject which has been made needlessly complicated by a superfluity of methods and an unnecessary number of proprietary preparations, many of which differ in little but the manufacturers' names.

DIFFERENCES BETWEEN COWS' MILK AND BREAST-MILK

THERE are fundamental differences between cows' milk and breast-milk which can never be overcome. Breast-milk is received by the infant warm and sterile, while cows' milk reaches the infant after some hours and is usually not sterile. The protein and fat of these milks is qualitatively different.

The main differences in composition of cows' milk and human milk can be found by turning to pp. 38–39. The question arises whether it is necessary in artificial feeding for cows' milk to be modified to make it as nearly like breast-milk as possible. The answer is that, because we cannot produce a mixture like breast-milk, we should concentrate on producing artificial feeds that are simple to prepare on which infants thrive. This may necessitate departing widely from the breast-milk standard. Cows' milk is composed of protein (caseinogen and lactalbumin), fat, carbohydrates and salts.

PROTEIN

When cows' milk reaches the stomach its caseinogen is coagulated by enzymes, forming casein which combines with calcium to form calcium caseinate. The resulting curds are rather coarse, but can be made finer in the following ways:

Heating, either by boiling or evaporation *in vacuo*, or in the process of drying, alters the structure of the caseinogen, so that it coagulates

43

into smaller curds. This is usually sufficient, but formerly it was sometimes thought necessary to peptonize the milk or to add sodium citrate. A similar effect can be achieved by the addition of a little cereal in the form of barley water.

If an infant's feed contains too much protein there is unlikely to be vomiting or diarrhœa, but the infant tends to become constipated. Occasionally semi-translucent, bean-shaped brown bodies are seen in the stools, which consist of protein curds insoluble in ether.

FAT

In early infancy there may be difficulty in the digestion and absorption of fat. The stomach empties more slowly when much fat is taken. The stools may be pale, bulky and greasy; fat " curds " are sometimes seen and these are soluble in ether. An excessive intake of fat inhibits appetite and may cause vomiting.

CARBOHYDRATE

Sugar. The fact that there is more sugar in human milk than in cows' milk suggests that the human infant has a relatively larger requirement than the calf. When cows' milk is used for artificial feeding, it is therefore sensible to add sugar to the feed. Contrary to expectation, there is no evidence that lactose is better for this purpose than dextrose or sucrose, so ordinary white sugar can be used. Dextrimaltose is especially well tolerated and can be used when necessary.

When too much sugar is given there is likely to be excessive gain in weight and the infant retains extra fluid in its tissues. Gradually such an infant becomes flabby and the abdomen is distended. There may be loose, frothy, acid stools (fermentation stools). On the other hand, when too little sugar is given, there is likely to be constipation and perhaps an unsatisfactory gain in weight.

Infant feeding can be simplified, as outlined on pp. 48–52, by using feeds with a standard energy value of 20 calories per oz. and it is a simple matter to raise the sugar content of cows' milk without altering its previous energy value which, like breast-milk, is approximately 20 calories per oz. It happens that 1 drachm by weight of sugar yields 14 calories, so 1½ drachms dissolved in 1 fluid oz. of water yields an approximately standard solution which can be added to cows' milk in any required proportion. That is to say, in the making up of a feed, 1 oz. of standard sugar solution can replace an equal volume of cows' milk and, similarly, 1½ drachms of sugar can replace a measure of full-cream dried milk, without altering the caloric value of the feed.

Since domestic teaspoons vary in size they are not reliable for measuring, and sugar measures designed to deliver 1½ drachms by weight seldom appear on the market. However, it is possible to have a particular teaspoon checked to show that it delivers approximately one drachm by weight and then to keep it as the measure for the sugar. Using such a teaspoon, it may be taken that when heaped it will be equivalent to 1½ drachms. Alternatively, the measure sold with a full-cream dried milk can be used; this when levelled off but not pressed down will contain approximately 1½ drachms of sugar by weight.

Starch. When an infant reaches an age of some 5–6 months, the sugar intake will have increased along with the rest of its food. The average infant, however, is not able to manage large quantities of carbohydrate in the form of sugar, and cereals should be commenced at this time. The starch contained in a cereal food, in process of digestion, is split into sugar, but since this process is slow, fermentation is not so likely to occur. Many infants who fail to gain when sugar is added to their feed will gain rapidly when a cereal product is substituted for a portion of the sugar.

COWS' MILK

DESIGNATED MILKS

THE grades of designated milks permitted by regulations in force in England and Wales are:

(i) *Raw Milk.*
   Tuberculin Tested Milk.
   Note that Accredited Milk (being the milk of a single herd) ceased to be permissible in 1954.

(ii) *Heat-treated Milks.*
   Pasteurized Milk.
   Sterilized Milk.

Under the regulations Tuberculin Tested Milk may be pasteurized and sold under the designations " Tuberculin Tested Milk (Pasteurized)."

Under Section 35 of the Food and Drugs Act, 1955, the Minister of Agriculture, Fisheries and Food and the Minister of Health jointly are empowered to make Orders specifying areas within which all milk sold by retail must conform to the requirements of the Milk (Special Designation) Regulations, 1960. Large areas of England and Wales have now been specified, and by the end of 1960 the milk supplies of over 98 per cent. of the population consisted wholly of " specially designated " milks.

DRIED MILKS

DURING the process of drying cows' milk, the casein curd is modified so that it is more easily digested by the infant than that of fresh cows' milk. Dried milks are made in two ways: either by pouring fresh milk on hot rollers, or by the spray process, in which it is dried by being forced through small jets into a hot atmosphere.

The advantages of dried milk are: (1) It is sterile and can remain so over long periods; (2) in the process of drying the caseinogen has been modified and has become more digestible than that of fresh milk; (3) it is easy to store a supply, which is a great advantage when travelling or when fresh milk cannot be properly kept; (4) the vitamin loss is very small.

NATIONAL DRIED MILK (full cream and half cream)

Dried milks are considerably more expensive than cows' milk itself, but in the United Kingdom a standard full-cream dried milk and a standard half-cream dried milk, both Government subsidized, are available at welfare centres at a special price. When reconstituted, the addition of sugar to each is advised. There are also many proprietary brands of dried milk which vary slightly in different ways. Usually a proprietary half-cream milk is already fortified with sugar so that the further addition of sugar is not required. Dried milks should be made up freshly, using the measure supplied. During manufacture, vitamin D is added to most varieties of dried milk. National dried milks contain an average of 90 to 100 i.u. of added vitamin D per ounce of powder, and therefore each measure includes 12–13 i.u. If the feed is made up according to the instructions, each reconstituted fluid ounce will contain about 10 i.u. of vitamin D. There is no addition of vitamins A and C. Orange juice or other source of ascorbic acid should therefore be given.

HUMANIZED DRIED MILKS

These are so made that when one measure is made up to 1 oz. of water the composition of the resulting mixture resembles that of human breast-milk. Cod-liver oil and fruit juice are given as well. Humanized dried milks are somewhat expensive and they are now used less frequently than formerly.

EVAPORATED AND CONDENSED MILKS

Cows' milk can be concentrated by evaporation *in vacuo* and the product can be sterilized by steam under pressure. The milk to be processed must be of good quality. The processing renders the casein curd more digestible and the fat globules smaller.

EVAPORATED MILK, which is unsweetened, can be used throughout the period of bottle-feeding. It gives results as good as those of the dried milks. In the United States, and also in other countries where this type of tinned product is popular, it is used more than dried milk. Reliable brands of evaporated milk are now available everywhere in the United Kingdom. Most brands have an addition of vitamin D_3, about enough to provide 33 i.u. per undiluted fluid ounce, equivalent to 500 i.u. per reconstituted quart. The standard products manufactured for the American and British markets are of different strength.

British standard evaporated milk has had 60–70 per cent. of the water removed and has a caloric value of 50–53 per fluid ounce so that a dilution of 1 part to 1½ parts of water is a " standard feed," equal to 20 calories per ounce, and also equal to full-cream whole cows' milk. American standard evaporated milk, no longer sold in the United Kingdom, is less concentrated and has a caloric value of 44 calories per fluid ounce. It is usually diluted with an equal part of water to make up the feed.

SWEETENED CONDENSED MILK consists of evaporated milk with sucrose added. The sugar helps to preserve it and it keeps longer after the tin is opened, but its high sugar content makes it unsuitable for routine use. Vitamin D_3 is incorporated. Its caloric strength is approximately 100 calories per fluid ounce and it can be reconstituted 1 in 5 to give a standard feed.

TABLE VI
SWEETENED CONDENSED MILK

	Undiluted	Diluted 1 Part Condensed Milk to 4 Parts of Water
Protein	9%	1·8%
Sugar	53%	10·6%
Fat	10%	2·0%
Calories	100 per fl. oz.	20 per fl. oz.

It will be seen from Table VI that the sugar content is too high and the fat unduly low for infant feeding. The amount of protein is also on the low side.

CEREAL PREPARATIONS

THE majority of the proprietary cereal foods are made up by adding them to cows' milk. Some require cooking, while others, such as Cow and Gate Cereal Food, Benger's Food, Pablum (U.S.A.), and Farex, need only be added to the warm milk mixture and allowed to stand. Cereal foods are used to introduce starch into the diet of the infant from about the fifth month, and they may also be used in the early months of life to thicken the food of babies addicted to rumination (see p. 59).

The average analysis of the cereal-containing preparations shows: protein 5 to 10 per cent., fat 2 to 10 per cent., carbohydrate 70 to 80 per cent. One to three heaped teaspoonfuls would be sufficient to add to the single 7-oz. feed of an infant.

Care should be taken not to give these cereal foods in excessive quantity or the infant is likely to become flabby and pale with a low resistance to infection.   Some cereal foods are deficient in vitamins, hence vitamin supplements are important.

The baby who will not tolerate sugar given as cane sugar or lactose will often take an adequate amount of carbohydrate in a preparation containing a mixture of dextrins and maltose (partly digested starch). Another may fail to gain weight on simple milk mixtures and will thrive at once when a little cereal is added to the diet.   At the period of weaning, a proprietary food may initiate with success the first attempt to give more than milk.

WATER

DILUTING a concentrated feed makes it more digestible, and water is necessary for metabolism.   More fluid is needed in hot weather and, if it is withheld, an infant may become dehydrated; the urine is concentrated and scanty, and the temperature rises (*see* pp. 94, 624, Dehydration Fever).   Extra water helps to correct constipation.

ENERGY CONTENT OF MIXTURES

IT has been noted (*see* p. 44) that an average sample of breast-milk contains 20 calories per fluid ounce and that cows' milk has a similar average caloric value.   In constructing infant feeds it is not difficult to arrange that a caloric strength of approximately 20 calories per fluid ounce is provided.   Feeds with this caloric strength can be called *standard mixtures*; their use greatly simplifies the feeding of infants up to about five months of age, when additional calories may be added without increasing the fluid volume.

METHODS OF ARTIFICIAL FEEDING

1. UNDILUTED COWS' MILK

THIS will be found unsuitable in practice except in some few cases. The majority of infants will tolerate it when acidified or citrated, but it is not the best method.

2. HUMANIZED COWS' MILK MIXTURE

To make up a mixture roughly similar in composition to that of human milk sounds most attractive.   As the infant requires more and more food, this mixture is increased in amount but not in strength. Some normal healthy infants thrive well on this, but there is a large number that finds the quantity of sugar too great and develops diarrhœa and flatulence.   This is easily explained.   The total amount of sugar offered in the day to the infant when very young is but small; as the child increases in size and its demand for food increases, the total quantity of sugar offered in the day also increases, and when the amount of added sugar in the day amounts to more than about 2 oz., diarrhœa frequently results, especially in warm weather.

3. SIMPLE DILUTION OF MILK, WITH THE ADDITION OF CARBO-HYDRATE

Method of choice.—The first step is to think in quantities necessary for 24 hours rather than in amounts necessary for individual feeds. The expected weight of the infant is much more help in calculating its food requirements than is its age, and while it may not lead to an exactly correct estimate it is the most useful basis we have. *The individual infant is a law unto itself and no rule can be set out which covers every case.*

CALCULATION OF THE FOOD REQUIREMENTS OF INFANTS

It is generally agreed that the daily requirement in calories for a healthy baby up to five months is 45 *to* 50 *calories per pound* (100–110 *calories per kilo*) *per day.* Human milk has an average caloric content of 20 calories per fluid ounce, so the quantity required is about $2\frac{1}{2}$ oz. per lb. (*see* p. 38). This volume can also be used as the guide to the approximate fluid requirement in average cool weather. The artificially fed baby will thrive on the same volume intake as the breast-fed one, and it has been explained that all feeds are best standardized to contain approximately 20 calories per fluid ounce (the same as breast-milk), such feeds being referred to as *standard feeds*.

The exact requirements of any given baby will be learned by individual study, but the requirements of an underweight infant should be calculated (as mentioned on p. 39) according to his expected weight rather than his actual weight.

EXPECTED WEIGHT

Method of Calculation	*Example*
Birth weight..........	Birth weight........7 lb. 3 oz.
Plus 1 oz. per day of life (excluding first 10 days) for 100 days.	Age........40 days. Therefore add 40 oz.
Thereafter the infant should gain 1 lb. per month up to the age of one year.	(less 10 oz.) i.e. 30 oz. ......1 lb. 14 oz.
	9 lb. 1 oz.

To Prescribe a Feed of Cows' Milk and Water

The expected weight of the baby having been calculated, the amount of feed required per day can be estimated. This amount, divided by the number of feeds, gives the size of each feed.

Example:—An infant of expected weight of 12 lb. requires about $12 \times 2\frac{1}{2} = 30$ oz. per day. It should receive five feeds, so each feed = 6 oz. Take 5 oz. of milk and add 1 oz. of standard sugar solution, that is $1\frac{1}{2}$ drachms of sugar dissolved in 1 fluid ounce of water, as described on p. 44.

TABLE VII

FEEDS FOR NORMAL BABIES OF AVERAGE WEIGHT FED ON NATURAL COWS' MILK

Age in Months	1	2	3	4	5	6
Approximate weight in lb. ...	$8\frac{1}{2}$	$10\frac{1}{2}$	12	$13\frac{1}{2}$	15	16
Number of feeds in 24 hours	5 or 6	5	5	5	5	5
Amount of cows' milk in oz.	$2\frac{1}{2}$ or 3	4	5	$5\frac{1}{2}$	$6\frac{1}{2}$	7
Level teaspoons of sugar ..	$1\frac{1}{2}$	$1\frac{1}{2}$	$1\frac{1}{2}$	$1\frac{1}{2}$	$1\frac{1}{2}$	$1\frac{1}{2}$
Boiled water in oz. ..	1	1	1	1	1	1

If it is decided to give a weaker feed, say milk and water in the proportion 2 : 1, which is commonly done during the first three months, then the feed will be constructed as follows:—

Cows' milk ....4 ounces (80 calories)   ) Total = 120 calories
Granulated sugar..3 drachms (40 calories)   }   or 20 calories per
Water ....2 ounces   )   ounce.

Before making the feed *cows' milk should always be boiled*. In order to protect the baby from vitamin deficiency, fruit juice and cod-liver oil, or its equivalent, should be given each day both summer and winter (for dose, *see* p. 42).

To Prescribe a Feed of Dried Milk

Most full-cream dried milks are so made that 60 grains by weight (delivered by the volume of one *level* measure) mixed with one fluid ounce of water reconstitutes as the equivalent of whole cows' milk with an energy equivalent of approximately 20 calories per ounce. Since the process of drying renders the protein more digestible, it is not necessary to dilute reconstituted dried milk with more than approximately 1 oz. of extra water with the corresponding amount of added sugar ($1\frac{1}{2}$ drachms).

Example:—An infant of expected weight of 10 lb. requires about $10 \times 2\frac{1}{2} = 25$ oz. per day. It should receive five feeds, so each feed = 5 oz. The feed will be constructed as follows:

Full-cream dried
  milk ....4 measures (80 calories)   ) Total = 100 calories
Granulated sugar..$1\frac{1}{2}$ drachms (20 calories)   }   or 20 calories per
Water ....5 ounces   )   ounce.

Fruit juice and cod-liver oil or its equivalent should be given both summer and winter.

TABLE VIII
National Dried Milk (Full-Cream)
Feeding Table for Normal Babies of Average Weight

Age in Months	1	2	3	4	5	6
Approximate weight of baby in pounds..	8½	10½	12	13½	15	16
Number of feeds in 24 hours	5 or 6	5	5	5	5	5
Number of level measures of milk powder	2½ or 3	4	5	5½	6½	7
Number of level teaspoons of sugar each feed	1½	1½	1½	1½	1½	1½
Ounces of boiled water ..	3½ or 4	5	6	6½	7½	8

DRIED MILKS WITH A REDUCED FAT CONTENT

The caloric value of a half-cream dried milk powder is less than that of a full-cream product and that of a skimmed dried milk is less again; however, different proprietary brands naturally vary slightly as between each other. The composition and caloric value of the reconstituted milk should be calculated from the information issued with the product, to confirm that the directions printed on the tin will give satisfactory mixtures. The manufacturer's measure should always be used to make up the feeds, because domestic teaspoonfuls vary in size and so does the volume of powder they deliver. Most of the proprietary brands of half-cream dried milk have the necessary amount of sugar already added, so that more need not be added when the feed is made up.

Attention should be given to the fact that National Dried Milk (half-cream) is sold without added sugar and therefore sugar should be added when making it up.

Fruit juice and " welfare " cod-liver oil 7–8 drops are given daily.

TABLE IX
National Dried Milk (Half-Cream)
Feeding Table for Babies of the Weights Indicated

Approximate weight of baby in pounds	6	7	8	9	10
Number of feeds in 24 hours ..	6	6 or 5	5	5	5
Number of level measures of milk powder for each feed	2	2½ or 3	3½	4	4½
Number of level teaspoons of sugar each feed	1	1	1	1	1
Ounces of boiled water	2½	3 or 3½	4	4½	5

TO PRESCRIBE A FEED OF HUMANIZED DRIED MILK

The feed, whatever its size, should be made up in the proportion of one measure to one ounce of water *but no sugar should be added*.

Evaporated and Condensed Milks

Sweetened evaporated milks, e.g. Nestlé's and Diploma, have a value of approximately 100 calories per ounce. A standard feed can be made up by diluting 1 in 5 but the sugar content of this will be too high for ordinary purposes (*see* p. 47).

Unsweetened evaporated milks, e.g. Ideal, Carnation, Libby's, have a value of about 50 calories per ounce and a dilution of 1 part of milk to $1\frac{1}{2}$ parts of water gives a standard feed equal to 20 calories per ounce. To the milk diluted in this manner an ounce of standard sugar solution can be added without disturbing the caloric value per ounce.

Example of a standard feed of unsweetened evaporated milk:

Evaporated milk ..	2 oz.
Water	3 oz.
Standard sugar solution ..	1 oz.

This can also be written as follows:

Evaporated milk ..	2 oz.
Sugar	$1\frac{1}{2}$ level teaspoonfuls
Water	4 oz.

Somewhat weaker mixtures are occasionally used during the first month. At six months of age, the mixture is sometimes strengthened by using equal parts of evaporated milk and water.

GENERAL DIRECTIONS TO MOTHERS AND NURSES

THE doctor can use the following directions when instructing a mother or nurse who is to feed an infant artificially:—

Calculate the approximate amount required by the baby according to his weight, allowing $2\frac{1}{2}$ oz. per pound of body-weight per day; the infant should be fed according to the " expected weight " and not according to the actual weight (*see* p. 39).

When given 6 feeds per day, i.e. 3-hourly feeding, the feeding times would be 6 a.m., 9 a.m., 12 noon, 3 p.m., 6 p.m., and 10 p.m.

When given 5 feeds per day, i.e. 4-hourly feeding, the feeding times would be 6 a.m., 10 a.m., 2 p.m., 6 p.m., and 10 p.m.

Quick feeding.—See that the hole in the teat is a good size, so that the baby can easily get the feed in ten minutes.

Breaking wind.—Hold the baby up before, during, and for twenty minutes after each feed until the wind is broken twice.

Vitamins.—Fruit juice and " welfare " cod-liver oil or its equivalent should be given daily from the age of one month (for dose *see* p. 42).

INFANT FEEDING IN THE SECOND HALF OF THE FIRST YEAR: THE INTRODUCTION OF MIXED FEEDING

At 5–6 months an infant weighs 15 to 16 lb. (it may even be heavier), and it is at this age that it is customary to introduce cereals into the diet, but this is an arbitrary choice and infants will do well on milk alone until about the ninth month.

THE PRELIMINARY STAGE

A month or more before the sixth month, it is well to offer bone and vegetable broth, thickened broth, homogenized vegetable purées, and lightly boiled egg (see p. 41). Such additions can be given before the milk mixture at the 2 p.m. feed. The quantities of newly tried foods should be small at first, i.e. 1 to 2 teaspoonfuls.

THE SECOND STAGE

The amount and consistency of the broth and vegetable purées is gradually increased and the infant is accustomed to feeding from a cup and spoon. Next a cereal feed is given, first at 10 a.m. in place of the previous bottle feed, and a week later at 6 p.m. In this way the outline of the future routine of three main meals begins to be established. The details of the diet offered can be seen in the diet sheets which follow. It is important that the vitamin supplements already being used should be continued.

DIET FOR BABIES AGED 5 TO 8 MONTHS (14 TO 18 LB.)

6 *a.m.*—Milk mixture,[1] 7 oz.

10 *a.m.* — A cereal,[2] 1–3 teaspoonfuls, made up with 4–5 oz. of milk mixture.[1]

2 *p.m.*—Milk, 5 oz., with broth,[3] 2 tablespoonfuls, and vegetable purée,[3] or egg yolk or scrambled egg or egg custard.

6 *p.m.*—Same as 10 a.m.

10 *p.m.*—Same as 6 a.m.

Babies will adapt themselves to changes if they are made gradually: dissimilarities in their tastes and appetites are natural. Raw milk must be boiled or pasteurized. Extra water may be given between feeds, and this is essential in hot weather. Give fruit juice (vitamin c) and " welfare " cod-liver oil (vitamins a and d) regularly.

[1] The milk mixture consists of boiled milk 5 oz., water 2 oz., and sugar 1 heaped teaspoonful, or whole-cream dried milk 5 measures, sugar 1 heaped teaspoonful and water 7 oz. (When cereal is being added reduce the amount of sugar by half.)

[2] The following prepared cereals are useful:—Farley's, Farex, M.O.F., Robinson's Groats or Barley, Robrex, Scott's Baby Cereal, Wheatex. Pay attention to the cooking directions because some need careful cooking, but Farley's, Farex, Robrex and Scott's Baby Cereal are ready cooked and M.O.F. is cooked in a minute or so.

[3] Bone and vegetable broth and vegetable purée can be made at home, but the varieties bought in bottles are safe and satisfactory—Brand's, Heinz', Libby's, Nestlé's, Trufood's; note that Scott's strained foods contain cereal as well.

Bone and vegetable broth is made as follows: 1 lb. chopped bones, 2 teaspoonfuls of vinegar, a pinch of salt, 1½ pints of water. Bring to the boil, skim, then simmer for one hour. Chopped vegetable and a piece of shredded liver is added during the cooking. Sieve and keep in a cool place.

To make thickened broth, take 1 tablespoonful of soya flour, 1 pint of vegetable stock, 1 teaspoonful of Marmite, sieved vegetables. Mix soya flour with stock and bring to boil. Add cooked sieved vegetables and flavouring during the cooking.

DIET FOR BABIES AGED 8 TO 12 MONTHS (18 TO 22 LB.)

On waking.—Give 1 tablespoonful fresh orange juice, tomato juice or grapefruit juice or 2 teaspoonfuls concentrated orange juice diluted with boiled water and sweetened with sugar, and a Farley's rusk. (No milk to be given at this time.)

8 *a.m.*—Give ½ to 1 cup of cereal made with milk and feed with a spoon. Give lightly boiled egg or crisp toast fried in bacon fat or grilled crisp bacon. Give rusk or toast with butter. 8 oz. of milk (this includes that made into cereal).

12.30 *p.m.*—1 heaped tablespoonful mashed potato and 1–2 table-spoonfuls sieved vegetables with 4 tablespoonfuls vegetable broth. The following may be added as the baby grows: pounded chicken, rabbit, sole, plaice, brains, scraped steak, liver. 1 to 3 tablespoon-fuls milk pudding or egg custard with fruit purées. Water to drink.

4.30–5 *p.m.*—Crust or rusk or thin brown or white bread and butter with grated cheese, honey, seedless jam or Marmite. Junket or custard with stewed fruit. 8 oz. milk (including that made into junket or custard).

10 *p.m.*—A small drink of boiled milk may be given if thirsty; this can be discontinued about the ninth month.

NOTE.—All milk to be boiled or pasteurized. Extra water as required. Give fruit juice and " welfare " cod-liver oil regularly. Feed by cup and spoon as soon as possible; bottles should be discontinued by the age of 9 months.

CHAPTER 5

Feeding Problems
in Infants and Young Children

THERE are many parts of the world where undernutrition is still the main problem in child health and, so frequently does it go hand-in-hand with diarrhœal, parasitic and other environmental diseases, that measures aimed at improving education, economic conditions and hygiene must have priority in the health programme. In countries where, as in Britain today, the general standard of living has risen, undernutrition is now seldom seen, although at the beginning of the present century, when smaller wage-packets spelt dear food, and when mothercraft and infant dietetics were then little taught, under-feeding and wrong feeding were all too common; almost daily, doctors and health workers had to propagate the fact that a sufficiency of food must be given and this in suitable, digestible forms.

Although the nutrition of children has so much improved, it would be a mistake to imagine that its problems have disappeared. Good-quality milk and plenty of the right kind of food are not the only things necessary; the teaching of mothercraft and good practicable advice about the problems which often arise during weaning, and afterwards, are also needed. Therefore, practitioners, health visitors and nurses should be thoroughly conversant with these aspects of child welfare because the guidance of mothers lies in their hands.

UNDERFEEDING

THE requirements of breast-fed infants are set out on p. 38 and those of infants fed artificially are on p. 49. In Britain, such knowledge is now readily available, yet ignorance persists in many quarters, and when an infant is being underfed it is usually due to lack of knowledge or commonsense on the part of mother, nurse or practitioner.

When underfeeding is suspected, the first step is to calculate whether the infant is being offered enough for his daily needs, and to enquire whether he seems satisfied and settles down to sleep after his feeds. The composition of the feed should also be checked and if possible the giving of a feed should be watched to observe details of technique and, in a suspicious case, to look for the physical signs of pyloric stenosis (see p. 180).

SYMPTOMS AND SIGNS

Failure to gain, or loss of weight is a constant sign of underfeeding. A strong infant will also show his hunger by sucking at his fists and by crying between feeds. Observed at feed-time, it can be seen that he sucks ravenously and will often swallow a considerable amount of air in the process. If this is not relieved by eructation, gurgling peristalsis may be heard and flatus may be passed before the feed is finished, perhaps with a loose and undigested stool. Eructation taking place after he has been put down usually results in vomiting; sometimes there is screaming because of colic (*see* Aerophagia, p. 58). In this way a vicious circle is often set up—hunger, ravenous feeding, aerophagia, vomiting, screaming, undigested stools and increased hunger (*see also* Underfeeding on the Breast, p. 37). Well-intentioned attempts to improve the infant's " digestion " by making him take his feeds more slowly or by making them more dilute have the effect of increasing the symptoms.

If the underfeeding goes on for a long time, loss of vigour gradually occurs, crying diminishes and hunger becomes less intense. This change is more abrupt if there is an intercurrent attack of severe diarrhœa. As the condition worsens, the signs of " marasmus " appear (also called " atrepsia," nutritional " atrophy," or nutritional " dystrophy "). At this stage the infant will be pale, wasted and apathetic, and the eyes set in a wizened face seem over-prominent. There is a virtual loss of subcutaneous fat, although the " sucking pads " in the cheeks are usually preserved. The loss of fat makes the skin seem loose and redundant and sometimes rough and dry. Dehydration may be present. Occasionally there is an increase of hair on the back. The motions are constipated and scanty, unless there is superadded enteritis. Sometimes the stools are small and frequent and dark green or grey in colour—the so-called " hunger stools."

UNDERNUTRITION RESULTING FROM DISEASE

Sometimes underfeeding is the result of disease, as in the following examples: *Pyloric stenosis* (*see* p. 180) can prevent much of the food taken into the stomach from reaching the small intestine; hence the infant will not gain weight until the obstruction at the pylorus has been overcome and the vomiting stopped. With a *hiatus hernia* (*see* p. 178) loss of food can occur. Congenital *heart disease*, especially when *cardiac failure* (p. 283) is present, can make it impossible for a baby to take feeds of adequate size. *Mucoviscidosis* (fibrocystic disease of the pancreas, etc.) (*see* p. 138) is another cause of undernutrition; also subacute and chronic infections, such as *pertussis* and *tuberculosis*.

OVERFEEDING

IN Britain and in some other western countries, overnutrition is just as common as underfeeding, for many of those who deal with infants equate bulk with health. There are wide variations in food tolerance. Some babies when overfed will take all that is offered, slowly becoming fatter and fatter. With others, appetite will fail, and if, in neglect of this, the baby is persuaded to finish the bottle either regurgitation occurs or an increase in the number of the stools. A wise mother can teach herself to gauge her baby's appetite and use this as a guide; but others are pleased to see the feeding bottle emptied; with a little encouragement baby will take a fraction too much at nearly every feed and become too fat.

SYMPTOMS AND SIGNS

Excessive gain in weight is the outstanding sign of overfeeding; the fat deposits gradually fill up and thus obesity is established. Subcutaneous fat is easily seen but it should be remembered that fat is also stored in other sites—in the thorax, around the peritoneum, the kidneys and the heart, also in the head and neck. A mother, feeling the firmness of the subcutaneous fat will often conclude that the muscles are themselves firm and well-developed, but the assessment of muscle-tone requires experience and practice, and a doctor used to the examination of children will find that the muscles beneath the fat are relatively thin and flabby, especially when a large proportion of the calorie intake is in cereal form.

ANOREXIA AND VOMITING

In small infants it is rather difficult to distinguish between thirst and appetite, because most of the fluid taken is in the form of milk, which the infant must have in order to satisfy his thirst. Although over-feeding may cause anorexia, thirst may make the baby suck, and, when this goes unrecognized, vomiting may occur.

ALTERED STOOLS

The frequency of the stools sometimes increases; they become " undigested " and are often green. Usually the buttocks become excoriated. Overfeeding with full-cream milk may provoke fat intolerance. The colour of the stools may become greyish or perhaps pale yellow; and the so-called " fatty curds," soluble in ether, may be present (see p. 44).

Overfeeding with Added Cereal. Milk is a physiological food for all mammalian young. Taking milk as a sole or main food, an infant can make optimum progress until about the ninth month. This food gives a proper balance during that period of dependence on the mother when rapid growth is occurring and plenty of first-class protein and a supply of minerals are needed for tissue-building. Cereal feeding is not a real physiological need, for if the calories in the early months of infancy come mainly from starches, these, after providing energy, favour the accumulation of fat rather than the building up of bone, muscle and other tissue. Thus, overfeeding with cereal imbalances the diet and results in a fat and often flabby baby who may be slow to throw off the common infections of the respiratory tract. A further stage of imbalanced feeding with cereal, at the expense of protein, will lead to *protein deficiency* and finally to the clinical syndromes of *protein malnutrition* (*see* p. 600).

FAULTS IN FEEDING TECHNIQUE

In these days when the choice of the feed and its correct composition are usually well understood, the symptoms of a so-called " feeding difficulty " arise from mistakes in feeding technique more often than from faults in composition. After details of the feed and the quantities offered have been checked, the mother should be asked to describe in detail the routine she follows at feed-time. It is even better to ask her to show how she feeds her baby, during which demonstration faults can be seen and corrected.

Aerophagia (Air-swallowing)

There is always some swallowing of air during feeds, whether from the breast or bottle. This is physiological, and an x-ray will normally show a bubble of air in the fundus of the stomach. The air is voided from the stomach by the process of *eructation*, which should take place easily as soon as the infant is sat up, aided perhaps by patting or rubbing of the back. If this is not properly done and the baby put to lie down too soon, he will be uncomfortable; vomiting occurs if he has to eructate lying down. Any air not released by eructation passes from the stomach into the intestine where it can cause distension and increased peristalsis. Gurgling peristalsis may be felt or heard. Discomfort and colic may result in attacks of screaming. Flatus, and perhaps a semi-formed and poorly digested stool, may be passed during the feed; when this happens at each feed weight gains will be poor.

Aerophagia, so common in infants reared on " Western " lines, is seldom a problem in countries where the mother, as in many Asian and African communities, normally carries her baby in a shawl on her back.

A common cause of excessive air-swallowing is the use of a teat with too small a hole. Mothers and nurses think that air is swallowed when too " fast " a teat is used, but this is a fallacy. With each sucking movement a little air is swallowed; if, say, 300 suctions are required to complete the feed, more air must necessarily be swallowed than for, say, 200 suctions through a larger hole. It is true that there may be gulping and spluttering when too " fast " a teat is used. The hole should be big enough to allow an actively sucking infant to take the entire feed inside 10 to 15 minutes, including a brief pause of about 1–2 minutes in the middle to allow for eructation. When the feed is finished, the baby should be held up, and patted, for approximately twice as long as the feed has taken, that is, for at least 20 minutes.

Prevention and Treatment of Aerophagia

1. Offer a sufficient quantity of food to meet the baby's needs.
2. See that he gets his feeds easily. If he is breast-fed, tell his mother not to check him unduly, explaining that, as milk does not have to be masticated, quick feeding does not cause indigestion. If he is on a bottle make sure that the hole in the teat is large enough to allow the milk to run easily at approximately one drop per second.
3. Allow the baby to eructate before beginning the feed; if held up for 1–2 minutes he will sometimes " burp " at this time. A second opportunity should be given when he pauses about half-way through the feed. Finally, when the feed is finished, hold him up for about twice the length of time he has taken to complete it.
4. When eructation is very slow, a carminative mixture may be effective, such as:

R Sodium bicarbonate	100 mg. (1½ grains)
Aromatic spirit of ammonia	0·9 ml. (1½ minims)
Compound tincture of cardamom	0·16 ml. (1½ minims)
Glycerin	0·3 ml. (5 minims)
Dill water .. .. to	3·67 ml. (60 minims)

Directions: Give 4 ml. (one teaspoonful) diluted with a little warm water after feeds.

Rumination (Merycism)

This is the term used to describe a habit developed by some infants of regurgitating a feed and re-swallowing a portion of it.

ÆTIOLOGY

Very often the food is a pleasant one, such as one of the sweetened condensed milks, and has been given in too dilute a form, so that the total feed is greater than the stomach can contain. The result is that natural vomiting occurs at first, but soon the infant acquires the trick of being able to regurgitate the feed at will. It has been said that some acute digestive disturbance may initiate the vomiting and that it continues afterwards as a habit.

CLINICAL PICTURE

In severe cases, the baby is very much under weight; thus at, say, six months he may weigh only 7 or 8 lb. The story is that from a very early age, a few weeks only, the infant brought up food in small amounts almost continuously from one feed to another. The pillow was always wet with vomit. In many cases, the regurgitation can hardly be called vomiting, but rather spitting. On close inspection the infant can be seen to hollow the tongue like a funnel, champing the jaws and struggling as if uncomfortable. Occasionally the back is arched. Suddenly the food wells up into the mouth, a small portion spilling from the corner and the remainder being slowly re-swallowed. This process is repeated over and over again until a considerable proportion of the food is wasted.

DIAGNOSIS

It is seldom that the clinical picture which has been described is seen by the physician, or even the mother, because the infant, often a girl, bright and clever, will not ruminate while anyone is present. The process is best studied by placing a screen round the head of the bed and peering over the top. The infant, when she thinks herself alone, will go through the process.

TREATMENT

There can be little doubt that rumination is a purely functional complaint. The spitting and vomiting will cease in the following circumstances:—

1. If between feeds the infant is watched and interested, held up to look out of the window, played with and talked to.
2. If the food is thickened with a cereal preparation, so that it is small in bulk and firm in consistency.
3. If, during the process of rumination, a drop of quinine solution is placed in the open mouth. The face of the child shows its disgust, and for the time being all efforts at rumination cease.

PROGNOSIS

Infants given to rumination usually gain weight rapidly on thickened feeds.

WEANING AND WEANING DIFFICULTIES

As soon as a baby begins to take any food other than milk, the process of weaning has begun. The verb " to wean " is derived from an Anglo-Saxon word " wenian "—to accustom; weaning should be a gradual process to accustom the infant to a variety of foods instead of taking only one.

Changing fashion during the twentieth century has done more than physiology to influence the age at which to start weaning. Formerly in Britain it was the custom to continue breast feeding until well into the second year; then the realization that such prolonged feeding on milk alone was a factor in the causation of anæmia led to a change of opinion in favour of earlier weaning, at first at about 9 months, and a decade or so later weaning from the age of 6 months came into fashion. Now there is a vogue to begin earlier, even at two months. When fashion and precept influence an important aspect of infant feeding, it is wise to see what guidance physiology can give. It can be accepted that milk is a complete food for young infants; but for how long? When infants are restricted wholly to a milk diet, anæmia from lack of iron is the first deficiency to appear. Milk contains only a trace of iron, but this mineral is stored in the fœtal liver during the latter part of pregnancy; the time taken for iron deficiency to manifest depends on how long the fœtal store lasts. Except in prematurely-born infants, iron-deficiency anæmia seldom appears until 9–10 months of age and it is wise to introduce iron-containing foods well before this age. It is interesting to note that among the various primitive peoples, whose custom it is to prolong breast-feeding into the second, third and fourth years of life, it is also the practice to give small quantities of the different foods taken by the other members of the family; thus, in primitive and natural settings, breast milk is an adjuvant and not a staple food after the first year of life.

Another reason why milk is unsuitable as the only food for the older infant is its bulk; it is so dilute that gain in weight becomes too slow towards the end of the first year. Dentition and the maturation of the intestinal enzyme pattern are also useful physiological guides. Most mammals suckle their young until some teeth are present. In infants, the date of eruption of the opposing incisor teeth (at six to nine months) approximate with what we know of the probable date of the maturing of the enzyme systems in the infant gut. Hence it can be concluded that milk should be the staple food until that age.

None of these arguments tells us when to begin the weaning. Perhaps the answer in part depends on the suitability and choice of the introductory foods available. In view of the physiological adaptability of infants, early mixed feeding is unlikely to be harmful, provided that a correct ratio between tissue-building and energy-producing foodstuffs is maintained. It should be remembered that an excess of starch-containing food upsets the balance of nutrition and tends to produce fat and flabby babies with impaired resistance to respiratory infections. Meat and vegetable broths and similar sources of mineral salts and protein are therefore indicated early in the programme of mixed feeding.

Weaning Difficulties

In weaning from the breast the *physical side* is a dual process, the infant becoming accustomed to a new diet while lactation is gradually brought to an end. But the *psychological implications* are also important. If birth is the first step towards independent existence, weaning is the second. The emotions engendered by breast-feeding, and to a lesser extent by bottle-feeding, are part of the foundations of the mother-child relationship. This implies that weaning is likely to be emotionally significant, and it is not surprising that the emotions caused by it vary from satisfaction in both partners to dismay, the latter chiefly in the mother.

The difficulty of weaning is refusal of new foods, acceptance of which is part of the process of getting used to new tastes and smells. Delayed dentition, mongolism, and anorexia caused by disease may be responsible, but it is usually predominantly psychological. Early weaning helps to prevent such trouble. It should be gradual and the object and emphasis placed on getting the new tastes and smells accepted. If, on the other hand, either consciously or unconsciously, the mother's idea is to maintain in the second six months, against nature, a rate of weight-gain only proper to the first five months, then only a placid baby will accept meal-times without resistance. An over-keen or anxious mother easily makes the mistake of pressing food on her unwilling baby and showing undue displeasure if it is rejected, whereas a calm one is often successful, perhaps because she is less put out when the baby disapprovingly spits out some new food which has been lovingly prepared.

Frequently the doctor has to help a mother whose infant of about nine months old is refusing his weaning diet, accepting only milk from a feeding bottle, and not gaining weight. He will at once think of faulty management, but organic causes need to be excluded. Sometimes the infant has as yet cut no teeth. By this age a cup and spoon should have been in use, for an infant of nine months need no longer be on a bottle. Having put this right, he can advise reducing the amount of milk offered in order that the baby may develop an appetite for other kinds of food. Reassurance is essential because the mother will be anxious, and she will need a warning that the first day or two of the new regime may be a time of unhappiness and tears.

IMPAIRED APPETITE AND REFUSAL OF FOOD IN CHILDREN

TRUE impairment of appetite is not uncommon. It may be a symptom indicative of infection, anæmia, or renal, hepatic or metabolic disorder. If organic disease is responsible the child will lose weight and soon become thin. On the other hand, with simple refusal of food the child is usually found to be plump and, with a gaining weight, there is obviously no real loss of appetite.

1. Food refusal is often part of a behaviour disorder; it is seen especially in spoiled children and only children. Refusal to eat at meals may be but one of several symptoms of " negativism." The young child may habitually give an emphatic answer " No " to a number of parental suggestions (*see* p. 24). The doctor should first give sympathetic consideration to the mother's problems, which may be found to go far beyond the single anxiety of the meal-time battles. He should give full reassurance and an explanation of the child's behaviour. The whole problem is discussed in Chapter 18.

2. It is easy to misjudge a child's true dietary needs, and therefore it is advisable within reason to let his appetite decide when he is hungry

and when he has had enough. Some mothers over-estimate how much a child should eat and will come to the doctor saying that " he hardly eats a thing," but this is contradicted by his energy, plumpness and evident health. Children vary in their dietary requirements, which depend upon age in relation to size, rate of growth, output of energy and intrinsic metabolic differences. It is not always easy for a mother to accept a rational explanation, but she may be convinced when, after weighing and measuring, it can be demonstrated that her child's weight is within the normal range in relation to his height.

CHAPTER 6

Feeding of Children in Health

In order that a child may be adequately nourished, it is necessary for him to receive a diet sufficient to cover his needs both in terms of growth and output of energy. Growth makes a particular call on protein, mineral salts, and vitamins. The protein for tissue-building is derived mainly from animal sources. It includes milk, cheese, meat, fish and eggs, but there is also valuable protein in soya flour and in the pulses. The essential mineral salts and the vitamins are widely distributed in most natural foods; the more foodstuffs are submitted to processes of manufacture, drying, storing and cooking, the greater will be the loss of these natural vitamins. It is right to utilize the protective foods available in the local produce of a country; and where these are neglected or wastefully used, there is scope for education in better food habits.

CALORIES

Children use up a great deal of food energy in their many activities and pursuits. Weight for weight their caloric needs are greater than those of adults; the total caloric intake of adolescents is actually higher than in most adults.

TABLE X
CALORIC REQUIREMENTS AT DIFFERENT AGES

Child	1– 3 years	1,200
Child	4– 6 years	1,600
Child	7– 9 years	2,000
Child	10–12 years	2,500
Adolescent girl	13–15 years	2,800
Adolescent boy	13–15 years	3,200
Adolescent boy	16–20 years	3,800
Adult woman (moderate work)		2,500
Adult man (moderate work)		3,000

PROTEIN REQUIREMENTS

The demands of growth and the repair of tissue require a generous amount of the proteins which contain the essential amino-acids. Up to about five years, a child can thrive on a total protein intake smaller than is required by an adult, yet he needs nearly as much first-class protein; after five years, a child requires about the same amount of protein as an adult but more first-class protein. It is to be noted that pregnant women and lactating mothers also have high protein requirements. In general, about fifteen per cent. of the caloric value of the diet should come from the protein intake.

CARBOHYDRATE AND FAT

The balance of the caloric needs is made up with carbohydrates and fats. Whilst individual and racial differences exist, approximately fifty per cent. of the caloric intake of children is taken as carbohydrate and thirty-five per cent. as fat. Yet there are individual peculiarities; thus some children can take less fat and more carbohydrate, while others are more tolerant of fats and require less carbohydrate. Fat has a high caloric value and is the vehicle for the fat-soluble vitamins, namely, vitamins A, D and K. Fat is somewhat more difficult to digest and its presence slows the emptying of the stomach; thus a little fat goes a long way and it is better not to give much of it when the appetite needs encouraging. Carbohydrates are more readily available for conversion into energy, and their metabolism also helps to complete the combustion of fat used for the production of heat and energy.

FLUID REQUIREMENTS

There is considerable variation in the fluid requirements of children of different ages. In the most general terms, children between the ages of one and three years, in a temperate climate, require 1,200–1,800 ml. of fluid per day; from the age of four to seven years the requirements increase to 1,500–2,000 ml., but great variations will exist in different environmental and exercise conditions.

VITAMINS

The precise requirements of individual vitamins necessary for normal growth and health are discussed in Chapter 10. In the United Kingdom children under the age of five years are offered, through the Welfare Clinics, " welfare " cod-liver oil containing vitamin A not less than 3,000 i.u. and vitamin D 400 i.u. to the drachm. Concentrated orange juice containing 50 mg. of vitamin C to the drachm is similarly available.

MINERALS

On a normal diet, a healthy child should not require any mineral supplements, except the premature infant for whom supplements of iron are essential (p. 81). The total requirements of two of the more important mineral salts (which are provided in a normal diet) are calcium 1·0–1·5 G. per diem, and iron 6–12 mg. per diem.

Diet Suitable for Children in the United Kingdom

The following specimen diet sheets, derived from those in use at The Hospital for Sick Children, Great Ormond Street, London, can be followed when using the kinds of food available in the United Kingdom.

Diet Suitable for a Child aged 1 to 2 years

On waking: Fruit or fruit juice.

Breakfast: A little porridge or cornflakes or Grapenuts or Cow and Gate
8 a.m. Cereal or Weetabix or Shredded Wheat served with plenty of milk and a little sugar. Toast or bread and butter, seedless jam, golden syrup or honey. Milk flavoured with cocoa or weak tea. Some children will prefer scrambled or coddled egg, chopped bacon and fried bread, sardine, a tablespoonful of creamed haddock or herring, or cod's or herring roe.

Dinner: Minced beef, mutton, Irish stew, liver, rabbit, chicken, steamed
12–12.30 p.m. fish or grated cheese; or meat soup thickened with sieved lentils; one tablespoonful of mashed potato and one tablespoonful of green or mashed vegetable. One or two tablespoonfuls of milk pudding, baked egg custard, blancmange, steamed sponge pudding, etc. In warm weather stewed fruit or fresh fruit salad from which the pips and skin have been removed. When dried fruits are given they should be soaked for six hours and then stewed. Water to drink.

Tea: Toast, rusks, or bread and butter, seedless jam, honey, golden
4–5 p.m. syrup or Marmite, or tomato, lettuce or cheese sandwiches. Fruit jelly or fruit salad; sponge cake, biscuits, apple. 8 oz. of milk to drink.

Diet Suitable for a Child aged 2 to 5 years

On waking: Fruit or fruit juice.

Breakfast: A little porridge or breakfast cereal with plenty of milk and some
8 a.m. sugar. In place of this in warm weather stewed fruit and milk. Crisp toast and butter or dripping. Then fried bread or egg or bacon or ham or fish. 8 oz. of milk including that given with the first course.

Mid-morning: Orange juice and a biscuit, or a cup of milk.

Dinner: Cutlet, mince, oxtail, stew, roast meat, offal, fish or grated cheese.
12–12.30 p.m. Potatoes cooked in various ways: baked or boiled in skins, chipped, mashed or riced. Carefully washed lettuce, watercress, cucumber, spring onions, tomatoes, beetroot, and grated raw carrot. All fresh and root vegetables in season steamed in very little water which should afterwards be added to soups and gravies. Dried peas and beans, tinned and frozen vegetables when fresh ones are not available. Bread and butter pudding with dried fruit, steamed puddings, milk puddings, baked apples, stewed fruit, custard, blanc-mange. Water to drink.

Tea: Toast or rusks with butter, jam, honey, golden syrup, black
4.30–5 p.m. treacle, Marmite, or sandwiches of tomato, lettuce, cheese, paste; or egg or baked beans on toast. 8 oz. of milk.

Diet Suitable for a Child aged 5 to 12 years

Breakfast: Fruit, orange juice or tomato juice. Porridge or cereal with milk and sugar. Sausage and potato, egg or bacon and tomato, ham, fish, fish cake, sardines on toast. Crisp, thin toast, butter, marmalade, a glass of milk or tea and milk.

Mid-morning: One-third pint of milk.

Dinner: Cutlet, stew, mince, oxtail, beef, chicken, fish, liver, rabbit, etc. Potatoes cooked in skins, roast or sauté. Salads containing lettuce, watercress, cucumber, spring onions, tomatoes, beetroot and grated raw carrot. Fresh and root vegetables in season. Baked or steamed puddings with custard sauce, baked bread pudding, pastry with jam or fruit, apple fritters, pancakes. Fresh raw fruit, or fresh fruit with custard or ice-cream, stewed fruit with milk pudding or custard. Water or a soft drink.

Tea: Bread or toast with butter, margarine or dripping; sandwiches with fish paste, cheese, egg or meat filling or jam, syrup, honey or Marmite; salads. Fruit, jelly, cake and biscuits as desired. Milk, or tea and milk to drink.

Supper: From about the age of 9 years most children require a light meal, such as bread and butter, sponge cake, biscuits, fruit.

Feeding of Children in Different Climates

The basic principles of nutrition as previously described apply through-out the world, but local climatic conditions, shortages of basic neces-sities, lack of hygiene, and ignorance of dietetic principles all raise their special problems in different countries.

TROPICAL COUNTRIES

In hot climates, the body requirements for heat production are inevitably reduced with a corresponding diminution of calorie intake affecting principally fat and carbohydrate. The protein requirements for tissue repair and growth are unaltered. Thus a Caucasian child entering a tropical climate will show some reduction in appetite, or alternatively, if the ingested food is excessive, a digestive upset may occur with vomiting or diarrhœa. Such an illness may be accentuated by the hot weather or by an associated intestinal infection.

For infants, special dried milks are available, such as Cow and Gate Dried Milk (tropical), which keep well in tropical climates and which are so constituted as to provide a relatively low fat content (2·3 per cent.). Powdered milks, such as Pelargon (Nestlé), which is a full-cream dried milk with added vitamins, and Eledon (Nestlé) which is a half-cream milk, are acidified with lactic acid and are also suitable for tropical countries.

The extra losses of water and sodium chloride in perspiration need special replacement by an increased fluid intake fortified by a small quantity of salt (half a teaspoon to the pint) to avoid the dangers of heat exhaustion (*see* p. 624). Young children have no way of indicating their special needs for extra fluid and salt. Steps must be taken to provide them, rather than additional milk feeds, when the infant is restless from what may be mistaken for hunger.

Infection from contaminated foods and drinks remains a serious problem in some countries. The apparent willingness of native servants to boil milk or water does not imply that this is always carried out unless constant supervision is exercised. The proper cleansing and sterilizing of feeding and cooking utensils requires equal attention.

In many parts of India raw cows' milk is not freely available, but where obtainable such milk should be boiled as should goats' milk. In many areas, mothers continue to breast-feed their children beyond six months of age whilst the more prosperous may make use of dried milks. Rickets and scurvy are seldom seen, but among the poor classes beri-beri is fairly common, although many alternatives to a polished rice diet are available.

WEST INDIES

The practice in Jamaica of supplementing breast feeding by feeds of " bush tea " from the age of a few weeks is potentially dangerous, in view of the risk of veno-occlusive disease of the liver which may follow the absorption of groundsel, a common ingredient of " bush tea." Cows' milk is in short supply, as are other first-class protein foods, such as fish, meat and eggs.

EAST AND WEST AFRICA

The special problem in these areas is one of protein deficiency (p. 600). Once breast-feeding is discontinued the protein intake of the child may become haphazard. Associated infestations, such as ascariasis, may be complicating factors. Better education and better availability of adequate protein for children between the ages of 6 months and 4 years of age will in due course abolish kwashiorkor, just as nutritional rickets has disappeared in the United Kingdom.

SOME GENERAL NUTRITIONAL PROBLEMS

The Thin Child

SOME children have been well nourished and then progressively lose weight, becoming thinner and thinner. Other children have always been thin and over-active, coming of a thin stock.

A thin child must be carefully examined to exclude organic disease as the cause of wasting. Inadequate feeding, nervous over-activity, prematurity, asthma, chronic naso-pharyngitis, tuberculosis, rheumatism, diabetes mellitus, and intestinal diseases, such as cœliac disease and fibrocystic disease, may all produce progressive wasting. Very rarely, a case of *progressive lipodystrophy* may be seen. As a rule, it is the upper half of the child that is involved in this condition; showing an almost entire absence of subcutaneous fat, the face, arms and chest present a picture of extreme emaciation, although the child feels energetic and well.

Children coming of thin stock are often naturally skinny. They are usually wiry, energetic, intelligent, and sometimes highly strung. The mother's complaint is that she " cannot get any flesh on him," he has " always been thin," although possibly quite a plump infant.

ÆTIOLOGY

A thin and underweight child may have a poor appetite or defective powers of assimilating food, especially fat, and tends to be over-active and to expend too much energy. The result of this is that the balance between the intake of food and the output of energy is too nearly equal. An attempt to increase the intake by the addition of cream, milk, butter and eggs produces increased anorexia, furring of the tongue, bad breath and even vomiting. The symptoms are accentuated by the common transient infections of childhood.

TREATMENT

Many thin children are full of energy and are in fact extremely healthy. In such instances and where physical examination is negative, the main treatment is to reassure the mother that her child is healthy and is growing as nature intended. Where the child shows symptoms of listlessness and excessive tiredness at the end of the day, treatment consists in *cutting down the child's output of energy* to the point where, with his moderate intake of food, he has a balance on the right side, so that he thrives and gains weight. This can be done by limiting the length of his day and arranging for a *midday rest*. *School or kindergarten* should be started early to provide rest and discipline. Carbohydrate, especially in the form of sugar, is sometimes well tolerated by such children, and powdered glucose or plain sugar is a useful adjunct to their diet. There is often an element of maternal anxiety, and it is important to explain to the mother that it is possible to overestimate a child's requirements in food. When appetite is lacking, persuasion to eat will sometimes defeat its purpose, but a change of environment brings about a satisfactory gain in weight.

Obesity

It is difficult to explain many cases of obesity. Some children will eat largely without becoming fat, while others will get plump on a similar intake; minor variations are not to be regarded as pathological. The body seems able to absorb and store up fat, but unable to call on it again. When fat is assimilated and is not burnt up, a vicious circle is formed. Fat is laid on, probably due to some metabolic error; once having become fat, the child is less active, and being less active, tends to put on more fat; this vicious circle continues. With the increased weight there is a tendency for the arches of the feet to give, and with painful feet there is even less inclination to activity. Sometimes genu valgum may develop (Fig. 4).

TYPES OF OBESITY

Obesity may be subdivided into *endogenous* (due to a more or less defined factor affecting storage) and *exogenous* (due to excessive caloric intake and inactivity). The latter is far commoner but there is no hard and fast line between the two main types.

The cases of *endogenous* obesity with a proven endocrine cause are rare. Cases of suprasellar cyst causing hypothalamic symptoms may show a greatly increased appetite and obesity. More often the precise defect is a matter of conjecture and the term *constitutional obesity* is suggested. When endogenous obesity occasionally follows encephalitis, meningitis, or hydrocephalus, it has been postulated that centres in the midbrain concerned with calorimetric control of the food intake are affected. Occasionally obesity is a sign of endocrine disorder (*see* p. 148).

The cases of *exogenous obesity* are more common in Jewish children. The onset is commonly at about 7 years and many patients normalize their fat metabolism after puberty. The condition is therefore probably functional.

TREATMENT

A careful history should be taken *to exclude organic causes*, e.g. encephalitis, meningitis, disease of the thyroid, pituitary insufficiency, and Cushing's syndrome (*see* pp. 148–150).

The *diet* should be regulated, and fat and carbohydrate reduced to a minimum. Limited fried food and not more than twenty ounces of milk a day should be given, and there should be a great reduction in bread, cereals, and potato. The child should have a full allowance of high-protein foods and vegetables. Sugar should be reduced to a minimum. Only three meals in the day should be allowed. Drinks of water need not be restricted. Fruit of all sorts may be given in moderate quantities in place of milk puddings (*see* diet, p. 72).

The full co-operation of the child and the parents (or school) is essential for success. It is well for the weight to be recorded once a week. It should be explained that the plan is to lose weight slowly but steadily, usually not more than a pound a week, and in the milder cases it is sufficient to keep the weight stationary while the child grows up to his weight. By these means a considerable degree of obesity can be righted over a period of some six months.

During the treatment the child should take plenty of exercise. At the beginning, active exercises to strengthen inadequate muscles will be valuable.

DRUGS

Thyroid extract is not indicated. Amphetamine, which increases activity and diminishes appetite, can be a useful aid.

PROGNOSIS

Without treatment, simple obesity, if not extreme, tends to clear up in adolescence. With methodical treatment excellent results are obtainable (Fig. 4).

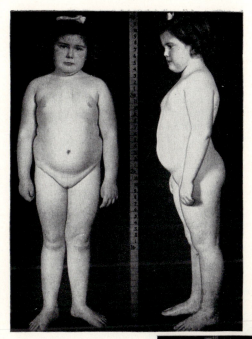

Fig. 4.—Simple obesity in a girl aged 5 years; and (*below*) after 9 months' dietetic treatment.

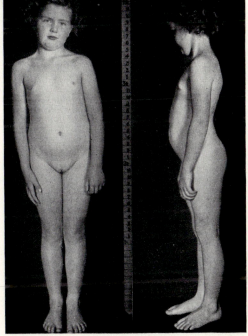

DIETETIC REGIME FOR OBESITY

The over-weight child must be given a diet consisting of all the food elements essential to maintain growth and health. At the same time, it should contain the minimum number of calories in order to reduce the child's weight. It is not *how much* the child eats, but *how many calories* are contained in *what* the child eats.

No hard and fast dietetic regime is given, but suggestions are made as to suitable articles of diet, which are given below.

Diet for Treatment of Obesity

Breakfast
1. Stewed or fresh fruit, apple, pear, orange, plums, rhubarb or grapefruit, etc.
2. One of the following:—
One rasher of grilled bacon, one boiled or poached egg (not more than three a week), portion of lean ham or tinned meat, or portion of smoked or white fish.
3. One thin slice of bread, or two Ryvita or Vita-wheat biscuits, or Plasmon oats, Limmits biscuits or Energen cereal products. Minimal helping of butter or margarine.
4. Weak tea and milk (6 oz.)

Mid-morning
Glass of orange juice with fresh fruit or one Energen biscuit; 6 oz. milk if not taken with breakfast.

Dinner
1. Average helping of lean meat with unthickened gravy, steamed or boiled fish.
2. Generous helping of lettuce, spinach, cabbage, cauliflower, celery, onions, parsnips, turnips, leeks, etc.
3. 4 oz. milk as junket or milk jelly, with helping of fresh or stewed fruit.
4. Water to drink.

Tea
1. Lettuce or tomato sandwich (thinly cut bread), or two Energen or Limmits biscuits, or two slices of Ryvita or Vita-wheat.
2. Cup of tea (milk 2 oz.).

Supper
1. Thin soup (meat or vegetable), or 1 oz. of cheese and salad, or slice of cold meat and salad.
2. One thin slice of bread and butter or margarine, or two slices of Energen bread, or two Ryvita, Vita-wheat or Limmits biscuits.
3. 8 oz. milk.

To be avoided
The following are to be avoided absolutely:—All fried foods, lard, suet, dripping, olive oil, ice-cream (occasional water ices only permitted), potatoes, extra sugar (only minimal amounts necessary in cooking permitted—aim at 4 oz. per week), confections, sweets and chocolate, jam, honey, treacle, cakes, sweetened condensed milk, bananas, thickened soups and sauces, cereals, including porridge, rice, etc., and special drinks such as Ovaltine and cocoa.

To be allowed
All fresh fruit (except bananas), stewed fruits, vegetables (except potatoes, haricot beans, baked beans and lentils). Fruit drinks (with only essential sweetening).
The child's co-operation over the diet is essential as well as the parents', and the principles must be explained at the start. A great incentive to the child is to have a pair of scales available for daily use.

CHAPTER 7

The Premature Infant

DEFINITION

By an agreed international standard intended to facilitate the comparison of statistics, any infant whose birth weight is $5\frac{1}{2}$ lb. (approximately 2,500 grammes) or less is considered to be immature or premature according to whether the estimated period of gestation is full-term or less. There are difficulties with such a definition. For example, the birth weight alone is a less sure indication of maturity than birth length; some full-term infants are of low birth weight and to assume that the average birth weight is the same for all races is incorrect. The average birth weight of Sinhalese babies is $6\frac{1}{4}$ lb., about 35 per cent. being $5\frac{1}{2}$ lb. or less; Indian and Japanese babies are also born smaller than babies born in the United Kingdom.

SIGNS OF PREMATURITY

The average weight and size of the fœtus at different periods of gestation are presented in the following table:

Fœtal Age	Weight in Pounds	Length in Inches
24 weeks	1·5	$11\frac{3}{4}$
28 ,,	3	$13\frac{1}{2}$
32 ,,	4	$15\frac{1}{4}$
36 ,,	5·5	$17\frac{1}{2}$
40 ,, (term)	7	$19\frac{1}{2}$ to 20

Immaturity of tissues and of enzyme systems gives rise to a variety of symptoms. The temperature is subject to wide fluctuations due to the inability of the regulating centre to cope with variations of external temperature. Immaturity of the respiratory centre, lungs, kidneys, gastro-intestinal tract, and liver may result in apnœic attacks, atelectasis, œdema, poor digestive function and more than the usual degree of neonatal jaundice. The deficiency of subcutaneous fat causes the skin to be wrinkled and the baby has the look of a little old man. There is excess of lanugo and deficiency of vernix caseosa. The bones are unduly soft and the nervous system is immature.

CAUSATION

The incidence of prematurity varies in different communities and social classes. In the United Kingdom 6–10 per cent. of births are premature. Major complications of pregnancy, especially pre-eclamptic toxæmia or ante-partum hæmorrhage, are associated with 30 per cent. of all premature births; other maternal diseases, such as diabetes or nephritis, are present in 10 per cent.; whilst multiple births (17 per cent.), fœtal deformity (5 per cent.), and premature induction of labour for rhesus incompatibility or disproportion

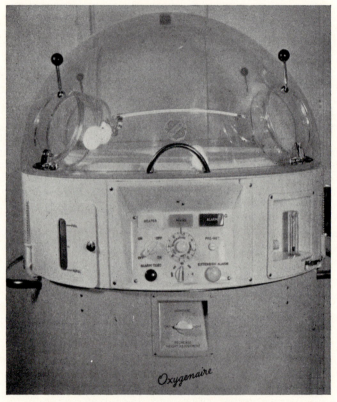

Fig. 5.—The Oxygenaire baby incubator.

(1–2 per cent.) are other well-recognized causes. In some 40 per cent. no medical reason for the premature onset of labour can be found. A significant factor is that premature births are slightly more common in mothers under twenty or over thirty-five years of age than in the other maternal age groups. Further, the prematurity rate increases as the economic scale is descended and in association with illegitimate births. Thus, in Chicago, the prematurity rate is about 5 per cent. in paying patients and over 11 per cent. in the impoverished negro classes. In communities where the diet is inadequate, the provision of dietary supplements for expectant mothers has been shown to reduce the incidence of premature births. The existence of constitutional causes, probably endocrine in nature, is shown by the not infrequent occurrence of recurrent premature labours without other obvious causes. There is an association between cigarette smoking during pregnancy and premature labour.

PREVENTION

The prevention of premature births will be greatly assisted by increased knowledge of their causation. At present prevention lies mainly in providing good antenatal supervision, including adequate nourishment for the mothers. *The adequate treatment of toxæmia of pregnancy is of particular importance.* Whilst some women can apparently continue to work almost up till the time of their confinement, it appears that in others premature labour will ensue unless they have adequate rest in the latter months of pregnancy.

SPECIAL HAZARDS TO THE PREMATURE INFANT

MORTALITY in premature infants is largely due to *functional immaturity* and this is greatest in the infants born after the shortest gestation periods, i.e. those of lowest birth weight. Thus, the chance of survival among infants of under 2 lb. at birth is almost nil, while those at the other end of the scale (between 5 and 5½ lb. at birth) have a survival rate of about 95 per cent.

TABLE XI

CAUSE OF DEATH IN PREMATURE AND FULL TERM INFANTS UNDER
ONE WEEK OF AGE

(From the Perinatal Survey, March 1958, organized by the National Birthday Trust)

Primary Diagnosis				5½ lb. and under	Over 5½ lb.
				%	%
Congenital Malformation	..	..	..	12·9	27·5
Hyaline Membrane	..	..	..	20·8	5·2
Atelectasis Only ..	..	..	..	12·2	1·7
Asphyxia (Intra-Uterine)	..	..	..	8·2	16·5
Trauma ..	..	..	..	6·3	19·9
Pulmonary Hæmorrhage	..	..	..	8·8	2·7
Pneumonia	..	..	..	6·1	7·9
Pneumonia (Intra-Uterine)	..	..	..	2·4	2·1
Infection Others ..	..	..	..	0·7	1·0
Intraventricular Hæmorrhage	..	..	..	8·5	1·4
Rhesus Incompatibility ..	..	..	..	2·2	7·6
Miscellaneous	..	..	..	1·7	3·4
No Anatomical Lesion ..	..	..	..	9·2	3·1

The immaturity of the central nervous system is shown by the sluggish responses of the centres in the medulla for respiration, heat-regulation, deglutition and coughing.   With few exceptions the cough reflex is inactive in premature babies of under 3 lb.   Immaturity of the circulatory system is shown by the sluggish peripheral circulation; that of the lungs by atelectasis and the increased tendency to hyaline membrane formation.   The digestive system and liver are immature but relatively less so than are the kidneys, in which both glomerular and tubular function are poor; urea and salt clearances are low and the infant has little power of concentration or dilution of the urine. Resistance to infection is also more slowly acquired and this is the reason why infection is a special danger.

The respiratory and metabolic acidosis which ensues from asphyxia (p. 89) forms a particular hazard, whilst the tendency to profound hypoglycæmia (p. 114) is a less common but most dangerous complication.   Despite all these physiological disadvantages, the adaptability of many premature infants to extrauterine life is almost mircaulous.

CARE OF THE PREMATURE INFANT

PLACE OF CARE

In most centres, it is considered desirable that premature infants with birth weights below 4 lb. should be nursed in special premature baby units.   This is not to say that adequate care cannot be provided elsewhere, but its organization may be difficult and the nursing time required is considerable.

It is obviously best that the infant should be born in the maternity unit to which the premature-baby unit is attached.   If the infant is born elsewhere, a portable incubator with oxygen should be available to transport the baby in a warmed ambulance to the centre, whither he should be accompanied by a specially trained midwife.

PREVENTION OF INFECTION

In domiciliary practice, respiratory and gastro-intestinal infections provide the greatest hazards, whilst in hospital practice the antibiotic-resistant *Staph. pyogenes* has become a special problem.   In the home no one with a respiratory infection should be allowed in the same room as the infant, and the greatest care should be taken to ensure that the feeds are prepared with meticulous attention to cleanliness.

In hospital, the strictest technique of aseptic nursing should be applied and handling should be reduced to a minimum.   Bathing has no therapeutic value.   In order to combat the special problems presented by the *Staph. pyogenes*, it is advised that all those attending premature infants should apply a barrier cream, such as chlorhexidine, to their hands after washing.

As the umbilicus is known to be a frequent reservoir of infection for *Staph. pyogenes*, the local application of a 1-per-cent. hexachlorophane dusting powder is of the greatest value as a routine measure.   An overtly infected umbilicus or the appearance of septic spots is an indication for isolation of the particular infant from other premature babies.

Premature infants should be spaced widely apart or nursed in separate cubicles. As the room temperature has to be maintained at high levels, ventilation becomes important and air-conditioning with a relatively high humidity (70%) provides the ideal answer.

THE FIRST FEW DAYS

Immediately after birth vitamin K, 1–2 mg., should be given (*see also* p. 84).

The clothing should be light and warmth maintained in other ways. An infant of low birth weight (under $3\frac{1}{2}$ lb.) should be nursed if possible in an incubator (*see* Fig. 5) without clothing. The temperature inside is thermostatically controlled and can be maintained between 85–90° F for as long as necessary. When a baby lies naked in an incubator it is possible to observe it very closely so that episodes of apnœa can be detected early and a stimulus, such as a gentle flicking of the skin, applied. The establishment and maintenance of respiration is discussed below.

BODY TEMPERATURE

The use of special low-reading (at least as low as 85° F) thermometers is essential in the care of the premature infant. The body temperature is very unstable and levels as low as 90–92° F (rectal temperature) are common. Judgement is required in deciding to what extent the infant's temperature should be raised by slowly increasing the external temperature. Below a *critical temperature* (the precise level varying with the humidity), the infant's oxygen consumption increases as the environmental temperature is lowered. Above the critical temperature lies a neutral temperature range in which the oxygen consumption is minimal. The maintenance of a body temperature of about 95–97° F is accepted as a reasonable compromise in many centres. A sudden fall in body temperature (without any change in environmental temperature) may be a sign of the onset of one of the complications of prematurity, such as infection (p. 79).

By contrast, the risk of hyperpyrexia due to faulty control of the incubator temperature remains an important reason for the regular taking of temperatures in premature infants.

Incubators also provide for increased humidity, which prevents undue loss of water vapour. High humidity is extremely advantageous to the lungs in certain circumstances (*see* p. 78).

When an incubator is not in use a cot should be prepared, its interior being kept warm (80° F) with hot-water bottles covered with blanket. The room temperature should be about 70° F. If the room is heated by gas, electricity or radiator, wet towels or bowls of water should be placed near the source of heat. In hospital, if air-conditioning and a thermostatically controlled temperature is provided, then the air should be humidified before entering the room.

RESPIRATION

THE first action after the birth of an infant is to ensure that there is a clear airway and that respiration is rapidly established. It is desirable that this should occur within one minute of complete birth and if breathing has not started within three minutes there is cause for serious concern. The treatment of initial apnœa and *asphyxia neonatorum* is discussed on pp. 89–92. Once respiration is established, the rhythm is often irregular and short periods of apnœa are common, but unless there is cyanosis these are not important.

Respiratory Distress Syndrome

IN some premature infants an expiratory grunt appears within a few hours of birth. The lower intercostal spaces and the sternum are sucked in on inspiration and the accessory muscles of respiration are brought into use. The respiratory rate begins to rise and cyanosis develops. Such infants either collapse and die about the age of forty-eight hours or begin to recover within the same period.

This condition, which is known as the *respiratory distress syndrome*, is almost entirely limited to premature infants and, whilst it may follow all types of delivery, it is rather more common after Cæsarean section and in the infants born to diabetic mothers.

At autopsy the lungs show atelectasis or incomplete expansion, and in a large number, but not all, of the cases *hyaline membrane* is found lining the alveoli. The extent of the membrane varies from case to case but shows no direct correlation with the severity of the symptoms. The membrane contains albumin and is thought by most workers to be the result of a capillary exudate into the lungs. The cause of the condition remains unknown, and it is to be noted that not all the infants who have had the clinical picture of the syndrome have hyaline membrane changes histologically. It is found only in lungs that have undergone some degree of expansion.

In recent surveys of mortality in premature infants, the respiratory distress syndrome with or without hyaline membrane has been the commonest cause of death in premature infants.

Treatment, since the cause of the condition is unknown, is symptomatic, the most important aspect being to supply sufficient oxygen and an atmosphere of high humidity. In severe cases, as a result of increasing carbon dioxide retention, a profound respiratory and metabolic acidosis develops together with a rise in the serum potassium. It is claimed[1] that clinical improvement follows the administration of intravenous hypertonic glucose and sodium lactate or carbonate. It is suggested that the glucose helps to replenish the depleted reserves

[1] Usher, R. (1961). *Pediat. Clin. N. Amer.*, **8**, 525.

of carbohydrate, especially of cardiac muscle and liver glycogen, while the alkali combats the danger of a falling blood pH. The value of this treatment is not yet finally established, but appears rational until the cause is known and prevention is made possible. Antibiotics are given to prevent secondary infection.

Neonatal Atelectasis

In addition to the infants who develop the *respiratory distress syndrome*, there are others whose respiration remains shallow from birth. Cyanotic attacks tend to occur from inadequate pulmonary ventilation, and recovery from these is slow. Occasionally, clinical examination or a chest x-ray will show evidence of unilateral atelectasis although more often the condition is bilateral. Secondary infection of the lung may complicate this state of primary atelectasis.

A primary failure of lung expansion of this nature may be due to bronchial obstruction with mucus, particularly in the unilateral cases; more commonly, it is the result of fœtal asphyxia whereby the depressed respiratory centre at birth fails to stimulate adequate respiratory movements. The respiratory centre may also be depressed by medication (such as pethidine) given to the mother shortly before delivery or by cerebral anoxia incurred during delivery. It is important not to overlook the rare cases of congenital diaphragmatic hernia (*see* p. 179) which clinically may resemble primary atelectasis.

The treatment is similar to that described for infants with the respiratory distress syndrome. In infants who are having repeated cyanotic attacks, or those in whom respiration is too shallow to maintain an adequate respiratory exchange, some pædiatricians use positive pressure respirators to enhance the normal respiratory movements of the infant or to produce entirely automatic respiration.

Neonatal Pneumonia

Neonatal lung infections may arise in four ways. In the first place, attention has been concentrated recently on the development of intra-uterine pneumonia, which is particularly likely to develop if the membranes remain ruptured (following either spontaneous or artificial rupture) for a considerable period before the onset of labour. In such circumstances, pneumonia may be well established by the time of birth. Secondly, infection may only too easily become superimposed in infants already suffering from the respiratory distress syndrome or neonatal atelectasis. Thirdly, due to poorly developed swallowing reflexes, inhalation pneumonia may develop, particularly in infants who have a tendency to vomit. Finally, the lack of resistance to infection makes the premature infant especially liable to primary pneumonia when directly exposed to infection.

The physician must learn not to wait until the classical signs of pneumonia are obvious, for by then the prognosis is always grave.

He must be prepared to act on minor indications—a falling body temperature (despite an unchanged environmental temperature), cyanotic attacks, œdema, the onset of vomiting, an increasing amount of mucus in the pharynx, reluctance to take feeds and an increased respiratory rate may all be warning signs. Later, focal signs will appear in the chest, among which localized showers of fine crepitations are pathognomic. Small areas of impaired percussion are not easily detected in premature infants. A portable chest x-ray (which may be used without removing the child from the incubator) may be most helpful.

Treatment consists primarily in the very early administration of antibiotics; indeed the prophylaxis of neonatal lung infections by this means in cases of the respiratory distress syndrome and neonatal atelectasis has already been mentioned.

The choice of antibiotic depends upon local conditions. In domiciliary practice, a combination of penicillin and streptomycin (for dosage, *see* Appendix I) is extremely valuable. In hospitals, where *Staph. pyogenes* known to be resistant to many antibiotics is prevalent, an antibiotic found to be potent against those particular strains should be employed. Oxygen should be given wherever dyspnœa or cyanosis is present and the airway kept clear by suction as frequently as may be indicated. If signs of peripheral circulatory collapse appear imminent, digoxin (for dosage, *see* Appendix 3) and steroids (*see* Appendix 2) should be added to the treatment. Much will depend upon the qualities of the nursing staff in regard to both the prevention and the treatment of neonatal lung infections of premature infants.

Pulmonary Hæmorrhage

One of the most dramatic complications and a potent cause of mortality in premature infants is that of a severe pulmonary hæmorrhage. This complication appears to be most common in infants where there have been serious complications of the pregnancy and, in particular, severe toxæmia or ante-partum hæmorrhage. The implication is that placental dysfunction had been present during the latter part of gestation.

An infant, who may have appeared to be in good condition during the first hours or days after birth, suddenly becomes collapsed and grey. A little blood-stained mucus may be sucked out of the pharyngeal passages. Despite all resuscitative measures the outcome is fatal. At autopsy there is found to be extensive hæmorrhage, usually into both lungs, disrupting the normal pulmonary structure.

The precise cause of this extensive pulmonary hæmorrhage is unknown, but there appears to be no correlation between it and the occurrence of more widespread hæmorrhagic disease of the newborn (p. 109).

NUTRITION

FEEDING

THERE are differing views concerning the ideal time at which feeding should be started; those in favour of delaying feeding stress the desirability of reducing early handling to a minimum and the danger of inhalation of stomach contents should regurgitation occur. On the other hand, it is suggested that symptoms of hypoglycæmia (p. 114) are more likely if feeding is long delayed. For this reason feeding is begun after about twelve hours in many centres, although at others a longer period of starvation is recommended unless the infant is restless.

The first feed should be 2–4 drachms (8–16 ml.) of sterile water. The smaller infants will be fed by tube, the larger ones by bottle, provided the swallowing reflexes are normal. In the case of very small infants a polythene catheter may be left in the stomach, the outer part being strapped to the head with adhesive tape. Certain centres are trying out the effect of intravenous feeding for the first few days of life of infants of extremely low birth weight.

THE FEEDS

The safest feed for a small infant is breast-milk. Progress is perhaps a little slower with this than with certain artificial milks, but it is surer. There are many alternatives, among which half-cream dried milk and diluted evaporated milk are of about equal merit.

In the first 24 hours of life, the infant requires 10 ml. (2½ drachms) of fluid per lb. of body-weight per day. This increases daily to 20 ml., 30 ml., 40 ml., 50 ml., 60 ml., 70 ml., 80 ml., and finally, by the tenth day, 90 ml. (3 oz.) per lb. of body-weight per day. These figures may also be used to calculate the basic requirements when intravenous fluid is required during the first days of life.

BREAST-FEEDING

As soon as the infant is able to suck vigorously without becoming exhausted, he is ready to feed at the breast. This is usually at a weight of about 4 lb. Until this stage, the mother's milk can be expressed and used for the baby.

VITAMINS AND OTHER SUPPLEMENTS TO FEEDING

Amino-acids, blood plasma, thyroid extract, testosterone, cortisone and eucortone have been advocated, but evidence of their value is chiefly negative.

Vitamin K should be given once (see p. 84). Vitamins A (3,000–4,000 i.u. daily) and D (400 i.u. daily) are given from the second week, and vitamin C (50 mg.) daily. Iron medication to prevent the anæmia of prematurity should be started at the age of two weeks. Colloidal iron, starting with doses of 0·06 ml. increasing up to 0·6 ml. daily, provides a suitable preparation.

Premature Baby Feeding Chart

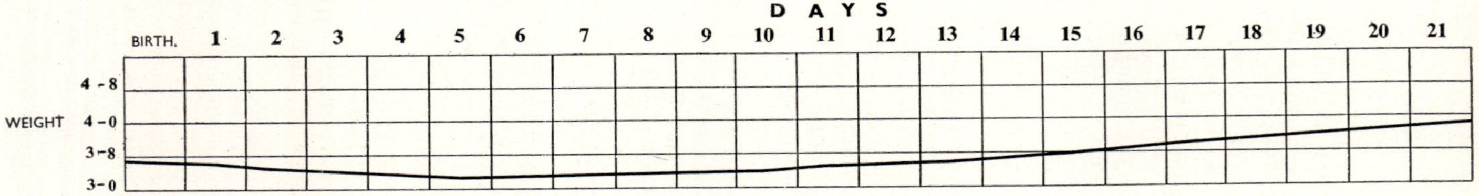

	BIRTH.	1	2	3	4	5	6	7	8	9	10	11	12	13	14	15	16	17	18	19	20	21
TYPE OF FEED			E.B.M. ¼ STRENGTH	E.B.M. ½ STRENGTH	E.B.M. ¾ STRENGTH	E.B.M.	"	"	"	"	"	"	"	"	"	"	"	"	"	"	"	"
AMOUNT OF FEED IN OUNCES	FEEDING COMMENCED 41 HOURS AFTER BIRTH			↑	↑	↑	↑	1	↑	↑	1¼	↑	↑	↑	↑	↑	↑	1½	↑	↑	↑	↑
								1			1¼							1½				
			½					1			1¼							1½				
			½	½	½	1	1	1¼	1¼	1¼	1½	1½	1½	1½	1½	1½	1½	1¾	1¾	1¾	1¾	1¾
			½					1¼			1½							1¾				
			½					1¼			1½							1¾				
			½	↓	↓	↓	↓	1¼	↓	↓	1½	↓	↓	↓	↓	↓	↓	1¾	↓	↓	↓	↓
DAILY INTAKE			2½	3½	3½	7	7	8	8¾	8¾	9¾	10½	10½	10½	10½	10½	10½	11½	12¼	12¼	12¼	12¼
CALORIES			12½	35	47½	140	140	160	175	175	195	210	210	210	210	210	210	230	245	245	245	245
CALORIES/LB			5	10	15	20	20	45	50	50	55	60	60	60	60	60	60	63	65	65	65	65

Fig. 6.—Feeding chart of a premature infant, one of many similarly managed, who was fed on expressed breast-milk (E.B.M.) in the quantities shown. The loss of weight recorded on the fourth day was only $3\frac{1}{2}$ oz. and birth weight was passed on the thirteenth day.

SPECIAL COMPLICATIONS IN THE PREMATURE INFANT

Retrolental Fibroplasia in Premature Infants[1]

RETROLENTAL fibroplasia is a retinopathy which may arise in premature infants, but seldom in those of more than 3 lb. The condition was described by Terry in 1942; before that it was not distinguished from " pseudoglioma." It has been shown that the use of oxygen in high concentration is responsible and that when oxygen is carefully restricted retrolental fibroplasia ceases to occur. In very young kittens it has been demonstrated that hyperoxia may cause vaso-obliteration of the immature retinal vessels and that, on transferring the young animal back to air, a disorderly growth of new retinal vessels follows, producing retinal changes analogous to the early stages of retrolental fibroplasia. The more mature retinal vessels of older kittens are not vulnerable in this way.

CLINICAL PICTURE

The earliest changes implicate the inner eye and usually appear between the third and the fifth weeks after birth, that is, at a time when detailed re-examination of small premature babies is still kept at a minimum. First, there is dilatation and tortuosity of the retinal vessels and, possibly, in this stage the condition is reversible. Retinal hæmorrhages may be seen. Then, new vessels appear upon the retina and adventitious twigs sprout forward into the vitreous. Progressive retinal œdema leads to *retinal detachment*. The active stage of the disease is usually over before the fifth month is reached. The end-results are those of organization and contracture; opaque, partially vascularized tissue forms behind the lens and there are radiating finger-like processes extending into the uvea (posterior synechiæ). The anterior chamber is shallow, and the eyes are small and deep set (microphthalmia), while the iris is usually atrophic. The condition is bilateral and causes complete or partial blindness; secondary nystagmus may develop. A high proportion of the affected children are later found to be mentally impaired.

DIFFERENTIAL DIAGNOSIS

The condition has to be distinguished from congenital cataract, congenital detachment of the retina, from glioma of the retina (which is usually unilateral), persistent hyaloid artery, and from " pseudo-glioma " due to metastatic uveitis occurring in older children.

Hyperbilirubinæmia of Prematurity

In the last decade it has been appreciated that jaundice due to erythroblastosis (p. 110) is not the sole cause of kernicterus (p. 113)

[1] Ashton, N., Ward, N., Serpell, G. (1953). *Brit. J. Ophthal.*, **37,** 513.
Forrester, R. M., Jefferson, E., Naunton, W. J. (1954). *Lancet*, 2, 258.
Owens, W. C., Owens, E. U. (1949). *Amer. J. Ophthal.*, **32,** 1 and 1001.
Terry, T. L. (1942). *Ibid.*, **25,** 230.

If unconjugated bilirubin is allowed to accumulate in the serum of small infants to levels of the order of 20 mg. per cent., whatever the underlying cause, the risk of kernicterus is considerable.

Thus, when the immature liver of the premature infant is unable to conjugate and excrete the normal bilirubin formed in the first week of life, this danger will obtain. It is necessary, therefore, to carry out frequent estimations of the serum bilirubin in any jaundiced premature infant and to perform a replacement transfusion if dangerous levels of bilirubin are reached (for details *see* p. 112).

Although the evidence available does not establish hard and fast limits, danger levels of indirect bilirubin vary with the birth weight, ranging from about 15 mg. per cent. in infants of under 3 lb. to 20 mg. per cent. in infants of 4 lb. The highest levels are frequently reached between the 4th and 8th days of life, after which they begin to fall spontaneously.

High dosages of vitamin κ analogues can give rise to intravascular hæmolysis and thus precipitate hyperbilirubinæmia. For this reason, prophylactic dosage of vitamin κ should always be restricted to a single 1 or 2 mg. injection. An adequate fluid intake for premature infants is probably one of the most important methods of preventing hyperbilirubinæmia. (For a description of other causes, *see* p. 95.)

Congenital Malformations *(see also* p. 97)

There is an increased incidence of congenital malformation in premature as compared with full-term infants. In the determination of precise figures, obvious difficulties arise in deciding what constitutes a minor malformation or what may be regarded as just a normal variation. Accepting these limitations, it appears that about eight per cent. of all prematurely live-born infants have a significant congenital malformation[1] as compared with an incidence of between one and two per cent. of all live-born infants.[2]

Other Complications

In this chapter a description is given of the complications to which the premature infant is particularly liable. The other complications which may affect both mature and immature newborn infants are described in Chapter 8.

PROGNOSIS IN PREMATURITY

The ultimate fate of a premature infant is difficult to predict. Most of the deaths occur within 48 hours of birth, especially in infants of under 3 lb., but there continues to be a slightly increased mortality rate at least until the end of the first year. For the others, the outlook depends upon their vitality, the care available and the presence or

[1] Corner, Beryl (1960). " Prematurity." London: Cassell.
[2] McKeown, T., Record, R. G. (1960). " Congenital Malformations." Ciba Foundation Symposium. London: Churchill.

absence of ante- or intra-natal complications. Infection takes its chief toll after the first two days, and this is now largely preventable.

Surviving premature infants show susceptibility to rickets and anæmia, and a slightly increased rate of respiratory infection during the first four years of life. There is a considerable morbidity from congenital defects; otherwise, premature infants appear in general to be as healthy as those born at full-term. But there are important reservations; low birth weight commonly figures in the early history of children with mental deficiency and of those with cerebral palsy, and in certain congenital anomalies.

CHAPTER 8

Neonatal Pædiatrics

Perinatal and Infant Mortality

SINCE 1900 a truly remarkable improvement in child health, with an impressive reduction in child mortality, has occurred in the socially developed countries of the world. Whilst this fall in mortality extends throughout the whole range of childhood, the improvement has been relatively less in the first week of life than at all subsequent periods. Thus, at the present time in the United Kingdom, more deaths occur in the first seven days of life than in the whole of the next seven years. Present research into the physiology of the fœtus and newborn infant, and a growing awareness of the adverse effects on the fœtus of the common complications of pregnancy and labour, including placental dysfunction, may well lead to a further reduction in the loss of life during the perinatal period.

It thus becomes necessary not only to consider the infant mortality (number of deaths under one year of age per 1,000 related live births) as a whole, but also the neonatal mortality figures (number of deaths under four weeks of age per 1,000 live births) as separate problems. In recent years, in order to correlate all the possible adverse results of pregnancy, attention has been directed towards the stillbirths (intra-uterine deaths after more than 28 weeks gestation) together with the deaths occurring immediately after birth, the two being combined as the *perinatal mortality* (combined stillbirths and infant deaths under seven days of age per 1,000 total births). By recording, in this way, the proportion of pregnancies which end fatally for the infant, a realistic assessment can be made of the standard of maternal care in a particular country or locality. The separate mortality figures for the 4–52-week age group give an indication of the subsequent standard of infant care during the first year of life. Whilst these latter figures have shown a twelvefold improvement in the United Kingdom during the past fifty years, there has been little alteration in the last two to three years; indeed, in 1959, a slight increase took place in the death rate in children between 6 and 12 months of age, compared with the previous year.

In determining the complete cause of death in a newborn infant, it is necessary to consider not only the morbid anatomical findings but also the abnormalities that may have existed in the intrauterine environment and during the course of the subsequent labour. Thus

TABLE XII
TRENDS IN INFANT MORTALITY AND PERINATAL MORTALITY IN THE
UNITED KINGDOM

(Registrar-General's Returns)

	Stillbirths (Per 1,000 Total Births)	Perinatal Mortality (Stillbirths and First Week Deaths Combined per 1,000 Total Births)	Neonatal Mortality (Deaths under Four Weeks of Age per 1,000 Live Births)	4–52 Week Mortality (Per 1,000 Related Live Births)	Infant Mortality (Deaths under One Year of Age per 1,000 Related Live Births)
1900	Not recorded				154
1906–10	Not recorded		40·2	76·9	117·1
1928	40·1	60·8	31·1	34·2	65·3
1950	23	38·2	18·5	11·3	29·8
1960	19·8	32·9	15·6	6·3	21·9

in a single infant, toxæmia of pregnancy, antepartum hæmorrhage, neonatal asphyxia, prematurity, atelectasis and neonatal lung infection may all have played a part. Classifications of causes of perinatal deaths which fail to take into account the triad of ante-natal, natal and post-natal factors must therefore be treated with reserve, and the same broad approach is required of the physician called upon to deal with the problem of the sick newborn infant. In terms of preventive medicine, the phrase " ante-natal pædiatrics " implies a positive approach to the problem.

Any consideration of perinatal mortality must therefore include ante-natal factors, such as toxæmia and eclampsia, ante-partum hæmorrhage, twin pregnancy, erythroblastosis, and also maternal diseases, such as chronic nephritis, diabetes or severe anæmia, and an undoubted tendency in some mothers to repeated spontaneous premature labour. Labour itself may have an adverse effect on the child due to disproportion, malpresentation, excessive sedation or anæsthesia administered to the mother, trauma resulting from the delivery, or asphyxia due to compression of the umbilical cord. Immediate post-natal factors include inhalation of liquor, or asphyxia neonatorum, usually the result of pre-existing ante-natal or natal complications). Congenital malformations of the infant, hæmorrhagic disease of the newborn, atelectasis and neonatal infections are among the common post-natal causes of mortality and morbidity in the newly born infant. In premature infants the respiratory distress syndrome (p. 78) and hyperbilirubinæmia of prematurity (p. 83) present special problems.

Reliable information concerning infant survival in all parts of the world is not yet available, but Table XIII provides some information regarding infant mortality in 1959 in Europe and North America.

TABLE XIII

COMPARISON OF INFANT MORTALITY RATES IN DIFFERENT COUNTRIES
FOR THE YEAR 1959

Country	Infant Mortality (Deaths Under One Year per 1,000 Live Births)
Sweden	16
Netherlands	17
New Zealand	20
England and Wales ⎱ Australia ⎰	22
U.S.A.	26
Scotland ⎱ Canada ⎰	28
France	30
Eire	32
Federal Republic of Germany	34
Italy	45

In many parts of the world it is still not possible to obtain accurate statistical information, but very much higher rates of infant mortality certainly exist at present in certain parts of Africa and Asia.

IMMEDIATE EXAMINATION OF THE NEWBORN INFANT

WHILST the detailed examination of the newly born infant need not have a high priority in the labour ward, it is essential to ensure that spontaneous respiration is immediately established. Virginia Apgar[1] has drawn attention to five objective signs which can be noted one minute after the birth of an infant and which give an indication of the need for immediate resuscitative measures; these signs may also give warning of subsequent complications during the neonatal period. The Apgar classification and method of scoring are set out in Table XIV.

METHOD OF SCORING

Sixty seconds after the *complete* birth of the infant (disregarding the cord and placenta), the following five objective signs are evaluated and each given a score of 0, 1 or 2. A score of 10 indicates an infant in the best possible condition.

A score of 3 or less is found in the great majority of infants who die in the neonatal period or who show severe respiratory or cerebral complications during this period. How much prognostic value may

Apgar, V. (1953). *Anesth. Analg. Curr. Res.*, **32**, 260.
Apgar, V., Holaday, D. A., James, S., Weisbrot, I. M., Berrien, C. (1958). *J. Amer. med. Ass.*, **168**, 1985.

TABLE XIV
APGAR CLASSIFICATION OF THE NEWBORN INFANT

Sign	0	1	2
Heart rate	Absent	Slow (Below 100)	Over 100
Respiratory effort	Absent	Slow Irregular	Good crying
Muscle tone	Limp	Some flexion of extremities	Active motion
Response to catheter in nostril (tested after oropharynx is clear)	No response	Grimace	Cough or sneeze
Colour	Blue Pale	Body pink Extremities blue	Completely pink

be ascribed to a low Apgar score in terms of permanent brain damage among the survivors cannot yet be fully assessed. Nevertheless an objective examination of this kind carried out routinely should ensure that there is no delay in initiating the active resuscitation of an asphyxiated infant.

Asphyxia Neonatorum

PATHOGENESIS

The term asphyxia neonatorum implies not only a state of hypoxia in the infant but also a degree of carbon dioxide retention. If this is continued for any length of time, a progressive reduction will also occur in the plasma pH. These three physico-chemical factors form the triad of asphyxia and cannot be considered except in association with each other.

Asphyxia neonatorum is in many cases a continuation of a pre-existing process, namely fœtal asphyxia, resulting from a state of placental insufficiency arising either before or during labour. Thus, infarction of the placenta, due to toxæmia of pregnancy or retroplacental hæmorrhage or inadequate placental supply to one member of a twinship, may give rise to fœtal asphyxia and distress which is later continued as asphyxia neonatorum. During labour, compression of the umbilical cord, which may prolapse or which may become twisted tightly round the neck of the child, may also give rise to an asphyxial state. On the other hand there may be no abnormality of placental supply, but factors within the infant may result in a failure to initiate respiration immediately after birth and thus cause asphyxia. Among such causes must be included depression of the respiratory centre by excessive use of drugs to promote analgesia or anæsthesia in the mother during labour. No single drug can be singled out, for almost all drugs used for these purposes can have a depressant action on the infant if given in sufficiently large quantities shortly before birth takes place. Infants with congenital cerebral malformations or infants suffering from cerebral damage incurred during the second stage of labour are also likely to fail to establish respiration and to develop progressive asphyxia. Finally, obstruction of the airway of the newly born infant by liquor or mucus remains one of the common and one of the most rapidly remediable causes of neonatal asphyxia.

CLINICAL PICTURE

Varying degrees of asphyxia neonatorum may be seen. In the mildest cases there may be minimal cyanosis of the extremities, whilst generalized cyanosis and ultimately an ashen pallor represent the more advanced stages. The lusty cry of the healthy newborn infant may be replaced by a weak cry, whilst in severe cases only occasional gasps may occur or there may be complete apnœa. This variation in the degree of depression of respiratory movements reflects the extent to which the respiratory centre is itself depressed. For it may be assumed that normal chemo-receptor mechanisms are actively stimulating the respiratory centre, and the progressive increase in the threshold stimuli required to produce an active response indicate the extent of this central depression.

The extent to which the infant is limp, with associated depression of normal reflex irritability, as shown particularly by the failure to react to pharyngeal suction, also indicates the severity of the asphyxia. Finally, the heart rate becomes progressively slower, a rate below 60 to the minute indicating the most profound neonatal asphyxia.

TREATMENT

If the infant does not show a normal cry followed by vigorous respiration immediately after birth, the posterior pharynx must at once be sucked out with a sterile mucus catheter. Usually this will have the effect of stimulating normal respiration. Where respiration still fails to occur, it is then ideally desirable that a doctor experienced in the art of laryngeal intubation should immediately pass a laryngoscope to the back of the tongue in order to suck out the larynx and upper trachea through a Magill 00 endotracheal tube, leaving the tube *in situ*. Subsequently, the lungs may be ventilated if necessary through the endotracheal tube (*see* p. 91). If such skilled help is not available, the infant should be nursed in the extreme head-down position whilst further efforts are made to remove any obstructive elements from the posterior pharynx by pharyngeal suction. Once the airway is clear, artificial respiration can be started if spontaneous breathing has still not commenced.

ARTIFICIAL RESPIRATION

It has recently been suggested that, in order to inflate the lungs after birth, the infant may augment the normal (negative pressure) inspiratory movements by a positive pressure mechanism. This mechanism has been demonstrated by Lind[1] by x-ray cinematography of the newly born infant, showing that the infant first fills the mouth and posterior pharynx with air and then, by a forced contraction of the pharyngeal muscles in the presence of an open glottis, forces air into the lungs. Such contractions of the pharyngeal muscles are synchronized with normal inspiratory movements of the diaphragm and chest wall.

Recent work by Cross[2] has demonstrated also the activity of Head's paradoxical reflex in the newborn infant. In contrast to the adult, the insufflation of air into the pharynx of the newly born infant initiates a reflex inspiratory gasp (as opposed to the expiratory movement initiated in the adult by the same stimulus).

Modern methods of artificial respiration have utilized a positive-pressure technique and James[3] has found that attempted inflation of the lungs with a positive pressure of not more than 30 cm. of water is a safe procedure. This positive pressure can be applied to the endotracheal tube by means of an anæsthetic bag with suitable manometer attachment, or directly from the mouth of an experienced operator through the endotracheal tube. In James's own hospital the latter technique is favoured. Such positive-pressure artificial respiration is continued until normal respiration is established or until it is clear that cardiac arrest has occurred.

Endotracheal intubation is a potentially traumatic procedure in inexperienced hands; where proper experienced help is not available, positive-pressure respiration may be carried out by direct mouth-to-mouth breathing. The operator should place a piece of gauze over the infant's face and then cover the infant's mouth and nose with his own mouth. An operator practised in this technique who has familiarized himself with a degree of respiratory effort which does not exceed a pressure of 30 cm. of water will cause no damage to the lungs of the infant nor does the risk of infection appear to be significant. Machines which produce a negative- as well as a positive-pressure phase of respiration, such as the Stephenson resuscitator, are very effective. Alternative methods of artificial respiration include Eve's rocking method.

It seems that the use in the past of intragastric oxygen, based on the assumption that absorption of oxygen occurred through the wall of the stomach into the blood stream, had no scientific basis. All resuscitatory efforts, whatever the method of artificial respiration used, must aim at increasing the concentration of oxygen reaching the alveolar membrane.

[1] Lind, J , Film (1960). *Arch. Dis. Childh.*, **35**, 416.
  Bosma, J. F., Lind, J., Gentz, N. (1959). *Acta pædiat. (Uppsala)*, **48**, Supplement 117.
[2] Cross, K. W. (1961). *Brit. med. Bull.*, **17**, No. 2, 160.
[3] James, L. S. (1960). Presbyterian Hospital, New York.

STIMULANTS

If the thesis is accepted that the chemo-receptors acting on the respiratory centre are already providing maximum stimulation, then additional stimulants are perhaps unlikely to be effective.

In certain circumstances, as when heavy sedation has been administered to the mother shortly before delivery, a stimulant is given to the infant; nikethamide 0·25–0·5 ml. may be used, or (particularly where the mother has received morphine or pethidine) nalorphine hydrobromide 0·5–1·0 mg. Vandid (vanillic acid diethylamide), one drop on the tongue is particularly useful for the apnœic attacks that occur in premature infants.

Atelectasis

Persistent atelectasis is a frequent sequelæ of neonatal asphyxia, due to the inadequate respiratory movements immediately after birth. The condition is commonest in premature infants and is fully described in Chapter 7, p. 79.

GENERAL EXAMINATION

ONCE the immediate problems following delivery are over, a detailed examination of the newborn infant can be carried out. *Cyanosis* due to persistent atelectasis or cyanotic congenital heart disease should be excluded. *Major congenital malformations*, such as cleft palate or hare lip, hypospadias, epispadias, imperforate anus, nævi, malformations of the limbs and skull, and mongolism, to mention only a few, should be excluded. It is particularly important to consider the possibility of *congenital dislocation of the hip*, which can be demonstrated as a limitation of abduction on the affected side; as the resistance to abduction is overcome a distinct click may be felt or heard (Ortolani's sign) as the forced abduction reduces the dislocation.

The doctor should examine the exterior of the body for bruising, and the bones for fractures and note whether the limbs move normally. The heart must be examined for congenital abnormalities, bearing in mind the fact that many infants have a transient systolic murmur in the second left interspace (probably due to a still patent ductus arteriosus) which disappears after a few days. The femoral pulses should be palpated to exclude coarctation of the aorta. *The tension of the anterior fontanelle provides valuable information:* a bulging, tense fontanelle indicates raised intracranial pressure due to hæmorrhage or cerebral œdema, whilst a sunken fontanelle suggests dehydration. A record of the *measurement of the head circumference* and the size of the fontanelle at birth may be of value in later months in the assessment of developing hydrocephalus. The eyes should be examined to exclude congenital cataract.

The presence of persistently forming mucus in the pharynx should raise the possibility of atresia of the œsophagus, particularly if there is a history of hydramnios (p. 98).

THE FIRST FEED

In some obstetric units it is the routine practice to pass a stomach tube to exclude *œsophageal atresia* and *tracheo-œsophageal fistula* (p. 177). If this has not been done, the first feed should always be of water and, if the infant chokes on the feed, nothing further should be given until the diagnosis has been excluded.

Vomiting

Vomiting in the newly born should always be regarded as significant. While it may prove to be due to a gastritis secondary to swallowed liquor or mucus (with rapid improvement after the stomach has been washed out), yet the possibility of serious causes exists, and cerebral damage or a congenital malformation of the intestinal tract, such as hiatus hernia (p. 178), partial obstruction from a malrotation of the intestine (p. 184), or complete obstruction from intestinal atresia (p. 185), must be considered. *Bile-stained vomiting* in the newborn always suggests intestinal obstruction until proved otherwise.

Meconium

The normal infant passes copious meconium during the first days of life. In the presence of *intestinal obstruction* either nothing is passed per rectum or, even though the obstruction is below the second part of the duodenum, a small quantity of pale mucoid material containing intestinal epithelial cells may be passed (p. 186).

Occasionally a mucus plug (p. 187) may be present in the lower bowel causing absolute constipation or even intestinal obstruction.

Urine

Concern is sometimes expressed because an infant has not passed urine for twelve hours after birth. The patency of the prepuce and meatus should be noted in boys and the genital orifice examined for congenital malformation in girls. The abdomen should be examined to exclude a large bladder with dilated ureters and renal pelves as is found in *congenital bladder neck obstruction* (p. 363). In such cases urine may dribble away rather than be passed in a proper stream.

In the great majority of cases, urine is passed normally before the end of the first twenty-four hours.

Loss of Weight

As a rule, an infant loses an ounce or more per day during the first four days. By the tenth day, however, this should have been regained and the infant may be even one or two ounces above the birth weight. From this time on, a gain of one ounce a day for the first 100 days is a guide to normal progress. Much of the early loss can be prevented by giving drinks of boiled water until the breast-milk comes in. When the milk appears early and is abundant, there may be little or no initial loss of weight.

Dehydration Fever

During the first two or three days of life no great harm comes from withholding fluid, because the infant's requirements are very small. Subsequently, fluid is needed and, if the breast-milk is slow in coming in, dehydration may develop, especially in very hot weather. Then the skin loses its elasticity and the temperature rises. A sudden loss of weight may be recorded. As the yield of breast-milk increases, the temperature subsides and the weight is recovered. Thus it appears that the temperature is produced by the infant's reaction to a shortage of fluid, and dehydration can be prevented by seeing that the infant gets an adequate amount of fluid during the period.

In the first 24 hours a full-term infant may be given about 1 oz. of boiled water per pound. In the second 24 hours the fluid intake should be a little more, on the third day $1\frac{1}{2}$ oz. per pound, and by the fourth day 2 oz. per pound on the average. These figures, of course, include whatever breast-milk the mother is able to give, the amount of which can be ascertained by test-feeds if necessary (*see* p. 38).

Anæmia

The newborn infant may occasionally show a greater or lesser degree of anæmia. This may be the result of *a hæmorrhage from the fœtal circulation into the placenta* prior to delivery. This origin for the anæmia can be confirmed by the demonstration of fœtal hæmoglobin in the maternal circulation in significant amounts. In severe cases, the infant may require a blood transfusion in the first hours after birth.

Enlargement of the Breasts (" Mastitis " Neonatorum)

Enlargement of the breasts is not uncommon in both male and female infants. This is not a true mastitis. It is caused by the lactation-stimulating hormone, believed to come from the pituitary gland, passing into the infant's circulation from the mother. A few drops of milk can often be squeezed from the nipples. No treatment is required and the breasts should be left alone.

Vaginal Bleeding

Vaginal bleeding is probably also caused by a hormone which, being secreted by the mother, affects the infant. This secretion stimulates the infant uterus, causing a transient menstruation. The condition is relatively rare, and no treatment is necessary.

JAUNDICE OF THE NEWBORN

JAUNDICE in the neonatal period always requires careful observation, particularly in premature infants, for although the majority of cases prove to be transient and benign this cannot always be decided in the early stages.

Jaundice due to Liver Immaturity (Physiological Jaundice)

The great majority of cases of neonatal jaundice are of this type. The cause of the jaundice appears to lie in the failure of the polygonal cells and the liver enzymes to deal with bilirubin in the first days of life, so that a mild jaundice becomes evident on about the third day. As hepatic enzymes become active, the jaundice fades and is usually not detectable by the end of the first week. The more premature the infant, the greater is the likelihood of liver immaturity although the correlation is by no means complete. In a minority of premature infants, and even fewer full-term infants, the accumulation of un-conjugated bilirubin may reach the danger levels at which deposition of bile in the mid and hind brain (kernicterus) occurs with irreversible consequences.

Apart from the danger of kernicterus and its attendant symptoms (p. 113), the infant may show transient lethargy and disinclination to feed during the period of the jaundice. The jaundice is not obstructive in character, the meconium showing a normal dark-green colour throughout.

Treatment consists of ensuring an adequate fluid intake and in the exclusion of the more serious causes of neonatal jaundice (*see* below). Replacement transfusion is indicated either on the grounds of hyper-bilirubinæmia alone (indirect serum bilirubin rising about 20 mg. per cent. in a full-term infant or to a somewhat lower danger level in premature infants—*see* p. 84), or because of symptoms of cerebral irritability with twitching movements of the limbs, athetoid movements or downward deviation of the eyes. The procedure (*see* p. 112) should take a minimum of three hours, in order to allow the return of bilirubin from the tissues to the plasma by diffusion and permit its subsequent removal from the plasma before the end of the transfusion. At least 200 ml. of blood per Kg. body weight should be used for the exchange transfusion.

DIFFERENTIAL DIAGNOSIS

Jaundice due to simple liver immaturity has to be distinguished from the other forms of neonatal jaundice.

HÆMOLYTIC TYPES OF JAUNDICE

Erythroblastosis (p. 110). Rhesus incompatibility should be recog-nized as early as possible in the pregnancy and certainly before the birth of the infant. In the infant, the jaundice is present at birth or develops shortly after; serology, including a Coombs test, will reveal the true state of affairs at once.

Where A/B/O incompatibility exists, the condition may not be suspected before birth. The early onset of the jaundice, its greater intensity and persistence than are found in simple liver immaturity, and the association of a mild degree of anæmia of hæmolytic origin should suggest the necessity for carrying out the necessary serological and hæmatological tests to confirm the diagnosis (p. 112).

Acholuric Jaundice (p. 337). In many families there is a history of acholuric jaundice. The jaundice may be present at birth or may develop at any time. The spleen is palpable and severe anæmia may develop. As in all hæmolytic jaundices, the stools remain dark and the urine normal in colour although containing an excess of urobilinogen. The appropriate hæmatological tests will confirm the diagnosis.

Rare Hæmolytic Anæmias (*e.g. Congenital Deficiency of Glucose-6-phosphate dehydrogenase* (p. 136), *Primaquine Sensitivity, Favism, Naphtha and Vitamin K Induced Jaundice*). It has recently been shown that naphtha and the water-soluble analogues of vitamin K (naphtha-quinone) in excessive dosage may cause a hæmolytic jaundice which may be particularly dangerous in premature infants, in whom an associated immaturity of the liver is likely to be present. This type of jaundice does not occur if the prophylactic dose of water-soluble vitamin K is restricted to a single 1·0 mg. injection. Infants with an inherited deficiency of glucose-6-phosphate dehydrogenase (p. 136) within the erythrocytes are most likely to be affected.

OBSTRUCTIVE JAUNDICE

Obstructive jaundice may also be present in the neonatal period but is distinguished by the presence of pale stools and bile-stained urine. The following varieties are seen:—

Congenital Atresia of the Bile Ducts or Bile Canaliculi (p. 218).

Inspissated Bile Syndrome (p. 219).

Neonatal Hepatitis (p. 218).

INFECTIVE FORMS OF NEONATAL JAUNDICE

Infective forms of neonatal jaundice, apart from the varieties of *neonatal hepatitis of viral origin*, can be distinguished by the presence of associated signs of general infection:

Portal Pyæmia following umbilical infection (p. 105). The presence of umbilical infection and the general symptoms of septicæmia and pyæmia in the neonatal period are present. The stools contain bile.

Syphilitic Hepatitis (p. 566). Other stigmata of congenital syphilis are usually found. The Wassermann reaction is decisive.

Cytomegalic Inclusion-body Disease (*see* p. 99).

OTHER CAUSES OF NEONATAL JAUNDICE

Galactosæmia (p. 131).

Cretinism (*see* p. 153).

Re-absorption of blood pigments after any internal hæmorrhage may create an undue demand on the immature liver, and transient jaundice may occur. This can occur following any internal hæmorrhage as a result of birth injury.

CONGENITAL MALFORMATIONS

THE incidence of congenital abnormalities among the general population is not accurately known, but it is probable that about 2·0 per cent. of all pregnancies which progress beyond the 28th week are associated with a major or minor fœtal anomaly (*see* Table XV). In some cases there is malformation of a vital organ, such as the heart, kidney or bowel, which is incompatible with life. In other cases the abnormality, although gross, may not involve such important organs and the infant's health is less impaired.

TABLE XV

ESTIMATE OF CONGENITAL MALFORMATIONS IN BIRMINGHAM[1]

The total births included 55,539 live births and 1,221 stillbirths

Type of Malformation	Incidence of Malformation (*per* 1,000 *Total Births*)
Anencephalus	1·96
Spina bifida (etc.)	3·00
Hydrocephalus	2·57
Mongolism	1·69
Cardiac malformations	4·18
Cleft lip and/or palate	1·94
Talipes	4·44
Dislocation of hip	0·67
All malformations	23·08

ÆTIOLOGY AND PATHOLOGY

Although no reason has yet been found to account for all developmental abnormalities, certain clear ætiological factors have been demonstrated. In the first place, there is a very large group which is *genetically determined* (*see* p. 20). Secondly, *mechanical factors* may be responsible, for example, abnormal intrauterine pressure (sometimes associated with oligohydramnios) exerted upon a part of the developing fœtus. Browne (1934)[2] has shown that such abnormalities are best understood if the infant is folded into the uterine position. A

[1] McKeown, T., Record, R. G. (1960). " Congenital Malformations." Ciba Foundation Symposium. London: Churchill.
[2] Browne, Sir Denis (1934). *Lancet*, 2, 969.

few of the cases of talipes equinovarus and pressure scars may perhaps be explained in this way.

The importance of maternal infection during pregnancy has been demonstrated in the case of rubella (p. 540). It has been shown that if the mother develops rubella between the 5th and 12th week of the pregnancy there is a considerable risk of the infant suffering multiple congenital defects. These include congenital cataract, deaf-mutism, congenital heart lesions, microcephaly, mental retardation, and dental defects. Apart from rubella, other maternal infections have not yet been shown to be ætiological factors, but the possibility needs exploring.

Drugs given to the mother may cause damage to the fœtus. The ectromelia and other congenital deformities of the infant that followed the use of thalidomide during the first trimester of pregnancy (p. 476) provide a tragic example. It is wise at present to regard all tranquillizing and new sedative drugs as potentially dangerous in pregnancy, particularly in the first trimester. Iodides taken by the mother may produce thyroid enlargement in the infant, and anti-thyroid drugs should not be administered in the last month of pregnancy unless absolutely essential. Androgens and progesterone may have virilizing effects in female fœtuses.

Maternal age may also be an important factor. The great majority of mongols are born to mothers over thirty-five years of age, although occasionally the mother may be very much younger. The finding of an abnormal chromosomal pattern (p. 19) in mongol children has already been mentioned. Congenital heart lesions and the rare deformity of duodenal atresia are found more frequently in mongols than in the general population.

Other causes of congenital deformity include *maternal diabetes*, in which condition very large infants are born (9–13 lb.) with an increased incidence of congenital deformity and neonatal mortality. The birth of very large infants may also occur to women, not diabetic at the time, but who develop the condition later. *Hydramnios* is frequently present in pregnancies associated with anencephalus and œsophageal atresia. It is suggested that the normal swallowing of liquor by the fœtus and resorption of the fluid by the placental circulation cannot occur in the presence of such malformations. Other causes, however, must also operate in the development of hydramnios, as it is not infrequently associated with the presence of congenital malformations not involving the upper intestinal tract and indeed with entirely normal births. Anencephaly is found particularly in female infants and in babies of blood group O mothers suggesting a particular genetic constitution. *Irradiation of the embryo* with radium or x-rays in large doses is associated with a liability to congenital malformation. The significance of *maternal nutrition* including especially deficiencies of vitamin A and riboflavine, particularly during the early months of pregnancy, as a cause of congenital defects is at present not clear; careful study of this subject may be informative.

A large group remains in which no definite ætiological factor can be demonstrated.

CONGENITAL INFECTIONS

AMONG infections acquired *in utero*, *congenital pneumonia* (p. 79), *congenital toxoplasmosis* (p. 413), *congenital tuberculosis* (a rare complication of pregnancy in mothers suffering from miliary tuberculosis) and *congenital syphilis* (p. 564) must be mentioned. It is likely that virus infections such as infective hepatitis may, when latent in the mother, be transmitted to the infant and emerge in the form of *neonatal hepatitis* (p. 219).

Cytomegalic Inclusion-body Disease

This is a virus infection (salivary gland or S.G. virus). The virus is of very low pathogenicity, except in young infants and debilitated subjects. When a mother is infected with S.G. virus, it may be transmitted across the placenta and will then manifest clinically with neonatal jaundice, skin hæmorrhage, and anæmia, possibly with involvement of lungs, central nervous system and retinæ. Characteristic inclusion-bearing cells are found in affected tissues.

BIRTH INJURIES

Caput Succedaneum

THIS is an œdematous swelling which forms normally in the soft tissues over the presenting part of an infant's head, and it is of no clinical significance. Occasionally, it hides a cephalhæmatoma. It disappears without treatment in the course of a week or two.

Cephalhæmatoma

This is an extravasation of blood beneath the pericranium, limited to the area bounded by the neighbouring sutures, and is due to pressure on the skull and scalp at birth. Asphyxia, congestion and hypoprothrombinæmia aid its formation.

CLINICAL PICTURE

Cephalhæmatomata are more likely after deliveries by forceps. An hæmatoma is felt as a soft fluctuating swelling with a definite margin which makes it feel rather like a depressed fracture. This sharp margin is due to elevation of the periosteum at the edge of the hæmatoma. Immediate and preventive treatment is to give vitamin K. Aspiration is not required, although the swelling, if large, may take several weeks to resolve. Occasionally a fracture is present in addition and, when this is suspected, an x-ray examination is advisable.

Fractures of the Skull

Fractures of the base of the skull are fortunately rare because the prognosis is always grave. The symptoms are those of intracranial hæmorrhage.

Fractures of the vertex are usually of the *fissure* type in which there are few signs, except perhaps bruising of the head or an overlying cephalohæmatoma, but they may occasionally be associated with the serious complication of subdural hæmatoma (p. 103). *Depressed fractures* are less common. Frequently there are no symptoms and the depression disappears spontaneously. It is only when there are neurological signs that a depressed fracture should be elevated. This should be done by a wide exposure so that the surgeon is able to see extradural or subdural collections of blood.

Fractures of the Long Bones

A fracture of the femur, humerus or clavicle may occur as a result of an unusual position of the infant or the use of undue force for delivery. As a rule, healing takes place readily, and there is no resulting deformity.

Hæmatoma of the Sternomastoid

This hæmatoma is probably due to the rupture of some of the muscle-fibres and vessels during birth, the sternomastoid being slightly over-stretched.

CLINICAL PICTURE

A few days after birth, a lump may be felt at about the middle third of the sternomastoid, or it may be noted that the child tends to keep the head tilted to one side, as if a torticollis were present, attention being drawn in this way to the extravasation of blood within the sheath of the sternomastoid.

PROGNOSIS AND TREATMENT

Complete recovery occurs as a rule, but occasionally slight torticollis may remain. The baby should be placed to lie on the affected side to produce counter-stretching. Gentle physiotherapy, in which the neck is put through the full range of movement, can be taught in order that the mother may carry out the treatment daily at home.

Facial Nerve Injury

The facial nerve may be injured by the blade of a forceps. Facial weakness appears within a few hours and soon reaches its maximum. Improvement then takes place and recovery is usually complete.

Erb's Paralysis

This is due to an injury of the brachial plexus. It is caused by a stretching or tearing of the upper cord (formed by the fifth and sixth cervical roots) of the brachial plexus during the process of birth. Acute flexion of the neck puts an undue strain on the brachial plexus, just as does pulling on the shoulders with the head firmly fixed.

The clinical picture is that of flaccid paralysis of the deltoid, supra- and infra-spinatus, biceps and supinator, so that the arm hangs by the side, fully pronated, with the hand in the position of a waiter's hand bent to receive a surreptitious tip.

TREATMENT

If the injury be slight, and due merely to over-stretching of the nerves and possibly some hæmorrhage into the nerve sheaths, recovery takes place spontaneously in the course of a few weeks. Where, however, the injury is extensive and the plexus has been torn across, an open operation may be contemplated but is seldom carried out. Meanwhile, every case should be secured in the position of rest. The arm is abducted at a right-angle from the trunk, and the forearm fully supinated, the elbow flexed, and the wrist dorsi-flexed. Fairbank's splint is used for this.

PROGNOSIS

All the mild cases and some severe cases clear up completely.

Klumpke's Paralysis

In Klumpke's paralysis the eighth cervical and first dorsal roots are injured, and there is weakness of the flexors and small muscles of the hand, with no power to grip. Damage to the sympathetic plexus gives rise to a Horner's syndrome on the same side.

Intracranial Injury and Hæmorrhage

Bleeding may occur into the meninges, into the cerebral substance and into the ventricular system. An extracerebral site of bleeding is commoner than an intracerebral one. Besides intracranial hæmorrhage, less serious complications at birth, such as cerebral congestion, œdema, and simple cerebral contusion are found.

The following types of intracranial bleeding may occur:

1. SUBDURAL HÆMORRHAGE

Bleeding occurs from the veins and sinuses, often in association with tears of the dural septa, and may give rise to unilateral or bilateral subdural hæmatoma (p. 103). If not fatal in the early stages such lesions may later cause serious sequelæ.

2. SUBARACHNOID HÆMORRHAGE

This type is unlikely to be fatal unless a major vessel is torn; recovery occurs within a few days. A minor degree of bleeding in the subarachnoid space is extremely common.

3. VENTRICULAR HÆMORRHAGE

This is likely to be immediately fatal. It is more common in the premature than in the full-term infant.

4. INTRACEREBRAL HÆMORRHAGE

This may consist of scattered or confluent petechial hæmorrhages; the prognosis depends upon the severity and extent of the bleeding. In severe cases in which recovery takes place despite extensive hæmorrhage, cysts may develop at the site of the old hæmorrhage, sometimes in continuity with the ventricular system. These are termed *false* porencephalic cysts as opposed to *true* porencephalic cysts which are of congenital origin.

ÆTIOLOGY

The following factors predispose towards cerebral hæmorrhage:
(1) Hæmorrhagic disease of the newborn (*see* p. 109).
(2) The type of presentation. Breech or occipito-posterior presentations are more dangerous, particularly in primigravida.
(3) Prematurity.
(4) Asphyxia.

SIGNS AND SYMPTOMS

If the bleeding has been very slight, or into one of the portions of the brain, such as the frontal or occipital lobes where immediate signs are not obvious, there may be no symptoms. However, if one of the great sinuses is torn across, there may be a gush of blood with consequent shock, white asphyxia, and death almost at once. There are several cardinal symptoms which indicate cerebral hæmorrhage:
(1) An inability to suck well.
(2) A fretful, high-pitched screaming cry.
(3) A defective swallowing reflex.
(4) A tendency to twitch or convulse. This may be postponed as late as the third or fourth day.
(5) Coma or semi-coma with the eyes wide open and staring.
(6) A tense fontanelle.

TREATMENT

If not already carried out as routine prophylaxis, vitamin K, 1-2 mg. in aqueous solution, should be given intramuscularly and repeated in twelve hours.

In the early stages it is important that the infant is kept quiet and handling reduced to a minimum. If there is doubt as to the infant's ability to swallow, tube feeding should be instituted. Severely ill or shocked cases should be nursed in an oxygen tent, particularly if cyanotic attacks are occurring.

Sedatives should be used while the stage of irritability lasts, chloral hydrate 60 mg. (one grain) three or four times a day for an infant weighing 7 lb. If convulsions are occurring, twice this dose of chloral may be given hourly until they are controlled. Alternatively, a barbiturate, such as Amytal 16 mg. (a quarter of a grain) may be given intramuscularly or by mouth at not more than eight-hour intervals.

Subdural Hæmatoma

The condition is usually bilateral. Following a subdural hæmorrhage, the symptoms of a space-occupying lesion develop, often after a delayed interval. The symptoms may be progressive over a period of several weeks since hæmatomata, though localized, increase in size. This increase is usually due to a combination of further hæmorrhage, leakage of cerebrospinal fluid through dural tears, exudation of serum, and transudation of cerebrospinal fluid due to increase in the osmotic pressure in the subdural space as the blood disintegrates. Thus, if the acute stage of the hæmorrhage is survived, chronic progressive symptoms develop.

It must be stressed that in some cases there may be no suggestive symptoms apart from a little vomiting, and the diagnosis has to be made on physical examination. In most cases, however, chronic vomiting and failure to gain weight are common symptoms in the early stages. As the size of the hæmatoma increases, irritability and lethargy develop. Later, convulsions or sudden attacks of collapse occur. Examination shows a pale anæmic infant with a tense fontanelle, limb rigidity, and, in the later stages, a head circumference above the usual serial measurements showing a more than normal increase. The optic fundi may show hæmorrhage and papillœdema. The differential diagnosis includes hydrocephalus and cerebral tumour, but difficulty during or soon after birth is suggestive of subdural hæmatoma.

The diagnosis is confirmed by exploring the subdural space, either by a needle through the lateral angles of the fontanelle or by burr holes, and the finding of bloodstained or xanthochromic fluid containing 1–2 per cent. of protein. Treatment by repeated aspiration will reduce the size of the hæmatoma, but if it has been present for any length of time it will be found that a fibrous membrane encases it. If this membrane is not excised it will later act as a constricting band around the brain, preventing its normal growth and giving rise to subsequent brain damage, sometimes associated with spasticity and epilepsy. For this reason excision of the whole subdural sac including the membrane is advised in all cases in which the subdural hæmatoma has been present for more than a few weeks.   Anæmia may require correction by blood transfusion.

INFECTIONS IN THE NEWBORN

THE infant inherits or acquires from its mother a temporary passive immunity to various infections, particularly measles and diphtheria, but not to coliform and pyogenic infections.   These infections often generalize rapidly;   therefore septicæmia is common, and may be overlooked.

(1) Infection may pass to the infant in the uterus through the placenta, e.g. syphilis, cytomegalic inclusion-body disease and toxoplasmosis.

(2) Via the liquor amnii, in cases where premature rupture of the membranes has occurred spontaneously or by surgical induction, followed by a delay in the onset of labour.

(3) During birth, the infant may become infected from the liquor or the maternal passages, as in ophthalmia neonatorum.

(4) After birth, nose, eyes, ears, umbilicus and skin are frequent portals of entry.

Shortly after birth an infant may show signs of ill-health.   The site of the infection may be obvious, such as in paronychia, conjunctivitis, umbilical infection or when the skin is infected and bullæ result.   On the other hand, there are often no external symptoms apart from a slight muco-purulent discharge at the umbilicus, and the correct diagnosis may be made only by the finding of a positive blood culture with a leucocytosis, or at post-mortem examination.   Staphylococcal and coliform infections are relatively frequent.

Neonatal Septicæmia

In the newborn infant, any generalized infection commonly causes listlessness, disinclination to feed, vomiting and loss of weight.   When there is diarrhœa, dehydration is likely.   The skin may show pustular or bullous lesions.   Pneumonia may occur, and peritonitis, empyema and meningitis may all ensue.   An examination of the urine may show some albumin, or pyelitis may be present.   In the later stages of septicæmia, anæmia, jaundice and cutaneous petechiæ may appear. The diagnosis should be suspected, however, at an earlier stage and should not be delayed until it can be made at a glance, by which time the prognosis has become grave in the extreme.   The temperature is not of diagnostic value, as it may be low, normal, or raised, and its height is not a gauge of the severity of the condition.

TREATMENT

The appropriate antibiotic should be administered in full doses once the type and sensitivity of the organism are known.   Until this information is obtained, a wide-spectrum antibiotic, such as tetra-cycline, is indicated, or methicillin or erythromycin in maternity homes where a *Staph. pyogenes* sensitive only to these latter anti-biotics is known to be endemic (for antibiotic dosage, *see* p. 656). Warmth, oxygen and intravenous fluids are necessary where de-hydration is marked, and feeding by stomach-tube is usually essential. Careful and expert nursing is of the greatest importance; breast-milk is the feed of choice. Where circulatory collapse is imminent or actually present, intravenous hydrocortisone becomes a vital part of the treatment (for dosage, *see* p. 660).

Neonatal Lung Infection (*see* p. 79)

Umbilical Infection

The umbilicus is the original source of infection in a large proportion of infants with generalized *Staph. pyogenes* infections (*see* p. 104). The cord does not shrivel and separate as it should. Usually, however, nothing is seen on examination beyond a slight moisture of the navel. If pus can be squeezed from the umbilicus it is likely that the obliterated umbilical vessels are heavily infected, but the next stage, *pylephlebitis*, can develop even when the umbilicus itself appears dry. From this stage, the signs and symptoms of neonatal septicæmia (p. 104), develop. Portal vein obstruction (p. 222) is a late complication.

Staphylococcal Infection of the Skin (Pyodermia)

Staphylococcal infection of the skin is especially common in the neonatal period. Usually it results in pustule formation and causes little constitutional disturbance, but even this simple type should not be taken lightly since metastatic abscesses or septicæmia can follow. More virulent staphylococcal infections (or occasionally streptococcal ones) may cause bullous lesions (*pemphigus neonatorum*), often starting in the napkin region. This type of lesion may spread rapidly over the body producing numerous bullæ which contain thin semi-purulent fluid. Delay in treatment may prove fatal. When a large part of the epithelium is shed the condition is called *exfoliative dermatitis* (Ritter's disease) (Fig. 7, p. 106).

Isolated cases of pyodermia may occur in infants born at home. When cases occur in neonatal nurseries, other sites of staphylococcal infection (conjunctivæ, nose or skin) are likely to be seen as well. Occasionally serious epidemics arise that necessitate closure of a nursery. These may be traced to a common source, often a carrier of virulent *Staphylococcus pyogenes aureus*.

PREVENTION OF INFECTION IN THE NEWBORN

IN the prevention of cross-infection within a maternity home, the following factors should be considered:

(1) Rooming-in of mothers and babies greatly reduces the serial handling of a number of babies by one member of the nursing staff, since the greater part of the handling of the individual baby is done by the mother.

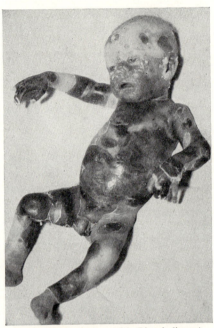

Fig. 7.—Exfoliative dermatitis (Ritter's disease). A post-mortem photograph of a 1-month-old baby showing an exfoliative type of "bullous impetigo" (pemphigus neonatorum) due to *Staphylococcus aureus*. The infection came from the mother, who had a septic finger. The nurse who handled the baby in hospital developed a septic finger as well.

(2) Overcrowding of babies inevitably leads to cross-infection.

(3) The use of hexachlorophane soap by staff and patients for washing and the use of chlorhexidine hand cream will greatly reduce the spread of *Staph. pyogenes* organisms from patient to patient.

(4) The use of 1 per cent. hexachlorophane dusting powder on the umbilical areas of all infants will reduce this potent reservoir of infection.

(5) The laundering of bed linen, towels and napkins should be of a standard that ensures that clean linen is free of pathogenic organisms.

(6) Isolation facilities should be available for mothers and infants exhibiting infections.

(7) The staff should be meticulous in their standards of hygiene, and nurses with clinical infections should not work in contact with newborn infants. There should be a constant awareness of the danger of neonatal infections. The close co-operation and advice of a bacteriologist is invaluable in maintaining standards.

THERAPY

At the first sign of infection (whether skin, umbilicus, conjunctivæ or nose), the patient should be removed from contact with other infants and the cause should be sought. Prompt treatment with antibiotics, as outlined in the treatment for neonatal septicæmia (p. 104), should be immediately instituted. Local treatment with a polybactrin spray and hexachlorophane powder is used for umbilical and skin infections; chlorhexidine and neomycin cream can be used for nasal carriers.

Paronychia

Infection round the base of the finger nails is relatively common as a skin manifestation of staphylococcal infection. Such lesions should be covered with a dressing and antibiotic treatment given.

Ophthalmia Neonatorum

ÆTIOLOGY

The commonest cause of ophthalmia was formerly the gonococcus, the disease being contracted as the child passed through the infected maternal passages. Now the *Staph. pyogenes* is found to be the usual cause. Occasionally other organisms, such as the pneumococcus, *E. coli*, or *Cl. diphtheriæ* are responsible.

CLINICAL PICTURE

On the second or third day the eyes become red and swollen, and begin discharging. Ulceration of the cornea is the most feared complication, with perforation and then destruction.

PROPHYLAXIS

This consists in efficient hygiene and early recognition of all forms of infection, especially in neonatal nurseries.

TREATMENT

At the earliest signs of inflammation or discharge (" sticky eye "), a conjunctival swab should be taken and then treatment commenced at once with saline irrigations. For established infections chloramphenicol ophthalmic ointment is an effective treatment. Oral antibiotics are indicated in the most severe cases (p. 650).

Urinary Infection

Urinary infections are one of the commonest and most under-diagnosed infections of infancy. Vomiting, fever and failure to thrive are the chief symptoms (*see* p. 365).

The diagnosis is made by examination of the urine, and careful abdominal examination occasionally discloses enlargement of the kidneys, ureters or a palpable bladder. At this age, males are affected just as often as females. For treatment *see* p. 366.

Neonatal Meningitis

The signs and symptoms may be less acute in the newborn than in older children. Vomiting and the clinical picture of slight cerebral irritation (p. 400) may be the only features. At times, convulsions are the leading symptom. Lethargy, staring eyes and a tense fontanelle should suggest the diagnosis even without evidence of neck stiffness and retraction. The diagnosis and treatment is fully discussed in Chapter 19, pp. 399–402.

Neonatal Tetanus (p. 427 and p. 593)

THERMAL DISTURBANCES
Neonatal Cold Syndrome

IF exposed to very cold external temperatures, the newborn infant may be unable to maintain its own normal body temperature. Thus, in times of very cold weather, if the nursery temperature is allowed to fall during the night to levels in the order of 35° F, a characteristic syndrome may develop. The infant becomes extremely lethargic and takes the feeds extremely slowly. Later no attempt may be made to suck at all. The extremities may become swollen and pink, the respiration rate may drop to less than 10 per minute and the heart rate fall to 60 beats per minute or fewer. The infant lies quite still and the peristaltic action of the intestine may cease. Oliguria develops. A firm sclerœdematous consistency may develop in the skin, which feels very cold to the touch. The rectal temperature is found to be between 77–90° F, depending on the severity of chilling.

Whilst a cold environment is undoubtedly the sole precipitating cause in some infants, it seems likely that the syndrome is more likely to develop if the infant is already suffering from an infection. In the fatal cases, pneumonia is often found at autopsy. Extreme cold may also occur in infants with brain damage.

PREVENTION

It is clearly of the first importance that all doctors and midwives should be aware of the possible development of the neonatal cold syndrome in times of very cold weather. Adequate heating should be available, both in domiciliary and hospital practice, to maintain the nursery temperature at 65° F (higher for premature infants) throughout the whole of the twenty-four hours.

TREATMENT

It is very important that the re-warming of the infant should be carried out extremely slowly. The use of a thermostatically controlled incubator is most useful in this respect. It is desirable that the infant's temperature should not rise more that 1° F every two hours. During the rewarming period, convulsions may occur which may sometimes be of hypoglycæmic origin. It is advisable, therefore, to estimate the blood sugar and to give glucose either by stomach tube or by slow intravenous drip if the level is below 60 per cent.

In view of the likely association with an infection, a broad-spectrum antibiotic, such as terramycin or methicillin should be administered (for dosage, *see* p. 656). In the most severe cases, with rectal temperatures below 80° F, ventricular fibrillation may develop and should be treated immediately with intravenous procaine amide.

Where deterioration occurs despite treatment, intravenous hydrocortisone (for dosage, *see* p. 660) should be given.

BLOOD DISORDERS

Hæmorrhagic Disease of the Newborn (Hypoprothrombin-æmia: Melæna Neonatorum)

THIS disease occurs in 0·5 to 1 per cent. of all infants. It appears to be due to deficiencies of various factors essential for blood coagulation. Although the majority of patients show a deficiency of prothrombin, other infants show varying degrees of deficiency of Factor VII, plasma thromboplastin and Factor X. It is not surprising that the efficacy of vitamin K in treatment is variable. In this respect, it is notable that premature infants are less responsive to vitamin K than full-term infants and that, in general terms, vitamin K_1 is rather more effective than vitamin K.

SYMPTOMS

Bleeding usually occurs between the second and fourth day of life. The commonest site is in the gastro-intestinal tract, giving rise to so-called *melæna neonatorum* or to vomiting of blood. Other sites of hæmorrhage are intracranial (with asphyxia or trauma), cutaneous or into the suprarenal glands. When there is melæenia neonatorum, an apparently healthy infant becomes blanched on the second or third day or later, and passes large, tarry stools filled with blood clots. Collapse and symptoms of hæmorrhage are present. *Post-mortem* nothing is found beyond petechial hæmorrhages into the gastro-intestinal wall. An infant may swallow maternal blood during the second stage of labour or may suck blood from the mother's cracked nipple, and then vomit or pass blood in the stool. These possibilities should be excluded before a diagnosis of melæna neonatorum is made.

PREVENTION

Vitamin K in a dosage of 1–2 mg. provides adequate protection against prothrombin lack if given at once after birth. In some centres this is given to all newborn infants, in others only to premature infants or those who have been subjected to difficult births, e.g. forceps. In some centres, vitamin K 10 mg. is given to all mothers at the commencement of labour.

TREATMENT

For the majority of patients 2 mg. of vitamin K_1 in aqueous solution, injected every twelve hours, is sufficient treatment. In cases of severe hæmorrhage or where fresh hæmorrhage occurs more than six hours after the first injection of vitamin K, additional treatment is indicated. Either whole blood or fresh-frozen plasma is effective in controlling the hæmorrhagic tendency, but whole blood is indicated if anæmia has developed.

Hæmolytic Disease of the Newborn (Erythroblastosis: Icterus Gravis: Hydrops Fœtalis)

ÆTIOLOGY

This is a hæmolytic anæmia, caused by blood-group incompatibility, affecting the fœtus or the newborn infant. Among the red-cell antigens, those of the Rh group are most commonly responsible. The Rh-positive red cells of the fœtus pass across the placenta into the blood of a Rh-negative mother, giving rise to an antibody response. The maternal antibodies so formed cross the placenta into the infant's bloodstream and attach themselves to fœtal cells (mainly to erythrocytes) causing cytolysis. This results in hæmolytic anæmia and jaundice, and sometimes damage to liver cells.

First children are seldom affected unless the mother has been sensitized by a previous transfusion of Rh-positive cells. In subsequent pregnancies, antibodies, which can be demonstrated in rising titre during the pregnancy, may develop in the maternal circulation. Once a child has been affected, if the father is homozygous Rh positive, it is likely that all subsequent pregnancies will be increasingly affected; if the father is heterozygous, there is an even chance that each subsequent pregnancy will be unaffected.

It not infrequently happens that although a Rh-negative woman gives birth to several Rh-positive children, erythroblastosis does not develop. In such cases it must be assumed that there is insufficient spill-over of the infant's cells into the maternal circulation to produce sensitization. Numerous sub-types of the main Rh group, known for recording purposes as C, D, E, c, d and e, have been identified. Of these, anti-D accounts for the great majority of cases and is the only maternal antibody routinely tested antenatally in most medical centres.

In addition to sensitization by Rh groups, it has been shown that hæmolytic jaundice can also occur as a result of A/B/O incompatibility. In such circumstances, the infant has inherited an A or B blood group from the father and sensitization may occur in the blood of an O group mother if fœtal cells cross the placenta.

Rh-negative women may become sensitized against Rh-positive cells not only in pregnancy, but also by transfusion of Rh-positive cells. Thus, in all blood transfusion work for Rh-negative females potentially capable of child bearing, care should be taken to ensure that Rh-negative blood is always used.

About 15 per cent. of the female population of the United Kingdom are Rh-negative. In the indigenous population of East and West Africa, the Rh-negative blood group is not found and thus hæmolytic disease of the newborn due to rhesus incompatibility is not seen.

CLINICAL FEATURES

These vary according to the severity of the process, which tends to increase with successive pregnancies.

Fœtal hæmolytic disease may cause (1) the birth of a macerated fœtus with cirrhosis of the liver, or (2) hydrops fœtalis:

(1) When the fœtus dies *in utero*, there is premature delivery of a macerated fœtus; the placenta is large and the fœtal liver shows cirrhosis.

(2) Hydrops fœtalis. When somewhat less severely affected, the fœtus survives longer and is then delivered, usually prematurely, either as an hydropic stillbirth or as an œdematous live birth. In the last case, death takes place in a few hours with increasing jaundice and anæmia. The placenta is large, œdematous and contains foci of erythroblastic activity. The viscera and blood of the fœtus also show erythroblastosis, particularly in the liver, and there is also evidence of damage to the polygonal cells.

Hæmolytic disease of the newborn takes the form of (1) icterus gravis neonatorum, or (2) anæmia hæmolytica neonatorum:—

(1) *Icterus gravis neonatorum.* Jaundice is present at birth or appears within hours. It is more intense and more persistent than the jaundice of simple liver immaturity. In mild cases, the fall in erythrocytes and hæmoglobin which normally takes place after birth is somewhat exaggerated, though insufficient to cause much anæmia. In more severe cases, jaundice is present at the time of birth and there is a more rapid fall in erythrocytes and hæmoglobin. The liver enlarges and sometimes the spleen is palpable. The grey matter of the hemispheres, midbrain, cerebellum and medulla may become bile-stained (kernicterus, *see* p. 113) and the ganglion cells degenerate. When this occurs, death may take place within a day or so. About 10 per cent. of infants surviving icterus gravis, in the days before replacement transfusion was routinely practised, later showed either mental deficiency, spasticity, rigidity or athetosis, but this incidence of kernicterus has now been greatly reduced.

(2) *Anæmia hæmolytica neonatorum* is a term used for cases in which anæmia develops without much jaundice some days after birth. Erythroblastæmia is less evident and kernicterus does not occur.

BLOOD PICTURE

There is an increasing anæmia as progressive hæmolysis occurs. Large numbers of nucleated red cells are present in the peripheral blood as a result of the hæmopoietic tissue response to the anæmia. (For normal blood picture at birth, *see* p. 324.) The serum bilirubin increases with the degree of hæmolysis. The direct Coombs' test, which shows whether the infant's cells have become sensitized against the circulating maternal antibody, is positive in Rh incompatibility.

In anæmia hæmolytica neonatorum, jaundice does not occur, either because the hæmolysis takes place slowly or because the liver function is more mature and adequate. In such cases anæmia develops insidiously and is often of a more chronic type.

CONFIRMATION OF DIAGNOSIS

In suspected cases the following tests are required and can be performed on a blood sample taken from the umbilical cord:—

(1) Coombs' test.
(2) Blood grouping.
(3) Hæmoglobin.
(4) Serum-bilirubin.

TREATMENT

Adequate antenatal supervision should provide warning of the birth of a potentially affected infant so that arrangements can be made for the baby to be born where facilities exist for prompt treatment.

There is no doubt that the disease gains momentum in the latter weeks of pregnancy. Where a rising titre of maternal antibodies is demonstrated between the 28th and 34th weeks of pregnancy, the medical or surgical induction of labour at the 37th week has much to commend it. In the most severe cases, where previous infants have either been stillborn or severely affected and an exceptionally high titre of maternal antibody is found at the 28th week of pregnancy with a rise at the 32nd week, induction may have to be undertaken even at this very early date if the infant is to survive.

The cord blood of the infant should be examined immediately after birth. It is the practice in some centres to undertake replacement transfusion in all infants in whom the Coombs' test is positive. In others, replacement transfusion is carried out only in Coombs'-positive infants who also show a reduction of cord hæmoglobin to 15 G. per cent. or below, or a level of serum bilirubin of 2·0 mg. per cent. or above. If immediate replacement transfusion is not carried out, serial measurements of haemoglobin and serum bilirubin are made and replacement transfusion undertaken during the next few days if the indirect bilirubin rises above 20 mg. per cent. or if significant anæmia develops.

The use of an icterometer,[1] a strip of perspex painted with five standard shades of yellow, which can be compressed against the tip of the infant's nose until the skin is blanched, is a rough guide to the degree of bilirubinæmia. Whilst it does not replace the necessity for direct estimations on the serum, it may reduce the number required.

Replacement Transfusion. It is estimated that by alternately recovering the infant's blood and injecting Rh-negative donor blood through the umbilical vein in equal quantities until 200 ml. of blood per Kg. body-weight has been donated, approximately 90 per cent. of the infant's blood will have been exchanged. Thus the majority of the circulating maternal antibody and the affected cells will have been removed. The time taken for this procedure should never be less

[1] Gosset, I. H. (1960). *Lancet*, 1, 87.

than one to two hours and preferably longer where jaundice is severe, in order to obtain a greater removal of bilirubin.

If the infant is anæmic at birth and associated heart failure is present with a high central venous pressure, it is desirable to use packed cells for the first part of the transfusion and to create a slight deficit in the circulating blood volume (by removing slightly more blood than the quantity injected) during the early stages.

The blood used should never be more than 4 days old, in view of the danger of a high level of serum potassium in blood stored for longer periods. After each 100 ml. of blood has been exchanged, 10 per cent. calcium gluconate 1·0 ml. should be injected intravenously to prevent a fall in the infant's serum calcium which might otherwise result from the combination of calcium with the sodium citrate present in the donor blood.

Additional replacement transfusions may be required if the level of serum bilirubin continues to rise. A level of 20 mg. per cent. of *indirect serum bilirubin* is taken as the critical level above which further replacement transfusion is carried out (direct or conjugated bilirubin appears to play no part in causing kernicterus). In small premature infants, slightly lower levels of indirect serum bilirubin may possibly cause kernicterus, so that replacement transfusion may be undertaken if the level reaches 15 mg. per cent.

FOLLOW-UP AND PROGNOSIS

After the initial dangers to the infant from acute anæmia and hyperbilirubinæmia are passed, a careful follow-up is desirable in the first instance to observe any further tendency to anæmia which may ensue in the next two months. If during this time the hæmoglobin falls to below 8 G. per cent., a simple transfusion is indicated. Oral iron (for dosage, *see* p. 331) should be given from the fourteenth day of life to try to prevent this development.

If an unchecked rise of *indirect bilrubin* far in excess of 20 mg. per cent. was present in the early stages, there is a real danger of deposition of bile pigment in vital centres of the brain (kernicterus). The full tetrad of symptoms of kernicterus is:

1. Athetosis.
2. Mental retardation.
3. High tone deafness.
4. Green discoloration and poor formation of teeth.

It is thus desirable that infants at risk after initial hæmolytic disease should be followed up over the next five years to assess particularly their neurological and intellectual status and hearing abilities.

TREATMENT OF A/B/O INCOMPATIBILITY

As mentioned above, hæmolytic disease of the newborn may some-times result from pregnancies involving a Group A, B or AB infant and a Group O mother. It is seldom of sufficient clinical severity to require replacement transfusion, but remains an important differential diagnosis in cases of neonatal jaundice and anæmia. For the exceptionally severe case in which replacement transfusion has to be carried out, Group O blood is used. It is to be noted that, in contrast to rhesus-sensitized cases, the Coombs' test remains negative in A/B/O incompatibility.

HYPOGLYCÆMIA IN THE NEWBORN

It has been known for many years that newborn infants, particularly those born to diabetic mothers, may have low levels of blood sugar without the development of clinical symptoms. In a few infants (mainly premature babies), convulsions and peripheral circulatory failure develop in association with profound hypoglycæmia. In such cases the blood-sugar level may be less than 10 mg. per cent. The symptoms are corrected by treatment with 20 per cent. dextrose given intravenously. Without such treatment, death may occur or permanent brain damage may be found in the survivors. Spontaneous hypoglycæmia in older infants and children is discussed on page 172.

CHAPTER 9

Vitamin Deficiencies

VITAMINS are organic substances concerned with many essential biological processes, including absorption and utilization of nutrients. They are effective in small amounts, do not themselves produce energy, and do not build tissue, but they form a necessary part of enzyme systems for the metabolism of protein, fat, and carbohydrate.

VITAMIN A

VITAMIN A appears to be necessary for normal growth and has a specific action on epithelial tissue, the normal coverings of the body, and the mucous membrane lining the important cavities and ducts of the glands. Its precursor is a yellow pigment known as carotene, which, when absorbed, produces vitamin A in the liver. Carotene is found in carrots, green vegetables, milk fat; vitamin A in fish-liver oil, such as cod, halibut or tunny, and in butter and eggs, liver and kidney. Heat does not readily destroy it. It is absent from vegetable oil. Vitamin A is stored in the liver.

The daily requirements are of the order of 2,000 i.u. for infants and between 3,000–5,000 i.u. for older children. Commercial cod-liver oil is standardized to contain not less than 600 i.u. per gramme. It is important, when assessing the value of a vitamin preparation for routine prophylactic use, to make sure that the vitamin-A content, as well as that of vitamin D, is adequate. The amount contained in human milk varies considerably with the maternal diet but is usually between 1,000–3,000 i.u. per pint.

Carotene may be present in the diet but not absorbed. This may occur when an excess of mineral oil (liquid paraffin) is given by mouth; the carotene is soluble in oil, and the latter is not absorbed. In a condition such as cœliac disease, where there is poor fat absorption, carotene may be lost in the fæces, along with the remainder of the intestinal fat.

Since vitamin A is necessary for the formation of visual purple, found in the rods and cones of the retina, its absence produces night-blindness. This vitamin is also necessary for the maintenance of columnar epithelium, and in its absence the epithelium undergoes metaplasia and keratinization. This produces xerosis of the conjunctiva (xerophthalmia) and ulceration of the cornea (keratomalacia). Xerophthalmia appears first as dry, rough, yellowish-white patches

115

on the bulbar conjunctiva (Bitot's spots); these are small and triangular and usually situated at first on the nasal side. The epithelium of the respiratory system, renal system, to a lesser extent the alimentary tract, and also the follicles of the skin are affected. The skin over the outside of the arms, particularly the upper part, may become dry and rough and is often called " toad skin." (*See also* p. 599.)

Vitamin A has been described as the " anti-infective " vitamin, but it has no direct antibacterial action. Clearly, if the mucous membranes are not healthy, through deficiency of this vitamin, local tissue-resistance may be impaired.

TREATMENT OF VITAMIN-A DEFICIENCY

Night-blindness shows rapid improvement under treatment. Halibut-liver oil, which contains about 30,000 i.u. per ml., may be given when a high dosage is required; alternatively, cod-liver oil provides 2,400 i.u. per 4 ml. If there is doubt about its absorption, preparations of vitamin A are available for subcutaneous injection. An adequate diet is the best prophylactic, but in the winter months, when the vitamin-A content of milk tends to fall, the routine administration of cod-liver oil is advisable for its vitamin-A as well as for its vitamin-D value.

VITAMIN-B COMPLEX

THIS is made up of various water-soluble vitamins, the absence of which produces a number of specific deficiency diseases including beri-beri, ariboflavinosis and pellagra. Multiple deficiencies may occur, producing a complex clinical result. The foods which contain a rich supply of these vitamins are wheat germ, yeast extract, eggs, meat (particularly pork and liver), nuts, bran, pulses, whole grain cereals and whole-meal bread, and leafy green vegetables.

VITAMIN B₁ (ANEURINE OR THIAMIN) (*see* p. 598)

VITAMIN B₂ (RIBOFLAVINE) (*see* p. 595)

NICOTINIC ACID (NIACIN) (*see* p. 600)

VITAMIN C

VITAMIN C (or water-soluble C) has been isolated as a colourless, crystalline compound—ascorbic acid. It is easily destroyed by heat and alkalis, and rapidly oxidized by atmospheric oxygen, and traces of copper. Among the best sources of vitamin C are: (1) *Citrus fruits*, such as grape-fruit, oranges and lemons. Bottled fruit juice is an excellent source of vitamin C, e.g. orange juice or rose-hip syrup. (2) *Vegetables*, such as broccoli, watercress, mustard and cress, sprouts. spinach, cabbage, tomatoes, cauliflower, turnips, parsnips and potatoes. Turnips or swedes can be cut up into small pieces and put through a press. The resulting juice, if used at once, is suitable for infants and children, but it does not keep. Potatoes, cooked in their jackets, constitute an excellent source. (3) *Summer fruits.* During the summer, red and black currants, raspberries, gooseberries and strawberries contain much vitamin c. During the winter months these fruits may be available bottled or tinned.

Infantile Scurvy

ÆTIOLOGY

Previously a veritable scourge among young children, scurvy has now almost disappeared from the United Kingdom, although it is still encountered in certain other countries. Its incidence is almost confined to artificially-fed babies receiving no fruit juice or other source of vitamin c, and it occurs between the ages of six months and one year. An acute infection may change a latent deficiency into a manifest one.

PHYSIOLOGY

Vitamin c is concerned in the formation of intercellular substance, and the integrity of capillary walls is diminished in states of deficiency. It is also concerned in the maturation of erythrocytes and the formation of bone and dentine; it plays an important role in tissue respiration.

PATHOLOGY

In scurvy, the infant ceases to grow, and widespread capillary bleeding occurs, particularly beneath the periosteum near the growing ends of long bones. If the incisor teeth have erupted, there may be submucous hæmorrhages opposite these teeth. Sometimes there is ecchymosis of the orbit or bleeding from some other site.

CLINICAL PICTURE

The first symptom is crying, and the mother notices that her baby dislikes being handled. He may cry with apprehension even when approached, because his bones are tender; when left alone, he is quiet and the limbs are kept at rest, the thighs separated and the knees bent (" frog-position "). The mother may also report that the urine has been " smoky " or red.

Even in early cases, x-ray changes are already fairly characteristic: slightly dense and irregular epiphyseal lines, " ringed " epiphyses and slight osteoporosis. Later on, swellings may be felt at the ends of certain long bones—characteristically at the lower ends of the femora. These swellings are subperiosteal hæmorrhages which will later become manifest in the x-ray. Microscopical examination of the urine always shows the presence of some degree of hæmaturia.

By seven months of age there are usually two lower incisors, and

5

about the base of these will be seen purple hæmorrhagic areas; the gums are swollen. An examination of the ribs shows that the sternum has become depressed and dislocated at the costo-chondral junction—that is, when the hand is passed out from the sternum towards the ribs the depression is reached, then the sharp tip of the rib is felt. This is quite unlike the beading in rickets, which is a smooth oval beading, with slight depression at either side, and not only at the sternal side, as in scurvy.

DIAGNOSIS

Vitamin-C Saturation Test. If a normal child is given a dose of 300 mg. of vitamin C, over the next two days the urine is found to contain large quantities of the vitamin. In cases of scurvy, this dose may have to be repeated daily for as long as a week before the urine becomes saturated with ascorbic acid.

DIFFERENTIAL DIAGNOSIS

Children who appear moderately well-nourished and cry incessantly may be thought to be suffering from acute osteomyelitis, especially if the swellings are large and the infant febrile. If the purpura is extensive, thrombocytopenic purpura may be suspected, or, if the subperiosteal hæmorrhage is mainly unilateral, a fracture or sarcoma may be suggested. Where the hæmorrhages are not very apparent, diagnoses such as teething or earache may be made. The clinical picture, however, is a very definite one: hæmorrhages about the gums, tenderness of the limbs with or without swellings, blood in the urine, backward dislocation of the sternum at the costo-chondral junction, and hæmorrhage beneath the periosteum. X-ray examination confirms the diagnosis in most cases.

PROGNOSIS

Properly treated, all cases of scurvy should recover completely. When the case is complicated by some infection, scorbutic infants resist the infection badly and the prognosis becomes less favourable.

TREATMENT

Scurvy can be cured in a dramatic way by giving ascorbic acid 300 mg. daily, or the juice of three oranges diluted with water and well sweetened with sugar. Potato-cream, made by adding the floury portion of the potato immediately beneath the skin to cows' milk, to the consistency of cream, is also effective. Six to eight teaspoonfuls of this should be given during the day.

PROPHYLAXIS

All infants from a fortnight old, whether breast- or bottle-fed, should be given fruit juice daily, two to four teaspoonfuls of orange or grapefruit juice, rose-hip syrup, black-currant purée or tomato juice, diluted with water and sweetened with sugar. Where infants refuse fresh orange juice, tomato or grapefruit juice, one-half to one teaspoonful can be added to each bottle, immediately before the bottle is given. Because ascorbic acid is destroyed by heat, the juice must not be heated.

VITAMIN D

THE two most important compounds with antirachitic properties are vitamin D_2 (irradiated ergosterol or calciferol), found in vegetables, and D_3 (7-dehydrocholesterol), found in animal fats. This vitamin can be formed in the fat cells of the skin by the action of the ultra-violet rays of the sun, and rickets will not develop unless both the antirachitic vitamin of the diet is deficient and at the same time the ultra-violet rays are absent. Vitamin D has a specific action in the absorption of calcium from the intestine; it also plays a part in the laying down of calcium in bone and in the re-absorption of phosphate in the renal tubules.

Some of the best-known sources are milk, cream, butter, egg yolk, cod-liver oil, halibut-liver oil and other fish oils. Vitamin D_2 (calciferol), the synthetic preparation, is available for those who cannot tolerate fish-liver oil, or where large concentrated doses are necessary.

Rickets

Simple nutritional rickets is a deficiency disease due to a lack of the fat-soluble vitamin D and/or an insufficient intake of calcium and phosphorus in the diet, leading to an imperfect calcification of the bones, most obvious at the sites of growth. In the United Kingdom, improvement in diet and education, together with the provision of cod-liver oil, have virtually eradicated all but the mildest degrees of rickets, but it may still be seen in some immigrant children.

AGE-INCIDENCE

The most active signs of rickets appear between the ages of six months and two years, but there seems no reasonable doubt that rickets is in process of development almost from birth onwards. The florid manifestations appear to be held off for at least three months and to be uncommon before six months.

ÆTIOLOGY

The two main causative factors of simple nutritional rickets are:

1. *Lack of Fat-soluble Vitamin D* (*see* above). The absence of this vitamin may be due to dietary deficiency or to lack of sunshine.

2. *Calcium Deprivation.* Even in the presence of sufficient vitamin and sunshine, rickets will result if the diet is so poor in calcium and phosphorus that too little is available for the needs of the body.

Usually, a pint of cows' milk daily provides sufficient of these minerals. Some of the sweetened condensed milks are so deficient in protein, fat, and calcium, and contain so much carbohydrate, that rickets may result from their use. A lack of vitamin D and calcium is accentuated by rapid growth. This is seen in premature babies and infants who are too fat.

There is present in wholemeal flour, and oat-flour, a substance (phytic acid) which has the power to combine and precipitate calcium, making it unavailable for use by the body. A diet relatively poor in calcium but which contains a large amount of phytic acid might well give rise to rickets.

PATHOLOGY

There is a failure of calcium deposition in the multiplying cartilage cells of the epiphyses and also in the freshly formed bone cells. Normally each maturing cartilage cell gives rise to another, and ultimately calcification and ossification take place. In rickets, this process becomes disorderly and the line of calcification is replaced by osteoid tissue. When healing takes place, a new line of calcification in the middle of the metaphysis can be seen, and ossification follows this process.

The proliferation of the cartilage can be seen clinically by an enlargement at the costochondral junctions and at the wrists and ankles.

CLINICAL PICTURE

The old saying that the rickety child has " the head of a philosopher, the chest of a greyhound, the legs of a grand piano and the tummy of a poisoned pup " is extremely apt.

As a rule, during the active stage of rickets pallor and anæmia are common, but there are exceptions to this. Sweating of the head is a feature and may be most striking. The muscles generally are soft, flabby and diminished. Rickets may be seen in fat babies as well as in undernourished ones.

Skeletal Manifestations. At first there is thinning along the suture lines (craniotabes), then the skull becomes thickened or bossed. The teeth may be late—often none appear until after one year of age—and when they do come the enamel may be poor. The bones of the legs bend so that the tibiæ and femora are bent either in or out, giving rise to knock-knees or bow-legs. The forearms are curved, because the child supports its weight on them when sitting. The anterior fontanelle is normally closed at about one year to 15 months; in rickets closure may be delayed past eighteen months.

Deformities of the Chest. Harrison's sulcus is a groove running round the chest at the attachment of the diaphragm, the pull of the diaphragm on the soft ribs having drawn them in at this point, causing the splaying out or eversion of the lower edges of the ribs. At the costo-chondral junctions beading is found, and these enlargements are as prominent on the inside of the rib as on the exterior. Postural defects, either kyphosis or scoliosis, are present. They are due to muscular weakness, however, as the curve is easily corrected if the child be picked up beneath the arms or placed on his face. If neglected, these deformities may become fixed.

Chemistry. Generally there is a reduction in the blood phosphorus (normal 4–5 mg. per cent.), together with increase in the alkaline phosphatase of about 50–60 King-Armstrong units (normal infants 10–22). Instead of a reduction in blood phosphorus, patients may show a low serum calcium (normal 9–11 mg. per cent.) with signs of latent or manifest tetany. Amino-aciduria can be shown chromatographically during the active phase of rickets.

Nervous Manifestations. Hyper-excitability of the nervous system, giving rise to overt or latent tetany, may appear in a case of acute rickets. This usually occurs in those cases in which the total serum calcium is reduced to below 8 mg. per cent. A reduction in the ionized fraction of the serum calcium is the determining factor.

Tetany (spasmophilia) manifests itself by:
1. Facial irritability or Chvostek's sign. When the cheek is tapped, so that the facial nerve is stimulated, the muscles innervated by it go into spasm.
2. Carpo-pedal spasm. The hands are held in the accoucheur's position, with the fingers fully extended, but slightly flexed on the palm, and the thumb adducted. The feet assume much the same position as the hands. Carpo-pedal spasm is a painful cramp. By inflating a sphygmomanometer cuff on the arm sufficiently to obstruct the circulation, the sign may be elicited in cases of latent tetany (Trousseau's sign).
3. Laryngismus stridulus (crowing). A spasm of the larynx may occur whenever the child is suddenly roused, frightened or annoyed. The breath is held, the face becoming blue, as in whooping-cough; then the larynx relaxes and a long-drawn inspiratory cry is heard. This is a dangerous condition and sometimes proves fatal.
4. Convulsions (*see* p. 453). Children with spasmophilia are liable to convulsions. The attacks may be precipitated by breath-holding, and by febrile illnesses.

DIAGNOSIS

The clinical diagnosis of mild rickets is extremely difficult. Since the bony malformations remain long after the condition has healed, the clinician is apt to diagnose rickets when in fact it is already cured. The presence of active rickets is confirmed by the x-ray appearances of the long bones and by chemical alterations in the plasma.

PROGNOSIS

Once the bony deformities are present in marked degree, they remain to a greater or lesser extent for some years. If the rickets is allowed to continue, stunting and dwarfing become obvious. The nervous manifestations, however, leave no residuum, so far as is known. The prognosis for life is excellent, though death occasionally results from *laryngismus stridulus* or from some acute infection.

TREATMENT

Dietetic. Cod-liver oil should be given and the diet should contain a sufficient quantity of protein, fat, phosphorus and calcium. To ensure this, plenty of milk should be given but not too much cereal food.

Medicinal. Whenever possible, vitamins should be given in their natural form. It is best, therefore, in supplying vitamin D, both for the prevention and cure of rickets, to give it as cod- or halibut-liver oil, rather than in synthetic preparations. In the United Kingdom, it is taught that protection is afforded by giving 400 i.u. of vitamin D daily, and double this dose or more can safely be given as treatment. It is necessary to give vitamin D to both breast-fed and artificially-fed infants (for dosage for those infants fed on dried milks fortified with vitamin D, see p. 42). Where cod-liver oil is not tolerated, one of the concentrated forms such as halibut-liver oil, or a synthetic preparation, may be substituted.

Sunshine. With due precautions exposure to sunshine is beneficial. An infant should have at least four hours in the fresh air every day.

Vitamin-resistant Rickets

As a rule, infantile rickets is cured by the age of $1\frac{1}{2}$–2 years, and it is very rare indeed to see a case of simple rickets after this age. Occasionally, however, an older child shows active rickets, and an x-ray and serum-phosphatase estimation will confirm the diagnosis. Further investigation shows that such children are failing to re-absorb phosphate from the renal tubule (a process in which vitamin D is concerned, p. 119). Thus, large quantities of phosphate are lost in the urine and the serum-phosphate level tends to be low, despite a normal intake of vitamin D. It will usually be found that these cases are particularly resistant to treatment with ordinary doses of vitamin D, and that they may show a fluctuating course with spontaneous periods of healing followed by relapse. Large doses of vitamin D, such as 100,000 i.u. daily, are usually effective treatment. This therapy, however, requires careful observation to detect early signs of *hypervitaminosis* D, such as anorexia, constipation, abdominal pain and loss of weight, together with a rising blood calcium. If such symptoms of overdosage are long-continued, renal failure due to calcification within the kidney will occur and even death. Certain cases of vitamin-D-resistant

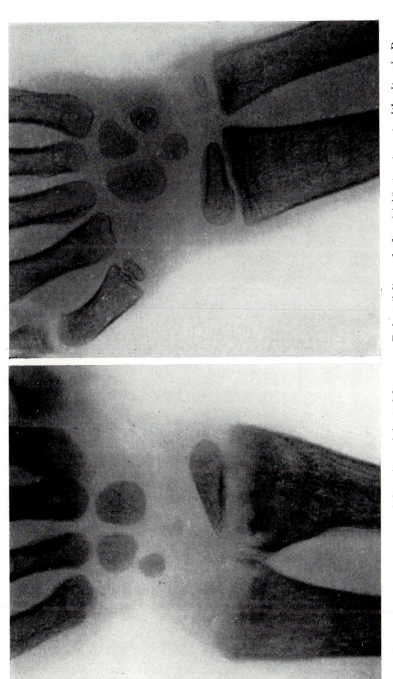

PLATE I. Vitamin-resistant rickets in a girl aged 3 years. Before (*left*): and after (*right*): treatment with vitamin D (25,000 i.u. daily).

rickets are thought to be genetically determined, inherited usually through a sex-linked gene.

Cœliac Rickets

This is dealt with under Cœliac Disease (*see* p. 143). It is sufficient to say here that while the child is not growing during the acute stage of cœliac disease, no rickets is to be found, although the bones show marked osteoporosis. Later, when the cœliac disease is rapidly improving and fresh growth is taking place, acute rickets may develop. Vitamin D, together with extra calcium, will forestall this.

Renal Rickets

This is dealt with under Renal Disease (*see* p. 375). It may occur at any age, even in infancy, but is commoner in those past the age of infantile rickets, that is, between 6 and 12 or 14 years. In an older child developing marked knock-knee and enlargement of the epiphyses at the wrists and ankles, the possibility of a renal lesion should be seriously considered. Examination of the urine and blood urea will help in the diagnosis. The treatment is greatly hampered by the underlying disease. Vitamin D, together with artificial sunlight, and alkalis, are usually indicated.

Other Forms of Metabolic Rickets

These are described in detail under Metabolic Disorders (p. 130).

VITAMIN K

THE importance of vitamin-K deficiency is discussed on p. 109

CHAPTER 10

Metabolic Disorders

FAILURE TO THRIVE IN INFANCY

MARASMUS, or wasting of unknown origin in infancy, was once a frequent diagnosis. In recent years causes of infantile wasting have been investigated, the pathology recognized, and treatment made possible, so that the incidence of " marasmus " has greatly diminished. Unfortunately, in the world population, starvation is still the commonest cause of wasting in infancy (*see* p. 55), despite the paradox that in " socially developed " countries there is over-production of food.

ÆTIOLOGY

In dealing with infants who are wasted, the physician has first to distinguish between (*a*) mismanagement of a healthy infant's feeds and (*b*) organic disease. In adverse home conditions the two may be combined as, for example, when infective gastro-enteritis is superimposed in an already underfed infant.

FEEDING MISMANGEMENT

Mistakes in feeding technique frequently account for an infant's failure to gain weight (p. 58), whilst rumination (p. 59) must also be considered. Investigation of infants who fail to thrive should be carried out on the following lines:

1. Make certain by calculation (p. 40) that the infant is offered sufficient fluid and calories for his expected weight. If the infant is breast fed, test feeding (p. 39) is necessary.

2. Watch a feed being given to ensure that the technique is satisfactory. Infants with micrognathos or nasal obstruction have particular difficulty in feeding (p. 224).

3. Observation, by an experienced district nurse or health visitor, of the daily routine at home will often show the reason for the infant's lack of progress.

4. A full history and clinical examination is necessary to exclude organic disease. Urinary infections remain one of the commonest

causes of poor progress in infancy and one of the most underdiagnosed; microscopy of the urine for pus cells should be a routine procedure.

ORGANIC DISEASE

The organic causes of failure to thrive in infancy are numerous and vary from common to very rare disorders.

Infective Disorders. In the United Kingdom, urinary infection, chronic naso-pharyngeal infection, chronic otitis media and mastoiditis, moniliasis, unresolved pneumonia, and gastro-enteritis are frequent causes; whilst tuberculosis, inadequately treated meningitis and congenital syphilis are less commonly found. In tropical countries, malaria, hookworm, and other intestinal infestations are important causes.

Dietary Deficiencies. In addition to general starvation, protein malnutrition (kwashiorkor, *see* p. 600) and the avitaminoses are prevalent in the underdeveloped countries of Africa and Asia.

Congenital Malformations. (*a*) Gastro-intestinal malformations including hiatus hernia, hypertrophic pyloric stenosis, intermittent duodenal obstruction, and Hirchsprung's disease impede normal alimentary function; (*b*) malformations elsewhere in the body, such as congenital heart lesions (particularly when heart failure occurs), mental retardation, and malformations of the kidneys and urinary tract, commonly give rise to nutritional failure in infancy.

Metabolic Disorders. Most of the metabolic disorders which interfere with nutritional progress in infancy are rare conditions. They may be divided into (*a*) those of genetic origin, such as fibrocystic disease, galactosæmia and glycogen-storage disease and (*b*) those not known to be genetically determined, including cœliac disease, idiopathic renal acidosis and hypercalcæmia of infancy.

Miscellaneous Disorders. The remaining causes of failure to thrive in infancy have widely differing origins; they include chronic accidental poisoning with heavy metals, such as lead and mercury (pink disease), neoplastic diseases, and birth injuries, including sub-dural hæmatoma.

Finally, there is still a small number of infants in whom the cause of their failure to thrive remains unknown, despite the most detailed investigation.

BIOCHEMICAL DISORDERS OF
GENETIC ORIGIN

THE introduction of new biochemical techniques, such as electrophoresis and chromatography, into clinical medicine has not only made possible a much wider understanding of many disease processes but has tended to integrate our knowledge of the pathogenesis of much that previously was diffuse, bizarre and apparently unconnected. The basic concept of an inherited inborn error of metabolism is not new; it was first suggested in 1908 by Sir Archibald Garrod. At that time, only four conditions, albinism, alkaptonuria, cystinuria, and pentosuria were included; now, many more disorders of this kind can be distinguished, although there is little doubt that the list is as yet incomplete. The majority are inherited as recessive characteristics, a few as dominant or incompletely dominant characteristics, whilst some are sex-linked in their transmission (*see* pp. 12–16).

BIOCHEMICAL DISORDERS OF INHERITED ORIGIN

Abnormal Amino-Acid Metabolism

  Albinism.
  Phenylketonuria.
  Alkaptonuria.
  Maple Syrup Syndrome.
  Argininosuccinic Aciduria.

Abnormal Renal Tubular Function

  Renal Glycosuria.
  Vitamin Resistant Rickets.
  Cystinosis.
  Cystinuria.
  Hartnup Disease.
  Lowe's Syndrome.

Abnormal Carbohydrate Metabolism

  Pentosuria.
  Galactosæmia.
  Fructosuria.
  Glycogen Storage Disease.

Endocrine Abnormalities

  Goitrous Cretinism.
  Adrenogenital Syndrome.
  Diabetes Insipidus.

Abnormalities of Plasma Proteins

  Agammaglobulinæmia.
  Analbuminæmia.
  Wilson's Disease.
  Afibrinogenæmia.
  Classical Hæmophilia.
  Christmas Disease.
  Other Coagulation Defects.

Abnormalities of Erythrocytes

  The Hæmoglobinopathies.
  Hereditary Spherocytosis.
  Congenital Porphyria.
  Congenital Methæmoglobinæmia.
  Glucose - 6 - phosphate - dehydrogenase deficiency.

Miscellaneous

  Congenital Hyperbilirubinæmia.
  Hypophosphatasia.
  Fibrocystic Disease (Mucoviscidosis).

All these conditions possess a common background in their pathogenesis, namely, an inherited deficiency of one or more essential components (usually enzymic) of particular biological processes. The effect in the body of such a biological failure varies greatly in each case. Some lead to disorders of growth or give rise to mental deficiency, whilst others endanger life itself.

The genetic origin of these disorders raises problems for the family doctor and pædiatrician called on to advise over family planning (*see* p. 470); the likelihood of better survival due to treatment will raise important eugenic considerations in treated patients in the not too distant future.

THE SIGNIFICANCE OF AMINO-ACIDURIA

The introduction of chromatography into clinical medicine has greatly increased our knowledge of the excretion of amino-acids in the urine. It is found that the normal person regularly excretes in the urine small amounts of many amino-acids, and that this follows a consistent pattern for the particular individual. The excretion of one or more amino-acids in excess may be due to various causes:—

1. *Simple Overflow Mechanism*

Where there is any inborn defect of protein metabolism, such as the inability to break down phenylalanine, the particular amino-acid will accumulate in excess in the plasma and will be excreted in the urine.

2. *Inherited Abnormality of Renal Tubular Function*

Certain inherited disorders relate specifically to renal tubular function. In cystinuria, for example, the renal tubule fails to reabsorb cystine (and certain other amino-acids) and persistent cystinuria therefore occurs, although the plasma level of cystine is never elevated and, indeed, tends to fall below normal.

3. *Secondary Effects on Renal Tubular Function by other Inherited Metabolic Disorders*

In other inherited metabolic disorders, such as galactosæmia and Wilson's disease, although the primary abnormality is unrelated either to amino-acid metabolism or renal tubular function, the secondary effects of the disorder include an interference with renal tubular action giving rise to a general non-specific amino-aciduria.

4. *Renal Failure*

As a consequence of severe widespread renal disease from any cause, generalized amino-aciduria is included among the other failures of renal function.

5. *Renal Immaturity*

In premature infants, a moderate amino-aciduria due to inadequate tubular re-absorption occurs. This may also be seen to a variable degree in full-term newborn infants.

INHERITED ABNORMALITIES OF AMINO-ACID METABOLISM

Albinism (*see* p. 499)

Phenylketonuria[1]

CHILDREN with phenylketonuria have an innate inability to metabolize the amino-acid phenylalanine. Although normal at birth, such

---

[1] Brimblecombe, F. S. W., Blainey, J. D., Stoneman, Margaret E. R., Wood, B. S. B. (1961). *Lancet*, 2, 793.

infants, when fed on normal protein foods, show during the first year of life a progressive mental deterioration ending in imbecility in all but a few instances. The disorder is transmitted as an autosomal recessive characteristic, with an incidence of about 1 in 20,000 births, i.e., about 50 new cases annually in England and Wales.

The defect lies in the absence of the liver enzyme, phenylalaninase, which is essential for the breakdown of phenylalanine into tyrosine. Its absence leads to the accumulation of phenylalanine in the serum, together with certain abnormal metabolic products, notably phenyl-pyruvic acid, which together with phenylalanine is excreted in the urine.

CLINICAL SIGNS

The majority of phenylketonuric children are blue-eyed, fair-haired and fair-skinned, with a predisposition to eczema. If untreated, they become mentally deficient by the age of two years, apart from a small group (amounting to two per cent. of all those affected) who retain normal intelligence. There is an increased tendency to epileptic seizures.

DIAGNOSIS

The diagnosis is suggested by the finding of phenylpyruvic acid in the urine. This can be demonstrated by the formation of a green-grey colouration when five drops of ferric chloride are added to 5 ml. of urine. Alternatively, a Clinitest with Phenistix (Ames) may be carried out, using a fresh specimen of urine or a freshly wet napkin. The diagnosis is confirmed by the demonstration of excess phenyl-alanine in the urine on chromatography and by a raised level of serum phenylalanine (normal 0·7–1·5 mg. per cent.).

If dietary treatment is to be effective in preventing mental deficiency, it must be commenced by the age of four to six weeks. Thus, the only way to make the diagnosis sufficiently soon is to carry out a routine test of the urine on all infants by the age of four weeks (the test is likely to be negative in the first few days of life, because insufficient accumulation of phenylalanine will have taken place in the serum for the abnormal metabolites to be present in the urine).

TREATMENT

The basis of treatment lies in the limitation of dietary phenylalanine to a level just adequate to provide for tissue growth and repair, but insufficient to allow abnormal accumulation of phenylalanine in the serum. In practice, this means that the main dietary protein has to be supplied as a synthetic casein hydrolysate of low phenylalanine content, apart from the very small quantity of normal protein food which will provide the basic phenylalanine needs. The details of the low phenylalanine diet are given in Appendix 7 (p. 684).

PROGNOSIS

The management of the phenylketonuric diet, which has to be continued at least throughout childhood, is difficult. If it is started by the age of six weeks and the serum level of phenylalanine kept below about 5 mg. per cent., then it is likely that normal intelligence will be preserved.

If treatment is started only later and after mental deterioration is already present, then the prognosis is less satisfactory. Nevertheless, there have been considerable improvements in the intelligence quotients of a few children, particularly those in whom mental deterioration had not been severe at the time that treatment was begun.

Alkaptonuria

In certain individuals, the urine, when first passed, is normal in colour but, if left to stand, turns brown and then black. In other respects the individual is quite healthy, although sometimes in old age the ligaments and cartilages also darken (ochronosis) and osteo-arthritis may develop.

The colour changes in the urine are due to the presence of the reducing substance *homogentisic acid*, which, when oxidized, gives rise to a black pigment. Homogentisic acid is an intermediate metabolic product in the breakdown of phenylalanine and tyrosine. Its appearance in excess in the plasma and subsequent excretion in the urine in certain individuals are due to an inherited failure to break down this substance to maleylacetoacetate, its normal degradation product.

This condition is inherited as a recessive characteristic and is thus only seen in individuals homozygous for the abnormal gene.

Maple-syrup Syndrome

This is a rare, recessively inherited disorder in which the urine has a curious smell reminiscent of maple syrup. The affected infants have been found to be mentally retarded, and death usually occurs in the first year of life. The plasma and urine contain an excess of the amino-acids valine, leucine and iso-leucine. The precise nature of the metabolic defect is not known nor is the cause of the curious smell of the urine.

Argininosuccinic-aciduria

Dent et al.[1] describe two mentally defective siblings who were found to be excreting this substance in their urine. It was also found in excess in the plasma and in even greater amounts in the cerebrospinal fluid. Argininosuccinic acid is an intermediate product in the ornithine cycle, and its appearance in excess in the cerebrospinal fluid is presumably due to an inherited defect of brain metabolism with which mental deficiency is associated.

[1] Allan, J. D., Cusworth, D. C., Dent, C. E., Wilson, V. K. (1958). *Lancet*, 1, 182.

INHERITED ABNORMALITIES OF RENAL TUBULAR FUNCTION

Renal Glycosuria (*see* p. 168)

Vitamin-resistant Rickets (*see* p. 122)

Cystinosis (Cystine-storage Disease) (De Toni-Fanconi-Debré Syndrome)

FAMILIAL cystinosis was recorded by Abderhalden in 1903 and by Lignac in 1924. That various defects of renal tubular function occur either with cystinosis, or sometimes without it, is being increasingly recognized, and it now seems probable that there are a number of genetic variants of the group as a whole which are included in the name De Toni-Fanconi-Debré syndrome.

The variety in which cystine is deposited in the tissues has a poor prognosis. It is usually inherited as a recessive character. The associated disturbances of renal tubular function include a generalized amino-aciduria, glycosuria and, in some cases, a failure of the kidney to conserve phosphate, with the consequent development of vitamin-resistant rickets (*see* p. 122). Other features include renal acidosis, potassium depletion and polyuria.

The symptoms may commence at about six to twelve months with failure to thrive associated with thirst, vomiting and polyuria. Attacks of severe vomiting with dehydration may occur. Later there is stunting of growth with evidence of rickets. The diagnosis may be suggested by the finding of glycosuria, amino-aciduria together with a renal acidosis, hypophosphatæmia, and hypokalæmia. In older children and adults, instead of rachitic-bone changes, a widespread osteomalacia is seen. The finding of cystine crystals in the bone marrow, lymph nodes, or cornea delineates cystinosis proper.

TREATMENT

Treatment consists in giving sodium citrate to correct the acidosis (*see also* p. 141) and potassium chloride if there is hypokalæmia. Vitamin-resistant rickets is treated with large doses of vitamin D (*see also* p. 122).

Cystinuria

This condition has been known since 1810 when Wollaston[1] first described the development of urinary calculi of this kind.

The disorder is now known to be due to an inherited abnormality (of varied genetic origin) of renal tubular function. Not only does the renal tubule fail to re-absorb cystine (the resulting excess of cystine in the urine giving rise to cystine stones) but there is an associated failure

[1] Wollaston, W. H. (1810). *Phil. Trans. B*, 223.

of renal tubular re-absorption of lysine, arginine and ornithine. Due to its relatively greater insolubility, cystine stones only are formed.

No primary symptoms occur, apart from the repeated formation of cystine stones throughout the renal tract, but, because of the recurrent formation of these calculi, life may be greatly shortened despite repeated surgical intervention.

In one form, the disorder is clearly inherited as a classical recessive genetic characteristic in which the heterozygotes show no detectable abnormality. In the other form, whilst the homozygote shows the fully established disorder, as in the classical recessive type, the hetero-zygote, on the other hand, may show a somewhat excessive and variable excretion of cystine and the other amino-acids without ever developing the full syndrome of calculus formation.

Hartnup Disease[1]

This is an exceedingly rare, recessively inherited disorder of renal tubular function. Whilst there is a generalized amino-aciduria of a characteristic type, there is also a particular disturbance of tryptophan metabolism, as shown by a greatly increased excretion of its indole derivatives—indolylacetic acid and indolylacetyl glutamine. No adequate explanation of this is known.

The symptoms include a pellagra-like skin rash of a photosensitive nature which is limited to exposed areas of the body, and cerebellar ataxia of a transient nature. The rash may improve on treatment with nicotinamide.

Lowe's Syndrome (see p. 523)

INHERITED ABNORMALITIES OF CARBOHYDRATE METABOLISM

Pentosuria (L-Xyloketosuria)

THIS condition is a curiosity rather than a disease. Individuals affected excrete large quantities of L-xyloketose throughout life. In other respects they are normal and healthy. There is no other disturbance of carbohydrate metabolism. The condition is usually found in Central European Jews and is inherited as a recessive genetic characteristic.

Galactosæmia

This disorder has assumed great clinical importance in view of the possible prevention by dietary treatment of the mental deficiency which otherwise occurs.

Milk sugar (lactose) is broken down in the intestine into glucose and galactose. After absorption, the galactose is acted upon by liver

---

[1] Baron, D. N., Dent, C. E., Harris, H., Jepson, J. B. (1956). *Lancet* 2, 421.
Milne, M. D., Crawford, M. A., Girao, C. B., Loughridge, L. W. (1960). *Quart. J. Med.*, **24**, 407.

enzymes to form eventually glucose-1-phosphate. In certain people, an enzyme, galactose-1-phosphate-uridyl-transferase, which is an essential enzyme for an intermediate stage of this process, is absent and galactose-1-phosphate accumulates in the blood, in the erythrocytes and tissues with serious and irreversible consequences.

SYMPTOMS

Following milk feeding in the first days of life, the accumulation of galactose-1-phosphate commences in these infants. The infant fails to thrive; there is vomiting and poor weight gain. The liver becomes pathologically enlarged and jaundice may develop. Convulsions and death may subsequently occur in the first months of life. In surviving cases, cataracts and severe mental impairment develop.

Such infants are found to be passing in their urine a reducing substance which can be identified as galactose. Due to renal tubular damage from the high levels of galactose, a generalized proteinuria and amino-aciduria is found. Examination of the red cells shows a high intracellular concentration of galactose-1-phosphate.

GENETICS

Those patients who show the fully established clinical disorder are homozygous for the abnormal gene. It is not uncommon to find that other members of his family show in a standard galactose tolerance test an impaired ability to deal with galactose. There seems little doubt that such individuals are heterozygotes for the disorder.

TREATMENT

The recognition of the disorder in the first weeks of life and the removal of normal milk from the diet effectively corrects the galactosæmia and prevents the development of permanent complications. Adequate substitutes in the form of specially prepared low lactose milks are available for infant feeding. It seems probable that this treatment must be continued throughout life, although the elimination of milk and its derivatives from the diet becomes less of a problem in the older child and adult than in infancy.

Fructosuria

The two forms of hereditary fructosuria are both very rare. In the first type, there is a recessively inherited failure of renal tubular re-absorption of fructose. The individuals never show clinical symptoms and the condition is usually detected at a routine examination of the urine when a reducing substance, later identified as fructose, is discovered.

In the second type[1] symptoms of hypoglycæmia, including sweating, pallor, vomiting and drowsiness, are found, associated with a high

[1] Froesch, E. R., Prader, A., Wolf, H. P., Labhart, A. (1959). *Helv. paediat. Acta.*, **14**, 99.

level of blood fructose, which is also excreted in excess in the urine. Such individuals also show a tendency to hypophosphatæmia although clinical rickets has not been reported. The exact cause of the disorder is not clear, but the condition is inherited as an autosomal recessive characteristic.

Glycogen-storage Disease

This is not a single disorder, but represents a group of diseases due to a number of different enzyme deficiencies in which glycogen metabolism is abnormal. The defects are inherited as recessive genetic characteristics. The two commoner forms are:

GLYCOGEN-STORAGE DISEASE OF THE LIVER AND KIDNEYS (VON GIERKE'S DISEASE)

After normal progress at first, these infants fail to thrive; there is vomiting and loss of weight. In the majority, convulsions occur and the infant dies under the age of two years. In a few instances the disease is more mild and adult life may be attained, although growth is stunted and the liver remains consistently enlarged. Such infants show marked hepatic enlargement, a tendency to hypoglycæmia when food is withheld, a flat glucose-tolerance curve, ketonuria and a gross excess of liver glycogen at liver biopsy and at autopsy.

The enzyme deficient in the liver is glucose-6-phosphatase, essential for the reaction:

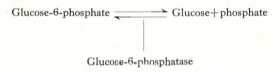

Glucose-6-phosphate ⇌ Glucose + phosphate

Glucose-6-phosphatase

The deficiency of this enzyme prevents the normal formation of glucose from glycogen, which consequently accumulates to excess.

GLYCOGEN-STORAGE DISEASE OF THE HEART

Infants affected with this form of abnormal glycogen metabolism develop heart failure, usually in the first months of life (see p. 283), and seldom survive beyond the second year of life. The heart is greatly enlarged and is found at autopsy to contain a gross excess of glycogen. An excess of glycogen may also be found in skeletal muscles.

The recessively inherited defect of glycogen metabolism responsible differs from that in von Gierke's disease, but its exact nature is not yet known.

TREATMENT

No treatment is effective, although glucagon may be tried, particularly in the hepatic type.

INHERITED ABNORMALITIES OF ENDOCRINE ORIGIN

Goitrous Cretinism (*see* p. 157)

Adrenogenital Syndrome (*see* p. 159)

INHERITED ABNORMALITIES OF PLASMA PROTEINS

Agammaglobulinæmia

BRUTON[1] (1952) first described a boy with a history of repeated severe infections who was unable to produce antibodies to standard immunizing procedures. His plasma proteins showed a complete absence of gamma-globulin.

Since then, children (almost always boys) have been described in whom bacterial infections, in addition to other non-specific infections, recur repeatedly and in whom standard immunizing procedures with bacterial toxoids provoke no antibody response. Electrophoresis shows a great reduction of plasma gamma-globulin, although the other plasma protein fractions are normal. Such children have a deficiency of lymph germ cells with a lymphocytopenia in the peripheral blood. The condition is almost completely confined to the male sex, and other males in the family may be affected. Inheritance is by a sex-linked gene which does not produce clinical effects in the female heterozygote.

It is likely that in the pre-antibiotic era none of these children survived childhood. Now, with the early use of antibiotics, together with repeated injections of gamma-globulin, it is possible that such individuals can survive, although the risk of overwhelming infections can never be far away. In such infants, vaccination may be a fatal procedure, since multiple vaccinial lesions which progress to gangrene (*vaccinia gangrenosa*) develop in some, but not all, of those vaccinated.

It appears likely that, in addition to complete absence of gamma-globulin, hypogamma-globulinæmia may also occur. This is seen as a transient form in the newborn and as an acquired form in adults.

Analbuminæmia

For completeness, mention must be made of a family[2] in which the serum of the siblings contained no albumin. The parents were second cousins. Of the two children, a boy and a girl, the girl suffered from slight œdema but was otherwise healthy, the boy had no symptoms of any kind. Both have reached adult life.

[1] Bruton, O. C. (1952). *Pediatrics*, **9** 722.
[2] Bennhold, H., Peters, H., Roth, E. (1954). *Verh. dtsch. Ges. inn. Med.*, **60**, 630.

Wilson's Disease (*see* p. 446)

Afibrinogenæmia (*see* p. 346)

Classical Hæmophilia (*see* p. 344)

Christmas Disease (*see* p. 345)

Other Coagulation Defects (*see* p. 345)

INHERITED ABNORMALITIES OF ERYTHROCYTES

The Hæmoglobinopathies (*see* p. 338)

Hereditary Spherocytosis (*see* p. 337)

Congenital Porphyria

THIS is a rare inherited disease in which the infant shows marked photosensitivity persisting from birth throughout life. Exposure to sunlight gives rise to marked erythema of the skin, progressing to blister formation and subsequent scarring. The red cells show an increased rate of hæmolysis. In ultra-violet light the bones and teeth produce a remarkable red fluorescence and the urine a typical reddish colour.

The disease is due to an enzyme deficiency in the synthesis of hæm from porphobilinogen. It is likely that the normal conversion of porphobilinogen into type-3 porphyrin is defective; instead, porphobilinogen is converted into porphyrin 1 in large amounts and this substance cannot be used for hæm formation. Therefore it accumulates in excess in the blood and tissues and is excreted in the urine. Its presence in the skin is responsible for the photosensitivity. The urine is found to contain uroporphyrin 1 and coproporphyrin 1 in excess.

The disease is found in individuals homozygous for the abnormal gene.

OTHER FORMS OF PORPHYRIA

The other varieties of porphyria are biochemically quite distinct from the congenital form. *Porphyria cutanea tarda* may indeed represent a group of differing abnormalities which show themselves clinically as photosensitivity and recurrent abdominal pain. The disease pursues an intermittent course. During the episodes the urinary output of porphyrins is increased; during the remissions the excessive output of porphyrin is seen in the stool.

Acute porphyria appears in late childhood or early adult life, with the acute onset of abdominal colic, peripheral nerve palsies and mental confusion (*see* p. 429). Photosensitivity does not occur. Porpho-bilinogen accumulates in the blood and is excreted in excess in the urine and stools. The attacks sometimes follow the administration of barbiturates and may be seen in the post-partum period. The disease is inherited probably through a dominant gene of incomplete pene-trance. The mechanism of the disorder is not understood.

Methæmoglobinæmia

This may occur both in an inherited and an acquired form. In either form the iron in the circulating hæmoglobin is present in the ferric state and is thus unavailable for the transport of oxygen. This gives rise to cyanosis and compensatory polycythæmia. The patients may show surprisingly little incapacity.

The acquired form may follow the giving of such drugs as acetanilide, phenacetin, and occasionally the sulphonamides. It may also follow the drinking of well-water with a high nitrate content.

The inherited forms are evident from birth, and one variety at least appears to be due to a defect in the synthesis of the globin fraction, which, in turn, predisposes to methæmoglobin formation. The precise mechanism is not understood. The type of inheritance varies; both a recessive and an incomplete dominant type have been described.

The presence of methæmoglobin may be determined spectro-scopically, thus confirming the diagnosis.

The administration of methylene blue and ascorbic acid permits the reduction of methæmoglobin with temporary abolition of the cyanosis. The methylene blue acts more rapidly and more com-pletely.

Glucose-6-phosphate-dehydrogenase Deficiency[1,2]

An inherited type of hæmolytic anæmia, with neonatal jaundice in the more severe cases, has recently been described in which a pro-portion of the red cells are found to be deficient of the enzyme glucose-6-phosphate dehydrogenase. This enzyme plays an essential part in a complex biochemical system within the red cell for the formation of reduced glutathione (GSH). The red cells deficient of the enzyme not only lack reduced glutathione but are unduly fragile.

Individuals affected may show an unusual degree of jaundice in the neonatal period, and variable degrees of hæmolytic anæmia, often of a drug-induced nature (*see* Primaquine Sensitivity, p. 137), follow.

The condition is genetically determined, but the precise type of inheritance is not yet clear. It is possible that two mutants of slightly different characteristics may exist, the one in Caucasian races, the other in negroes.

[1] Dern, R. J., Weinstein, I. M., Le Roy, G. V., Talmadge, D. W., Alving, A. S. (1954). *J. Lab. clin. Med.*, **43**, 303.
[2] Marks, P. A., Banks, Julia, Gross, Ruth T. (1962). *Nature*, **194**, 454.

PRIMAQUINE SENSITIVITY[1]

It has been known for some years that the administration of the antimalarial drug primaquine may in certain individuals produce hæmolytic anæmia. It appears that these individuals have inherited the particular red-cell enzyme deficiency of glucose-6-phosphate dehydrogenase described on p. 136. Hæmolysis occurs only when primaquine is administered and does not occur spontaneously. Such sensitivity to primaquine is inherited by about ten per cent. of American negroes. It may be less common among Caucasian races. It seems probable that *favism* (hæmolytic anæmia after eating fava beans) is due to the same inherited defect. The relationship of primaquine-sensitive hæmolytic anæmia to the hæmolysis that occurs in the newborn infant following the administration of excessive quantities of water-soluble *vitamin K analogues* (*see* p. 96) or the accidental ingestion of *naphtha* may be similar.

Hæmolysis may also follow the use of sulphonamides, furadantin, phenacetin, phenylhydrazine, sulphones, and PAS.

MISCELLANEOUS METABOLIC DISORDERS OF INHERITED ORIGIN

Congenital Hyperbilirubinæmia

SEVERAL rare, inherited metabolic anomalies give rise to persistent familial jaundice.

One variety is known as Gilbert's Disease[2] in which intermittent episodes of jaundice occur throughout life, although the first attack in some individuals may not occur until adult life. The bilirubin in the serum is unconjugated and the jaundice is non-obstructive in character. The majority of these patients suffer little disability and lead normal lives. The condition is thought to be inherited as a dominant characteristic of incomplete gene penetrance.

A more serious variety of familial jaundice has been described[3] in which the majority of the affected infants developed fatal kernicterus (p. 113). A few infants have survived, appearing to be free of symptoms apart from persistent jaundice. As in Gilbert's Disease, there is a persistent increase in the indirect serum-bilirubin level.

It appears that both conditions may be due to an inherited deficiency of the enzyme, bilirubin glucuronyl transferase, essential for the formation of bilirubin glucuronide from indirect bilirubin. It may be that the severe form in which kernicterus occurs represents the homozygous form of the disease.

Another inherited defect in bilirubin metabolism was described by Dubin and Johnson[4] in 1958. Here a normally conjugated bilirubin is ineffectively excreted from the liver cells, giving rise to an accumula-

[1] Tarlov, A. R., Brewer, G. J., Carson, P. E., Alving, A. S. (1962). *Arch. intern. Med.*, **109**, 137.
[2] Gilbert, A., Lerebouillet, P., Herscher, M. (1907). *Bull. Soc. méd., Paris*, **24**, 1203.
[3] Crigler, J. F., Nazzar, V. A. (1952). *Pediatrics*, **10**, 169.
[4] Dubin, I. N. (1958). *Amer. J. Med.*, **24**, 268.

tion of conjugated bilirubin. Symptoms include an intermittent, low-grade jaundice, abdominal pain, weakness, nausea and vomiting, anorexia, and diarrhœa. Signs may include an enlarged liver, dark urine and pale stools. Other than for the elevation in conjugated bilirubin and an abnormal retention of bromsulphalein, there appears to be little change in biochemical parameters. Both oral and intra-venous cholecystography show non-visualization of the gall bladder. Grossly, the liver appears enlarged, smooth, and dark green or black. Microscopically, a coarsely granular, brown pigment with a centro-lobular distribution is characteristic. No treatment is known or indeed indicated since the defect is compatible with a long life.

In the neonatal period these conditions have to be distinguished from the more common causes of jaundice (p. 95).

Congenital Hypophosphatasia (Osteoblastic Dysplasia)

This rare disorder is believed to be an hereditarily determined congenital metabolic fault in bone formation. Osteoblastic functions are or the bone matrix is defective, the bone trabeculæ are thin and the matrix hypoplastic (? osteoblastic dysplasia). There is a deficiency of alkaline phosphatase in the serum and in the matrix of growing metaphyseal cartilages, which may be due to non-use of phosphatase substrate. Thus, in the urine of a two-month-old infant suffering from hypophosphatasic rickets an unusual amino-acid (phosphoe-thanolamine), which can act as a substrate for phosphatase[1], was found.

Clinical Picture. When the disease is seen in early infancy, the usual symptoms are anorexia, vomiting and wasting. The epiphyses are enlarged, the ribs beaded, and the skull may be paper-thin. An x-ray shows irregular decalcification of the bones and a very wide gap at the cranial suture lines. Later, the cranial sutures may close prematurely. The metaphyses are markedly decalcified and a periosteal reaction occurs.

In older children, skeletal deformities resembling rickets occur, also poor calcification, premature shedding of the first teeth and a persistently low serum alkaline phosphatase, usually 3–7 King-Arm-strong units.

Treatment. There is no curative treatment. Intensive therapy with vitamin D has been given in some cases; however this is contra-indicated if hypercalcæmia is present—a not uncommon complication of the disease, especially in infancy.

Fibrocystic Disease of the Pancreas (Mucoviscidosis)

This condition was brought into prominence by Andersen in 1938. It is an inherited condition of a recessive type in which abnormal mucus is secreted. Throughout the body the mucus glands produce

---

[1] McCance, R. A., Morrison, A. B., Dent, C. E. (1955). The excretion of phosphoethanolamine and hypophosphatasia. *Lancet*, 1, 131.

a thick viscid substance which obstructs their ducts, causing dilatation, stasis, infection and subsequent fibrosis. The term mucoviscidosis is sometimes applied instead of the more usual *fibrocystic disease*. The condition occurs probably a little more frequently than cœliac disease.

PATHOLOGY

The extent of the disease varies from case to case since the lesions are progressive. In early cases not all mucus secreting glands in the body are necessarily affected. The pancreas, however, is always involved, and at least minor changes are present in the lungs in all but a few. Greatly dilated ducts containing mucus, surrounded by fibrosis, leaving only the islet cells unaffected, are the characteristic pancreatic changes. In the lungs, the bronchial wall is first damaged in a similar fashion, the subsequent infection producing dilatation of bronchi with surrounding patches of collapse and emphysema in alveolar tissue.

CLINICAL PICTURE

There are three main clinical types of the disease:

Meconium Ileus. Mucus is a normal constituent of meconium. Secretion of viscid mucus due to fibrocystic disease results in meconium becoming solid in consistency along the whole length of the intestine, with resulting ileus and paralytic intestinal obstruction in the first few days of life. Perforation of the intestine may sometimes occur *in utero* giving rise to *meconium peritonitis*. Thin layers of calcification may appear within a short time.

Gastro-intestinal. There is a second type in which chronic diarrhœa or the passage of loose, offensive, pale and bulky stools occurs. Such stools are found by microscopy to contain an excess of fat globules, sometimes with undigested meat fibres and starch granules, because of the lack of digestive enzymes.

These cases usually present between the third and eighteenth month of life. The child, despite the diarrhœa or offensive stools, has a voracious appetite and vomiting is unusual. There is a failure to gain weight; the child becomes wasted and flabby, and often shows an umbilical hernia or a prolapse of the rectum.

Respiratory. Sooner or later respiratory infections occur, progressing to bronchiectasis with widespread collapse and emphysema. Acute or chronic infections, such as pneumonia, are frequent. These symptoms usually present between the sixth month and second year and thus they overlap with the gastro-intestinal symptoms already mentioned.

DIAGNOSIS

Patients with fibrocystic disease produce more concentrated sweat than normal individuals. This observation is utilized in the various tests devised to estimate the concentration of sodium in the sweat. In the fibrocystic child the sodium concentration is usually above 60 mEq/litre; it is below this figure in the normal controls.

The diagnosis is confirmed by duodenal intubation and the demonstration of viscid juice with greatly reduced or absent tryptic properties. This serves to distinguish it from cœliac disease and other wasting syndromes. A word of warning is necessary before the diagnosis is irrevocably accepted on the result of examination of duodenal juice. In infants who have recently undergone severe illnesses, a temporary suppression of pancreatic activity may occur, giving rise to a type of duodenal juice which is temporarily similar to that found in fibrocystic disease. Once the infant has recovered completely from the original illness, the character of the duodenal juice reverts to normal.

PROGNOSIS

Although incurable, the disease can be treated and, in favourable circumstances, a fairly normal existence can be followed, but the prognosis in individual cases depends on the severity of the symptoms and the age at which they appear. Thus, in *meconium ileus* death usually occurs within the first week; when wasting, diarrhœa and pulmonary symptoms appear during infancy, the outlook is bad and it is difficult to prevent recurrent attacks of pneumonia; irreversible bronchiectasis is likely to occur. In other cases, the outlook has been greatly improved by diet, pancreatin and antibiotic treatment.

TREATMENT

Meconium Ileus. Successful attempts have been made at laparotomy to wash out the inspissated meconium from the bowel. Nevertheless, the bad prognosis from the generalized disease remains.

Intestinal and Respiratory Types. For the absent digestive enzymes replacement therapy in the form of pancreatin granules (containing triple-strength pancreatin, B.P.) can be given with meals, 5–15 grammes according to age; with quantities such as this, fat-absorption and nitrogen-retention can be significantly increased. The diet should be as nourishing as possible with a high protein content. Fatty foods should be avoided. It is advisable to give extra vitamins and iron. For the respiratory component, tetracyclines as prophylactics should be started as early as possible, preferably before any respiratory infection has occurred, and continued on a long-term daily basis. Acute infections should be treated intensively with the antibiotic appropriate to the sensitivity of the organism. The diminished vital capacity in these children makes the use of oxygen advisable in all but minor pulmonary infections. Inhalations of three per cent. saline through a humidifier help to liquify the viscid mucus in the respiratory tract.

BIOCHEMICAL DISORDERS NOT OF GENETIC ORIGIN

Idiopathic Renal Acidosis of Infancy[1]

THIS condition was not known until 1935, when the clinical features were described by Lightwood. These features consist of loss of appetite, vomiting, constipation, hypotonia and failure to thrive. The condition is due to a defect in tubular function, namely, inability to conserve sodium bicarbonate causing the paradox of acidæmia (low plasma bicarbonate, 8 to 18 mEq) and the passage of alkaline urine (high urinary bicarbonate). There is usually also a rise in plasma chloride (105 to 120 mEq) which may be compensatory. Pronounced acidosis also causes polyuria and this, together with anorexia and vomiting, is responsible for recurring episodes of dehydration. In this stage death may occur; at autopsy medullary calcification will be found in the kidneys, a result of the metabolic disturbance. Occasionally this nephrocalcinosis is dense enough to show in an x-ray film taken during life.

TREATMENT

The mildest cases undergo spontaneous recovery; others improve in a remarkable manner as soon as the acidæmia is overcome; sodium lactate, sodium bicarbonate and sodium citrate are each effective. At The Hospital for Sick Children, Great Ormond Street, a modification of Albright's solution is used (sodium citrate 100 G.; citric acid 60 G., water 1,000 ml.: 90 to 180 ml. daily, in divided doses with the feeds). The treatment is continued until the appetite is normal and the weight is steadily rising. A watch must be kept on the plasma-chloride and bicarbonate levels. Apart from the risk of intercurrent infection, the ultimate prognosis is excellent; a few weeks or a few months sees the end of the disorder, after which renal function shows no residual abnormality. This, together with the absence of rachitic or osteomalacic changes, marks the condition off from Albright's type of nephrocalcinosis which is also characterized by acidæmia. The latter occurs in older children and adults and has a poor prognosis.

Idiopathic Hypercalcæmia[2]

This is a disorder starting in the first year of life, commonly between three and seven months of age in artificially fed infants. Anorexia, vomiting, failure to gain weight and constipation are the symptoms, and sometimes there is thirst and polyuria as well. Dehydration and spikes of fever may occur. Leucocytes and epithelial cells are found in the urine. Sometimes mild urinary infection accompanies the

[1] Lightwood, R., Payne, W. W., Black, J. (1953). Infantile renal acidosis. *Pediatrics*, **12**, 628.
[2] Lightwood, R. (1952). *Arch. Dis. Childh.*, **27**, 302.

disorder. Recognition turns on finding an increase of calcium and urea in the blood.

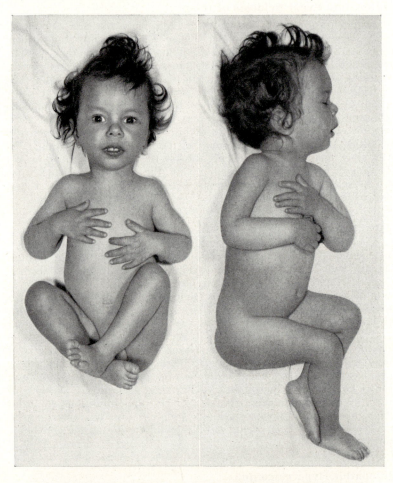

Fig. 8.—Idiopathic hypercalcæmia, a severe type with osteosclerosis. This girl, aged 2 years, had prolonged hypercalcæmia, azotæmia and osteosclerosis. The abnormal facial appearance is well shown in the photographs: prominent forehead, depressed nasal bridge, low-set ears, pouting lips and protruding upper incisor teeth.

ÆTIOLOGY

High intake of vitamin D has been responsible in many of the cases. The calcium content of cows' milk, being about 3–4 times that of human milk (*see* table on p. 38), is another factor, but the varying tolerance of different infants to vitamin D is equally important. At present, almost nothing is known about the mechanism by which unneeded vitamin D is inactivated. In a small proportion of cases the disorder appears to be present from birth; there is a characteristic facies and the heart shows a systolic murmur. Mental retardation may be present.

TREATMENT

Currently, a diet containing little or no calcium and liberal amounts of fluid is recommended. Added vitamin D and administration of alkalis should be avoided until the hypercalcæmia has disappeared. The high level of calcium can also be reduced by cortisone.

PROGNOSIS

Most of the cases are relatively benign, recovery taking place in a few weeks to a few months, but about one-fifth are more severely affected, and there may be permanent damage to the kidneys and physical and mental retardation. Nephrocalcinosis may occur. In the severe cases the bones become osteosclerotic.

Pyridoxine Dependency

A small proportion of infants who develop infantile spasms (p. 456) can be given dramatic relief from their attacks if treated with pyridoxine 5 mg. daily. Such infants clearly require a larger intake of pyridoxine than that needed by the normal child. It is probable that this represents an abnormality of the enzyme system involved in the metabolism of tryptophan, in which system pyridoxine plays an integral part.

Cœliac Disease

This is a condition of intestinal malabsorption of fat, carbohydrate and minerals, perhaps dependent on defective enzymic activities in the mucosal cells of the duodenum and jejunum.

ÆTIOLOGY AND PATHOLOGY

The failure of fat absorption in cœliac disease is related to the presence of wheat and rye flour, and in particular the husk or gluten fraction of the flour, in the diet. Withdrawal of these flours from the diet causes an immediate improvement in the steatorrhœa and the general condition of the patient.

CLINICAL PICTURE

The complaint is usually that the child is failing to thrive and lacks appetite. Without treatment, dwarfing occurs, a child of two or even three years weighing only 15 or 20 lb. and being proportionately small.   The abdomen is large and the rest of the body wasted (Fig. 9).

On palpation of the abdomen, the liver is not usually felt, but fæcal masses may be present.   The buttocks are wasted, and the child resembles one with abdominal tuberculosis.   The Mantoux and tuberculin patch tests, however, are negative.

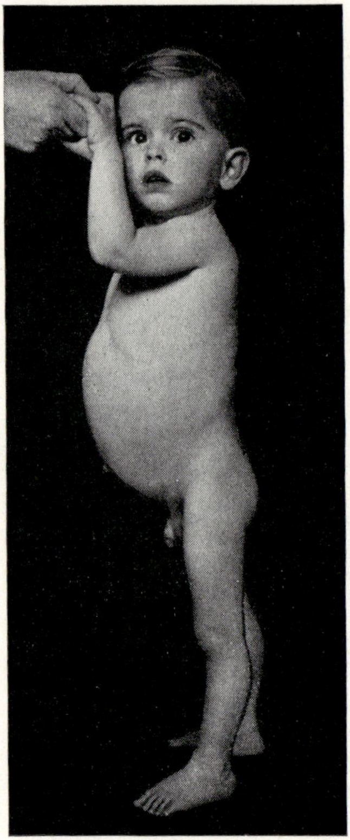

Fig. 9.—Cœliac disease.

Stools.   These are large, pale, offensive, and often putty-coloured; they suggest an excess of fat present as soaps. Bouts of looseness may alternate with constipation.

On a known fat intake, the amount of fat excreted in the stool is measured if possible over a nine-day period.   A normal child will absorb over 90 per cent. of the dietary fat, but in cœliac disease the amount absorbed may be as low as 50–70 per cent.   In infancy the normal figure may be slightly lower. Serial balance studies provide a good index of progress.

The duodenal juice shows normal tryptic activity.

Alimentary Tract.   A barium meal shows an unusual flocculation of barium along the length of the small intestine.

Jejunal biopsy[1] during the active stage of cœliac disease shows a characteristically flattened appearance of the jejunal mucosa, which can be shown to revert, in serial biopsies, to normal, following dietary treatment.

Carbohydrate Metabolism.   The oral glucose tolerance curve is a flat one in cœliac disease.   The child does not absorb carbohydrate properly from the bowel.   This can be demonstrated by the giving of oral glucose, after which the normal rise in the blood sugar level does not occur.   If the glucose is injected intravenously the normal rapid rise occurs.

Vitamin A Absorption Test.   A fasting blood specimen is withdrawn, after which 7,000 i.u. of vitamin A per kilo of body-weight is given orally.   Specimens of blood are then withdrawn 2 hours and 5 hours after the administration.

[1] Shiner, M. (1956).   *Lancet*, 1, 85.
    Crosby, W. H., Kugler, H. W. (1957).   *Amer. J. dig. Dis.*, **2**, 236.
    Cameron, A. H., *et al.* (1962).   *Quart. J. Med.*, **21**, 125.

The vitamin-A content of the blood in a normal child rises to an average maximum of 130 units in three to seven hours; in both cœliac disease and fibrocystic disease of the pancreas, the rise attains a maximum of between 10 and 20 units in a similar time.

Anæmia. In the majority of cases a hypochromic anæmia is found; occasionally macrocytic anæmia, responsive to folic acid, is present.

COURSE AND PROGNOSIS

The present-day treatment of cœliac disease with a gluten-free diet makes for a shorter and less dangerous illness than in the past. Without such treatment a young child with cœliac disease is likely to show chronic malnutrition for many months, with periods of painfully slow improvement interrupted by distressing relapses. Under such circumstances, the mortality rate was about 20–40 per cent. But with a gluten-free diet the symptoms of cœliac disease usually diminish steadily, provided that any conditioned dietary deficiencies (e.g. of iron, calcium or vitamin) are treated concurrently. Premature relaxation of gluten-free diet will result in a return of symptoms together with mal-absorption and steatorrhœa; therefore cœliac disease should not be regarded as cured until the stools are normal on a normal diet. This may take several years to achieve.

TREATMENT

General. In the more active stage and before the disorder is under control, the patient should be nursed in bed. He is usually inactive, miserable and " difficult," especially until his capricious appetite picks up and the stools improve. Possible contributing factors, such as anæmia or a conditioned vitamin deficiency, will need attention. During exacerbations there may be great wasting, and dehydration and collapse may appear; then intravenous fluid and electrolyte therapy may be essential to save life; often a blood transfusion marks the turning point to recovery.

Diet. The essentials in dieting are the exclusion of wheat and rye gluten-containing foods from the diet, together with a liberal allowance of protein. In severe cases, it is necessary to commence with just a milk diet (*see* below). As the child improves, a gluten-free diet may be introduced.

Where relapses occur, due to intolerance of some portion of the diet or more probably to parenteral infections, such as nasopharyngitis, it may be necessary to return to a milk diet temporarily.

Initial Milk Diet

Skimmed milk (such as separated Cow and Gate or skimmed Trufood) 6–8 ounces every four hours (five feeds in all).

Fruit juices *ad lib.*, diluted and sweetened as necessary.

Gluten-free Diet

As soon as possible the child is established on the wheat and rye gluten-free diet described in Appendix 6.

Vitamins.   The fat-soluble vitamins are not absorbed satisfactorily, and vitamins A and D should be given in concentrated form and in higher dosage than usual.   Abedec, being water-soluble, is suitable.

Anæmia.   As the majority of cases show a hypochromic anæmia, iron should be given in the form of ferrous sulphate, 90 mg. twice daily to a two-year-old.   In severe cases, however, a fresh blood transfusion has a most beneficial effect upon the general condition as well as upon the anæmia.   Folic acid is used for the rare cases with macrocytic anæmia, with dramatic effect.

FOLLOW-UP

A continuous record of the height and weight is an important part of the long-term supervision, together with a check on the hæmoglobin level.

Lack of satisfactory progress usually indicates a failure to keep to the diet.

CHAPTER 11

Endocrine Diseases

ENDOCRINE disorders in childhood give rise to complexities which, because of their interference with active skeletal, gonadal and general physical growth, are additional to those seen in adults. Premature or delayed closure of epiphyses, with subsequent alterations in final stature, also have their effect. Thus, the endocrine lesions occurring in children and in adults produce in both varying clinical pictures. For a more detailed account of the endocrinology of childhood than can be given in this chapter the reader is referred to the classic text-book of Lawson Wilkins.[1]

PITUITARY DISORDERS

PITUITARY disorders have to be considered in relation to lesions of the anterior pituitary lobe, posterior lobe and hypothalamic areas, and as combined lesions. Secondary effects may occur from adrenal, thyroid and gonadal changes, as a result of the primary pituitary disorder, and vice versa. For this reason, a general description will be given of disorders, such as gigantism, obesity, dwarfism, and infantilism, which result partly from secondary endocrine disturbances in addition to strictly pituitary disorders. Most commonly, pituitary disease is due to hypofunction of the whole or part of the gland, with failure to secrete pituitary hormones, but occasionally hyperfunction occurs, as in the acidophil tumour of the anterior lobe (giving rise to gigantism in childhood and acromegaly in adults) and the basophil tumour of the anterior lobe (producing Cushing's syndrome).

A brief summary of normal pituitary activities[2] is provided in the following table:

HORMONES PRODUCED BY THE ANTERIOR PITUITARY LOBE

Growth hormone	Direct action on tissues (may occasionally have a diabetogenic effect when secreted in excess).
Adrenocorticotrophic (ACTH)	Stimulates growth of adrenal cortex and production of its hormones.
Thyrotrophic (TSH)	Stimulates growth of thyroid gland and production of thyroxin.

[1] Wilkins, Lawson (1957). " The Diagnosis and Treatment of Endocrine Disorders in Childhood and Adolescence." Springfield, Illinois: Thomas.
[2] Mason, A. S. (1961). " Introduction to Clinical Endocrinology." Oxford: Blackwell Scientific Publications.

Gonadotrophins
   Follicle Stimulating   ⎫
      hormone (FSH)   ⎬   Stimulates growth of gonads,
   Luteinizing hormone ⎭   their hormone production and
      (LH)   reproductive processes.

Luteotrophin   Stimulates lactation.
   (Prolactin)

HORMONES PRODUCED BY THE POSTERIOR PITUITARY AND
ITS NEURAL CONNECTIONS

Oxytocin   Stimulates uterine contraction.
Vasopressin   Inhibits water diuresis.
(Anti-diuretic hormone ADH) To a lesser extent stimulates vaso-
                             constriction.

The hypothalamus and posterior pituitary also exert a regulatory influence on the control of sleep, appetite, body temperature, carbohydrate balance, and, to some extent, sexual function.

Gigantism

This is a rare condition in childhood, although it may be seen more commonly in adults as acromegaly. Hypersecretion of growth hormone by the anterior lobe of the pituitary gland causes an excessive growth of the bony skeleton and the viscera. Such over-action of the anterior portion of the pituitary may be the result of an adenomatous growth of the acidophil cells. An x-ray of the pituitary fossa may show an enlargement and help to establish the diagnosis.

Thus, for true pathological gigantism, an excessive activity of the anterior-lobe eosinophil cells of the pituitary during the active growth period is necessary. Gigantism may be classified as (1) the simple hereditary type, and (2) the endocrine group. In the hereditary type, this undue stimulus appears to run in families. The endocrine group may be subdivided further into (*a*) hyperpituitary gigantism, due to excessive secretion of growth hormone, in which general overgrowth is the characteristic feature, though, in some instances, localized overgrowth in the form of acromegalic changes may be in evidence too; (*b*) hypogonadal (decrease of sex-gland activity) gigantism, where the particular factor favouring overgrowth is the markedly delayed closure of the epiphyses. In these individuals, the growth curve in adolescence is prolonged beyond the normal and often far into adult life. It must be stressed that this variety is exceptional; more often, growth hormone is also deficient.

Adiposity

The exact part played by the hypothalamus and pituitary gland in the ætiology of all types of adiposity is often difficult to evaluate. Whilst a few types of obesity may be definitely ascribed to reduced hypothalamic or pituitary function, in the majority, other factors are more often predominant. Genetic inheritance clearly plays a part in many cases, whilst other endocrine diseases, such as a tumour of the suprarenal cortex, hypothyroidism and hypogonadism are less frequent causes. How far these conditions produce adiposity by secondarily affecting pituitary function is not yet decided. It must be admitted also that when all possible influences, such as overeating and excessive carbohydrate intake, have been taken into account, there remains a group of obese children in whom the cause is quite unknown (*see also* p. 69).

As a general guide, it is useful to recall that obesity associated with a height above average is seldom due to serious endocrine disturbance. In such tall and obese children, constitutional and genetic influences predominate in the ætiology. On the other hand, obesity in children of unusually short stature should be regarded with considerable caution, since it is likely that hypothalamic and pituitary function may be depressed. This may be due to a pituitary or parapituitary tumour, to encephalitis, cerebral birth injury, or congenital malformation. Such cases of hypopituitarism may also show secondary depression of thyroid activity due to the diminished output of thyrotrophic hormone (p. 154). Obesity associated with short stature is also seen in Turner's syndrome (p. 163) and in pseudohypoparathyroidism (p. 158).

The part played by pituitary dysfunction is therefore complex. In addition to the variations already described, the following eponymous forms of pituitary obesity are also recognized:

FRÖHLICH'S SYNDROME

In 1901, Alfred Fröhlich described a boy of fourteen, with marked obesity and hypogonadism, who was found to have a craniopharyngioma. Since that description was written, much confusion has arisen as to what is meant by the term "Fröhlich's syndrome." To avoid any confusion with other forms of obesity, the name should be applied only to children with obesity and hypogonadism due to hypothalamic or pituitary disease. Dwarfism and diabetes insipidus (*see* p. 151) are features of the syndrome which may be present but are not essential to the diagnosis.

If these criteria are followed, the syndrome is found to be a rarity. Intrasellar and suprasellar tumours, such as chromophobe adenoma or craniopharyngioma, third ventricle tumours, internal hydrocephalus, or encephalitis, have all been found as causative factors. Focal neurological signs and evidence of raised intracranial pressure may be present as results of a tumour.

LAURENCE-MOON-BIEDL SYNDROME

This syndrome includes obesity and hypogonadism, but in addition polydactylism, *retinitis pigmentosa* and mental deficiency are also present. It is genetically determined by recessive inheritance.

6

CUSHING'S SYNDROME[1]

Cushing's syndrome is not common in children. As in adults, the underlying lesion may be an adrenal cortical tumour (adenoma or carcinoma), a basophil tumour of the anterior pituitary, either adenomatous or carcinomatous, a thymus carcinoma, or an ovarian arrhenoblastoma. Whichever of these tumours is present, the diagnostic pathological lesion of Cushing's syndrome—namely, degranulization and hyalinization of the basophil cells of the anterior pituitary—is present. In all cases, hyperfunction of the suprarenal cortex also occurs.

Clinically, the findings may be summarized as including adiposity, plethora, hirsutes, hypogonadism, hypertension, polycythæmia, hyperglycæmia and glycosuria, rarefaction of bone, particularly in the vertebral column, and marked lassitude. Purple *liniæ distensæ* may be very marked on the thighs, hips and breast regions. In the urine there is an abnormal output of 17-ketosteroids and of 11-oxysteroids.

Dwarfism

By dwarfism is meant a failure of skeletal growth with no alteration in sexual growth and maturity. If hypogonadism subsequently persists beyond puberty in association with dwarfism, the term infantilism is applied. Pure dwarfism as opposed to infantilism is rarely of endocrine origin, but a brief description of the common causes will be given. Dwarfism may be associated with *a low birth weight* despite a full gestational period.[2] Several varieties of *low birth weight dwarfs* are described, including a bird-headed type with a beaky nose, receding chin and often subnormal intelligence; other varieties of low birth weight dwarfs include a dominantly inherited type, with normal intelligence, and a recessive variety, often with low intelligence; a further type shows assymetry between the two sides of the body; finally a marked disparity between the birth weight of twins may sometimes persist, the smaller twin remaining stunted in growth and sometimes intellectually retarded.

Inherited skeletal diseases, such as *achondroplasia*, *dyschondroplasia* and *osteogenesis imperfecta*, give rise to gross stunting of stature. *Acquired skeletal disease*, such as the various forms of *rickets*, and spinal diseases, including *spinal caries* giving rise to spinal deformity, are important causes.

Metabolic disorders, including cœliac disease, fibrocystic disease, ulcerative colitis, Crohn's disease, glycogen disease and chronic renal disease, have all been found to cause stunting of growth. Certain of the more severe forms of *congenital heart disease* also give rise to growth impairment. In the past, *chronic infections*, such as tuberculosis and congenital syphilis, were causative factors.

[1] Wilkins, Lawson (1962). *Arch. Dis. Childh.*, **37**, 1.
[2] Black, J. (1961). *Ibid.*, **36**, 633.

Endocrine causes of dwarfism include *precocious puberty* (*see* p. 161), which, although at first associated with rapid growth, subsequently gives rise to premature closure of epiphyses preventing any further increase in stature.

Cretinism (*see* p. 153), if not treated early, may lead to permanent stunting of growth. True *pituitary dwarfism* is an uncommon condition which should be diagnosed only when clear evidence of pituitary disease or dysfunction can be demonstrated.

PITUITARY DWARFISM

This rare disorder may be due to a pituitary or parapituitary tumour such as a craniopharyngioma, to compression from internal hydrocephalus, or to brain damage or encephalitis. Finally, there remains the type that results from a primary failure of pituitary function. Infantilism will occur when, as a result of one of these processes, a failure of growth hormone production is subsequently combined with a failure of sex hormone production at the time of puberty. Signs and symptoms of a pituitary or parapituitary tumour may be present and must be looked for in all cases (p. 452). In the prepuberal period, the only endocrine deficiency associated with hypopituitary infantilism may be a mild degree of hypothyroidism, which can be confirmed or excluded by special tests (p. 155).

Idiopathic Dwarfism. Where all possible factors have been examined, both endocrine and general, there remains a group of small children who are perfectly proportioned and healthy in every respect.

TREATMENT

The underlying cause of the dwarfism should be treated whenever possible. Recent work[1] on human growth hormone, although not yet fully available for general clinical practice, is encouraging. At present, such nitrogen-retaining hormones as 1-dehydro-methyltestosterone appear to offer some limited value in stimulating growth. Treatment with sex hormones (p. 164) is an essential factor after the normal age of puberty. They should not be used indiscriminately but only in such cases of hypogonadism in which all hope of naturally occurring growth has ceased. If given prematurely, large doses of androgenic hormones may inhibit the secretion of intrinsic hormones and can certainly cause premature closure of epiphyses, thus removing the possibility of any further natural growth that might have occurred. Where investigation has shown that there is associated hypothyroid function (p. 156), replacement therapy with L-thyroxine sodium should also be given.

Diabetes Insipidus

In normal health about ninety-nine per cent. of the water filtered by the renal glomeruli is reabsorbed by the renal tubule, only one per

[1] Medical Research Council (1959). *Lancet*, 1, 7.
Leading article (1963). *Brit. med. J.*, 1, 1035.

cent. remaining to be excreted as urine. Failure of active re-absorption results in the syndrome of diabetes insipidus with its principal symptoms of polyuria and polydipsia. In infants, severe dehydration may develop.

Renal tubular re-absorption of water is regulated by an anti-diuretic hormone (vasopressin) elaborated by the posterior pituitary and its connected neural pathways. Damage to any part of this system by a brain tumour, encephalitis, or brain injury may lead to failure of formation of antidiuretic hormone and hence to diabetes insipidus.

In addition, genetic forms of diabetes insipidus are found which fall into two entirely separate groups. The first group consists of patients whose symptoms respond to replacement therapy with vasopressin (*vasopressin-sensitive diabetes insipidus*). Such patients, whose disorder is usually inherited as a dominant or occasionally sex-linked charac-teristic, have presumably an innate inability to form adequate amounts of antidiuretic hormone.

The second group of patients fails to respond to treatment with vasopressin and appears to have an inherited dysfunction of the renal tubules which interferes with the re-absorption of water (*vaso-pressin-insensitive or nephrogenic diabetes insipidus*). Such a disorder is inherited as a sex-linked characteristic and is confined to the male sex.

CLINICAL PICTURE

The child remains small and stunted. There is great thirst, and much urine is passed. Many pints of fluid may be drunk and passed each day. The urine is pale and of low specific gravity but other-wise normal.

TREATMENT

Replacement therapy with posterior pituitary extract is effective treatment, except for patients with the nephrogenic type of diabetes insipidus. The maintenance dose varies in individual cases but is usually of the order of vasopressin tannate (5 units), 1·0 ml. in oily solution, daily. Some patients prefer to take vasopressin powder in the form of snuff.

Progeria

This is an extremely rare condition in which the child, at or shortly after birth, has the appearance of senility, and may be carried off by intercurrent disease. The condition was named by Hastings Gilford. The child is small, hairless, wrinkled, and has the appear-ance of an elderly person. The intellect may be impaired. No specific endocrine changes can be made out and the condition seems to be one of premature ageing of the tissues.

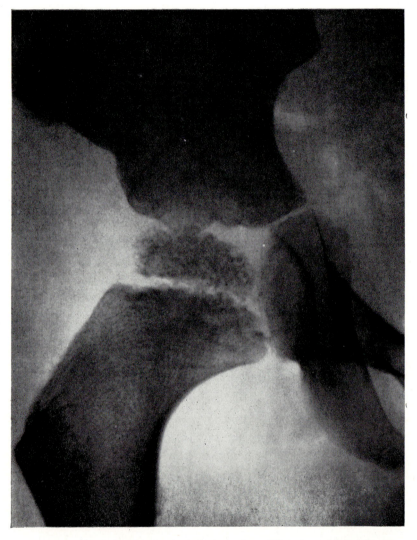

PLATE II.   Epiphyseal dysplasia in hypothyroidism in a child of 8 years
who had not received treatment.

Simmonds's Disease (Panhypopituitarism)

This disease is spoken of more in relation to the failure of pituitary function in adult life than in childhood. In the younger patients, there is deficient secretion of all anterior pituitary hormones with consequent poor growth, failure of closure of epiphyseal centres and absence of secondary sexual characteristics. Evidence of hypothyroidism and subnormal adrenal cortical function (p. 159) is often also present. The cause is usually a septic embolus cutting off the blood supply to the anterior pituitary. It is rare in childhood. Treatment consists of the combined use of thyroid, cortisone and androgens, such as 1-dehydro-methyltestosterone, in an attempt to provide replacement for the deficient endocrine secretions.

THYROID DISORDERS

Hypothyroidism

THIS condition may be present from birth or acquired at some later date; in the former case it is termed cretinism and in the latter myxœdema. Diagnosis is possible at the age of a few weeks. The sex distribution is equal. The great majority of cretins show a relative reduction or complete absence of thyroid tissue. Usually, there is no familial history, and no cause, except that it is a congenital malformation, can be offered. There may be a history of prolonged neonatal jaundice.

Hutchison[1] has described the rare occurrence of familial goitrous cretinism and found it to be a recessively inherited condition in a family of itinerant tinkers (see p. 157).

CLINICAL PICTURE

The cretin is pale and has a yellow-tinged, rough, dry skin. The hair is straight, dry and sparse; the cry is hoarse and low-pitched; the tongue is greatly enlarged and protrudes from the mouth continuously, because it is actually too large for the mouth to contain (Fig. 10). The child is slow in all his movements, the smile comes and goes slowly, and the mentality is greatly retarded. He is very backward in learning to raise his head and sit up and, if untreated, it may be several years before he can walk. He is inclined to make snorting noises with his nose. The temperature is subnormal, the hands and feet being cold, and the pulse slow. He is chronically constipated. The growth of the skeleton is slow, and he is dwarfed in size. An x-ray of the wrist will show marked delay in the appearance of the centres of ossification (see Appendix 5). Dysgenesis of the epiphyses of the humerus, femur and tibia is of diagnostic importance, the epiphysis being formed by multiple foci of calcification. The teeth are late in appearing and, when they do appear, tend to be carious. The thyroid gland cannot be felt, but it is seldom that cretinism is

[1] McGirr, E. M., Hutchison, J. H., Clement, W. E. (1959). *Lancet*, 2, 823.

accompanied by other evidence of congenital malformation, except occasionally congenital dislocation of the hips. The abdomen is large, and a well-marked umbilical hernia develops.

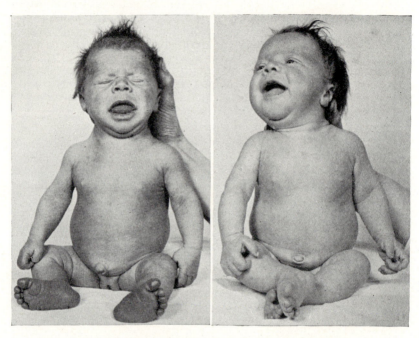

Fig. 10.—A typical cretin, aged 8 weeks, with an umbilical hernia. *Left:* **Before treatment,** *Right:* **Four weeks later—the umbilical hernia is much smaller.**

An excess of fat accumulates in the subcutaneous tissues, especially about the shoulders (supraclavicular pads), just as in the hibernating bear; fat is also laid down in many other parts of the body, such as the tongue and the subcutaneous tissues.

DIAGNOSIS

Simple laboratory investigations are not of great help in early diagnosis, the specific changes from the normal being found only in those cases in which the diagnosis is already obvious on clinical grounds. In such cases, the blood cholesterol is found to be raised to 250–300 mg. per 100 ml. or higher, and the ECG reveals a low-voltage tracing.

In the clinically less obvious cases, such as those in which a component of hypothyroidism is associated with hypopituitarism or in other patients with only minimal features of hypothyroidism, more specialized investigations may be indicated.

Protein-bound Iodine. The amount of protein-bound iodine in the plasma reflects the functional efficiency of the thyroid gland. The level is greatly raised in hyperthyroidism and is reduced below normal in hypothyroid states. Unfortunately, its determination is extremely difficult and prone to error. It is therefore not used in routine laboratory practice, although undertaken in a few special centres. The normal range of protein-bound iodine in the plasma is 3·5–8·0 microgrammes per 100 ml., but may be raised as high as 25 microgrammes per 100 ml. in hyperthyroidism or reduced almost to zero in hypothyroidism.

Thyroid-stimulating Hormone. The principal controlling factor of thyroid function is the thyrotrophic hormone (TSH) secreted by the anterior pituitary. Whilst most cases of cretinism are the result of a congenital absence of thyroid gland substance itself, there are some patients in whom hypothyroidism is a secondary result of a primary pituitary failure and inadequate output of TSH. In such cases there are likely to be other evidences of hypopituitarism (p. 151) in addition to hypothyroidism. By contrast, patients with familial goitrous cretinism (p. 157), in whom there is an enzymic failure of thyroxine production within the thyroid gland itself, show a TSH level greatly above normal which accounts in turn for the goitrous condition. The biological estimation of TSH is a complex technique and is not available in routine laboratory practice. The measurement of protein-bound iodine before and after the administration of a test dose of TSH will indicate whether the endogenous output of TSH is adequate or whether a degree of hypopituitarism is present.

Radioactive-iodine Uptake. The use of iodine[131] to measure the extent to which the thyroid gland takes up iodine may be a useful examination where the diagnosis is in doubt. In normal health, between 20–50 per cent. of an orally administered dose of iodine[131] taken up by the thyroid in twenty-four hours. Values above and below these limits are indications of hyperthyroidism and hypothyroidism respectively.

There is a natural reluctance to use radioactive substances in the investigation of small infants, even in the very small doses necessary for this diagnostic test, and it is the usual practice to employ such techniques only where the diagnosis is in doubt.

PROGNOSIS

In cretinism, this is a matter of great difficulty, as it depends largely on how early and how efficiently the child is treated. There are, however, a few cases in which there is mental deficiency despite very early treatment. Where cretins are treated late and inefficiently, they tend to lag some distance behind the normal child, failing to catch up or reach normal intelligence. A good proportion, taken in hand early and properly treated, become completely normal.

TREATMENT

Treatment must be started immediately the diagnosis is made and must be continued for the rest of the patient's life. L-thyroxine sodium is the preparation of choice, and, for an infant a few months old, the dose should be 0·05 mg. daily. This is slowly increased, week by week, until the greatest dose is reached which the infant can tolerate without diarrhœa and without undue loss of weight. The dose varies with the age of the child and with the individual patient. A child of one year may tolerate 0·1–0·15 mg. daily and a child of five years 0·1–0·3 mg., but there is a big variation. The signs of recovery are that the constipation ceases, the cold hands become warm, the dry hair soft and even curly, the increased subcutaneous tissue disappears, the skin is soft and loses its yellow tinge, becoming pink and white. The rate of the heart's action should be normal for the child's age. The voice ceases to be hoarse and is clear and infantile. The tongue is small and does not protrude from the mouth, the mentality is quickened, and the baby smiles and obviously appreciates his surroundings (Fig. 10).

When too much thyroxine is being administered there is a tendency to tachycardia, looseness of the bowels, undue loss of weight and an elevated temperature. The child is nervous and fearful, and there are attacks of palpitation, with sudden fainting fits probably accompanying the palpitation. In infancy, diarrhœa is the earliest and most important sign that the dosage of the drug is excessive.

After the administration of thyroxine there is rapid mental and physical development and a greatly increased growth of the bones, which brings in its train the danger of rickets. It is essential, then, that the diet should be carefully investigated and adjusted, and that cod-liver oil should be administered at all times along with the thyroxine.

Once the diagnosis of cretinism has been made, it must be stressed to the parents that replacement therapy with thyroxine will be necessary for the rest of the patient's life and that under no circumstances should it be stopped. It is a wise precaution to provide the parents with a photograph of their child in the untreated state which they can show to any doctor who may at a later date suggest stopping the treatment.

JUVENILE MYXŒDEMA

Except for the later onset this resembles cretinism but it is more rare.

Occasionally, an infant is born normal and in the first few years of life has some acute illness or local inflammation in the region of the thyroid which is followed by the development of typical myxœdema. Such cases react rapidly to treatment.

Goitre

PUBERAL GOITRE

It is common at puberty, especially in girls, to find some enlargement of the thyroid gland but without signs of hyperthyroidism. At the onset of each menstrual period, the neck enlarges, and the child tends to be emotionally unstable and to flush unduly easily. No treatment is necessary, and with the establishment of puberty the condition seems to right itself.

ENDEMIC GOITRE (DERBYSHIRE NECK)

This is an extremely rare condition in the British Isles, although cases have been reported, especially from Derbyshire, Somerset and Gloucestershire. It is said that a deficiency of iodine in the soil and water is the causative factor. Iodized salt used with food prevents the disease.

In such cases, the thyroid may occasionally undergo cystic changes, and in a proportion of these the child may show signs of L-thyroxine insufficiency.

GOITROUS CRETINISM

Rare metabolic errors impede thyroid function; one type has a recessively inherited deficiency of dehalogenase, an enzyme essential for the formation of thyroxine. A large goitre may develop, due to the stimulus of thyrotropic hormone. Replacement treatment with thyroxine is required and the goitre may require surgery.

THYROTOXICOSIS (GRAVES'S DISEASE, EXOPHTHALMIC GOITRE, HYPERTHYROIDISM)

This is not very common in childhood, but as puberty approaches it becomes more frequent. Females are affected at least twice as often as males. Infants are rarely affected.

The ætiology is not known, but in a proportion of cases the condition appears to be hereditary.

The clinical picture is similar to that seen in adults, namely, flushing, tachycardia, sweating, tremor, extreme nervousness and exophthalmos. The appetite may be large, and there is a loss of weight.

In older children, the treatment is similar to that for adult thyrotoxicosis; in general, surgical treatment is to be avoided initially and an attempt made to stabilize the patient with carbimazole or methyl thiouracil. Only if an adequate trial of medical treatment is unsuccessful, or if pressure symptoms threaten, is surgery to be contemplated in childhood. In the post-puberty hyperthyroidism of adolescent girls, nothing short of surgery is likely to be effective.

DISEASES OF THE PARATHYROID GLAND

Hypoparathyroidism

IDIOPATHIC hypoparathyroidism is a rare disease in childhood. There is a fall in the blood calcium level to as low as 4–6 mg. per 100 ml., with a slight rise in blood phosphorus to 5–10 mg. per 100 ml. The outstanding symptom is tetany, which may in severe cases progress to epileptiform convulsions. Cataracts may occasionally develop. Treatment with high doses of calciferol (50,000–100,000 units daily) may be required to restore the calcium to a normal level; such treatment may have to be continued for life. Symptoms of hypervitaminosis D (*see* p. 122) must be carefully watched for.

Pseudohypoparathyroidism

In this condition, there are symptoms additional to those already described in idiopathic hypoparathyroidism. These may include stunting of growth with adiposity, thickening of the bones of the cranial vault, shortening of the metacarpal bones, soft tissue calcification, and mental backwardness. In the opinion of Dr. Albright, the disorder is due to several genetic defects occurring simultaneously.

Hyperparathyroidism

Parathyroid tumours giving rise to hyperparathyroidism are occasionally encountered in childhood. Decalcification of the skeleton occurs, with the development of multiple areas of osteitis fibrosa, often with cyst formation. The blood calcium is raised to 15–20 mg. per 100 ml., with an increase in the alkaline phosphatase level, and a fall in blood phosphorus to 1–2 mg. per 100 ml.

Removal of the tumour cures the condition, but tetany may develop (*see* above), which requires treatment with high dosage of calciferol.

DISEASES OF THE ADRENAL CORTEX

A DESCRIPTION of the normal function of the adrenal cortex is given in Appendix 2.

Hyperfunction of the adrenal cortex is responsible for the following small but important group of diseases in childhood.

1. Adrenogenital syndrome (p. 159).
2. Cushing's syndrome (p. 150).
3. Hypercorticalism from neoplasm (p. 160).

The adrenogenital syndrome is caused by a recessively inherited inborn error of metabolism which interferes with the formation of hydrocortisone.

In Cushing's syndrome, there may be hyperplastic or carcinomatous changes in the adrenal cortex in association with degranulization and hyalinization of the basophil cells of the anterior pituitary. In hypercorticalism alone, either hyperplastic or carcinomatous changes occur in the gland but without secondary effects in the pituitary. The cause is unknown.

Hypofunction of the suprarenal cortex may occur as an acute or chronic condition. The acute form is seen as a hæmorrhage into the suprarenal cortex, occurring in such a condition as meningococcal septicæmia and giving rise to the Waterhouse-Friderichsen syndrome (*see* p. 403). Chronic hypofunction, due to tuberculosis or atrophy of the adrenal cortex, is extremely rare in childhood.

The Adrenogenital Syndrome

Whilst dysfunction of the suprarenal cortex may occur as a result of simple hyperplasia, or adenomatous or carcinomatous change, it is now recognized that the majority of cases in childhood and particularly in infancy are due to a recessively inherited enzyme deficiency. The absence of this enzyme results in a failure of hydroxylation in the final stage of hydrocortisone production. Thus the precursor, hydroxy-progesterone, accumulates in excessive amounts and its breakdown product, pregnanetriol, is excreted in excess in the urine. The low level of hydrocortisone production stimulates increased ACTH secretion from the pituitary, and this in turn gives rise to hyperplasia and hyperfunction of other areas of the suprarenal cortex and, in particular, androgen formation, associated with an abnormally high urinary excretion of 17-ketosteroids.

As this process can occur in fœtal life, females may by the time of birth already show evidence of pseudo-hermaphroditism as a result of the excessive androgen production. In the male, enlargement of the genitalia is not usually obvious at birth, but develops later.

In the female there is marked enlargement of the clitoris and labia majora. At birth the appearance may be mistaken for a penis and bifid scrotum, the urethral opening at the base of the clitoris being confused with hypospadias. In other cases, the changes only become noticed during childhood with increasing enlargement of the clitoris and a general configuration more reminiscent of a boy than a girl.

Other evidence of excess androgen formation is soon evident; growth is excessively rapid, the bone age is far in advance of the chronological age, muscular development is very marked, and pubic hair appears at an early age. At the time of puberty, secondary female characteristics do not develop; indeed, the voice may deepen and hirsutes appear on the body.

Careful examination of the external genitals together, when possible, with injection of Urografin into the small vaginal orifice to obtain contrast radiography of the uterus and Fallopian tubes should confirm the diagnosis. Occasionally laparotomy may be necessary, but it must be appreciated that these children may suffer, in addition to the excess of androgen secretion, from a subnormal secretion of hydro-cortisone, and thus laparotomy may precipitate an Addisonian crisis.

Hypoadrenalism may also occur spontaneously or from infection.

In young infants, in whom pseudo-hermaphroditism in the female or excessive virilism in the male has not been noted, *adrenal insufficiency* may cause great difficulty in diagnosis. The infant refuses feeds and appears limp and apathetic. Vomiting occurs. A mistaken diagnosis of pyloric stenosis may be made. The infant fails to gain weight and may suffer from intermittent diarrhœa. Pigmentation may develop particularly around the genitalia. Occasionally acute crises may occur with collapse, pallor, sweating and even convulsions.

Electrolyte examination shows the characteristic changes of a high level of serum potassium and reduction of the normal sodium and chloride levels. The urinary excess of 17-ketosteroids and pregnanetriol has already been mentioned.

TREATMENT

In females, this depends to a large extent upon the age of the child when first seen. If seen in the first months of life, attempts should be made to restore feminine characteristics. The older treatment of partial adrenalectomy, combined with a plastic operation upon the external genitals, was unsatisfactory. In recent years, treatment with cortisone has been found to suppress the excessive androgen production, with consequent reduction in virilism and hirsutism, and a return to female characteristics. In this way also the symptoms of adrenal insufficiency are corrected. Life-long replacement therapy is essential and in those patients who show *adrenal insufficiency* (*salt losers*) must include the administration of extra salt as well as steroids.

If the child is seen after the age of one year, considerable care has to be exercised before any treatment is undertaken. In cases in which a female child has been brought up as a male, the psychological consequences of attempting to restore her to her proper sex may be disastrous, suicide being not uncommon in such circumstances.

In male children, just sufficient cortisone should be given to suppress the abnormal virilization and to permit the normal masculinization to occur.

Female Hypercorticalism in Postnatal Life

Postnatal hypercorticalism is usually due to the development of a neoplasm, either adenomatous or carcinomatous. Sexual precocity is the outstanding feature, but other additional signs, such as hirsutes, an advanced bone age and excessive growth, may suggest an adrenal tumour. The differential diagnosis between the different forms of sexual precocity, and their treatment are discussed on p. 161.

Male Hypercorticalism

In the male, hyperfunction of the adrenal cortex can produce two entirely different clinical pictures:

(1) Both cortical hyperplasia and neoplasm are likely to cause virilism. Thus, even in infancy, there may be marked enlargement of

the penis and scrotum together with the appearance of hirsutes. Growth may be excessive at first but terminates prematurely, owing to early closure of the epiphyses. Muscular development is remarkable, giving rise to the term "infant Hercules." Despite the enlargement of penis and scrotum, the testes do not progress to adult size and spermatogenesis does not occur. Although an adrenal carcinoma is an uncommon cause, it should be excluded by a pituitary suppression test, using prednisone or cortisone. Carcinomatous origin can also be differentiated from simple hyperplasia by the excessively high levels of 17-ketosteroids in the urine which may rise to 200 mg. per 24 hour specimen. With carcinoma, the outlook is grave.

(2) In extremely rare instances an excess of œstrogens is secreted, and femininization occurs. Such changes only develop in males in whom puberty has already occurred.

Cushing's Syndrome. (*See* p. 150.)

Phæochromocytoma

This adrenaline-secreting tumour of the suprarenal medulla is a great rarity, causing hypertension in the affected subjects. It usually occurs in adults.

GONADS

Precocious Puberty

THIS condition is far commoner (in the proportion of about 3:1) in girls than in boys. The cases may be divided into two groups, namely, true precocious puberty, in which spermatogenesis or ovulation takes place, and those with advanced secondary sex changes but in which true sexual maturity does not occur, the latter sometimes being called pseudo-precocious puberty.

TRUE PRECOCIOUS PUBERTY

In this group, in which true sexual maturity is reached at an unusually early age, are found about two-thirds of all the cases. The single commonest type has been called *constitutional precocious puberty*. These children show no abnormality whatever apart from an early onset of puberty, and there is often a history of early onset of the menarche in the mother. Since they are in all other respects healthy children, the avoidance of secondary psychological upset due to their preco-

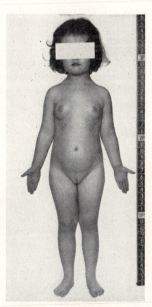

Fig. 11.—A child of 3½ years old. Precocious puberty due to a neoplasm in the region of the hypothalamus.

cious development is the only important aspect of their management. These cases are almost entirely female. As well as starting at an early date, menstruation continues beyond the usual age of the menopause.

Other causes of true precocious puberty are rare. They may be due to the effect of a cerebral tumour, or a meningitis, involving the hypothalamus and leaving the pituitary gland intact.

Treatment. Because these children find themselves different from other children, secondary psychological upset requires careful handling. Boarding school is to be avoided. It must be remembered that they are capable of conception, a pregnancy having been recorded in such a child at the age of five years.

PSEUDO-PRECOCIOUS PUBERTY

In this group, despite the development of secondary sex characteristics and growth of the penis or clitoris, no spermatogenesis or ovulation occurs. It is to be noted, moreover, that the testes remain of pre-puberal size.

Hyperplasia or neoplasm of the adrenal has already been mentioned as an important cause (*see* p. 160). Other rarer causes are granulosa-cell tumour of the ovary, and interstitial-cell tumour of the testis.

A greatly raised urinary excretion of 17-ketosteroids is suggestive of an adrenal tumour, and its site may be located by peri-renal insufflation of air together with a lumbar aortogram or by intravenous pyelogram. The rare granulosa-cell tumours of the ovary are almost always palpable on bimanual examination.

Where laparotomy is being undertaken to confirm the presence of a tumour, or to excise a known tumour, the dangers of adreno-cortical insufficiency, which may be associated, must be allowed for and prevented by treatment with systemic hydrocortisone acetate (*see* Appendix 2).

Undescended Testes

In most mature infants, the testes have already descended into the scrotum at the time of birth. Sometimes, however, they are retained in the abdomen (*cryptorchidism*) or in the inguinal canal; while a testicle lies in its normal course of descent but keeps above the scrotum it is called a *retained testis*. A retained testis is almost certain to reach the scrotum spontaneously some time before puberty and, therefore, no treatment is required, either operative or hormonal.

Often retained testicles are visible in the inguinal canal and it is possible to manipulate them into the scrotum, only for them to retract again from a cutaneous stimulus. Such testes are called *retractile*. But since they can remain out of sight in the inguinal canal, a careful examination is required before the doctor pronounces that they are undescended, and this diagnosis should never be given if the testes can be pushed into the scrotum with the boy either standing or lying. The trick is to force the testis down with one hand from above while catching it from below with the other.

Sometimes a testis in its course of descent misses its way for anatomical reasons and reaches an abnormal position. It is then described as *ectopic*. Often inguinal hernia is present as well, and both conditions require operation. Hormonal treatment cannot correct a mechanical displacement.

TREATMENT AND RESULTS

Orchidopexy is advised at about eight years of age, and is usually an anatomical success, but functional results need to be considered. If the testis is intra-abdominal until adolescence, fertility may be normal in vases of unilateral cryptorchidism, but this depends on the other testis because there is no spermatogenesis in the retained testis; if both testes are retained until adolescence, sterility is the rule. Even if operation is undertaken before puberty in bilateral cases, there is likely to be either sterility or subfertility. Nevertheless, operation in cryptorchidism is to be advised because without it there is an increased risk of malignant disease of the testis, the neoplasm being usually very deadly, and a retained testis is liable to torsion. It is also important for psychological reasons that the patient should have the testes brought down into the scrotum. The value of endocrine treatment, using pregnyl or testosterone, has not been established and this treatment is now seldom used. It has, too, some disadvantages; testosterone accelerates epiphyseal union, and there is perhaps also a risk of permanent damage to the testes, even when the hormone is given before puberty. Moreover, there are obvious objections to anticipating the changes of puberty before the normal age.

Female Hypogonadism

A primary form of hypogonadism has been described by Wilkins, and gonadal deficiency occurs in Turner's syndrome (*see* also p. 164, Fig. 12, and pp. 18–19). Hypogonadism may also be caused by bilateral ovarian disease. There is amenorrhœa, and lack of genital and mammary development. The epiphyses close late and the girl is sometimes very tall, but she may be very short (*see also* Turner's syndrome, below). Secondary hypogonadism is usually caused by hypopituitarism, or severe and prolonged wasting diseases.

TURNER'S SYNDROME

This rare syndrome consists of ovarian agenesis with failure to develop secondary sex characteristics. It is associated with stunted growth, congenital webbing of the neck, cubitus valgus, and other congenital abnormalities, such as coarctation of the aorta. Neonatal œdema may be the first symptom. Recent work has shown that there is a basic abnormality in chromosomal pattern in these patients (*see also* p. 18); only 45 in place of the normal 46 chromosomes are present, the missing chromosome being one of the female X chromosomes, giving in this respect the pattern XO instead of the normal XX. This is probably due to non-disjunction of the sex chromosomes at the primary stage of cell division (meiosis). The ova produced in this way would either carry a chromosome pattern O or XX. If the former type of ovum is fertilized by a Y-bearing sperm, theoretically an individual with a sex chromosome pattern YO would be produced. In practice no such individual has been identified as yet, and it is thought that this combination is lethal *in utero*. Fertilization by an X-bearing sperm produces an individual with an XO sex chromosomal pattern and Turner's syndrome.

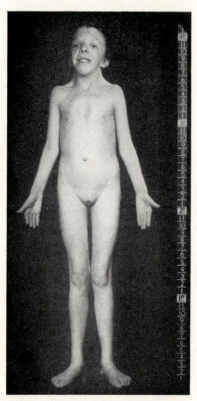

Fig. 12.—Turner's syndrome (gonadal deficiency, cubitus valgus, and webbing of the neck) in a child of 14 years. The syndrome is often associated with abnormalities of the aorta, such as coarctation, etc. This patient had a loud systolic murmur at the base of the heart, possibly due to congenital aortic stenosis.

Fertilization of the XX type of ovum by a Y-bearing sperm, giving rise to the sex chromosome pattern XXY, is seen clinically as Klinefelter's syndrome (p. 165). Fertilization by an X-bearing sperm would produce the pattern XXX. Such females have been identified; they show retarded mental development and, on ovarian biopsy, deficient follicle formation.

Male Hypogonadism

Primary cases are caused by disease affecting both testes, e.g. cryptorchidism, mumps, syphilis, or by castration. The symptoms are those of eunuchoidism, and gigantism may occur (*see* p. 148). Primary testicular degeneration has also been described. Secondary hypogonadism can be caused by hypothyroidism, and by pituitary or hypothalamic disease (Fröhlich's syndrome, p. 149). The direct treatment of male hypogonadism is by gonadotrophin, or by testosterone or methyltestosterone. This should be carried out with great care and only after hormone excretion studies have been performed.

Klinefelter's Syndrome

This syndrome is most commonly recognized at the time of puberty or in adult life. It consists of poorly developed testes, gynæcomastia, poor growth of facial hair and a persistence of the high-pitched voice of childhood. The abnormal chromosomal pattern in these patients is described on p. 164.

Gonadal Tumours

The granulosa-cell tumour of the ovary and the interstitial-cell tumour of the testis give rise to precocious sexual development (*see* p. 161). The granulosa-cell tumour is usually palpable on bimanual examination, but laparotomy may be necessary to confirm the diagnosis. In the case of each tumour, the correct treatment is excision.

Pseudo-hermaphroditism and True Intersex

The investigation of a patient whose genital development deviates from the normal is no longer limited to a delineation of the gonadal and genital-tract structure. Recent advances have made possible a much more extensive assessment upon which treatment and prognosis may be based. This may need to include:

The genetic sex (by chromosomal investigation and nuclear sex examination).

The gonadal sex (by biopsy).

Delineation of the genital tract (by contrast radiography or laparotomy).

Hormonal output (biochemical).

Psychological attitude of the patients to their own accepted sex status prior to investigation.

Such patients fall into three groups: females with some male characteristics (female pseudo-hermaphrodites); males with some female characteristics (male pseudo-hermaphrodites); and the very exceptional patient with both ovarian and testicular tissue (true intersex).

FEMALE PSEUDO-HERMAPHRODITISM

The great majority of such cases prove to be examples of the adreno-genital syndrome, which has already been fully described (p. 159). Very rarely, an adrenal tumour, either adenomatous or carcinomatous, may develop in childhood giving rise to symptoms of Cushing's syndrome (p. 150) with virilizing features in the female. Congenital malformations of the external genitalia, suggestive of the male but with female, genetic sex gonads and hormonal output, may occur if virilizing drugs are given to the mother during pregnancy.

MALE PSEUDO-HERMAPHRODITISM

Male pseudo-hermaphrodites form a more complex and heterogeneous group than their female counterparts. The majority are familial and genetically determined.

In the first group, the external genitalia may appear completely feminine in infancy, but at some stage, a gonad (testis) may be felt in what had been taken for the labia majora or in the inguinal region. Genetic sex by chromosomal or nuclear cytology confirms the basic male sex of the patient. If the testicles are intra-abdominal or pass unnoticed, the child may be accepted as female up till the time of puberty. At puberty, testicular feminization may occur with normal breast development, but characteristically no pubic hair appears and menstruation in the absence of a uterus cannot develop. At this stage, investigation, which may need to include laparotomy, will reveal the presence of testes.

In the second group, the external genitalia are ambiguous, but the patient is usually accepted in the early years as female. At puberty, the excess of physical strength, general body configuration, and male pubic hair pattern, may cast doubts about the sex. Investigation at this stage will reveal male genetic and nuclear sex, the diagnosis being confirmed by the finding of testes at laparotomy and biopsy.

Between these two groups there are many intermediate individual examples. The pattern of genital-tract configuration as shown by contrast radiography is also very variable. It is not possible in the early years to predict whether testicular feminization, as described above, will occur at puberty or whether virilizing changes will develop.

TRUE INTERSEX

There are a few exceptionally rare individuals in whom both a testis and ovary are found. In such cases the external and internal genitalia may also have features of either sex.

TREATMENT

In all these patients over the age of one year, the most important factor in determining treatment is the patient's own psychological sex acceptance and adaptation. Attempts to impose a change of sex upon an individual carry a heavy risk of severe mental illness and even suicide. Only where the patient demands a change of sex from that previously accepted should appropriate treatment be undertaken.

The treatment of the adreno-genital syndrome has already been fully described (p. 160). In male pseudo-hermaphroditism, each case must be treated on its individual merits once the patient's psychological needs are understood. The procedures necessary will include plastic operations on the external genitalia, and, in appropriate cases after the age of puberty, removal of gonads and replacement hormone therapy where the psychological sex acceptance is at variance with the gonadal sex.

THYMUS

THE thymus gland increases slowly in size up to the age of puberty, and then regresses. Extremely wide variation in size is found in normal children. Various symptoms have been attributed to its enlargement. Among these symptoms are sudden death, thymic asthma, collapse and fainting, and breath-holding attacks. There is little scientific evidence to support these opinions. In the past, a diagnosis of status thymo-lymphaticus was often made at autopsy in children who had died suddenly. This also has been generally discarded by pathologists.

Occasionally, a much enlarged thymus is seen in a child who is wheezing and has obvious respiratory distress. Abscess formation in the thymus from a pyogenic organism must be excluded, also other infections and leukæmia by a blood-count. Actual tumour formation in the thymus should also be kept in mind (thymoma). The extremely rare thymic carcinoma may be associated with Cushing's syndrome (*see* p. 150). In myasthenia gravis, benefit may sometimes be obtained from removal of the thymus. For the possible role of the thymus in auto-immunity, *see* p. 321.

DISEASES OF THE PANCREAS

Diabetes Mellitus

DIABETES is slightly more common in females than males and is inherited as a recessive characteristic. Nevertheless, environmental factors appear to be involved in the exact timing of the emergence of clinical symptoms. Diabetics should be warned, if they marry into families in which the disease is known to be present, that there is a risk that their children may be affected. If they marry another diabetic, it becomes almost certain. In childhood the disease is rare, particularly under the age of one year.

CLINICAL PICTURE

The child is noted to be losing weight rapidly, to have an intolerable thirst and to be passing water too frequently and in excessive quantities. Enuresis of recent origin should raise suspicion. Vulvitis is a fairly frequent initial complaint in girls. Other symptoms are tiredness, irritability, and hunger, but this last occurs in only one-sixth of the cases. In about 15 per cent. the onset of the disease appears to follow an acute infective disease, or a septic infection. Occasionally, the first indication of the disease is the onset of coma or a pre-coma state. Examination of the urine shows the presence of a reducing substance, which is glucose, and there may be diacetic acid and acetone. On examination of an untreated diabetic, the tongue may be red and clean, the skin dry, and the palms of the hands and soles of the feet slightly yellow. A sweetish acetone smell is often present in the breath. The child is rapidly reduced to extreme emaciation.

BLOOD-SUGAR CURVE

An examination of the blood-sugar of a normal child shows that the resting blood-sugar is about 100 mg. per 100 ml. After a meal, or following the ingestion of glucose, it rises to 180 mg. per 100 ml. within half an hour, and within one and a half hours has fallen to normal, or nearly so. The blood-sugar curve of a diabetic, on the other hand, may start higher, say 150 mg. per 100 ml., and after the ingestion of sugar or a meal rise steadily to 250 or 350 mg. per 100 ml.; it may even go much higher or remain there for an hour or more, settling much more slowly than the normal (Fig. 13).

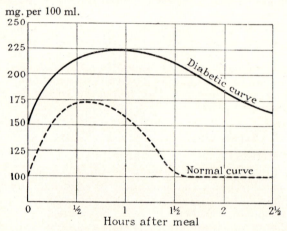

Fig. 13.—Blood-sugar curve of a normal child and of a diabetic child.

From this it may be seen that the sugar content of the blood in diabetic children is much higher than in non-diabetic children and, being above the sugar-threshold of the kidney, leads to a constant leaking of sugar into the urine.

RENAL GLYCOSURIA

Occasionally, children are found who have sugar in the urine yet whose sugar-tolerance curve and blood-sugar turn out to be quite normal. These have a low threshold for sugar, allowing it to pass out into the urine at a lower level than normal.

DIABETIC COMA

A child with diabetes is always liable to coma, and this may set in rapidly. The onset may be due to several causes; the commonest is an acute infection, the next most frequent are vomiting following a bilious attack, insufficient dosage of insulin, and gross departure from the prescribed diet. Yawning, drowsiness, irritability and vomiting may herald the onset. Later, air-hunger is marked, and complete unconsciousness occurs. The skin is found to be dry and dehydration may be found. The plantar responses are extensor. The breath smells of acetone.

HYPOGLYCÆMIA

If too large a dose of insulin is given, the child becomes pale and lifeless; occasionally, he is irritable and extremely emotional. He is seized with shakiness of the hands and giddiness and, if the condition is not checked, severe convulsions with unconsciousness supervene. Other common symptoms are sweating, abdominal pain, hunger, headache, double vision, squint or actual temporary blindness. Not infrequently the attack starts abruptly with sudden unconsciousness, or a fit. As a rule the plantar responses are flexor. When using a long-acting insulin, hypoglycæmic attacks may occur in the early morning. Difficulty in waking up at the usual time is a warning of this.

PROGNOSIS

Before the introduction of insulin, the life of the diabetic was short. Now it appears that, with adequate treatment, the disease is compatible with a normal life. The risk of long-term complications, however, cannot be disregarded (*see* p. 172), diabetic retinitis and diabetic nephropathy being especially important sequelæ of the disease when it commences in childhood. From a short-term point of view, with the institution of proper treatment, the child puts on weight, develops, and appears normal mentally and in every other respect.

TREATMENT

When the diagnosis of diabetes mellitus is first made, it is essential that the child should be admitted to hospital for the initial stabilization treatment. Later, maintenance treatment can be carried out at home, provided the domestic arrangements are adequate. Residential schools are available in certain cases for diabetic children.

Diet. For initial stabilization the child is put to bed, and is offered a diet containing a caloric value calculated from the following formula: A child aged one year is offered a diet containing 1,000 calories; for each succeeding year of age up to ten years an extra 100 calories are offered. After the age of ten years an extra 200 calories are offered for each succeeding year of age.

Up till the age of five to six years growth requirements as compared with energy requirements are relatively greater than in the older age groups, and until that age relatively more protein is required. The proportion of carbohydrate, protein and fat recommended is as follows:

RATIO IN GRAMMES

	Up to 6 Years of Age	At 10 Years of Age
Carbohydrate	.. .. 2·5	3·5–4·0
Protein	.. .. 1·0	1·0
Fat ..	.. .. 1·0	1·0

After the initial stabilization has been carried out, Payne recommends a fairly free diet for children over the age of ten years. It is clearly more convenient for a school child to be fed on ordinary foods if possible. The line-ration diet system as devised by Lawrence is a useful standard, but is not easily applicable to small children.

Insulin. For initial stabilization of an untreated diabetic the child should be started on a diet as outlined on p. 169, and soluble insulin (5 units twice daily for the smaller children and 10 units for larger children) should be given initially. The urine should be tested every four hours, and the dose of insulin increased until the glycosuria and ketosis are controlled. For children who present in a more advanced stage of the disease, much larger doses of insulin are necessary (*see* diabetic coma, p. 171). At this stage it is often found that the child is hungry, and the amount of diet and consequently the insulin should be accordingly increased. Modifications to the amount of food at individual meals (particularly carbohydrate), and alteration in the times at which the insulin is injected, may be required before satisfactory stabilization is achieved.

After a satisfactory diet adequately controlled by soluble insulin has been established, a trial of a delayed-acting insulin (intermediate or long-acting lente insulin) may be made, but it is not always possible to achieve adequate control on a single daily injection. Minor adjustments in the amount and type of insulin are likely to be necessary to achieve satisfactory insulin coverage for the whole twenty-four hours, and minor episodes of hypoglycæmia may have to be treated (*see* p. 172) whilst stabilization is being carried out.

In older children, it is found that with suitable instruction the patients soon achieve an understanding of the condition and the necessity for the insulin, learning quickly to carry out injections themselves.

After initial stabilization, the question arises as to whether attempts should be made to eliminate hyperglycæmia and consequently glycosuria for the whole of each twenty-four hours. This is not advised, because in practice it is found that such attempts are usually attended by episodes of hypoglycæmia and that the patients are more comfortable if allowed to have a trace of glycosuria. On a long-term policy the effect of long continuing hyperglycæmia in the ætiology of the complications of diabetes has to be considered. In practice, therefore, glycosuria should be reduced as far as is possible without producing episodes of hypoglycæmia.

DIFFICULTIES IN MANAGEMENT

Certain gross errors are apt to be made in calculating any diet.

1. The composition of the various foodstuffs may obviously vary greatly. For example, the difference in food content between a bitter and a sweet orange, a ripe and an unripe apple, old and new potatoes, fat and lean meat, may be a source of error.

2. The presence or absence of infections must be considered. A slight tonsillitis or cold causes an increased output of adrenaline, and a consequent increase in the blood-sugar and depletion of the sugar stores. Extra insulin must be given to counteract this action of adrenaline. Failure to do this will result in ketosis, and sometimes coma. On this account it is most important that all sources of sepsis be treated in the diabetic child. Septic tonsils or teeth should be removed.

3. The site of insulin injection should be varied each day. There is a danger, if the same site is used repeatedly, that necrosis of tissue may occur and that subsequently the absorption of insulin from that particular site may be variable. In this way, periods of apparent instability of control may occur, for which more complex explanations may be sought. Routine instructions to diabetics and their parents should always include mention of this danger.

4. The amount of exercise taken in the day is important. With much exercise more of the blood-sugar is used up. Less insulin need then be given. It will be apparent, therefore, that regularity in the amount of exercise and excitement is necessary if the dose of insulin is to be the right one and attacks of hypoglycæmia are to be avoided.

5. It has been found that the onset of puberty may greatly alter the insulin requirements of a diabetic child and considerable difficulty may sometimes be encountered in attaining adequate stabilization over this period.

OPERATIONS ON DIABETIC CHILDREN

Provided adequate care is taken, operations may safely be performed on diabetic children according to the ordinary surgical indications. Four to six hours before the operation, soluble insulin together with sufficient glucose to equal the caloric value of the corresponding meal (usually breakfast) is given. One to two hours before, a further dose of glucose corresponding to the next meal (lunch) is given. After the operation, glucose and soluble insulin are given, again corresponding to the normal routine. The normal diet is resumed as soon as possible.

TREATMENT OF DIABETIC COMA

The basic treatment consists of intravenous fluid to overcome dehydration, insulin in large doses, glucose to prevent ketosis, and treatment for shock. Five per cent. glucose saline alternating with normal saline, in equal quantities, should be given intravenously and injections of soluble insulin four-hourly until improvement occurs. The urine reaction to sugar and frequent estimations of the blood sugar give a guide to the exact amount of insulin to be given at each interval; 20–40 units are likely to be required in the initial stages, decreasing as the urine becomes free from sugar. Metabolic acidosis can be assessed by estimation of the serum electrolytes and corrected by the addition of M/6 lactate (p. 196) to the intravenous infusion. As the metabolic acidosis improves, the serum potassium may fall; therefore once dehydration has been overcome, potassium chloride (0·5 G. four-hourly) should be given by mouth or even intravenously (p. 196) if vomiting still persists. Thereafter, restabilization must be carried out with insulin, given at six-hourly intervals at first, and a diet containing plenty of fluids and a known quantity of carbohydrate.

TREATMENT OF ACUTE HYPOGLYCÆMIA

If the child is in the early stages of an attack, sugar will rapidly stop the trouble. From 4 to 8 lumps should be given by mouth and the effect noted. In more severe cases, glucose 50 G. is given by stomach tube or intravenously in 20 per cent. solution.

OTHER COMPLICATIONS

Growth in a well-stabilized diabetic child differs little from that of normal children. There may be a tendency to skin infections in uncontrolled diabetics. The serious significance of diabetic retinitis, leading to blindness, and diabetic nephropathy (almost always fatal within three years) as complications of childhood diabetes has already been mentioned. The vascular changes of adults are not seen in childhood.

Diabetic children appear to have no greater tendency to acquire tuberculosis than normal children, but, once contracted, the disease is poorly withstood. Vaccination with BCG is therefore advisable for all in whom tuberculin-testing gives negative results.

Spontaneous Hypoglycæmia (*See* also p. 114)

Spontaneous hypoglycæmia may have different origins. The insulin-secreting islet-cell tumour of the pancreas is a well-known but extremely uncommon cause. Other cases are of unknown ætiology and are probably due to a variety of causes. One form is undoubtedly familial and appears to be recessively inherited.

In the most severe type, convulsions, indistinguishable clinically from other forms of status epilepticus, may occur in the first two years of life, progressing to brain damage or a fatal outcome from hypoglycæmia, unless active treatment is undertaken. Thus, estimation of the blood-sugar is desirable in all sustained epileptic seizures in early childhood to exclude this possibility. Blood-sugar levels below

30 mg. per 100 ml. are not infrequently found. Immediate treatment of the attack with intravenous injections of hypertonic glucose is urgent to try to prevent brain damage.

In a slightly less severe form, spontaneous hypoglycæmia may give rise to recurring episodes of unconsciousness in which the child is seen to become pale and then collapse. The period of unconsciousness is usually considerably longer than that seen in a simple vaso-vagal seizure. A low blood-sugar level during such an episode confirms the diagnosis.

In the milder form, episodes of hypoglycæmia may give rise to nausea, vomiting and abdominal pain. In such an attack the child may sometimes become confused and irritable. These episodes may occur after a period of fasting or may occasionally be *reactive* in type. The latter occur after a meal and are presumably due to an over-secretion of insulin following the initial glucose absorption that has commenced after the meal.

It was found by Cochrane[1] that in one group of patients episodes of spontaneous hypoglycæmia could be induced by the injection of leucine (leucine-sensitive hypoglycæmia). The test is carried out by giving leucine in doses of 0·15 gramme per Kg. body-weight or casein in a dose of 1·5 gramme per Kg. body-weight, after which serial measurements of the blood-sugar level are made.

In patients with islet-cell tumours, increasingly severe and frequent episodes of hypoglycæmia occur which are unresponsive to treatment with steroids. In such cases laparotomy is essential. Any palpable tumour of the pancreas is removed, but if none is found partial pancreatectomy is performed.

In cases of idiopathic hypoglycæmia, prolonged steroid therapy (*see* Appendix 2) is the treatment of choice when the attacks are severe. The dosage should be reduced to the minimum level adequate to suppress the attacks and may need to be continued for six to twelve months. In many of the idiopathic cases there is a natural tendency to spontaneous cure within two or three years.

[1] Cochrane, W. A., Payne, W. W., Simpkiss, M. J., Woolf, L. I. (1956). *J. clin. Invest.*, **35**, 411.

CHAPTER 12

Diseases of the Alimentary Tract

VOMITING or disturbance of bowel habit provides valuable evidence in the diagnosis of many disorders of the alimentary tract. Careful inquiry and observation will elicit information which might otherwise be overlooked. Alteration of bowel habit or absence of bowel actions may often have as much, and sometimes more, clinical importance than the passage of abnormal stools.

VOMITING

The *type of vomiting* (for example, projectile vomiting as in pyloric stenosis, vomiting when the child is lying down as in cases of hiatus hernia, or effortless vomiting as occurs with raised intracranial pressure) should be noted, also the approximate amount of the vomit and its time relationship to meals or to other symptoms. It is taught that in acute appendicitis abdominal pain precedes vomiting, but this is by no means the invariable history with small children in whom the first appearance of abdominal pain may not have been recognized by those in charge of the child.

The *vomitus* should be examined. *Bile-staining* suggests intestinal obstruction; after the first few days of life (p. 109), *streaks of fresh blood* together with mucus indicate hiatus hernia, or may be found when acute gastritis occurs secondary to pyloric stenosis. In older children hæmatemesis is rare; it is found in local disorders of the œsophagus, such as a hiatus hernia giving rise to secondary œsophageal ulceration, or where portal obstruction has caused the formation o œsophageal varices; peptic ulceration must not be overlooked, whilst acute gastric erosion is sometimes seen after taking aspirin. The swallowing of a sharp-edged foreign body by a toddler or mentally defective child may also cause hæmatemesis. General hæmorrhagic diseases, such as leukæmia, may cause gastric hæmorrhage in addition to bleeding in other parts of the body. In the investigation of all cases of hæmatemesis, the possibility that the blood had come originally from the back of the nose, and had been subsequently swallowed and then vomited, will indicate the need for a thorough examination of the nose and throat.

A vomit is acid in reaction because of the presence of normal gastric secretions, but in œsophageal atresia (p. 177) " the vomit " (that is, the liquid regurgitated from the blind upper œsophageal segment) will be alkaline.

Whenever poisoning is suspected, the vomit or gastric aspiration must be saved for analysis.

ABNORMAL STOOLS

Pale grey, bulky, greasy, offensive stools are found in mal-absorption syndromes such as cœliac disease.   In fibrocystic disease, the characteristically offensive odour is due to the presence of undigested protein in addition to the excess fat.   Where liver disease or biliary obstruction prevents bile from entering the intestine, the stools are white in colour.

Whilst green stools may be considered normal in a breast-fed infant who is gaining weight, in artificially-fed infants they indicate intestinal hurry and possible infection, particularly when unformed and accompanied by the passage of mucus.   Very small green stools are sometimes found in underfed infants, the so-called " hunger stools ".

In gastro-enteritis, the stools may be loose and yellow initially. As the disease gains momentum, they become green and watery, and finally contain blood and mucus.

Black stools are found in patients taking iron, bismuth, or charcoal, or they may denote blood; the term " tarry stools " indicates the typical appearance when altered blood is present in large amounts. After the first few days of life (p. 109), melæna may be the result of the general hæmorrhagic disorders and particularly Henoch-Schönlein purpura, or may be due to a local condition, such as œsophageal varix, peptic ulcer or ulcerated Meckel's diverticulum.   Blood which is unaltered and accompanies or streaks the outside of a formed stool may come from an anal fissure.   Hæmorrhoids and rectal polypi are not common.   Blood and mucus are found in ulcerative colitis and dysentery.   The " red-currant jelly " stool of intussusception is characteristic but it is a late manifestation.

Mucus suggests that there is irritation of the bowel; when it appears on the outer surface of the stool only, it denotes colitis rather than enteritis; in the latter the mucus is intimately mixed with the stool. Vigorous purgation such as the use of castor oil will give rise to the passage of much mucus due to acute irritation of the bowel wall.

Pus is present when there is inflammation of the bowel wall, as is found in typhoid and dysentery infections.   The various worms which may be found in the stools are described in Chapter 27.

CONGENITAL ABNORMALITIES
OF THE ALIMENTARY TRACT

FOR a general discussion of the ætiology of congenital deformities, see p. 97.

Hare-lip

This is occasionally an inherited condition exhibiting male sex-linkage.   The inherited form is seen both with and without associated cleft palate.   The deformity may be unilateral or bilateral, and may involve the lip only or extend upwards and backwards to include the floor of the nose and the alveolar ridge. In bilateral cases the pre-maxilla is displaced forwards.

Hare-lip, with or without cleft palate, occurs three times more commonly in boys than girls; whereas cleft palate alone is seen slightly more frequently in girls, in the proportion 3 girls to 2 boys.

When a normal couple have a child with hare-lip, the risk to their subsequent children is in the order of 1 in 20[1]. If one parent has hare-lip, the chance of a first child being affected is about 1 in 50. If an affected person already has a child with a hare-lip, the chance of a subsequent child also being affected is at least 1 in 10. These estimates are, however, based on a narrow survey.

Early repair of hare-lip is usually advised unless infection is present or there is a medical contra-indication to prolonged general anæsthesia. A suitable age for operation is often between two and three months. If necessary a second plastic operation can be carried out later at perhaps the age of four to five years.

Cleft palate

This may occur by itself or in association with hare-lip. The genetic inheritance of the combined lesion has already been mentioned above. Where cleft palate exists alone, a proportion of the cases are due to a dominant gene of low penetrance. Other cases are not genetically determined, as for example in the rubella syndrome (p. 540) and probably in the Pierre Robin syndrome (p. 224). Where the parents are normal and one child is affected, Fraser Roberts states that the chance of a further child developing a cleft palate is about 1 in 80. If the family has another relative with a cleft palate, the chance is increased to 1 in 10. In families where one parent is affected, the chance that a child may also show cleft palate is again about 1 in 10. Where both a parent and a child are already affected, the chance of involvement for further children is increased to 1 in 6.

The cleft may vary considerably from a small defect in the soft palate, which causes little disability, to a complete separation of the hard palate combined with a hare-lip. With extensive lesions, considerable difficulty may occur in feeding due to the inability to suck and to nasal regurgitation.

TREATMENT

With the co-operation of an orthodontist, it is possible to fit a prosthesis to cover the defects in both the hare-lip and cleft palate. In some cases breast-feeding has been successfully established. If such help is not available, spoon feeding is usually the method of choice, although a large number of infants with cleft palate alone feed successfully from an ordinary feeding bottle.

[1] Fraser Roberts, J. A. (1959). " Introduction to Medical Genetics." London: Oxford University Press.

Plastic repair is usually undertaken at between a year and eighteen months of age and should be followed by speech therapy. Close dental and orthodontic supervision is essential.

Pierre Robin Syndrome (*see* p. 224).

In this condition a cleft palate is combined with retrognathos and backward displacement of the tongue. In the most severe cases respiratory obstruction occurs shortly after birth and immediate treatment is required.

ŒSOPHAGUS

THE congenital anomalies of the œsophagus include tracheo-œsophageal fistula, stenosis, and diverticulum. True congenital stenotic lesions are extremely rare, compared with the acquired lesions associated with hiatus hernia.

Tracheo-œsophageal Fistula

This is a rare condition in which the most frequently seen abnormality consists of an œsophagus in which the central portion is absent, the upper segment ending in a blind pouch and the lower part having a fistulous communication with the trachea. Due to œsophageal obstruction, much mucus collects in the pharynx despite repeated clearing by a mucus catheter, and this should suggest the diagnosis. When such infants are first fed, immediately the upper œsophageal segment is filled, spill-over occurs with choking fits and cyanosis. Repeated attempts at feeding lead inevitably to inhalation pneumonia.

If the pregnancy was complicated by hydramnios, suspicion may have been aroused before the birth of the infant (p. 98), whilst in the remainder the diagnosis should be suspected at or before the first feed. Once the suggestion has been made, no more feeds should be given until further investigations have been carried out. The practice at some centres of giving boiled water rather than milk to all new-borns as the first feed has much to commend it. The diagnosis is confirmed radiologically by the careful introduction of a radio-opaque tube into the œsophagus as far as the obstruction. Under the x-ray screen a small quantity of Dionosil may then be introduced to outline the upper segment and is then aspirated before the tube is withdrawn.

In the best hands, operation produces excellent results, unless additional congenital abnormalities incompatible with life are present.

Either the fistula is closed and a direct anastomosis of the two ends of the œsophagus carried out, or, if the gap between the two ends of the œsophagus is too great, the upper end is exteriorized to allow drainage of respiratory secretions, the fistula is closed, and the lower end of the œsophagus tied off and a gastrostomy performed.   At the age of one year a continuous œsophagus can be fashioned by means of a colon transplant.

In the management of an infant with tracheo-œsophageal fistula, it must be remembered that associated congenital defects are common and that in particular there may be an associated atresia of the small intestine (p. 185) which will also require surgical correction.

Œsophageal Hiatus Hernia

In addition to the more severe degrees of diaphragmatic hernia, varying degrees of laxity of the œsophageal hiatus, formed by the crura of the diaphragm, are found.   In such cases, retraction of the œsophagus and the proximal part of the stomach may take place through the hiatus and give rise to the condition of apparent short œsophagus.   Reflux of gastric contents into the true œsophagus is then likely to occur, through an incompetent cardiac sphincter, when the patient is lying flat.   Irritation and ulceration of the lower end of the œsophagus is produced in this way with excessive mucus formation, hæmorrhage (hæmatemesis or melæna) and spasm simulating an œsophageal stricture.   Fibrosis of the œsophagus can ultimately follow, producing a true stricture and a true shortening of the œsophagus.

SYMPTOMS

Vomiting of mucus and feeds is usually present from birth, sooner or later associated with hæmatemeses.   The vomiting occurs particularly when the child is laid flat.   Difficulty is found in taking solids from the time of weaning.   There are definite periods of remission and exacerbation, sometimes of weeks in duration.   In severe cases there is failure to gain weight and considerable wasting, with associated anæmia from the hæmatemeses.   Screening with barium swallow, if carefully done, will show the abnormality; as part of this investigation the child should be positioned with the head right down so that reflux of gastric contents into the œsophagus can be observed.

TREATMENT

The infant should be fed in the erect position and kept sitting up on pillows between feeds.   Special nursing chairs in which the older infants may be maintained in a part sitting position are most useful. The feeds should be thickened with Benger's Food or Nestargel. Iron or blood transfusions may be necessary for the anæmia.

A number of cases improve spontaneously with this treatment, but if the condition has persisted to the age of nine to twelve months, surgical repair is indicated in view of the likelihood of fibrotic contracture of the œsophagus with stricture formation later in childhood.   The surgical results are excellent.

Œsophageal Stenosis

This may occur as a congenital lesion (*see* p. 177), as a result of a hiatus hernia, or as a result of trauma from the swallowing of a corrosive poison, usually a strong acid or alkali.

In each case, dysphagia, profuse mucus, vomiting immediately after swallowing, and the ability to take fluids but not solids are the outstanding symptoms. In the acquired cases, the lesion is often progressive. Patients with severe lesions become wasted to a degree that resembles *anorexia nervosa*.

Œsophagectomy and replacement of the stenosed portion by a colonic transplant has become a surgical possibility. In less severe cases, repeated dilatation of the stricture with bougies may be helpful.

Cardiospasm (Achalasia)

This condition is rare in childhood and symptoms do not appear usually before 5 years of age. It has to be distinguished from the other causes of œsophageal obstruction already described. It is considered to be due to a neuro-muscular inco-ordination of the cardiac sphincter. Certainly there is a constriction at the lower end of the œsophagus with dilatation above it which can be demonstrated radiologically by barium swallow.

Treatment with nitrites results in transient relief of the spasm. Inhalation of octyl nitrate takes effect in 60–90 seconds. Dilatation with mercury bougies is helpful and the child can learn to carry out this treatment himself. Œsophageal wash-outs with a solution of sodium bicarbonate are indicated if much œsophagitis is present. Operative treatment consists in incision of the muscular coat of the œsophagus (Heller's operation) and is most successful.

Diaphragmatic Hernia

This is more commonly seen on the left side than on the right, the usual sites being in the postero-lateral region of the diaphragm.

In severe cases, in which a large proportion of the abdominal contents pass into the thorax, symptoms are present from birth. Respiratory embarrassment and cyanosis, which is typically relieved by altering the infant's position, are usual symptoms accompanied by intermittent vomiting and a failure to thrive. Considerable areas of pulmonary collapse are common. Thus, the chest signs will include areas of collapse associated with unusual patches of hypersonance and borborygmi due to the presence of intestinal viscera.

In less severe cases, no symptoms or only occasional unexplained attacks of vomiting may be present. The first sign of the presence of such a hernia may arise from strangulation; this produces profound shock, with symptoms of acute obstruction, and usually ends fatally.

The diagnosis of diaphragmatic hernia can be confirmed radio-logically by straight x-ray and barium study, if necessary; at the same time the site of the diaphragmatic defect can usually be localized.

TREATMENT

Nixon and O'Donnell[1] stress the necessity for immediate operation, medical treatment being of no avail in this condition. This is absolutely essential in the severe cases presenting at birth.

Eventration of the Diaphragm

In this condition, the diaphragm is intact but is deficient in muscle, the deficient area varying in extent from case to case but usually occurring on the left side. In the severe cases, the symptoms are similar to those of diaphragmatic hernia, except that strangulation does not occur. In other cases, few symptoms may be produced. X-ray will reveal paradoxical movement of the diaphragm on the affected side and barium studies will confirm the true state of affairs. In severe cases, the possibility of surgical intervention should be carefully considered.

Congenital Pyloric Stenosis

This disorder is not really congenital but develops soon after birth. The muscle sphincter guarding the exit from the stomach becomes thickened, so that food cannot leave the pylorus. Symptoms of obstruction then occur.

Pyloric stenosis is far more common in males than in females, with a ratio of 6 or 7 males to each female. The initial symptoms occur most frequently at the end of the second week after birth. Occasionally, however, the vomiting commences sooner, or as late as the tenth week. Quite often the patients are found to be the first children of young mothers.

Although an incomplete dominant sex-linked inheritance is un-doubtedly an ætiological factor, all the data cannot be fitted to any simple genetic hypothesis, and the probability is that early post-natal environmental factors play an additional part.

PATHOGENESIS

The pylorus is enlarged mainly because of hypertrophy of the circular muscular fibres. On section, the mucous membrane is seen to be folded and tight, and often a ball of it blocks the gastric end of the pyloric canal. The thickened pylorus forms a mass, firm, round or oval, and the muscle-fibres on incision are hard and in some cases feel almost cartilaginous. Usually, there is associated gastritis. Microscopically, the circular muscle-fibres of the pylorus are seen to be greatly hypertrophied and thickened.

[1] Nixon, H. H., O'Donnell, B. (1961). " The Essentials of Pædiatric Surgery." London: Heinemann.

SYMPTOMS AND DIAGNOSIS

As a rule, the infant seems to thrive up to the age of two weeks, when projectile vomiting commences. The vomit is large and often consists of more than one feed. It contains curdled milk and mucus, and is occasionally tinged with blood. A day may pass with only one vomit, but the next day several vomits immediately following on the feeds usually occur. The infant wastes but remains surprisingly bright. He has an eager, hungry look and gnaws at his hands. Marked constipation occurs. Often, the vomiting is attributed to the food being unsuitable; a new food or method of feeding is tried, with what appears to be success for a day or two; then the vomiting recommences. The diagnosis rests on:

1. The history of repeated large projectile vomits.
2. Obstinate constipation.

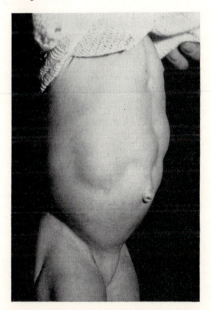

Fig. 14—Visible peristalsis in pyloric stenosis.

3. Vigorous gastric waves passing from left to right across the abdomen (*see* Fig. 14).
4. The palpation of a pyloric tumour.

Pyloric obstruction should always be suspected by the physician when vomiting has been persistent and constipation obstinate; the infant should be given a feed and gastric waves watched for. The mere " standing out " of the stomach is insufficient, as this occurs in so-called

7

pylorospasm. Waves the size of a small tangerine orange may be seen passing from left to right across the abdomen. Very often two waves may be seen at the same time; the more wasted the baby, the clearer the peristalsis. Vigorous waves will be seen in every case of true pyloric stenosis if the infant is observed for any length of time. During the feed, if the abdomen is palpated, a pyloric tumour can almost always be felt, sometimes superficial, sometimes deep in the abdomen, immediately to the right of the right rectus, high up and just beneath the liver margin. X-ray confirmation of the diagnosis is seldom necessary and is somewhat undesirable (if operation is to follow), but if there is real doubt a barium meal will show a delay in the gastric emptying time, and a narrow pyloric canal may be outlined (silver wire appearance).

With simple pyloric spasm, the vomiting is intermittent and there may be remissions of several days; constipation is present but less persistent than in pyloric stenosis. Gastric waves are never vigorous and no pyloric tumour is left. X-rays may show a prolonged spasm which later relaxes in the prepyloric region.

TREATMENT

The choice is between medical and surgical treatment. To make the diagnosis certain, however, may take one to two days, and during this uncertain period gastric lavage relieves the infant of the retained food and tends to prevent gastritis. The vomiting, if long continued or severe, causes loss of water, chloride and some potassium, which will require correction by means of subcutaneous or intravenous fluid. In such cases, it is important that the correct amount of electrolyte is given since the renal function of a small infant is too immature to control readily a disturbed fluid and salt balance. Thus, overdosage of intravenous saline may convert a dehydrated infant into an œdematous one by virtue of salt retention. For this reason, repeated examinations of the plasma-chloride level give the best indication of how far the chloride deficit has been corrected, and once a figure approaching the normal has been achieved only one-fifth normal saline should be used. If facilities for this estimation are not available, it is usually a safe practice to give half-strength saline for the first twenty-four hours of the infusion, followed by one-fifth normal saline in 4·5 per cent. glucose for the remainder (for details of the calculation of the quantity of parenteral fluid to administer, *see* p. 196).

Medical Treatment. In Scandinavia especially, medical treatment has been very successful; in most centres in this country, however, operation is chosen in the majority of cases. The treatment consists of gastric lavage carried out once or twice daily, careful feeding, and the use of an atropine preparation. The feed selected is usually a simple one, such as breast-milk or an artificial feed which forms a fine curd (for example, evaporated milk) thickened with Benger's Food or Nestargel. Atropine methylnitrate (Eumydrin) may be given in the form of 0·6 per cent. alcoholic solution, one drop increasing to 3 drops being given 20 minutes before each feed, or as 0·1 mg. lamella (Pylostropin), from 1–3 lamellæ being given under the tongue at similar intervals. Scopolamine methylnitrate may be used with similar effect. Toxic symptoms are shown by erythema or hyperpyrexia. It may be necessary to keep up treatment for many weeks; during this time the utmost care and attention and the most expert nursing are necessary as infections are not well withstood. In most centres in Great Britain, medical treatment is reserved for mild cases or for those infants who do not develop symptoms until the sixth to eighth week of life.

Surgical Treatment. Where the child is only two to four weeks old, and especially when breast-fed, surgery provides a much more rapid method of treatment and produces excellent results. In preparation for the operation serum electrolytes should be checked. Saline and glucose are administered subcutaneously or intravenously, depending on the degree of dehydration present (*see* p. 196). The stomach is washed clean with normal saline an hour before the operation. The arms and legs of the infant should be enveloped in cotton-wool, lightly bandaged on to prevent cooling, and the child is then placed on a T-splint. Either local or general anæsthesia can be employed with equally good results in experienced hands.

Rammstedt's operation consists of splitting the circular fibres of the pylorus. The folded pyloric mucosa can then herniate, thus relieving the obstruction and allowing the food to pass through. It is a short operation, taking less than 10 minutes. The infant, when returned to its cot, must be kept warm.

POST-OPERATIVE CARE

Feeding should be recommenced four hours after the operation. At first only glucose and one-fifth normal saline should be offered, one drachm hourly for two hours, followed by two drachms hourly for four hours. Thereafter the feed should be increased to half an ounce hourly. The feeding schedule should always be interrupted to give the infant a complete rest between midnight and 6 a.m. Usually, about 16 hours after the operation, dilute feeds (one-eighth strength dried milk or quarter strength breast-milk) should be commenced, one ounce being given at two-hourly intervals. The amount and strength of the feeds and the intervals between them should be gradually increased so that a breast-fed infant will resume normal three- or four-hourly breast-feeding 24–36 hours after operation, an artificially fed infant returning to a normal feed usually about 12 hours later.

The child should be discharged from hospital at the earliest opportunity, 48 hours after operation being the rule in some centres. While the infant remains in hospital, the use of cubicles and all aseptic precautions to prevent cross-infection are essential.

Post-operative vomiting should be treated by gastric lavage once or twice daily. If dehydration is still present further subcutaneous or intravenous fluid may be necessary.

PROGNOSIS OF SURGICALLY TREATED CASES

Many series of 100 or more cases with little or no mortality are on record. David Levi (1941) operated on 100 consecutive breast-fed infants without a death. With good nursing and freedom from cross-infection, there is extremely little mortality.

NEONATAL INTESTINAL OBSTRUCTION

A NUMBER of conditions, mainly due to congenital malformation, can give rise to intestinal obstruction in the first days of life.

For this reason, vomiting, and particularly bile-stained vomiting, in the newborn should always be regarded as significant until proved otherwise. The other cardinal symptoms are upper abdominal distension and complete constipation or a greatly reduced passage of meconium; in cases of obstruction below the ampulla of Vater, the meconium is light in colour and consists mainly of desquamated intestinal epithelium.

The outlook for many of these patients has been greatly improved by technical advances in surgery and particularly by the maintenance of fluid and electrolyte balance during the pre-operative and post-operative periods. For more detailed consideration of these and other abdominal surgical conditions in childhood the reader is referred to such authors as Gross, Nixon and O'Donnell, Swenson, and White and Dennison.[1]

Duodenal Obstruction and Atresia

Atresia may be due to some developmental error in the duodenum, associated with partial or complete absence of its lumen. It is of interest that this condition is much more frequent among mongols than in normal children.

Obstruction is commonly due to duodenal compression or constriction of the duodenum by abnormal peritoneal bands in association with incomplete rotation of the intestine; here, there is no special association with mongolism.

SYMPTOMS

In atresia, vomiting of bile-stained fluid in large amounts after every feed is the rule from birth. Constipation is complete, and only a little light coloured material is obtained by washing out the

[1] Gross, R. E. (1953). "The Surgery of Infancy and Childhood." Philadelphia and London: Saunders.
Nixon, H. H., O'Donnell, B. (1961). "The Essentials of Pædiatric Surgery." London: Heinemann.
Swenson, O. (1958). "Pædiatric Surgery." New York: Appleton-Century-Crofts.
White, M., Dennison, W. M. (1958). "Surgery in Infancy and Childhood." Edinburgh: Livingstone.

lower bowel.   Where there is only stenosis, very small quantities of
food may find their way through.   The bowel distal to the obstruction
is undilated throughout its whole length.   X-ray shows a dilated
stomach and first part of the duodenum with a fluid level.

Mild degrees of duodenal stenosis may pass unnoticed until later
in childhood, when repeated attacks of vomiting, which may be
mistaken for bilious attacks, develop.   Barium meal will reveal the
diagnosis in most instances, but in others it can only be made at
laparotomy.

Incomplete rotation of the intestine may give rise to duodenal
obstruction due to bands or adhesions.   In infancy, the clinical
picture is in many ways like that of congenital pyloric stenosis; there
is marked vomiting with constipation, the infant fails to gain weight,
and is restless and crying.   The outstanding differences from pyloric
stenosis are the presence of bile in the vomit and the fact that the
vomiting usually starts from birth.   On examination, waves can be
seen passing from left to right across the epigastrium, but they pass far
out into the right flank.   The pylorus cannot be felt in such cases.
A barium meal confirms the diagnosis.   In older children, recurrent
bouts of bilious vomiting occur as in cases of duodenal stenosis.

In some cases of malrotation the partial obstruction from bands is
suddenly converted into an acute surgical emergency by the development of volvulus (p. 186).

PROGNOSIS AND TREATMENT

The outcome in cases of atresia is poor in the presence of mongolism.
The possibility of a second atresia distal to the first must not be
forgotten.   The post-operative management involves either intravenous therapy (p. 196) and gastric suction or feeding *via* a tube
passed through the anastomosis at the time of operation.

The cases which react best to surgical treatment are those in which
the obstruction is due to bands or adhesions which can be relieved
by direct operation.   Gastro-enterostomy may be necessary where the
bands cannot be freed.   In every case a laparotomy should be performed and the child given the advantages of surgical treatment.

Intestinal Atresia

Some cases of intestinal atresia are probably the result of a volvulus
occurring in fœtal life when the mid-gut is still outside the abdominal
cavity.   In such circumstances the portion of the mid-gut involved
undergoes aseptic necrosis and the two ends of the viable intestine
become sealed off.   This theory is of practical importance in the
planning of the subsequent surgical repair, since the blood supply in
the loop of mesentery proximal to the atretic end is often inadequate.
Thus it is essential that the surgeon should resect the proximal loop of
dilated bowel above the atresia before carrying out the anastomosis.

When the atresia is high up in the jejunum the picture may be indistinguishable from duodenal atresia. When the ileum or large bowel is affected, there is a picture of progressive vomiting of feeds and mucus, abdominal distension and absolute constipation except for the occasional passage of a little desquamated intestinal epithelium. If large numbers of squamous epithelial cells are present in the intestinal excretion, it can be said with certainty that complete atresia is not present, because such cells can only have come from the œsophagus or mouth (Farber's test). X-ray in the erect position shows distended coils of gut with fluid levels present. Clinically the condition may resemble meconium ileus (*see* p. 139).

The earlier the diagnosis is made the better will be the chance oɩ surgical cure. The maintenance of the fluid and electrolyte balance by intravenous therapy has greatly improved the survival rate of these infants. It is to be remembered, on the surgical side, that the atresia may be multiple and associated with congenital malrotation of the gut.

Volvulus

When the gut returns to the peritoneal cavity from the umbilical cœlome, it does so in an orderly manner—jejunum first, cæcum and colon last. Occasionally there are faults in this process which may result in abnormalities of rotation and of mesenteric fixation. A malrotated gut is liable to volvulus which may be partial and recurrent, or complete.

In volvulus there is twisting of a loop or loops of intestine. Though rare, it is most likely to occur as a complication of congenital malrotation of the gut, the usual site of obstruction being the duodeno-jejunal junction. Another cause is abnormal fixation of a loop of ileum by a persistent vitello-intestinal duct. Acute volvulus by twisting of a freely movable cæcum or loop of sigmoid colon is still rarer. Volvulus may sometimes occur in an abdomen full of adhesions following previous operations.

CLINICAL PICTURE

In acute cases the classical symptoms of obstruction are present, i.e. vomiting, pain, collapse. Blood may be present in the stool. Occasionally there are recurrent cases which undo themselves and pass for periodic bilious attacks extending through the first years of childhood (p. 212). In such cases, however, the abdomen is full and distended rather than scaphoid as in an ordinary bilious attack.

TREATMENT is surgical.

Meconium Ileus (p. 139).

Hirschsprung's Disease (p. 209).

Both these conditions may present as neonatal intestinal obstruction and must be considered in the differential diagnosis.

Intestinal Obstruction from Meconium Plug

Occasionally a plug of meconium in the rectum or distal part of the colon may become so solid as to obstruct the intestine. This diagnosis must always be considered in cases of low intestinal obstruction. Thus the passage of a catheter into the rectum followed by rectal and colonic washouts may relieve the condition without recourse to surgery. Occasionally, when the plug is higher in the colon, there is no alternative to laparotomy.

Imperforate Anus and Rectal Atresia

This may be due to a failure of absorption of the anal plate; only a narrow bar may separate the anal dimple and the rectum. In the majority of cases, it is associated with a greater or lesser degree of failure of development of the rectum.

The condition should be recognized at birth or certainly within the first 24 hours when it is realized that no meconium has been passed. An idea of the extent of the lesion may be gained by taking an x-ray of the inverted infant so that the air in the bowel collects in the highest possible point, a metallic marker denoting the position of the anal dimple.

The type of surgical procedure to be adopted depends upon the extent of the lesion. After an initial colostomy has been carried out, most patients require a major perineal operation at a later stage. It is useless to create an artificial anus without a sphincter and therefore the sphincteric muscle must be located. It is to be noted that fistulous communications with the genito-urinary system are frequently found in cases of rectal atresia. There may also be congenital malformations in other parts of the body.

Ectopic Anus

Occasionally the anus has an ectopic orifice, including the various perineal, vulval, and vaginal types. In addition, a normally positioned anus may have a fistulous communication with the vagina, or very rarely with the urethra or bladder in the male. The treatment is surgical.

INFECTIVE DISORDERS OF THE MOUTH

Moniliasis

Thrush is an infection of the mucous membrane and submucous tissues by *Monilia albicans*, the spores of which project from the surface and give the characteristic white appearance. Colonization by *Monilia* is favoured by oral antibiotics, notably those of the tetracycline series. Feeding utensils or *Monilia* vaginitis in the mother may be the source of infection. Thrush is rare, except in young infants, unless there is a predisposing cause, such as leukæmia, or unless antibiotics have been given.

CLINICAL PICTURE

The tongue, roof of the mouth and inside of the cheeks have a white, patchy or furred appearance, as if the infant had just been drinking creamy milk, and thin clots had been left sticking to the mucous membrane. An attempt to wipe these off, however, shows the patches to be firmly adherent to the tongue or cheek. The infection may be accompanied by vomiting and diarrhœa. In severe cases it may spread to the œsophagus and give rise to dysphagia. In other cases the infection may involve the larynx and cause symptoms of respiratory obstruction. Extension into the lungs may also occur.

TREATMENT

Oral thrush is treated by freshly prepared 1 per cent. aqueous solution of gentian violet or alternatively Dequadin paint applied to the mouth after feeds and until one week after the last spot has gone. Generalized infections require systemic nystatin (for dosage *see* p. 656). Antibiotics, by disturbing the normal bacterial flora of the mouth, favour the growth of *Monilia* organisms and are contra-indicated. Vitamin-B preparations encourage normal bacterial re-colonization. The possibility of vaginal thrush in the mother and re-infection from that source should be remembered.

Herpetic Stomatitis (Aphthous Stomatitis)

This is due to herpes simplex virus, and is often associated with herpes labialis. It may be very mild, causing a slight temperature only, with vesicles on the mucosa and tongue which rapidly give place to white or grey ulcers. There is usually some gingivitis. Very often, however, the infection is severe, accompanied by a high fever and much salivation, with secondary infection of the tongue, gums and mucosa. The child, usually aged from one to three, is unable to eat. There is loss of appetite, sleeplessness and general misery.

It is a self-limiting disease subsiding usually within seven days. Glycerin of borax B.P.C. has a soothing effect, whilst the local application of gentian violet, although not affecting the virus, may prevent secondary infections. Chemotherapy and antibiotics are to be avoided. Plenty of fluid is essential.

Herpes Labialis

Recurrent herpes labialis, particularly in association with any respiratory infection, may occur in children or adults in whom a chronic carrier state with the herpes simplex virus has occurred. Such infections are extremely difficult to eradicate, but it is said that, as some cross-immunity exists between the vaccinia virus and the herpes simplex virus, vaccination is sometimes helpful.

Herpangina (*see* p. 561).

In this condition a vesicular eruption develops on the posterior third of the tongue and palate and on the back of the pharynx due to infection with the *Coxsackie* B virus.

Geographical Tongue

This is a common condition and seems to have little significance. The tongue shows areas where the surface is pink and normal, interspaced with areas which are slightly raised and greyish. The shape of the normal areas may be round, or have a serpiginous edge, hence the name " geographical tongue." The cause of the condition is not known. Certainly it is not, as a rule, accompanied by ill-health and no treatment is required.

CONSTIPATION

Chronic Constipation

The term constipation is correctly applied when the stools are so hard that straining is caused and perhaps there is pain on defæcation. Constipation is also present when defæcation is incomplete and fæces are allowed to accumulate in the rectum. Sometimes, when the rectum is almost impacted, spurious " diarrhœa " occurs and fæcal soiling is then common. Infrequent defæcation, the bowels moving easily perhaps every other day, is no more abnormal than a habit of diurnal action of the bowel.

Chronic constipation is a feature of certain organic disorders such as cretinism and juvenile myxœdema. Local conditions, such as anal stenosis, have also to be considered. In addition the following causative factors must be remembered in cases of chronic constipation.

CONSTIPATION IN THE BREAST-FED INFANT

True constipation is less common than infrequent normal defæcation. The following are amongst the causes of constipation:

An insufficient intake of fluid, especially during the summer months. In addition to the breast, the child should be offered 4 to 6 oz. of water daily, either from a bottle or with a teaspoon from a cup.

Faulty training. The training to pass motions into a chamber should begin as soon as the child can sit up.

If the child has an *anal fissure* he fears defæcation. Ung. hamamelidis should be pressed into the anus both before and after a motion, and the motion kept soft with paraffin emulsion. Some toddlers have been so frightened by the pain that they still refuse to defæcate, and it may be necessary to give a preparation, such as bisacodyl, in a dosage sufficient to make a bowel action each day inevitable.

A certain number of children suffer from *congenital anal stenosis*, that is, the anus is actually too small and requires careful slow dilatation. This is best done by inserting a finger lubricated with soft paraffin. It should be done gently and with sedation if necessary.

In the *starved* or *underfed infant* constipation is often one of the first signs of failure of the milk supply.

CONSTIPATION IN THE ARTIFICIALLY-FED INFANT

The above remarks are also applicable in great measure to the artificially-fed infant, but in addition some other points must be stressed. The higher the proportion of protein in the diet, the more alkaline and constipated are the stools. On the other hand, the more fat and sugar present, the higher is the acid content, and the more likely the child is to have diarrhœa and sore buttocks.

When an infant is inclined to be constipated and the dietary sugar and fat content are not unduly high, a slight increase is indicated. For the occasional attack of constipation, a teaspoonful of cream of magnesia given first thing in the morning should be sufficient.

Puréed fruit and vegetables added to the diet may be helpful.

CONSTIPATION IN THE OLDER CHILD

Constipation in the older child has various causes and in its severest forms may be associated with overflow incontinence of fæces.

Faulty training in infancy. Insufficient care may have been attached to the emptying of the bowel or insufficient time devoted to this act, with the result that it is put off and neglected, with subsequent constipation. To correct this state of affairs, regular habits must be established, the child " sitting down " at the same time daily and, if unsuccessful, repeating the process later in the day. Poor housing with one lavatory shared by many families may be an important factor.

In the older child at school, it is essential that sufficient time be given for proper attention to the bowels.

Anal fissure or *hæmorrhoids* occur in some children. In all cases where pain is complained of, a careful examination should be made and the appropriate treatment applied. Following an anal fissure fear of painful defæcation may persist for months or years, and the consequent inhibition of normal action results in chronic constipation, often with overflow incontinence of fæces. Emotional maladjustment may be a result rather than a cause.

Chronic constipation of this type may have to be distinguished from Hirschsprung's disease, although the degree of abdominal distension is usually less. Rectal examination is decisive, for in Hirschsprung's disease the rectum is small and empty (*see* p. 209), whilst with chronic constipation the rectum is greatly dilated and filled with hard fæces.

The normal child who is getting *insufficient food*, or a diet low in cellulose, will tend to be constipated. The diet should contain wholemeal bread and cereals of all kinds, and especially vegetables and fruit, and a liberal supply of each of the last two should be present in every child's diet. It is seldom that green vegetables or raw or cooked fruit are given too freely, the great tendency being to provide children with an insufficient quantity of these items in the diet.

The diet of many children is *deficient in fluids*, especially in summer-time. In this way the motions become dry and crumbly. Drinks of water should be given on waking and, during warm weather, even between meals, and every child should drink from one pint to a pint and a half of fluid daily as a minimum. Quantities less than this will tend to produce a dry intestinal content.

MEDICINAL TREATMENT

Emulsion of petroleum and agar can be given to older children for a few weeks, but purgation should be avoided in cases of simple constipation, as it tends to leave the child more constipated than before.

In long continued cases of constipation in which the colon is loaded, following anal fissure or poor training, initial treatment with enemata is required. Repeated small enemata should be given until the colon has been emptied. A useful purgative for this type of case is:

Neostigmine Bromide	..	..	..	10 mg. ($\frac{1}{8}$ grain)
Magnesium Sulphate	..	..	..	1·3 G. (20 grains)
Paraffin Emulsion 50%	..	..	..	3·5 ml. (1 drachm)
Water	..	..	..	7·0 ml. (2 drachms)

Two teaspoonfuls are given twice daily and the dose is adjusted until a soft easy bowel action is achieved daily. This is maintained for several weeks during which time the atonicity of the bowel disappears and the dose is then gradually reduced as normal bowel action is established.

A methylcellulose-containing preparation or similar-acting compound, such as Normacol or Isogel, which helps to increase the bulk and water content of the stool, is valuable in the recovery stage.

DIARRHŒA IN INFANCY AND CHILDHOOD

CLASSIFICATION OF DIARRHŒA

1. *Infective diarrhœa:* (a) Due to known dysenteric organisms such as Sonne, Flexner, Shiga and the Newcastle bacillus. Also infestation with *Giardia lamblia* (p. 632). (b) Epidemic gastro-enteritis of infancy due to specific types of *Esch. coli* or viral infections.

2. *Dietetic diarrhœa* (due to over-feeding, particularly on fat and carbohydrate).

3. *Symptomatic diarrhœa* (e.g. diarrhœa secondary to some parenteral infection, such as otitis media, tonsillitis, pyelitis or pneumonia, which causes an accompanying intestinal upset).

The proportion of each group among the cases of diarrhœa in any summer, in any country, will depend upon the climate and hygienic conditions. Infective diarrhœa is commoner in hot, dusty climates than in temperate zones. In the United Kingdom there has been a welcome reduction in the mortality from gastro-enteritis since adequate precautions against cross-infection have been taken and the principles of correction of the electrolyte and fluid balance have been more widely understood.

Persistent diarrhœa is found in ulcerative colitis (p. 203) and in the low-grade, but persistent, entero-colitis which may follow an acute gastro-enteritis.

Dysentery

Infants and children are affected in dysentery epidemics in similar fashion to the adult population, except that small infants withstand these infections very poorly, and even such mild infections as Sonne dysentery may have a high mortality if a group of neonates (as in a maternity unit) is infected. In most cases, the disease runs a short course of fever and diarrhœa for 3 to 5 days, with blood and mucus in the stools and copious vomiting in those more severely affected. Dehydration and electrolyte depletion (p. 193) may ensue.

TREATMENT

In cases of dysentery, the treatment of choice is Sulphatriad and oral streptomycin. Neomycin may be tried in resistant cases (for dosage, *see* Appendix 1, p. 646). The correction of dehydration and electrolyte depletion in the more severe cases is described on p. 194.

Epidemic Gastro-enteritis of Infancy

Epidemic gastro-enteritis of this type is almost entirely confined to infants. Although older children and adults can carry the infecting organisms, they are not usually affected clinically. In some epidemics, pathogenic strains of *Esch. coli*, such as 055 and 011, have been isolated. On the other hand, they are by no means always found and it is suggested that some cases are viral in origin. Another theory suggests that any strain of *Esch. coli* may be pathogenic to an infant who has not previously been in contact with that strain and has inherited no passive immunity to it from his mother. Thus, many strains of *Esch. coli* might in the appropriate circumstances become pathogenic and give rise to infection.

It is of considerable interest that breast-fed infants very rarely suffer from epidemic gastro-enteritis, the mortality and most of the morbidity being confined to artificially fed infants.

Blood and mucus are occasionally present in the stools, but *post mortem* little or no inflammation of the small or large bowel is found. The liver is fatty, there is cloudy swelling of the kidneys and enlargement of the mesenteric glands. A terminal broncho-pneumonia is common.

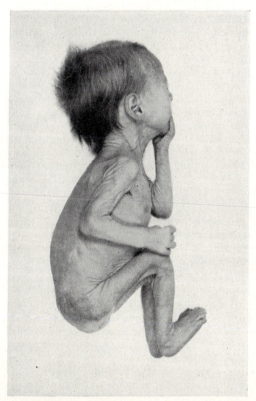

Fig. 15.—A female infant, 10 weeks old, showing pronounced wasting after a diarrhœal illness.

CLINICAL PICTURE

A previously perfectly healthy child develops acute diarrhœa and vomiting, with rapid dehydration, the skin becoming inelastic, the tongue furred and the fontanelle depressed; the stools finally consist of watery fluid. There is a low blood pressure and peripheral circulatory failure may develop.

In association with the dehydration, there is considerable biochemical disturbance, due to the loss of sodium, chloride and potassium, giving rise to a secondary metabolic acidosis.

PREVENTION

Since infantile gastro-enteritis is so highly infectious and potentially fatal, meticulous care must be taken to prevent its spread. This applies to any institution of any kind that accepts responsibility for a number of infants.

All infants admitted to an institution should be isolated from the remainder until it has been shown that they are not suffering from diarrhœa and that their stools do not contain pathogenic *Esch. coli* organisms. The greatest care should be taken to ensure that feeds are prepared under sterile conditions.

In hospital, separate gowns should be worn for the handling of each infant, and soiled linen and napkins must be transferred to a special sluice for disposal. The staff should be meticulous in their hand-washing technique before and after handling each infant.

When a case of clinical gastro-enteritis or a positive excretor of pathogenic *Esch. coli* organisms is encountered, the patient should be nursed away from uninfected infants in a cubicled isolation ward or in a hospital block dealing especially with infectious fevers.

TREATMENT

Deaths from gastro-enteritis in infancy are due to dehydration and electrolyte disturbance rather than to toxæmia. The most important aspect of treatment is the restoration and maintenance of fluid and electrolyte balance. The technique of treatment depends upon the severity of the symptoms.

(1) *Mild Cases.* Where gastro-enteritis is recognized early, or where the symptoms are so mild that dehydration has not occurred, it is sufficient to stop all milk feeds and to give the infant boiled water by mouth; this may be made more palatable by the addition of orange juice and glucose. The likelihood of vomiting is further diminished by giving small amounts at frequent intervals rather than larger four-hourly feeds. The infant should receive a minimum of 150 ml. of water per Kg. of expected body-weight (2½oz. per lb.) per day; details of the smaller requirements of infants in the first week of life are described on p. 81. To this total is added a further 300 ml. (10 oz.) of fluid to counteract the fluid loss from the intestinal tract. In mild cases, milk feeds can be re-introduced after twenty-four or forty-eight hours.

(2) *Moderate Cases.* Where there is evidence of slight or moderate dehydration, it may be necessary to supplement the oral fluid intake outlined above by means of subcutaneous fluid, for which purpose half-strength Hartmann's solution, made isotonic with dextrose, may be used as the standard solution. Where laboratory estimations of the serum electrolytes have helped to provide additional evidence of the extent of the loss of sodium and chloride from the gastro-intestinal tract, appropriate modifications may be made in the con-

centration of electrolytes to be given in the subcutaneous fluid. Thus, to infants in whom marked depletion of serum sodium and chloride has been demonstrated a proportion of the subcutaneous fluid is given as normal saline or normal Hartmann's solution; whilst for infants in whom the loss is primarily of water, without reduction of the reserves of sodium and chloride, a proportion of the subcutaneous fluid may be provided as 0·18 per cent. saline in 4·5 per cent. dextrose or as one-fifth normal Hartmann's solution made isotonic with dextrose. In this way, the contrasting complications may be avoided of *water intoxication* (see p. 196), due to the administration of parenteral fluid containing insufficient concentrations of electrolytes, on the one hand, and of *œdema from salt retention* caused by an excessive intake of parenteral sodium chloride, on the other. In more severe cases, repeated estimations of the serum electrolytes are needed to achieve satisfactory control during the period of rehydration.

Absorption of subcutaneous fluid is facilitated by the addition of Hyalase (1·0 ml.) to the infusion; by this means, 300 ml. of fluid may be given over a six- to twelve-hour period in addition to the oral fluids. Where vomiting persists despite the substitution of water for milk by mouth, a trial may be made of intragastric drip feeding. Where skilled nursing is in short supply, this technique is considerably safer than unsupervised intravenous fluid therapy, to which, in moderately severe cases, it provides a suitable alternative; in the most severe cases there is no choice but intravenous therapy.

In all cases the loss of potassium from the intestinal tract should be corrected by giving potassium chloride (0·5 G.) orally twice or three times a day.

After twenty-four hours of treatment with intragastric feeding, or water and subcutaneous fluids, the infant is usually able to retain the total daily fluid requirement given orally. This means that a moderate case has been converted into a mild case and can be treated as such (*see* under (1), p. 194).

(3) *Severe Cases.* Where severe dehydration is already present and where the clinical picture is complicated by peripheral circulatory failure, all oral feeding is stopped and immediate intravenous fluid is essential. The basic fluid requirement, 150 ml. per Kg. of expected body-weight per day, is given intravenously. This is supplemented, in the first twenty-four hours, by an additional allowance for correction of the dehydration. The amount varies with the weight of the infant but may be between 300 and 600 ml. of fluid in addition to the normal daily requirement; the greater part of this supplement can be given in the first six hours of treatment. After one to two days on intravenous therapy alone, clear fluids are slowly re-introduced by mouth, the total daily requirement being divided at first between the oral and the intravenous routes. Subsequently, the infant is given the full total daily requirement, as clear fluids, orally, and this is followed later by a careful re-introduction of diluted milk feeds.

It is usually preferable for intravenous fluid to be given by scalp vein; alternatively, the internal saphenous vein is exposed at the ankle and a fine polyethylene tube is inserted. The fluid is run through a special vacolitre attachment, calibrated in single ml. units, so that the calculated amount of fluid (usually between 10–30 ml. each hour) may be given accurately. A record of the intravenous fluid intake should be recorded on an hourly basis.

(4) *Selection of Intravenous Fluid.* The choice of intravenous fluid depends upon the extent to which electrolyte disturbance has been incurred either from vomiting or diarrhœa, or both. In some cases there may be considerable loss of chloride from intense vomiting, whilst with diarrhœa loss of base (sodium) may give rise to severe metabolic acidosis. Diarrhœa may also cause a serious loss of potassium. Thus, the choice of solution is governed by the type of electrolyte disturbance that is present. In most cases, during initial resuscitation, some normal saline or normal Hartmann's solution may be required in quantities varying between 200 and 500 ml. depending upon the weight and maturity of the infant.

The initial phase is followed by the correction of the metabolic acidosis, and at this stage 0·18 per cent. saline in 4·5 per cent. dextrose, rather than Hartmann's solution, should be the basic intravenous solutions so that the required amount of sodium lactate solution to be added can be easily calculated.

The normal bicarbonate content of the plasma in infancy is 20–25 mEq/litre or 40–65 vols. per cent. of CO_2. In severe acidosis the figure may be reduced to as low as 6–10 mEq/litre or 13–22 vols. per cent. of CO_2. In general terms 4 ml. of M/6 sodium lactate per Kg. of body-weight will raise the plasma bicarbonate by about 1·0 mEq/litre, or 2·2 vols. per cent. of CO_2. It is considered advisable to add only the amount of M/6 sodium lactate solution which will raise the plasma bicarbonate to the lowest normal figure. The calculated amount should be added to the intravenous solution.

Potassium depletion is an important consideration in all cases of gastro-enteritis. The giving of additional potassium may cause a dramatic improvement in the clinical condition and is an essential part of treatment in all but the mildest cases. Potassium loss can usually be corrected by giving 0·5–1·0 G. of potassium chloride by mouth daily. In very severe cases with persistent diarrhœa it may be given intravenously, but only after the dehydration has been corrected and a good flow of urine re-established. It should be given intravenously in quantities of not more than 3 mEq per Kg. of body-weight per day and can be added to the general intravenous infusion.

(5) *Water Intoxication*[1]. Whereas dehydration is easily recognized, this is not true of the opposite condition, water intoxication, which

[1] Hill, F. S. (1954). "Practical Fluid Therapy in Pediatrics." Philadelphia and London: Saunders.

TABLE XVI

HARTMANN'S SOLUTION

(Liquor Ringer-Lactatis) (Supplement to B.P.C. 1934.   Part III, Formulary 1941)

Lactic acid	2·4 ml.	(23 minims)
Solution of sodium hydroxide	A sufficient quantity to neutralize the lactic acid	
Sodium chloride	6·0 G.	(52½ grains)
Potassium chloride	0·4 G.	(3½ grains)
Calcium chloride	0·2 G.	(1¼ grains)
Distilled water to	1,000·0 ml.	(20 fl. oz.)

develops when the quantity of water in the body is greater than the quantity of electrolytes and solutes.   This can happen when dilute electrolyte solutions, for example, glucose, are given by intravenous and other routes in excess of requirements.   The danger is greatest in young infants, in cases of adrenogenital insufficiency, and in oliguria from any cause.   The administration of water and a low intake of sodium and potassium causes a fall in serum electrolytes.   Then, when the extracellular fluids become *hypotonic*, water moves into the cells and this causes progressive cellular dysfunction; a woody œdema of the skin and muscles is characteristic of this stage.

Water intoxication is a dangerous condition and its recognition is apt to be deferred.   The affected child may give a deceptive impression of well-being, because any wasting is hidden and the child may have a good colour.   The outstanding symptoms are in the nervous system and usually appear before the interstitial spaces expand sufficiently to produce pitting œdema.   Convulsions and signs of respiratory failure then draw attention to the gravity of the situation.

The diagnosis can be made in a child who has been energetically rehydrated on the following data: Clinical picture; calculation of the amount of fluid administered; output of urine; condition of the skin; undue heaviness of the limbs; and the fact that there has been a dramatic increase in weight in the last 6–18 hours.   The diagnosis is confirmed by finding a reduction in serum electrolytes.

Immediate treatment is to stop fluid administration.   If convulsions are occurring, hypertonic saline is indicated in quantities just sufficient to relieve the symptoms.   Should the respirations become shallow, or perhaps cease, mechanical respiration is required.   Anoxia is the main danger for it may cause permanent cerebral damage.

(6) *Re-introduction of milk feed.*   (1) Breast-milk if obtainable. (2) Half-cream dried milk, with or without lactic acid (e.g. half-cream Lacidac, Cow and Gate Ltd.).   (3) Boiled milk, with or without lactic acid (babies over 6 months dislike lactic acid milk).   (4) Unsweetened evaporated milk.

The strength of the feed is gradually increased from quarter to half and, finally, to full strength. Sugar should be carefully introduced when a half-strength milk mixture is reached. The speed at which the strength of the feeds can be increased varies; a recurrence of vomiting or diarrhœa will indicate the need for temporary return to clear fluids.

(7) *Warmth and oxygen* should be available for all seriously ill infants. Where circulatory collapse occurs, hydrocortisone should be given intravenously in full amounts (for dosage, *see* p. 660). Methedrine 0·5 mg. intramuscularly is given to correct the fall in blood pressure.

(8) *Antibiotics.* Neomycin and colomycin are the antibiotics of choice. They are given orally (for dosages, *see* p. 655).

Dietetic Diarrhœa

Badly balanced feeds, such as those with a high-fat or unduly high-sugar content, are usually responsible.

CLINICAL PICTURE

Unlike infective gastro-enteritis, the onset is slow and insidious. There is at first a failure to gain in weight and a tendency to refuse food, with finally a slight rise in temperature. The infant is not very ill in the initial stages but, unless the error in diet is corrected and the management improved, the condition may change into mild dehydration. At first, curds or frothy motions are passed; later, with increased peristalsis, the stools become bright green or resemble chopped spinach and burn the infant's buttocks. Vomiting may or may not be a feature.

TREATMENT

In slight and early cases, the feed should be corrected and special attention given to preventing ærophagia. In more severe cases, the milk feed should be stopped for 24 hours, at least the same volume of quarter-strength saline being given in its place. After this period of rest, it is usually possible to re-introduce a suitable feed.

Symptomatic Diarrhœa (Parenteral Infection)

The commonest cause is a respiratory infection. Often there is coryza or otitis media—quite unsuspected. Pyelitis may show itself only as gastro-enteritis. Too often the attention of the mother and doctor is diverted by the diarrhœa, and the real cause is overlooked.

It is obvious, therefore, that a thorough clinical examination, including the ears and urine, should be made in every case of gastro-enteritis. Why an infection in some other part of the body should cause diarrhœa is not understood.

The first step is to treat the underlying infection. Secondly the infant should be taken off its feeds and put on to quarter-strength saline by mouth only. The treatment of dehydration and the re-introduction of a normal diet has been described on pp. 194–198.

OTHER GASTRO-INTESTINAL DISORDERS

Peptic Ulcer

Although peptic ulceration of the stomach or duodenum is still primarily a disorder of adults, an increasing number of cases are being recognized in adolescents and older children. It is difficult to say whether this represents a true increase in incidence or more accuracy in diagnosis. In this age group, the pain may not be as typical of peptic ulceration as in the adult and an onset with hæmatemesis or melæna with little previous history of abdominal pain is not un-common.

It is to be remembered also that a silent peptic ulceration may be a complication of steroid therapy, symptoms only occurring when actual perforation occurs.

Small erosions giving rise to minor hæmatemesis may occur in acute gastritis from such cases as aspirin sensitivity. Aspirin is a not in-frequent cause.

Medical treatment of the acute episodes is similar to that employed in adult medicine; the emotional background may provide the reasons for the disease and suggest ways in which recurrences may be pre-vented (*see* Chapter 18).

Acute Appendicitis

This is the most common, and may be the most serious, of all the inflammatory abdominal conditions. Early diagnosis is of the utmost importance.

ÆTIOLOGY AND PATHOLOGY

Appendicitis may occur at any age. Under three years of age, the diagnosis is more difficult and the mortality higher. There is no sex predominance. By some it is claimed to be due to an infection gaining entrance to the blood-stream, possibly through the mucous membrane of the bowel or through the tonsils, and passing directly to the appendix. Others contend that it is a local abscess, starting in the lymphoid tissue of the appendix, due to kinking or blocking of the appendicular lumen; occasionally, threadworms filling the appendix may be associated with a typical attack. There is ground for believing that in some cases there may be connection with respiratory tract infections, as in schools and institutions. Once the organ has become inflamed it may be distended and congested; this inflammation may extend through the walls to the peritoneal coat and set up local or general peritonitis. In a very virulent or severe infection, local gangrene may develop, with perforation, the fæcal contents of the appendix finding their way directly into the abdomen. Where the omentum becomes adherent in the region of the appendix, the area becomes shut off and an abscess may form.

SYMPTOMS AND DIAGNOSIS

The chief symptoms are *abdominal pain* accompanied by *vomiting, with tenderness and rigidity of the lower right rectus at McBurney's point.* The clinical picture varies with the site of the appendix and the stage of the disease. When the appendix is retrocæcal, the clinical picture is often atypical, pain and tenderness being much less marked than in the average case and located, perhaps, in the loin. Often the symptoms are so slight that they are taken for an ordinary bilious attack. Fever is not constant but is usually present, especially in the smaller children, and is rarely above 100·8° F unless perforation of the appendix and peritonitis are present. Pelvic appendicitis in small children often commences with diarrhœa and may, particularly in times of influenza epidemics, easily be mistaken for an attack of enteritis. In every case a rectal examination should be made. In doubtful cases the very greatest importance should be attached to the time of onset of the pain. Pain which precedes vomiting is significant; pain which follows vomiting, especially if much retching has occurred, is of rather less diagnostic significance. Tenderness and rigidity or spasm of the abdominal muscles, coupled with abdominal pain, make the diagnosis complete.

Where diagnosis has been delayed, the eyes are sunken and the tongue furred and dry. The pulse is raised out of proportion to the degree of fever and is bounding. As a rule, constipation is obstinate, but occasionally there may be a tendency to small infrequent motions.

DIFFERENTIAL DIAGNOSIS

Usually the diagnosis is easily made, but occasionally appendicitis may be mistaken for a *bilious attack*. In such cases the absence of abdominal pain, with tenderness and rigidity, should be of some help. In the retrocæcal type, however, there is a close similarity between the two, and a rectal examination will help to decide the diagnosis. *Migraine* in childhood, with marked abdominal symptoms, may simulate appendicitis. *Diaphragmatic pleurisy* and *right-sided pneumonia* may present a similar picture in the early stages, but the general appearance of the child should here assist the diagnosis; the face is flushed, the respirations are increased, and a rectal examination does not reveal tenderness. *Prodomal infective hepatitis* can be a difficulty.

Inguinal and mesenteric adenitis, when the group of glands deep in the inguinal region on the right side become inflamed, may be difficult to distinguish from appendicitis. The general systemic upset is less marked as a rule, and colicky pains tend to pass off rapidly. Fortunately, this condition is rare. *Infection of the right kidney* may simulate appendicitis closely, but an examination of the urine should settle this point. In *general peritonitis due to the pneumococcus*, tenderness is present throughout the whole abdomen, toxæmia is extreme, and pain has not been limited at any time to the right iliac fossa. Only by local examination and consideration of the child as a whole can a differential diagnosis be made; laparotomy may decide the diagnosis. *Acute follicular tonsillitis* and *acute otitis media* are sometimes accompanied by colicky pains about the umbilicus (*umbilical colic*). The mode of production of these pains has not been satisfactorily explained, but they are universally recognized. With the subsidence of the tonsillitis the pain disappears. *Henoch's purpura* (p. 342) must also be considered.

PROGNOSIS

The sooner the diagnosis is made and treatment instituted, the better the prognosis. Once general peritonitis has supervened, the mortality rises, especially in children under the age of six. With early diagnosis and efficient surgical treatment, the mortality is less than 1 per cent., but it rises when peritonitis is already established.

TREATMENT

The treatment is surgical. Antibiotics are a valuable part of the post-operative management of cases where peritonitis is present.

Chronic or Recurrent Appendicitis

The question whether true chronic appendicitis occurs in childhood is debatable. Probably, the term *recurrent appendicitis* is much nearer the truth, but even recurrent appendicitis must be considered rare.

SYMPTOMS AND CLINICAL PICTURE

After a mild or subacute attack of appendicitis, with fever, pain, vomiting and tenderness, the symptoms may subside and the whole illness may be regarded as merely a bilious attack. Some weeks or even months later there may be a recurrence, this time possibly with sharp, stabbing pains or nausea, coated tongue, lassitude and a low, " grumbling " temperature. The temperature may never have properly settled between the first attack and the second, although on examination between the exacerbations there is little or nothing to be found. Such recurrences may go on for some months or even years before the child is seen in one of the attacks and a diagnosis is made.

DIFFERENTIAL DIAGNOSIS

Some of the conditions which may simulate recurrent appendicitis are inflamed abdominal glands, tuberculous or otherwise, pyelitis, intermittent hydronephrosis, calculus, ulcerated Meckel's diverticulum, a partial volvulus, recurrent intussusception, follicular tonsillitis with so-called umbilical colic, or cyclic vomiting attacks. It is only by keeping such conditions as these in mind and excluding each, when possible, that a correct diagnosis can be made.

In a series of suspected cases submitted for x-ray examination, no very real help was obtained. The barium certainly passed readily into the majority of normal appendices, but where it did not, no definite evidence of disease was necessarily found at operation.

Very often the question of appendicitis is raised in children with recurrent abdominal pain (see p. 210), particularly where other members of the family have had appendicitis recently.

Chronic constipation in childhood, giving rise to vague abdominal pain, and quite often severe colic when purges are used, is often mistaken for recurrent appendicular trouble. Such a child, put on a proper régime with suitable treatment, rapidly loses his symptoms (see p. 189).

Primary Pneumococcal Peritonitis

This is now a rare disease, seen more often in girls than boys, especially between the years of three and seven. It was much commoner among the poor than the well-to-do. It has been shown that the majority of the patients have previously suffered from vulvo-vaginitis and that virulent pneumococci may be obtained from the vagina in such cases. The infection starts in the pelvis and is probably the result of an ascending infection from the vagina, through the genital tract.

CLINICAL PICTURE

Both before and at the onset of the infection, there is diarrhœa. Abdominal pain varies and may be misleading; usually, the pain is less than would be expected and it may be slight or absent. The onset is acute, with high fever and delirium suggesting pneumonia. At this stage there is usually septicæmia with a positive blood culture. Later, there is abdominal discomfort or pain, with a gradually increasing tumidity of the abdomen, which is tender. The temperature continues high for some days and tends to settle gradually. The full and tumid abdomen gradually becomes more doughy, and loculated areas of pus may be made out. The intestines are matted together and may show ladder patterns.

DIFFERENTIAL DIAGNOSIS

The acute onset may suggest appendicitis, and it is with this in mind that operation is generally undertaken. Again, if the condition has gone on for a few days, the picture may somewhat resemble typhoid fever, with delirium, a tumid, slightly tender abdomen and diarrhœa. The sudden onset, the delirium and the presence of pus in the peritoneal cavity, and the fact that the patients as a rule are girls should point to the correct diagnosis.

TREATMENT

It is probably wise, despite the availability of antibiotics, to make a small incision, recover the organism and insert a drainage tube. Penicillin in full doses is the drug of choice.

PROGNOSIS

Those cases in which a residual abscess forms recover completely when this is drained. The mortality before the days of chemo-therapy was about 50 per cent. but is now greatly reduced.

Secondary Pneumococcal Peritonitis

This rarely follows on a pneumonia but should be still included among the possible complications of pneumonia. It may be accom-panied by pneumococcal infections of other serous cavities such as the middle ear, pleura and pericardium. It may appear during the œdematous phase of the nephrotic syndrome.

Colitis

Acute entero-colitis or acute infection of the intestinal tract with pathogenic organisms has already been mentioned in the description of infective diarrhœa (p. 191). The characteristic of this condition is the presence not only of mucus but also of blood in the stools, and *post mortem* there is often a definite ulceration of the mucous membrane of the bowel. In all cases of long-standing diarrhœa without severe constitutional upset, *giardiasis* (*see* p. 632) should be thought of and the cysts sought in the stools.

Chronic Ulcerative Colitis

This is comparatively rare in childhood; it may commence in infancy but is usually seen in older children. There is usually a history of bouts of loose stools, containing blood and mucus, at intervals, over a prolonged period. Occasionally, a case is seen which follows immediately on what appears to be an acute dysenteric infection. Until a fulminating episode occurs, some children may be surprisingly well nourished, particularly those with regional colitis confined to a small area in the colon. On the whole, however, such patients are wasted, anæmic and fail to thrive. Recurrent jaundice is a rare complication.

Patterns of emotional stress, comparable to those seen in adult patients with ulcerative colitis, are found in Indian children. In others, the child's temperament and the environmental background appear no different from that of many healthy children.

Recently Truelove[1] has suggested that milk may play a part in provoking attacks and relapses in some patients with ulcerative colitis.

[1] Truelove, S. C. (1961). *Brit. med. J.*, 1, 154.

DIAGNOSIS

This can best be made by sigmoidoscopy, followed by barium-enema examination. A tuberculin test should always be made. As a rule, the sedimentation rate will be found to be high, and a blood-count shows well-marked anæmia.

TREATMENT

The long-term responsibility for the management of a patient with ulcerative colitis is not an enviable one. On the one hand, it is suggested[1] that without operation 1 in 5 of all such patients will eventually develop colonic carcinoma; on the other hand, it is likely that adequate surgery will involve the formation of a permanent ileostomy for the patient. The problem of eventual development of carcinoma, however, is not the immediate question in childhood; indeed, it may be that this incidence is somewhat exaggerated if all cases including the least severely affected are included.

In the first instance, therefore, the line of treatment is medical with recourse to surgery only if the progress of the disease cannot be adequately controlled.

Medical Treatment. All but the mildest cases should be treated by rest in bed initially, and sedation with phenobarbitone should be given (dosage, *see* p. 664). The diet should be of a low residue type and a therapeutic trial of a milk-free diet (*see* above) may be attempted.

In fulminating cases, a blood transfusion followed by intravenous therapy may be an essential preliminary to other lines of treatment. For such severe episodes it is essential also to start the patient on full treatment with systemic ACTH or corticosteroids (for dosage, *see* p. 660) together with sulphasalazine (dosage, *see* p. 648). In less severe attacks sulphasalazine may first be tried alone; if no improvement occurs, local treatment to the rectum and colon by means of daily retention enemata containing prednisolone 21-phosphate (for dosage, *see* p. 660) should be tried in addition. If an improvement is still not attained, systemic corticotrophin or prednisone should be given as in the more fulminating cases. Surgery may be indicated if these medical measures fail to control the progress of the disease (the types of procedure are described below).

Long-term Management. About equally good results are obtained in maintaining patients in clinical remissions by long-term treatment either with sulphasalazine or with local retention enemata containing hydrocortisone or prednisolone 21-phosphate.[2] In this connection the real dangers of prolonged steroid therapy to any patient must be borne in mind (*see* p. 661); thus, no patient should be left on prolonged systemic steroid therapy unless there is no satisfactory alternative. It is wise to continue with a low residue diet and with maintenance treatment with phenobarbitone.

[1] Slaney, G., Brooke, B. N. (1959). *Lancet*, 2, 694.
[2] Watkinson, G. (1961). *Brit. med. J.*, 1, 147.

Surgery. As has been indicated, the decision when to employ surgery in ulcerative colitis is an extremely difficult one. A progressive course to the disease despite all the medical measures previously suggested is a clear indication, but it is equally important that the patient should not be allowed to have become so ill as to make the surgical procedure unduly hazardous. A simple ileostomy may be carried out as an emergency measure in seriously ill patients. For long term surgical cure (a problem more for the adult than the child patient) total colectomy with a permanent ileostomy seems to be the treatment of choice at present.

MECHANICAL DEFECTS

Inguinal Hernia

By far the commonest site of rupture or hernia is in the inguinal region. Here, there is a continuation of the peritoneum down into the scrotum or towards the labia. This type of hernia is present in a proportion of 9 males to 1 female.

CLINICAL PICTURE

As a rule, inguinal hernia is present at birth, or shortly after birth, and is first noticed as a swelling in the scrotum, much more marked when the infant is crying. When the child is quiescent the lump seems to disappear. It may be present on one or both sides. On examination, slight pressure will often replace the hernia with a gurgle, showing that it contains bowel. The size of the hernial ring can be ascertained by passing the little finger up the inguinal canal, Occasionally, a hydrocele accompanies or is mistaken for a hernia.

Irreducible Hernia. Should the rupture become firm and tense, the following procedure should be attempted. The infant is laid on a pillow with the head considerably lower than the buttocks. A feed is given to quieten him. When quite quiet and sucking, gentle pressure is exerted over the mass and an effort made to replace the rupture. Force must not be used or the gut may rupture. In a proportion of cases the hernia does not reduce and operative treatment is necessary.

Strangulated Hernia. Where an inguinal hernia is associated with pain and symptoms of intestinal obstruction, immediate surgical treatment is indicated.

TREATMENT

Surgical repair is necessary; many surgeons are now prepared to operate on all cases in the early months of infancy, unless some medical contra-indication exists. One of the authors has seen an infant who had twice undergone operation for repair of an inguinal hernia and in which the hernia had recurred a third time; the presence of marked hypotonia due to undiagnosed cretinism had not previously been appreciated. Other causes of hypotonia and persistent cough must be looked for and dealt with before operation is carried out.

Umbilical Hernia

This is common in African races. Sex incidence is equal. It tends to spontaneous cure. By the age of two years the umbilical hernia has disappeared in most cases, while in the remainder it is much reduced in size. In infancy, efficiently applied strapping, or a rubber truss, is probably helpful. Hypotonic, flabby, weakly children, such as cretins and mongols, tend to have widely separated rectus muscles and umbilical hernia. Children with rickets, cœliac disease and, indeed, any general disease giving rise to flabby musculature are also liable to umbilical hernia. The treatment of the general condition of such children is essential if a spontaneous cure of the hernia is to be expected. If the rupture persists after the age of five years, surgical treatment should be undertaken.

Intussusception

ÆTIOLOGY

Intussusception is slightly more frequent in boys than in girls, and is commonest between the ages of 6 and 18 months, although it may occur at any age. The patients are usually vigorous, strong children. Food indiscretions have long been considered the primary cause, acting, it is thought, by causing a gastro-enteritis which inflames the lymphoid tissue, especially about the cæcum. The nodule of lymphoid tissue serves as a starting-point from which the intussusception moves forward. A polypus or congenital malformation, such as a duplication of the bowel or Meckel's diverticulum, will also act in the same way. Zachary and Potter[1] have shown that cases of intussusception may coincide with outbreaks of adenovirus infection. These viruses have been found in the fæces and the mesenteric lymph-nodes in a significant proportion of patients but are not the only cause of the condition.[2]

VARIETIES

The most common form is the ileocæcal in which the ileum becomes invaginated into the cæsum, passing up the ascending colon and onward. The next most common is the ileo-colic; then the purely enteric intussusception of the small intestine only. Finally, there is the pure colic type.

CLINICAL PICTURE

A well-nourished child, usually breast-fed, between the ages of 6 and 9 months, suddenly vomits and screams with colic; he looks grey

[1] Zachary, R. B., Potter, C. W. (1961). *Proc. roy. Soc. Med.*, **54**, 1018.
[2] Knox, E. G., Court, D. M., Gardner, P. S. (1962). *Brit. med. J.*, 2, 692.

and ill. The attack may pass off, to be followed quickly by another and yet another at varying intervals of a few minutes. Very often this is followed by a stool containing blood and some mucus, which may be repeated. In some cases the appearance of blood and mucus in the stools is a late finding and its absence should not preclude the making of the diagnosis at an earlier stage. Between attacks of pain the child may appear quite bright, although not himself. Careful palpation of the abdomen reveals a sausage-shaped mass, usually lying transversely across the abdomen. The mass may be soft and difficult to feel, but with continued palpation it hardens under the hand, so that it is unmistakable. On rectal examination, the end of the mass may be felt if it has travelled round to the sigmoid, but usually nothing can be discerned. On withdrawal, however, the finger is covered with blood and mucus. If any doubt exists a barium enema will reveal the lesion, provided that the colon is involved. Such an examination may sometimes reduce an intussusception.

PROGNOSIS

If the case is taken early, the outlook is excellent, but the mortality rises steeply after 24 hours. After 48 hours the outlook is bad.

DIFFERENTIAL DIAGNOSIS

The commonest mistake is to confuse an acute entero-colitis with intussusception. In the former, blood and mucus are present in the motions, the child is collapsed and there may be vomiting. The attacks of pain are not so severe nor so frequent. The temperature is high. An examination reveals no mass and the motions are frequent, although small. Other conditions to be excluded are Henoch's purpura and abdominal tuberculosis.

TREATMENT

The treatment in most centres is still surgical and should be instituted at once, but in expert and careful hands non-operative reduction by barium enema under screen control may sometimes succeed.

Recurrent Intussusception

This usually occurs in older children, but may be found in infants. A child may have attacks of abdominal pain at intervals for some weeks, and on examination a mass is found. Meanwhile, motions are passed and blood is unlikely to be present. In this group the intussusception is usually secondary to some other lesion, such as a polypus, an inflamed appendix, Meckel's diverticulum or an inflamed Peyer's patch. The treatment is surgical.

Meckel's Diverticulum

The persistence of a Meckel's diverticulum in extrauterine life may give rise to varied symptoms. In the first place, if ectopic gastric mucosa is present in the diverticulum, ulceration may occur which will give rise to periodic pain occurring shortly after meals. As a result of such ulceration, there may be hæmorrhage with repeated episodes of melæna of varying severity. Sometimes there is actual perforation with general or localized peritonitis. If abnormal mesenteric bands attached to the diverticulum are present, intestinal obstruction or volvulus may occur (*see* p. 186). The diverticulum may also be the leading point of an intussusception.

In all these conditions laparotomy is required.

Volvulus

This condition is most commonly the result of a congenital mal-rotation of the intestine and is described on p. 186.

Acute Intestinal Obstruction due to Adhesions

In children who have had previous abdominal operations, such as appendicectomy, acute obstruction, with vomiting and abdominal distension, is a rare complication resulting from the presence of adhesions from the first operation.

Prolapse of the Rectum

INCIDENCE

Prolapse of the rectum is quite common, the incidence being about equal in the two sexes. It may occur at any age, but is most frequent between one and three years.

ÆTIOLOGY AND PATHOLOGY

A general lack of muscular tone is an important predisposing cause and, contrary to expectation, diarrhœa accompanies the prolapse almost as often as constipation. Prolapse is frequent in cases of cœliac disease and cystic fibrosis of the pancreas. With constant, frequent stools there is much loss of the intrapelvic fat, especially in the ischio-rectal region. The rectum is not supported properly, the sphincter becomes lax and there is a protrusion at the anus, at first very slight, but finally a large extrusion, as big as a tangerine orange, may be seen. Bleeding from this surface and ulceration are common, and there may be difficulty in replacing the mass.

The condition is particularly troublesome in children with lesions of the sacral plexus, such as a lumbar meningo-myelocele or sacral dysgenesis, in which permanent cure is not possible.

TREATMENT

The mass may be replaced by covering it with a piece of clean lint or muslin, placing the whole hand over it and gently pressing. Once the mass is replaced, the buttocks should be strapped tightly together. The stools should be kept soft by giving liquid paraffin emulsion to prevent straining and recurrence of the prolapse. This treatment should be continued for some months to allow the *sphincter ani* to recover its tone where this is possible. Treatment should be given at once for the underlying causes. The injection of sclerosing agents, such as one per cent. phenol in almond oil, into the peri-rectal tissue is now seldom required.

Hirschsprung's Disease: Congenital Megacolon

ÆTIOLOGY

This rare, inherited congenital malformation consists of a developmental defect of the parasympathetic ganglion cells in the wall of the terminal colon. With few exceptions it affects males and has an incidence of about 1 in 20,000 to 1 in 30,000 births. It may appear in more than one member of a family, and in affected families the predicted incidence is about 1 in 5 for males, although very small for females. The exact mode of inheritance has not been determined (partial male-sex limitation).

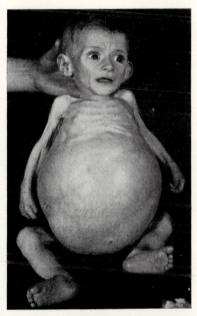 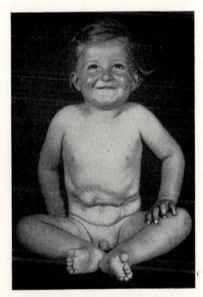

Fig. 16.—*Left:* **Hirschsprung's disease in a 5-month-old boy who was treated by rectosigmoidectomy.** *Right:* **The patient aged 1 year and 9 months.**

PATHOLOGY

The ganglion cells of the intramural plexus of the colon normally transmit impulses which relax its circular muscle. In Hirschsprung's disease, these nerve cells are absent from a segment of narrowed colon extending upwards from the rectum for a variable distance. Exceptionally, this segment is longer, extending even to the splenic flexure and beyond, but usually it is only a few inches. The lack of parasympathetic function means that there can be no co-ordinated peristalsis in the narrow segment, and unopposed sympathetic action causes tonic contraction. Above the aganglionic segment there is an active type of megacolon, with dilatation, hypertrophy and often visible peristalsis.

CLINICAL PICTURE

The severity of the symptoms depends on the length of the aganglionic spastic segment of colon. The long-segment variety comprises not more than 10 per cent. of cases and in these death from obstruction may take place in the neonatal period unless surgical treatment is undertaken. The short-segment type is less dangerous but there is more or less intractable constipation with increasing distension; much gas collects in the colon and peristalsis is very active (Fig. 16). There may be attacks of obstruction. Growth is likely to be stunted and there may be anæmia. The rectum is small and usually empty. This is a diagnostic point of some importance, differentiating the condition from the forms of secondary constipation, due to poor training, in which the rectum is greatly dilated and full of hard fæces. The passage of a tube from the rectum into the enlarged colon often results in much flatus. Characteristically, the stools are fragmented and narrow in calibre. The spasm of the distal segment of colon and its length of involvement can be shown if the initial flow of a barium enema is closely observed by fluoroscopy.

TREATMENT

This consists in the removal of the defective innervated distal segment of colon and rectum (rectosigmoidectomy). Mild cases have been treated with fairly large, divided doses of liquid paraffin, enemata, and the use of the flatus tube at intervals when required. Radical operation is more satisfactory.

FUNCTIONAL DISORDERS

Recurrent Abdominal Pain

THERE are few commoner symptoms in pædiatric practice than recurrent abdominal pain. For a full description of the problem the reader is referred to the account by Dr. John Apley.[1]

[1] Apley, J. (1959). "The Child with Abdominal Pains." Oxford: Blackwell Scientific Publications.

To some extent the referral of all discomfiture to the abdomen must be deep rooted in the minds of all children. That the abdomen may continue after infancy to be a centre for gratification or distress is not surprising. Only as the body image enlarges and the individual becomes more concerned with his own diverse physical potentialities may certain organic pains be referred to their rightful locality in the body and stress reactions become related to more selective functions.

It has been shown by Apley and others that in not more than five per cent. of children complaining of recurrent abdominal pain is any organic cause detectable. This means, however, that the physician consulted about the pain has a duty to diagnose accurately this small but important proportion of his patients with varying organic diseases. In this group will be included such diverse conditions as recurrent appendicitis, mesenteric adenitis whether of tuberculous or viral origin, peptic ulcer either in the stomach, duodenum or Meckel's diverticulum, colic from severe constipation, pain caused by over-enthusiastic purgation by the parents, urinary infections and other urological disorders, spontaneous hypoglycæmia, abdominal migraine, referred pains from spinal disease and muscular strain or traumatic fat necrosis in the abdominal wall, to mention only a few. There is also the group of children whose tastes in food are catholic and whose eating speed is remarkable; that such children should suffer from time to time from indigestion and colic is perhaps not always more than they deserve.

The sifting out of this group of children with organically determined abdominal pain is less formidable than might appear at first sight. The basic principles of medicine apply: a careful unhurried account of the history, given in their own words first by the parents and separately by the child, followed by a full physical examination, including an examination of the urine, will provide the essential information in the great majority of patients. The information thus obtained will enable the physician to divide his patients into three groups: (1) A few who probably have organic pain and will need further investigation along orthodox lines; (2) a large number in whom the pain is probably not organically determined but who will need handling in the manner described below; and (3) a third group about whom the physician is undecided. It may be said, perhaps unkindly, that the size of this third group varies inversely with the time expended in taking the history and carrying out the examination.

If after one or more consultations the physician considers that a child's abdominal pain is not organically determined, then a plan of campaign must be made. In the authors' opinion it is wrong at this stage for the doctor to prescribe a bottle of medicine, for, if he does, he has committed himself to prescribing a succession of bottles of medicine and his patient to a succession of visits to the surgery. The patient and his family may come to terms with the abdominal pain, but only at the expense of establishing it as a powerful element in their lives with its own totem pole, decorated with a chemist's label, as a constant reminder on the mantelpiece.

It seems preferable, when confronted with this situation, to try to assist the family towards an awareness of the causes of stress and anxiety within the child and the family. A normal child of six or seven has basic needs in terms of love, security, discipline and a daily routine, as well as the material essentials of life. He needs to be treated not like a television set which can be switched off and forgotten when not required, but as a human being.

When listening to the child's and the parents' own words or when visiting the home, the wise physician will come to know how far his patient's situation measures up to the ideal. By tactfully directing his questions, he may help the parents to see what special problems in the home life may be affecting the child. Parents who have had the opportunity of discussing home difficulties with a doctor whom they trust can achieve greater insight into the basic needs of the child.

If there is bullying at school, a word to a good head teacher may work wonders.

Growing up may be a painful process at all stages, recurrent abdominal pain at six or seven years old is sometimes not the worst of it. Where the home situation is irremediable the doctor must try to help the child to a state of relative independence of mind at an earlier stage than usual; great help may be found through youth clubs and similar organizations. Where there is evidence of more complex emotional disturbance in addition to the abdominal pain, the help of a psychiatrist should be sought. The indications for seeking such advice are discussed in Chapter 18.

The Periodic Syndrome (Cyclical Vomiting Attacks)

Most children have occasional " bilious " attacks, but there are some who appear to have a constitutional pre-disposition to suffer periodic spells of vomiting, often in association with other symptoms (fever, headache, furred tongue, pale stools, abdominal pain or sore throat). There may be a history of a similar pre-disposition in one or other of the parents, or of migraine, or motion sickness. The child himself may be over-excitable or easily fatigued. Clearly this is a very ill-defined syndrome, and each case needs individual study before a diagnosis can be made and acted upon.

If it be accepted that such a pre-disposition can occur, then, after taking a careful history, it may be possible to analyse the symptoms and make a presumptive diagnosis. Perhaps physical examination will yield confirmatory evidence, but more often the doctor will need to examine the child during an attack, looking for signs of infection in the nose, throat, ears, urine or elsewhere.

The term *cyclical vomiting* was formerly applied to cases with a variety of possible causes, and this diagnosis was too often made, perhaps without recognizing the presence of an evanescent sore throat or other infection. Later it became the fashion to use the name " acidosis " or " acetonæmic " attacks, regardless of the fact that there was seldom a true acidosis or even much acetone in the blood. The current term, *periodic syndrome*, has the advantage of not suggesting a single entity or one causation. It is now also agreed that ketone bodies are formed whenever vomiting has occurred. This is because oxidation of fat cannot be completed except in the presence of glucose and without glucose, ketone bodies are formed; these pass into the blood and appear in the urine. Clinical examples of ketone production are starvation, fever, vomiting, the hypoglycæmia of von Gierke's disease (glycogen-storage disease of liver), and diabetic coma (when, despite hyperglycæmia, glucose is not available for cell metabolism).

Vomiting, then, is an important cause of ketosis but there is no evidence that ketosis can produce vomiting. Thus, in patients fed on ketogenic diets, no symptoms occur other than anorexia from the high caloric value of fat and its effect in slowing the emptying-time of the stomach. Therefore, it is clear that recurring attacks of vomiting, fever, and other symptoms cannot be put down to ketosis and that the cause of the periodic syndrome must be sought elsewhere.

DIAGNOSIS

The commonest cause of a vomiting attack is an acute infection. Examples of this are ordinary sore throats and tonsillitis, otitis media, urinary infections and virus infections, including influenza. Vomiting may also occur from fatigue, either physical or nervous, and this is often recurrent. Dietetic indiscretions may be responsible, and some children are more easily upset than others. Then, too, it is believed that bilious attacks in childhood can be the equivalent of migraine at a later age; in such cases headache gradually replaces the vomiting.

Before accepting the diagnosis of the periodic syndrome, it is essential that the possibility of more serious causes for the symptoms should be excluded. In many cases a barium meal examination is desirable to exclude intermittent duodenal obstruction from a duodenal valve or malrotation of the intestine. Recurrent urinary infection must also be excluded. Where effortless vomiting occurs or headache is a feature, the possibility of a cerebral tumour must never be overlooked.

TREATMENT

During an acute attack, the child should be put to bed. A careful clinical examination should be made to ascertain the cause of the vomiting, the temperature being taken and the urine examined. Any infection should receive the appropriate treatment. The child may be helped by phenobarbitone or chlorphromazine (for dosage, *see* p. 664) and frequent sips of glucose and water are given.

8

Dehydration. The vomiting may be so severe that an intravenous drip of saline and glucose, or Hartmann's solution with glucose, is required, in which case all fluid by the mouth should be withheld.

It is a mistake, particularly in younger children, to take such cases lightly. If the vomiting is allowed to continue, collapse and death may occasionally follow. The possibility that some additional abdominal condition may co-exist must not be forgotten.

Sips of glucose fruit juice drinks should be given as soon as the child is retaining fluids. Glucose sweets should be offered. Sometimes carbohydrates in the form of dry biscuits or crisp toast, with honey or jam, are retained best.

To prevent attacks, sources of infection, such as bad teeth, septic tonsils, and nasal obstruction, should be overcome. It is a mistake to keep such children on a low-fat diet, particularly a milkless one, as they tend to contract more frequent infections and the teeth may suffer further damage.

These children require much rest and a short day. Kindergarten school is often a great success in conserving energy.

Migraine

Migraine in young children often passes undiagnosed. There are various theories of its causation, and certainly it is highly familial, passing from one generation to another and alternating with asthma, hay fever and eczema in some individuals. The following are said to be factors in its production:

1. Infections—particularly of the naso-pharynx or urinary tract.
2. Eye strain.
3. Fatigue.

SYMPTOMS

The term " abdominal migraine "[1] is sometimes used to explain abdominal pain, accompanied by vomiting and headache, which recurs every few weeks. Fever is usually present. As the child approaches puberty the headache is accentuated. He complains of pins and needles in the fingers and tongue, and the vision is affected. A hemicranial headache is common, and dislike of light and violent vomiting follow. The whole thing may last a few minutes or some hours.

DIFFERENTIAL DIAGNOSIS

The greatest care must be exercised to ensure that some serious organic disease does not occur under the guise of migraine. Brain tumour with papilloedema, hypertension, recurrent pyelonephritis from some abnormality of the genito-urinary tract, and congenital aneurysm of the circle of Willis must all be excluded.

[1] Farquhar, H. G. (1956). Abdominal migraine in children. *Brit. med. J.*, 1, 1082.

TREATMENT

Ergotamine tartrate may be given, and a suitable dose for a child aged 6 years is a 1-mg. tablet given at the very commencement of an attack and repeated in half an hour if there is no relief. Such treatment should not be repeated frequently over long periods. Phenobarbitone in ¼-grain doses given twice daily over a period of several months may be helpful in breaking the vicious circle of repeated attacks. No treatment is entirely effective.

HEPATIC CONDITIONS

Jaundice

JAUNDICE can be classified under the following headings:

1. OBSTRUCTIVE HEPATIC JAUNDICE

This is unusual in childhood, as stone in the common bile-duct, growth in the pancreas, or glands pressing on the common bile-duct are comparatively rare. The condition is seen in the newborn as a result of congenital obliteration of the bile-ducts or canaliculi.

2. TOXIC AND INFECTIVE HEPATIC JAUNDICE

The best example of this is epidemic infective hepatitis. Spirochætal jaundice (Weil's disease) is another. Phosphorus- and chloroform-poisoning also come into this group.

3. HÆMOLYTIC JAUNDICE

In this group evidence of hæmolytic anæmia is present in the blood. The urine contains an excess of urobilin and bile is present in the stools in excess amounts. The commonest examples in childhood are hæmolytic disease of the newborn, and acholuric familial jaundice in the United Kingdom and the various hæmoglobinopathies in the Mediterranean, Africa and South-East Asian countries.

CAUSES IN INFANCY

In infants the commonest types of jaundice are:
Simple icterus neonatorum (*see* p. 95).
Hæmolytic disease of the newborn (*see* p. 110).
Icterus due to liver infection secondary to umbilical sepsis (*see* p. 104).

Rare causes include:
Congenital obliteration of the bile ducts (*see* p. 218).
Inspissated bile syndrome (*see* p. 219).
Neonatal hepatitis (*see* p. 219).
Congenital syphilis (*see* p. 564).
Congenital spherocytosis (*see* p. 337).

Glucose-6-phosphate-dehydrogenase deficiency (*see* p. 136).
Galactosæmia (*see* p. 131).
Familial hyperbilirubinæmia (*see* p. 137).

CAUSES IN CHILDHOOD

In older children the commonest types are:

Infective hepatitis (*see below*).
Congenital spherocytosis (*see* p. 337).
The hæmoglobinopathies (*see* p. 338).

Rare causes include:

Cirrhosis of the liver (*see* p. 220).
Liver tumours (*see* p. 223).
Plasma-cell hepatitis (*see* p. 217).
Familial hyperbilirubinæmia (*see* p. 137).

Infective Hepatitis

Two forms of this condition can be distinguished: *epidemic infective hepatitis* and *homologous serum jaundice*. The epidemiology of infective hepatitis suggests that the stools contain the virus and that infection is transmitted by direct contamination of food. In children, clinical attacks usually seem to be sporadic, but in schools and other institutions the disease may assume epidemic form.

INCUBATION PERIOD

This appears to be about a month, although in some cases it is shorter, or prolonged to two months. Serum hepatitis, with almost identical clinical manifestations, develops after an injection which contains or is contaminated with icterogenic serum from another patient. In such cases the incubation period is of the order of 100 days. Pooled serum and convalescent serum carry this risk when given to patients. Gammaglobulin fractions, when prepared under proper conditions, do not.

AGE INCIDENCE

Children above the age of six years and young adults are more commonly affected, although occasional cases are seen between the first and second year of life.

CLINICAL PICTURE

The onset may be sudden, with headache, fever and malaise. Vomiting and quite severe abdominal pain are also frequent. At this stage there is no definite clue to the disease and it is often termed " gastric influenza." In three or four days, or longer, depending on the severity of the symptoms, jaundice appears first in the sclerotics and then becomes widespread, and bile is obvious in the urine. As a rule, the diagnosis is easily made by the seventh day. The liver and sometimes the spleen are palpable, and the stools become light and, finally, almost white. The level of direct bilirubin rises sharply in the serum and the alkaline phosphatase, which is normally 5 to 15 units, is as high as 40 units, falling to normal by the second or third week.

Dislike of food, with nausea and vomiting, may continue for two or three weeks. The tongue is coated and the patient feels low and dispirited. As a rule, the temperature has subsided within a week. Convalescence is slow and it takes in all about 6 weeks to make a clinical recovery.

TREATMENT

The patient should be put to bed and kept there until the appetite has returned, the stools and urine are normal in colour, and all traces of jaundice have disappeared. The bowels should be kept open with some mild vegetable or saline aperient.

Diet. This should be low in fat and high in proteins and carbohydrates. Glucose, especially in the form of fruit drinks, should be offered, and eggs and butter excluded during the acute and sub-acute stages.

From the nature of the liver lesion, it is obvious that some weeks may pass before that organ has completely recovered. A period of convalescence should therefore elapse before a child is sent back to resume strenuous school life.

PROGNOSIS

Although the majority of cases make a complete recovery from the disease, a small percentage progress to subacute necrosis (yellow atrophy) of the liver.

Plasma-cell Hepatitis[1]

This is a rare hepatic reaction in older children and adolescents with symptoms basically similar to infective hepatitis, but less acute in their onset and very much slower to disappear. The plasma proteins show a grossly raised level of the gammaglobulin. Liver biopsy shows the presence of giant plasma cells within the parenchyma. The condition may be part of a systemic disease akin to lupus erythematosis, and joint pains and skin rashes occur. The course of the disease may be modified by treatment with corticosteroids, but the prognosis is poor.

Acute or Subacute Yellow Atrophy

This is a rare disease which starts like an attack of ordinary epidemic hepatitis. The symptoms, however, become much more severe, with headache, delirium, vomiting diarrhœa and high fever.

[1] Grossman, A., Rosenthal, I. M., Szanto, P. B. (1962). *Pediatrics*, **29,** 933.

ÆTIOLOGY

The disease is commoner in older children and young adults. Some cases follow anæsthesia and phosphorus poisoning, others upon what appears to be an acute hepatitis; the virus of homologous serum jaundice may also be responsible. Toxic hepatitis progressing to necrosis has followed the use of certain tranquillizing drugs.

PATHOLOGY

The liver-cells show acute necrosis, with an attempt, if the case lasts any length of time, at regeneration, budding out being most noticeable in the region of the bile canaliculi.

CLINICAL PICTURE

The child, who has been drowsy and vomiting, becomes gradually delirious and jaundiced, the urine being deeply bile-stained and the motions pale and frequent. What was at first thought to be infective hepatitis is now seen to be a graver illness. Delirium is present. The liver, which at first was easily palpable, shrinks rapidly beneath the costal margin, and the spleen cannot be felt. There is a tendency to hæmorrhages in the mucous membranes and purpuric patches on the skin. Air-hunger and coma rapidly supervene, death taking place in the severe cases.

Congenital Obliteration of the Bile Ducts or Bile Canaliculi

Shortly after birth, the infant is seen to be slightly jaundiced and at first may be considered to be suffering from the jaundice of liver immaturity only. Then it is noticed that the jaundice is becoming more and more marked, the stools continue light in colour, and the urine is deeply stained with bile. The sclerotics have an icteric tinge. The spleen is always palpable, and the liver, which is down several fingers' breadth below the costal margin, is hard and resistant on palpation. The hæmatological and serological changes which characterize hæmolytic disease of the newborn (p. 110) are not present. The most notable change in the liver-function tests is the very high serum alkaline phosphatase, characteristic of obstructive jaundice. The conjugated bilirubin and alkaline phosphatase levels are greatly raised. The flocculation tests show varying degrees of abnormality. The serum-transaminase levels are less raised than in neonatal hepatitis but the differences are not sufficiently constant as to be of diagnostic value. The main differential diagnosis is from neonatal hepatitis.

PATHOLOGY

The liver is involved in every case. In some cases, the obliteration of the bile is extra-hepatic, but in others only the intra-hepatic bile canaliculi are involved. The gall bladder is usually shrunken and empty. The liver shows a diffuse unilobular and intra-lobular cirrhosis.

TREATMENT

After a reasonable period of observation, usually about four to eight weeks, during which time a number of infants with neonatal hepatitis or the inspissated bile syndrome will have improved spontaneously, the child should be given the chance of surgery. In a minority, a plastic operation on the common duct is possible. At worst, an adequate biopsy specimen can be obtained to determine the type of intra-hepatic pathology. In general, however, the prognosis with or without surgery is poor.

Neonatal Hepatitis

Infants with prolonged jaundice, dating from soon after birth, will be suspected at first of Rh incompatibility and, when this has been excluded, congenital obliteration of the bile-ducts will be considered, especially if there is acholia. Sometimes, however, cases closely resembling congenital biliary obstruction in nearly all their features may suddenly recover spontaneously. Biopsy of the liver in such cases has shown that the condition is one of hepatitis and the bile-ducts are normal except for containing inspissated bile. In some the histological diagnosis is extremely difficult since fair numbers of large plasma cells may be seen even in the presence of biliary obstruction. For this reason it is recommended that the taking of the liver-biopsy specimen should be combined with laparotomy, when a full examination of the biliary apparatus may be made. This procedure is usually carried out when the infant is four to eight weeks old.

The liver-function tests differ from those in congenital atresia of the bile ducts, in that the alkaline phosphatase is somewhat less raised, the serum-transaminase levels are higher and the flocculation tests more abnormal. The pattern may not be sufficiently clear to permit a clear differentiation on these tests alone.

In general terms about sixty per cent. of patients make a good recovery from neonatal hepatitis. The remainder die or progress to cirrhosis. Infection with the virus of infectious hepatitis or that of homologous-serum jaundice[1] is believed to be responsible in some cases; there may be a history of such infection in the mother.

Inspissated Bile Syndrome

It is doubtful whether this constitutes a separate disease entity. It seems probable that in any severe case of neonatal jaundice bile may become inspissated in the canaliculi, particularly when stasis is present. Such a state of affairs may well be present, for example, in severe cases of hæmolytic jaundice due to rhesus incompatibility, for

---

[1] Stokes J., Jr. (1951). *Amer. J. Dis. Child.*, **82**, 1951.

short periods of time. It is certainly also seen in neonatal hepatitis and in biliary atresia. Treatment with corticosteroids (for dosage, *see* p. 660) sometimes appears to act dramatically; it must be recalled, however, that sixty per cent. of the patients with neonatal hepatitis recover spontaneously without treatment.

Cirrhosis of the Liver

Cirrhosis is not a disease but the end-result of different disease processes. It may develop early or late; it has been found in new-born infants, or it can develop in early childhood or later.

There are hereditary types (e.g., Wilson's disease—hepatolenticular degeneration, p. 446), there are cases due to hepatitis, to chronic congestion (cardiac cirrhosis), those due to infiltration (galactosæmia, Gaucher's disease), to biliary obstruction, to hæmolytic disease of the

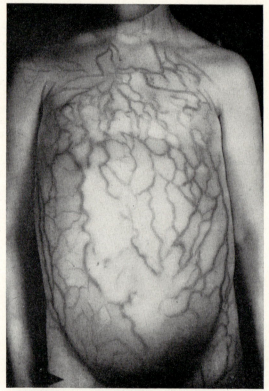

Fig. 17.—An infra-red photograph showing anastomotic venous channels. This patient had hepatic cirrhosis and post-cirrhotic primary carcinoma of the liver. *See also* Fig. 19, p. 222.

newborn, to mucoviscidosis, to bilharziasis, and to severe nutritional
deficiencies (e.g. kwashiorkor).   In many cases the cause is unknown.
In the United Kingdom cirrhosis is rare in children, but in certain
tropical countries nutritional cirrhosis (p. 601) is common.

PATHOLOGY

A multilobular cirrhosis may be found with hypertrophy and
proliferation of liver cells.   Macroscopically there is a nodular
appearance (hobnail liver) (Fig. 18).

Other cases, presumably dating from a congenital biliary obliteration, show a biliary cirrhosis with an enlarged, firm, granular liver,
which shows proliferation of bile canaliculi and peri- or intra-lobular
cirrhosis.

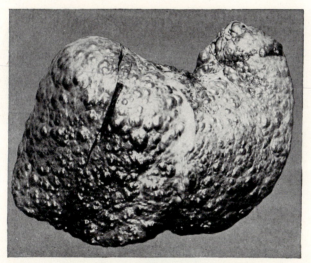

Fig. 18.—Hepatic cirrhosis in a child aged 6½.

SYMPTOMS

The onset is insidious.   The child remains vaguely unwell.   Growth
is less than normal and the child tires easily.   Anæmia is present and
transient episodes of jaundice may occur.   Spider nævi may develop
on the face and on the fingers.   The signs of portal hypertension may
appear (*see* p. 222).   There is progressive depletion of serum albumin,
due partly to defective synthesis as a result of liver damage and partly
to loss of protein into the ascites which accumulates when portal
hypertension is present.

Ultimately, after a varying and indefinite period, sometimes years,
the child develops jaundice, ascites, œdema, delirium, twitching, and

before death passes into coma; but, if portal hypertension is present, death from œsophageal or gastric hæmorrhage is more likely.

Portal Hypertension

As a result of hepatic cirrhosis, other liver diseases, or of portal thrombosis (*see* p. 105), obstruction of the portal vein may occur. This gives rise to ascites and evidence of a collateral circulation for the portal vein. Thus, large veins appear over the abdomen (*see* Fig. 17, p. 220). Œsophageal veins dilate and may form varices which in turn may bleed giving rise to hæmatemesis. The spleen enlarges. Partly from the disturbed liver function and partly from the loss of protein into the ascitic fluid, hypoproteinæmia may develop giving rise to generalized œdema.

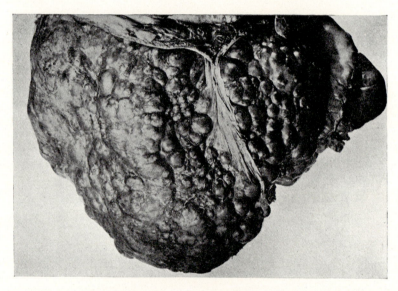

Fig. 19.—A markedly cirrhotic liver from the case depicted in Fig. 17, showing nodular hyperplasia with extensive primary carcinomatous change. The patient, aged 7, presented as a case of hepatic cirrhosis with portal obstruction. The neoplastic changes were widely distributed in the liver and masses of malignant cells filled the main hepatic veins and extended into the inferior vena cava.

TREATMENT

In cases where the signs of portal hypertension and obstruction predominate over the signs of liver failure, it is reasonable to consider the operation of porto-caval anastomosis to relieve the obstruction. As a preliminary to such a procedure, venograms and measurements of the portal pressure may be required. The operation should be undertaken only at a surgical centre familiar with this special work.

Syphilitic Pericellular Cirrhosis (*see also* p. 566)

This cirrhosis follows syphilitic hepatitis. Infection is conveyed from the mother *via* the umbilical veins direct to the infant's liver. The majority of stillborn syphilitic infants show this change.

The pathological appearance in the early stages is one of diffuse round-cell infiltration, resembling miliary gummata. This causes complete loss of the normal histological pattern and gives rise to diffuse pericellular fibrosis.

Tumours of the Liver

The very rare primary liver tumour of childhood is usually a hepatoblastoma. It is an embryonic tumour showing varying degrees of differentiation. Primary carcinoma is even more rare but is not unknown in children, the majority of cases showing pre-existing cirrhosis.

The symptoms are variable, but progressive enlargement of the abdomen, due to the rapidly growing tumour, and an ominously excessive weight gain are often the first signs. Jaundice is variable. Portal obstruction develops in some cases. Bleeding into the skin and mucous membranes may occur.

Death occurs within two or three months of the appearance of symptoms.

Secondary Growths of the Liver

The liver will be involved in the general invasion of leukæmia and lymphadenoma. Secondary deposits also occur, particularly from adrenal tumours (neuroblastoma), embryoma of the kidney and lymphosarcoma.

DISEASES OF THE GALL BLADDER

DISEASE of the gall bladder is rare in childhood. Apart from the well recognized *congenital obliteration of the bile ducts*, malformations include the *choledochus cyst* which may obstruct the flow of bile and give rise to an obstructive jaundice. In both cases the treatment is surgical.

Gall stones in childhood are found most commonly in cases of congenital spherocytosis (*see* p. 337) and are of the pigment variety.

Rarely *acute cholecystitis* may occur with severe vomiting, fever and right epigastric pain. Such cases are commonly mistaken for a high retrocolic appendicitis or sub-phrenic abscess, the true pathology being found at laparotomy.

CHAPTER 13

Diseases of the Respiratory System

DISORDERS OF THE UPPER RESPIRATORY TRACT

CONGENITAL MALFORMATIONS

Choanal Atresia

THIS is a rare malformation; the infant is born with a septum extending across the posterior nares. It may consist of fibrous tissue but in some instances contains actual bone substance.

Despite the complete nasal obstruction, the infant makes abortive attempts at nasal breathing, thus becoming cyanosed and asphyxiated. This is terminated by a fit of crying, when at once normal oxygenation is restored. Once the crying ceases, the infant again becomes cyanosed. Breathing is also complicated by the accumulation of secretions behind the atretic septum. The diagnosis is confirmed by the finding of an obstruction to the passage of a nasal tube.

Emergency operation is essential to perforate the septum, after which a nasal catheter is passed to maintain the airway. Without such treatment a fatal outcome is not infrequent.

Micrognathos and Retrognathos

Underdevelopment of the lower jaw is often associated with a degree of posterior displacement of the tongue, with intermittent obstruction of the posterior pharyngeal airway. Respiratory difficulties are particularly obvious during feeding because the infant cannot co-ordinate breathing with swallowing. Added difficulties in feeding are due to the tendency for the nipple or teat to be placed under the tongue.

Such infants breathe more easily in the prone position. The feeding problems are overcome by spoon feeding or even tube feeding in the most severe cases. Spontaneous improvement occurs by the age of three months.

Pierre Robin Syndrome

The association of a posterior cleft in the palate with marked under-development of the lower jaw may make it possible for the tongue to be withdrawn so far backwards as to obstruct the airway, and an infant will quickly suffocate after birth unless the tongue is drawn forwards. Lying in the prone position may be helpful but is not in itself sufficient to maintain a clear airway.

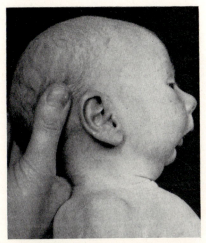

Fig. 20—Micrognathia in a suckling infant.

The tongue should be held forward, preferably by means of a stitch inserted anteriorly, until the plastic operation of fixing the tongue to the floor of the mouth and securing it by stay sutures around the mandible can be carried out.

The general problems of hare lip and cleft palate are discussed on pp. 175–177.

UPPER RESPIRATORY INFECTIONS

Acute Rhinitis (the Common Cold)

ÆTIOLOGY

Recent work has confirmed the supposition that the common cold is usually due to a filtrable virus. It has been shown that such viruses can be transferred by droplet infection. The incubation period is two to five days. Coryza is highly infectious, and passes rapidly from one child to another. A " cold " appears to confer on the individual very little immunity to a second or subsequent attack. Because of this, repeated colds can and do affect susceptible subjects.

CLINICAL PICTURE

Such infections are usually a cause for concern only in very young or debilitated children. In the tiny infant there may be very little local reaction (that is, not much sign of a cold) but symptomatic diarrhœa may result (*see* p. 198). The infection may spread to the larynx or ears. In premature infants and other small children whose resistance to infection is low, what commences as a simple cold may become complicated by secondary infection with other organisms and may progress to broncho-pneumonia. In such children colds should be carefully watched and antibiotic treatment commenced if physical examination suggests that the infection is extending. In an average case, in two or three days the secretions become thicker and less profuse, and gradually the inflamed nasal mucous membrane subsides. The whole process takes about a week.

Allergy should be borne in mind; sometimes so-called " colds " are in fact attacks of rhinorrhœa and not true virus infection. In allergic rhinitis (p. 267), sneezing is, as a rule, excessive and the temperature is not raised.

TREATMENT

Individuals with colds, in contact with small infants and particularly the newborn, should be encouraged to wear masks if complete segregation is not possible.

One grain of powdered aspirin may be given three times a day to a feverish infant. As previously mentioned, a careful watch must be kept for serious respiratory or aural complications and antibiotics administered to small or premature infants at the earliest indication.

Acute Tonsillitis

This is usually due to a Lancefield Group A hæmolytic streptococcal infection. Occasionally a staphylococcal or virus infection may be the cause. As a rule, tonsillitis is acquired by droplet infection from some other individual.

CLINICAL PICTURE

The onset is sudden; the first symptoms may be those of the common cold—lassitude, fullness in the nose and throat, headache and shivering. The throat is sore, and the child often refuses to eat or drink. It is, however, unusual for a child to complain of sore throat before the age of five or six years. Most parents fail to realize this, and are much surprised when the diagnosis of tonsillitis is made. In every case of illness in an infant or child, it is necessary, therefore, to examine the throat carefully.

It will be noticed that the anterior pillars of the fauces are inflamed and œdematous, and that the tonsils themselves are dark red and engorged. At intervals, over the tonsil itself, protruding from the crypts, small points of pus will be seen, perhaps from four to a dozen on each side in a severe case. Very often the tonsillar glands at the angle of the jaw are enlarged, but they may not be in the first or second attack. The tongue is coated, and tends to be dry; the breath is unpleasant. There may be a short cough, or a continual clearing of the throat, particularly in nervous children. If solid food is taken there is often a tendency to retch and vomit. The temperature is high, and the face flushed.

In infants there may not be a violent reaction to the infection. Much less is to be seen locally, but the general upset is greater and more widespread.

In three or four days there is a decided improvement, and by the tenth day the throat condition has largely cleared. Much, however, will depend on the age of the child and the nature of the infection.

COMPLICATIONS

The complications of upper respiratory infections are many and varied, and are of the utmost importance. *Sinusitis, bronchitis* or *pulmonary collapse* very commonly follow infection of the nose or throat. *Otitis media* is a direct result. *Umbilical colic* is often associated with sore throats. It is difficult to explain the ætiology of this, but it is probably due to enlarged mesenteric glands, caused either by enteral infection which has passed through the intestinal wall to the glands, or by infection reaching the abdominal glands by way of the bloodstream. It is much more likely to be the former.

Vomiting Attacks. Besides having an acute sore throat or catarrh of the nose, the child may suffer severe vomiting. Acetone may be found in the urine or smelt in the breath. Constipation, or, on the contrary, diarrhœa may occur. If the infections appear over and over again at regular intervals a wrong diagnosis of cyclical vomiting may be made (*see* p. 212).

Rheumatism and acute nephritis are usually preceded by a hæmolytic streptococcal throat infection. In this respect, the Lance-field Group A Griffith type 12 streptococcus has been shown to be associated particularly with outbreaks of nephritis. In acute rheumatism no restriction to a single type of hæmolytic streptococcus has been found but it is always a member of Group A.

Peritonsillar Abscess. This is uncommon before the age of four or five (*see* p. 228).

Retropharyngeal Abscess. This is most often seen in the first few months of life (*see* p. 228).

Upper respiratory infections undoubtedly precipitate *asthmatic attacks* in allergic children.

TREATMENT

In cases of acute tonsillitis the child is best in bed, as there he is less likely to become chilled and can less easily convey his infection to others. The temperature of the room should be about 60° F, and cross-ventilation is desirable. A nose and throat swab should be taken to detect the organism. When this has been done, and if the temperature is raised and the throat shows a moderate or severe degree of inflammation or exudate, the appropriate chemotherapy should be prescribed (for more details, *see* Appendix 1). In mild cases aspirin should be given every four hours and a potassium chlorate and phenol gargle B.P.C. may be helpful in children old enough to co-operate.

Retropharyngeal Abscess

Usually this occurs in infants who are under the age of one year. Subsequently the retropharyngeal lymph glands atrophy. The condition is most frequently seen in debilitated and under-nourished children, in whom a history of pharyngitis usually precedes infection of the retropharyngeal glands. The symptoms increase over several days until one of the retropharyngeal glands breaks down, causing an abscess in the lateral walls of the pharynx.

SYMPTOMS

There is often some fever, but occasionally this is very slight. Swallowing is increasingly difficult; the child tends to hold the head backward. The breathing is noisy and, since the pharynx is obstructed, mucus tends to drain from the mouth and nose. There is usually a swelling due to a gland at the angle of the jaw on the affected side. A careful examination of the pharynx reveals the swelling and, on palpation, fluctuation may be felt. A soft tissue x-ray of the neck reveals the forward displacement of the larynx.

PROGNOSIS AND TREATMENT

Very often such abscesses drain themselves, the pus either being coughed up or swallowed. When discovered, the abscess should be opened and suction applied. It is most important that the head should be held vertically down during this procedure so that the pus will drain into the mouth and nose from whence it can be removed by continuous suction to prevent inhalation. Relief is immediate, and recovery rapid. Penicillin should be administered in full doses.

Peritonsillar Abscess (Quinsy)

This may occur in children from four to five years of age and upward. The inflammation commences deep in the tissues, usually behind the tonsil, pushing it forward. There is difficulty in swallowing, much pain and high fever. Pus is formed and must be evacuated by incision, or the abscess will burst and drain spontaneously. Early administration of penicillin may prevent pus formation, and is indicated in all cases.

Acute and Chronic Sinusitis

Every acute naso-pharyngeal infection is bound to spread to the nasal accessory sinuses, for they are lined by an extension of the mucous membrane of the nose. Usually, the inflammation of the sinuses subsides with general recovery, but, if an ostium becomes blocked, exudate may accumulate under tension in the cavity and acute sinusitis may thus be initiated. More often, chronic sinusitis results from partial, but not complete, obstruction, or from severe infection even with an adequate ostium.

ACUTE ANTRITIS

Acute inflammation of the antra may occur during a severe cold or other upper respiratory infection. The temperature is raised, there is severe headache, and there may be pain localized over the affected antrum. An x-ray will show opacity of the sinus. One object of treatment is to induce shrinkage of the swollen nasal mucosa so that the ostium opens and drainage is established. Ephedrine ½-per cent. nasal drops in normal saline are indicated for this purpose. Hot inhalations, using menthol and friar's balsam, may give some relief. The second and more important object of treatment is to overcome the infection as soon as possible. Prompt chemotherapy or antibiotic treatment may do this. If the infection persists, a swab should be taken in order that the sensitivity of the causative organism can be tested.

CHRONIC ANTRITIS

The chronic condition is often the outcome of repeated colds which have failed to clear up completely, or may depend upon a large mass of adenoids partly obstructing the nasopharynx. The child has a stuffy, " catarrhal " nose, and persistent postnasal discharge. Such discharge into the throat causes chronic cough, and may lead to bronchitis, pulmonary collapse or even bronchiectasis. Headaches and a gastritis as a result of swallowed mucopus are common. Because of the mucopus the child may vomit in the mornings and refuse breakfast. Later in the day the appetite improves. Frequently, otitis media may result from a spread of infection along the Eustachian tube. Transillumination and x-ray will show opacity of the antrum. In a proportion of cases the chronic antral infection is associated with an allergic reaction of the nasal mucous membrane, as seen in hay-fever, and rhinorrhœa.

Treatment of mild antral infection is on general lines. Oral antihistamines together with steam inhalations are valuable, and a change to sea air is of the greatest help, although bathing is forbidden. Adenoids causing nasal obstruction should be removed. Failing improvement from these measures and in more severe cases, antral lavage is frequently followed by most satisfactory results. Obviously, further upper respiratory infections may lead to inflammation of the antrum again, and colds must be avoided as far as possible and treated strenuously when they do occur.

Washing out the antra or sinuses by Proetz displacement is most beneficial in selected cases.

Cervical Adenitis

This is one of the commonest sequels of tonsillitis, and may run a recurrent course in small children.

ACUTE CERVICAL ADENITIS

After an acute naso-pharyngitis, usually due to the hæmolytic streptococcus, the tonsillar glands enlarge at the angle of the jaw, and become extremely painful. Shortly after this, other glands in the neck may enlarge, the swellings being unilateral or bilateral. At the slightest movement of the head, intense pain is felt. The tongue is furred, and the temperature high and inclined to swing; it will be down in the morning and up in the evening. Some cases are accompanied by otitis media or mastoid disease, and in other cases the glands may break down and form abscesses.

Swabs should be taken to exclude any possibility of diphtheria and, despite the acute onset, a single case in a household may prove to be tuberculous. An intradermal tuberculin test should be done if there is any doubt about the ætiology.

Penicillin is indicated in full doses. As a result of this treatment, it is now unusual for these glands to require incision.

Chronic or Recurrent Cervical Adenitis

After a first acute streptococcal infection, a three-year-old child may have persistently enlarged cervical glands which may become intermittently tender and fluctuate in size for at least six months.

In a child of five to seven years of age, chronic tonsillar infection is associated with persistent cervical gland enlargement and failure to gain weight.

A chronic streptococcal cervical adenitis has to be distinguished from a tuberculous adenitis (p. 585) and glandular fever of the chronic remittent type (p. 349). Leukæmia (p. 347) and Hodgkin's disease (p. 351) may also have to be excluded. The presence of glands elsewhere, splenomegaly, anæmia, and the appropriate investigations will usually resolve the diagnosis. Tuberculous glands are often the most difficult to distinguish.

INDICATIONS FOR REMOVAL OF TONSILS AND ADENOIDS

TONSILLECTOMY is now performed less frequently than in the past. The main reason for this lies in the realization that simple enlargement alone is seldom a justification for surgery. There is a natural tendency for the tonsils to regress in size after the age of 7–10 years. Sometimes the indications are chiefly for adenoidectomy and this operation may be done without removal of the tonsils. There is, however, the possibility that the tonsils will require removal later.   Therefore the double operation is more commonly performed.   The main indications for operation are:

   (i) Persistent nasal obstruction due to enlarged adenoids.
  (ii) Recurrent otitis media and/or middle-ear deafness associated with recurrent tonsillitis or nasal discharge and obstruction.
 (iii) Recurrent tonsillitis (more than three attacks a year) with cervical adenitis or loss of weight.
  (iv) The rare occurrence, in small children aged 1–3 years, of acute difficulty in breathing or swallowing due to enlarged tonsils.
   (v) Repeated sore throats after acute nephritis or acute rheumatism, despite prophylactic penicillin therapy.
  (vi) Tuberculous cervical adenitis.

It is not uncommon for more than one of these indications to be present in the same patient.

DISEASES OF THE EAR

Otitis Media

EARACHE in the child is most commonly due to viral or bacterial infection of the middle ear, and involves the tympanic membrane or surrounding parts.   The inflammation, however, may be in the Eustachian tube, causing an obstruction of the passage of air to the middle ear and bulging or retraction of the drum.   Foreign bodies in the external auditory meatus, such as wax, peas and beads, may also give rise to earache, and earache is quite common after the operation for removal of tonsils and adenoids.

Otitis media is a common complication of coryza, influenza, measles, scarlet fever and diphtheria.

CLINICAL PICTURE

Simple otitis media is preceded by a viral infection of the naso-pharynx.   The child has a cough, and there is a discharge from the nose, generally with some fever.   The infection spreads from the Eustachian tube to the middle ear, the temperature rises and pain is felt in the ear.   The infection is usually bilateral.   Examination shows no bulging of the drum, and, in the absence of secondary bacterial invasion, the earache subsides with the viral infection.

In suppurative otitis media, the drum of the ear is red, has lost its lustre, and bulges.   The temperature rises rapidly, reaching 104°–106°, with a varying degree of irritability, nausea, anorexia, vomiting and diarrhœa.   If no treatment is instituted, in 24 to 48 hours, during which time the pain waxes and wanes, the drum will burst, releasing a purulent discharge.   Accompanying the infection of the middle ear, there may be an infection of the mastoid process.   The infecting organism varies, *Staphylococcus aureus*, streptococcus, pneumococcus and *Hæmophilus influenzæ* being the most usual.

In the infant with otitis media, suspicion may not fall on the ears merely from observation. The drums should be examined in every case. The child often shows toxæmia and may even behave as in meningitis, holding the head back and screaming at intervals. Very frequently, there is an accompanying naso-pharyngitis and cervical adenitis. A baby's action in putting its hand to its ear cannot be taken as a sign of earache, as a healthy infant will often do the same thing.

TREATMENT

Earache in children should always be taken seriously, and a careful examination made of the drums. If wax is present, the ear should be gently cleaned out with a ring probe. If the drums are red, and early bulging is detected, paracentesis should be undertaken.

Following myringotomy or spontaneous rupture of the drum, great care should be taken that the external auditory meatus is not allowed to become infected by the discharge from the ears, as an eczema may develop, giving rise to a chronic otitis externa. To prevent this, toilet to the ear is carried out by dry mopping of the ear followed by the application of spirit drops:

> Boric acid, 0·5 G. (8 grains)
> Alcohol, 8 ml. (120 minims)
> Water, 8 ml. (120 minims)

Once the nature of the organism and its severity is known, the appropriate antibiotic can be administered. In the meantime penicillin should be given in full doses. Inadequate chemotherapy without myringotomy is potentially a highly dangerous treatment. A dormant and masked infection may smoulder on for several weeks until evidence of mastoid involvement becomes obvious.

Acute Mastoiditis

This condition may accompany acute otitis media. In the infant its onset can be very rapid, and within 24 hours the clinical picture may be complete. The infection usually spreads from the middle ear to the mastoid antrum, infecting the mastoid cells. The organisms are the same as in acute otitis media.

CLINICAL PICTURE

The child becomes drowsy and lethargic, and may vomit repeatedly. The temperature is high, accompanied by headache. Very often, with the onset of mastoiditis the earache ceases and the child may appear quite bright at intervals, although generally drowsy. Careful examination may reveal a slight œdema over the mastoid process, or the œdema may be marked, with forward displacement of the ear. Occasionally, however, no œdema is present and there is little or no tenderness over the mastoid.   Redness and swelling of the posterior wall of the external auditory meatus help the diagnosis in such cases. X-rays may show clouding of the mastoid air cells.   Leucocytosis is usual.

TREATMENT

Surgery is required for those cases in which the infection is well advanced and those which do not respond to antibiotics.   Chemotherapy should be started at once, penicillin or a tetracycline being given until the sensitivity of the causative organism is known, after which the appropriate antibiotic may be started.

Complications.   Occasionally, infection or thrombosis of the lateral sinus, meningitis (*see* p. 399) or cerebral abscess (*see* p. 415) occur.

PREVENTION OF OTITIS MEDIA AND MASTOID DISEASE

Early removal of infected tonsils and adenoids is the best prophylaxis for those patients in whom earache has been associated with sore throats or recurrent deafness.   Inadequate chemotherapy may mask a dormant otitis media, particularly if associated with absent or inadequate drainage of the middle ear due to closing over of a spontaneous perforation of the drum.

Serous Meningitis (Otitic Meningitis)

During the course of an acute otitis media or mastoid infection, signs of meningitis may occur.   Headache, drowsiness, and vomiting, with or without neck rigidity, may be present.   The differentiation between meningitis and cerebral abscess (p. 415) may be very difficult in the early stages.   Where an abscess is well established, focal neurological signs of cerebellar dysfunction and the presence of papilloedema clarify the position.

In early cases where no papilloedema is present, a lumbar puncture may be done, care being taken to remove only the minimum of fluid necessary to allow the laboratory investigations to be carried out.

If the fluid shows an increase of cells and a raised protein content, a paracentesis should be performed, or an exploration of the mastoid is indicated.   If this has already been done on one side, it may need to be done on the other, and a search for a further source of infection should be made in the region of the mastoids.   Chemotherapy with sulphonamides and penicillin should be given in full doses (Appendix 1) until the precise sensitivity of the organism is known.

Otitic Hydrocephalus (Benign Intracranial Hypertension)

Symptoms and signs of raised intracranial pressure may develop after an ear infection; here again the possibility of an intracranial abscess will need exclusion (*see* p. 415).   In some cases, however, there has been a thrombosis of one or more of the cerebral venous sinuses which, by interfering with the absorption of cerebrospinal fluid, causes a rise in intracranial pressure.

CLINICAL PICTURE

Headache is present, occurring in attacks. Sometimes there is internal strabismus and diplopia (sixth cranial nerve). Papillœdema is always seen but there are no localizing signs in the nervous system. The cerebrospinal fluid is normal but its pressure may be as much as 300 mm.

TREATMENT

Regularly repeated lumbar-puncture drainage is necessary—at first daily or every other day, then less frequently, a chart of the pressures being kept. With this treatment the symptoms disappear, the papillœdema clears away and the prognosis is excellent.

DEAFNESS

THE prevalence of deafness in childhood has not always been appreciated. It seems probable that nearly 10 per cent. of children suffer from deafness, either of an intermittent or permanent nature. The great majority of cases are of the intermittent type due to suppurative otitis media and Eustachian obstruction secondary to naso-pharyngeal infection. Effective treatment of aural infections (p. 232) will greatly diminish the incidence of permanent sequelæ in this group.

In addition, there are a number of causes of permanent deafness which may be present at birth or which may develop shortly afterwards. It is of the greatest importance that such patients should be detected early so that treatment may be started, if possible, at the age range during which speech would normally be acquired. The commoner causes of deafness include:

PERMANENT

Hereditary
Congenital—Congenital malformations of the ears.
            Rubella syndrome (p. 540).
            Congenital syphilis (p. 564).
Acquired — Perinatal asphyxia and birth injury.
            Kernicterus (p. 113).
            Iatrogenic (dihydrostreptomycin).
            Meningitis (particularly in infancy).
            Infections of the middle ear (p. 231).

INTERMITTENT

Middle-ear Infections (p. 231).

DIAGNOSIS

The parents' suspicion of deafness in an infant remains both the commonest method of case finding and the most reliable evidence of deafness. Such suspicion should never be dismissed lightly. Some parents are less observant and, particularly with infants at special risk (i.e. those who fall into the ætiological groups mentioned on p. 234, including all premature infants), routine observation during infancy should always include simple testing to exclude deafness.

Complete deafness is very rare. The majority of children retain some residual hearing but this may not be uniform throughout all tonalities. In particular, selective high-tone deafness is both common and easily overlooked in the first years of life. Even in the most severe cases, islands of residual hearing are usually found to exist in some frequencies.

Testing infants or small children is a patient and time-consuming task which cannot be hurried. The child must be relaxed and in-apprehensive. The room must be soundproof. For initial screening tests, little apparatus is required; this should include three pitch pipes of different frequencies representing the higher, middle and lower registers of normal hearing, and other simple equipment to represent familiar sounds of different frequencies such as rustling paper, a rattle and a drum. The child's attention should be engaged whilst an assistant out of sight of the child produces the various sounds. The examiner should be in a position to observe the child's face and reactions to the sounds. In addition to the detection of qualitative loss, some impression of quantitative loss of hearing may be obtained by varying the intensity of the sounds and their distance from the child.

The diagnosis of deafness in small children is not infrequently com-plicated by the possibility of mental backwardness. Some retarded children can in fact hear but do not bother to listen. A detailed history and an examination of their comparative developmental progress in skills not involving hearing is therefore essential. In such children the exclusion of associated deafness can be extremely difficult.

Suspicions of deafness should always be aroused by any child who is late in talking, and steps taken to exclude it before any arrange-ments are made for speech therapy.

Some children with isolated high-tone deafness, and particularly those of high intelligence, may escape attention until after they have entered school. Although speech may be unintelligible to them they are self-taught lip readers. At school they may get into trouble because of their apparent " fidgetiness " which is in fact their natural tendency to turn to face each person in the classroom who may be speaking. Their inability to lip read and write at the same time brings out a particularly poor performance in dictation. In most children over the age of five, hearing can be tested by normal audio-metric methods.

TREATMENT

Modern hearing aids have greatly improved the possibilities of cultivating the residual hearing of deaf children. The teaching of such children, however, remains a highly skilled technique involving speech therapy, lip reading instruction, and special educational methods. Above all, the child must not be allowed to feel cut off from his family and the rest of society as a result of his deafness. A deaf child shut off from the normal communication with the family and society may easily develop emotional and behavioural difficulties. Advice at an early stage from experienced teachers of deaf children and entry to a nursery school that caters for such child is of the utmost value. Children deaf at birth or in early infancy should be brought, by their first birthday or as soon after as possible, to a centre where such treatment is available.

DISORDERS OF THE LARYNX

Laryngeal Papilloma

WHETHER laryngeal papillomata are present from birth is not known, but the first symptoms often appear at the age of about 2 or 3 years. Simple papillomata are usually found growing from the vocal cords, or wall of the larynx close to the vocal cords; frequently they are multiple. When removed they tend to recur repeatedly, but ultimately, usually in adolescence, they disappear spontaneously.

The onset is very gradual, the voice being slowly lost. There is usually only a huskiness at first, then gradually complete loss of voice occurs. Later, symptoms of inspiratory and expiratory obstruction appear, which may become acute and threaten suffocation.

Treatment is largely surgical; direct diathermy or piecemeal removal may be necessary. There is a risk of producing laryngeal stenosis. If obstruction is present, tracheostomy should be done prior to removal. Radiotherapy should be avoided.

Congenital Laryngeal Stridor

This is found more commonly in girls than in boys, and it is present from birth. It may occasionally be associated with underdevelopment (hypoplasia) of the mandible (micrognathia). In such cases, the tongue appears to fall back and give rise to the inspiratory stridor. Laryngoscopic examination may show a narrowing and flabbiness of the aryteno-epiglottic folds, which tend to collapse and obstruct inspiration.

Very shortly after birth, a noise on inspiration is noticed. It is a crowing noise accompanied by an indrawing of the intercostal spaces and of the episternal notch, worse when the child is roused than when quiescent. The physical condition is, as a rule, excellent and the mentality normal. The voice and cry are clear. The condition must be differentiated from papilloma, where the voice is hoarse and the symptoms come on some time after birth, and from laryngismus stridulus, associated with rickets.

As a rule, the symptoms pass off about the age of one year, and certainly by two years, and there is no further sign of the condition. No active treatment appears to be of any benefit nor does it seem necessary in the majority of cases.   In severe and persistent cases, however, x-ray of the neck to outline the lumen of the larynx, and direct laryngoscopy, should always be performed to exclude papilloma or other congenital malformation, such as a laryngeal web or congenital stenosis.

Croup

This term is commonly applied to five different conditions:

(i) Simple laryngitis: spasmodic croup (laryngitis stridulosa).

(ii) Laryngeal diphtheria (*see* p. 550).

(iii) Laryngismus stridulus (*see* p. 121).

(iv) Acute epiglottitis.

(v) Acute laryngo-tracheo-bronchitis.

Spasmodic Croup

ÆTIOLOGY

Spasmodic croup is caused by the same types of infection as other upper respiratory infections, but there is extension of the infection. There is swelling and congestion of the vocal cords, which impede their function.   In children, it is very often accompanied by a greater or lesser degree of spasm of the laryngeal muscles.

AGE-INCIDENCE

Spasmodic croup most commonly occurs between the ages of 6 months and 3 years.

CLINICAL PICTURE

During the afternoon the child may have a slight cough and be a little feverish.   After being put to bed he awakes and attracts attention by his crowing inspiratory stridor, which is accompanied by inspiratory recession of the sternum and intercostal spaces.   All the ordinary and extraordinary muscles of respiration are overacting.   Such an attack will commonly last for one to four hours.   The general constitutional upset is not great, and immediately the attack is over the child seems himself again.   Spasmodic croup appears, therefore, to consist of two separate factors: first, the simple laryngitis and, secondly, the nervous spasm of the larynx.   The latter is the more important in producing the clinical picture.

DIFFERENTIAL DIAGNOSIS

It is necessary to differentiate between laryngeal diphtheria, laryngismus stridulus (a symptom of tetany), acute epiglottitis, acute laryngo-tracheo-bronchitis and a foreign body. In *laryngeal diphtheria* the constitutional upset is severe and the colour grey. The onset is seldom sudden, often occurring in the morning or during the day. An examination of the throat shows, as a rule, accompanying pharyngeal diphtheria or nasal diphtheria. When there is any doubt whatever, antitoxin should be administered at once. In *laryngismus stridulus* the stridor is inspiratory and, between attacks, the breathing is quiet. Signs of rickets are usually present.

In *acute epiglottitis* (below) there is commonly a preceding respiratory infection. The stridor is progressive but in the early stages is indistinguishable from simple laryngitis. Laryngoscopy, which will reveal the obstruction of the airway by the œdematous epiglottis, may be the only certain way to differentiate this potentially fatal condition from the mild inflammation and secondary laryngeal spasm of simple laryngitis.

Acute laryngo-tracheo-bronchitis (*see* p. 239) is a rapidly progressive condition. In severe cases, complete bronchial or laryngeal obstruction from the viscid secretion produced causes death from asphyxia, unless tracheostomy or intubation is carried out. Signs of bronchial involvement are usually present. The condition often occurs in epidemics.

A *foreign body* in the larynx may be unsuspected by the parents but must be excluded by direct laryngoscopy in cases of persistent stridor.

TREATMENT

The provision of a high humidity is the most important aspect of treatment. Either a steam tent is made or the child is placed in an oxygen tent with a humidifier attachment, such as the Croupette (Airshields). A sedative, such as phenobarbitone or chloral, should be given (for dosage, *see* p. 664). Tracheostomy or intubation is indicated in patients who continue to show acute spasm for more than a few hours, particularly if the cyanosis and obstruction are progressive over this period. Children tend to tire suddenly and get acute cardiac dilatation. Laryngitis should therefore be taken seriously in all but the mildest cases. Allergy should be borne in mind as a possible ætiological factor.

Laryngismus Stridulus (*see* p. 121)

Diphtheritic Croup (*see* p. 550)

Differentiation between this form of croup and acute epiglottitis is sometimes extremely difficult. If there is any doubt, diphtheria antitoxin should be administered at once. It may be necessary to perform a tracheostomy in severe cases. A detailed description of the treatment of diphtheria is given on p. 552.

Acute Epiglottitis

Acute inflammatory œdema limited to the epiglottis will cause a rapidly progressive inspiratory stridor, which in severe cases can progress to death from obstruction. The child's colour may be deceptive, because cyanosis will develop only when the occlusion of the epiglottis is complete. In all children with croup, in whom this diagnosis cannot be excluded, immediate indirect laryngoscopy should be carried out. The œdema is seen to be restricted to the epiglottic region, so that in all severe cases of this kind, tracheostomy, which will completely relieve the obstruction, is indicated forthwith.

Supportive treatment, including antibiotics, is similar to that for acute laryngo-tracheo-bronchitis.

Acute Laryngo-tracheo-bronchitis

This is an acute inflammatory infection which often occurs in epidemic form. In several epidemics influenza virus has been the causative organism, in others the *Hæmophilus influenzæ*, whilst in the remainder varied organisms have been found. The disease has now become a more common cause of death in children under two years than the notifiable infectious diseases. The inflammatory reaction produces a dry, viscid exudate which the child is unable to cough up. This, together with the œdematous reaction in the larynx, trachea and main bronchi, so obstructs the airway that suffocation may occur. There is intense inspiratory stridor with indrawing of the lower inter-costal spaces, and peripheral circulatory failure may develop. The mortality is high, particularly in children under two years of age.

Emergency tracheostomy may be necessary, after which repeated sucking-out of the trachea and main bronchi through the tracheostomy tube is required to maintain an airway. Less severe cases may not need surgical intervention. In all cases, high humidity and oxygen are absolutely essential, and can be provided by using the Humidaire (obtainable from Oxygenaire Ltd.), or alternatively the Croupette (obtainable from Air-Shields Ltd.).

Immediate treatment with a tetracycline or synthetic penicillin should be given until the sensitivity of the infecting organism is known. Dehydration, which tends to make the secretions even more viscous, must be prevented by means of an adequate fluid intake.

DISORDERS OF THE LOWER RESPIRATORY TRACT

Congenital Cystic Disease of the Lung

CONGENITAL cystic disease of the lung is a very rare condition. It seems possible that in the past infants with staphylococcal pneumonia (p. 245) may have been so diagnosed. In older children, tension cysts may develop in asthma, and, in severe bronchiectasis, large areas of lung may progress to a multiple-cyst formation. It is extremely difficult to prove that any particular instance is of congenital rather than acquired origin.

Agenesis of the Lung

In very rare circumstances, a lung or a portion of a lung may fail to develop. Whilst this may in some cases be compatible with a full span of life, absence of larger areas gives rise to cyanosis from birth and death in infancy. The symptoms may be thought to be due to primary atelectasis until bronchography reveals the true state of affairs. There may be other associated congenital abnormalities.

Neonatal Atelectasis (see p. 79)

Hamartoma of Lung

This term is used to describe a " tumour " formed by an aggregation of incompletely differentiated tissues, among which blood vessel tissue can usually be seen. Such " tumours " may be found in any part of the body and are usually discovered in the lung as a chance finding by x-ray. Further investigation and possibly excision may be necessary to exclude a malignant tumour.

Foreign Body in a Bronchus

The accidental inhalation of a foreign body into a bronchus is a not uncommon happening in small children. Peanuts are particularly dangerous, but other objects, such as solid food, small toys, brooches and pieces of coal, may all be involved.

If the trachea is obstructed, immediate treatment to prevent suffocation is essential. The child must be held upside down whilst the back is vigorously slapped. There is seldom time to organise bronchoscopy and if all else fails an immediate tracheostomy is carried out, in the hope that the obstruction is restricted to the larynx.

Where the foreign body has passed directly into a main or lobe bronchus and the occurrence has not been witnessed by an adult, the true state of affairs may not be recognized. The child presents with a persistent dry cough and wheezy respirations. The absence of fever in the early stages is an important diagnostic point. The subsequent course varies; either the cough and wheeziness persist over several days, completely unaffected by treatment, or reactive œdema of the bronchus gives rise to increasing bronchial obstruction with increased inspiratory and expiratory stridor, dyspnœa and cyanosis. Localizing signs either of pulmonary collapse or of ball valve emphysema (due to the fact that air can get past the obstruction into the lung but cannot be exhaled) are the usual signs found in the chest.

The diagnosis is confirmed either by the finding of a radio-opaque foreign body on x-ray or by bronchoscopy. Removal can usually be effected through a bronchoscope; if this is unsuccessful, a thoracotomy must be carried out. In cases where the diagnosis has been delayed, lung abscess (p. 255) and, in the long term, bronchiectasis (p. 256) are serious complications.

Bronchitis

ÆTIOLOGY

A healthy child may develop acute inflammation of the trachea and bronchi as a result of a virus or bacterial infection, such as the *Hæmophilus influenzæ*. An ill, debilitated child is more likely to develop bronchitis, especially as an extension from an infection in the upper respiratory tract. The overweight child with an infected naso-pharynx also tends to develop bronchitis by an extension of this infection. Bronchitis commonly follows the naso-pharyngitis which accompanies measles, whooping-cough, influenza and scarlet fever. Some children develop what is termed bronchitis while they are teething, but it is a matter of doubt whether this is true bronchitis or merely a " cough " due to an excess of saliva collecting around the larynx. Close contact in overcrowded living rooms is probably an important factor, particularly in undernourished children.

PHYSICAL SIGNS

On examining the chest of an infant or young child with bronchitis, the following physical signs may be found. Anyone standing near the child may observe the prolongation of expiration and hear wheezing breath, and the hand on the chest detects the same wheeze. There may be high- or low-pitched rhonchi, as heard with a stethoscope. If the smaller tubules or bronchioles are affected, and especially if the exudate is profuse and thin, moist sounds, both fine and coarse, are present. Both lungs are involved, and usually the distribution is diffuse.

CLINICAL COURSE

In most cases, bronchitis has two definite consecutive stages, namely, a dry stage, when the surface is congested and inflamed, and a second stage, when there is much mucus secretion and moisture. With some infections, the bronchioles seem to stream, just as the nose does, from the beginning. With other infections, there seems to be a period of dry inflammation, during which the cough is short and hacking and accompanied by pain, followed later by a period of moistness or looseness, when much relief is obtained from coughing up the mucopus or bronchial exudate. The temperature is almost invariably raised in bronchitis to 100° or 101°F. The respirations are increased. The cheeks are flushed, and the child is drowsy and irritable. In asthmatic children, there is bronchial spasm, so that prolonged expiration and the characteristic expiratory rhonchi are added to the clinical picture. These expiratory rhonchi are often sibilant or " piping".

TREATMENT

The child should be nursed in a temperature of about 60° F, and during the dry stage an atmosphere of high humidity is most helpful.

Where the cough is dry, hacking and unproductive, and examination of the chest shows high-pitched rhonchi with a minimum of moist sounds, the air can be further moistened by the use of a steam kettle. Oil of eucalyptus or compound tincture of benzoin in the kettle will help to produce an antispasmodic effect.

The indications for chemotherapy depend upon the severity of the infection, the constitution of the child, and the type of organism. In general, the majority of cases do not require such treatment. For weakly children, however, the disease may be cut short and complications avoided by a course of sulphonamide, penicillin or a broad-spectrum antibiotic (*see* Appendix 1). Fluids should be given liberally. The following mixture is helpful where bronchospasm is present in infants:

Tinct. Belladonna	.. .. ..	0·15 ml. (2½ minims)
Ephedrine Hydrochloride	.. ..	8 mg. (⅛ grain)
Potassium Iodide	.. .. ..	60 mg. (1 grain)
Benzoic Acid Solution ..	.. ..	75 mg. (1¼ minims)
Concentrated Anise Water	.. ..	0·1 ml. (1½ minims)
Liquorice Liquid Extract	.. ..	0·15 ml. (2½ minims)
Syrup	.. ..	0·6 ml. (10 minims)
Water	.. ..	to 4 ml. (60 minims)

Give 4 ml. 6-hourly.

Acute Bronchiolitis

When considering infections of the lower respiratory tract, it must be understood that the principal site of infection may be located in the trachea and main bronchi (acute laryngo-tracheo-bronchitis), the medium bronchi (acute bronchitis), the finer bronchioles (acute bronchiolitis) and the alveoli (pneumonia).

In practice, inflammation is seldom restricted to one section alone, but extends both up and down the bronchial tree, although maximal in one particular segment. The clinical picture varies according to which site is predominantly affected.

In acute bronchiolitis or suffocative bronchiolitis, there is widespread inflammation of the terminal bronchioles with the production of a sticky, glairy exudate which obstructs the air-flow to and from the alveoli.

This type of infection is particularly common in small children and in infants still has a significant mortality. It is normally of viral origin, but in some cases the *Hæmophilus Influenzæ* may be responsible. Secondary bacterial infection, usually of staphylococcal origin, may supervene.

CLINICAL PICTURE

The onset is rapid, and by the end of twenty-four hours the child is severely ill. The outstanding features are tachypnœa, with indrawing of the lower intercostal spaces and restlessness. The accessory muscles of respiration come into action as the condition progresses. There is cyanosis, which may be deceptively light in view of the severity of the illness. The child may quickly become collapsed, with associated pallor and limpness. The cough is dry and tends to be repetitive when it occurs.

Examination of the chest reveals no impairment of percussion and the signs on auscultation, which may be limited to scattered fine râles, give little indication of the widespread respiratory obstruction. Despite the relative paucity of physical signs, the condition will often progress to a fatal conclusion in children under two years of age if adequate treatment is not given.

TREATMENT

Treatment is urgent and great vigilance is required in the nursing of these patients. Oxygen should be given in sufficient concentration to overcome restlessness and cyanosis. In this respect, the placing of a child in an oxygen tent may at best only raise the oxygen concentration to 30–40 per cent., and additional oxygen through a face mask may be required for short periods. It is also important to place the child in an atmosphere of high humidity, either by the use of steam or by a humidifier. If oxygen is to be administered simultaneously, the Humidaire or Croupette humidifier may be used to provide a fine mist. In severe cases with generalized toxæmia, there is a place for digoxin in view of the possibility of cardiac failure. It should be introduced cautiously, the full digitalizing dose (see p. 667) being given over a forty-eight hour period.

Antibiotics are advisable in the form of tetracycline or penicillin. If there are signs of collapse, then steroids should be given either by intravenous or intramuscular injection, hydrocortisone acetate in doses of 25 mg. every six hours being suitable for a child of twelve months. After forty-eight hours the dose should be gradually reduced.

It is of the greatest importance to maintain the fluid intake of these infants, as dehydration will tend further to dry the secretions. As the child begins to improve, the secretions become rather less sticky and may be coughed up into the main bronchi and trachea to obstruct the airway at those levels. At this stage, gentle postural drainage or suction at the back of the pharynx, which also stimulates the cough reflex, will help to clear the airway.

After recovery from the acute stage, there may be localized segments of pulmonary collapse which resolve less rapidly and which can become the site of secondary bacterial infection (pneumonitis).

Pneumonia

Pneumonia may be classified as follows:

(i) BRONCHO-PNEUMONIA:

(a) Primary bacterial. — Pneumococcus, streptococcus, staphylococcus, Friedlander's bacillus and *Hæmophilus influenzæ*.

(b) Primary viral. — Viral infections, including influenza A, B and C, psittacosis and ornithosis, adenovirus, ECHO virus, strep. M.G., and the rickettsia of Q fever.

(c) Mixed bacterial and viral infections.

(d) Staphylococcal pneumonia of infancy.

(e) Secondary (i.e. following acute infectious fevers, such as measles and whooping cough). — Similar flora to primary bacterial broncho-pneumonia.

(ii) LOBAR PNEUMONIA: — Pneumococcus (95 per cent.), streptococcus, staphylococcus, and Friedlander's bacillus.

(iii) ASPIRATION PNEUMONIA: — Gastric contents, lipoid or kerosene, and foreign body.

The classification of pneumonia is not as clear cut in clinical practice as this table might suggest. Each type merges into the other and mixed viral and bacterial infections are not uncommon. Primary bacterial pneumonia and classical lobar pneumonia are less common than in the past, due, presumably, to the improved nutrition of children and possibly to a change in virulence of the organisms responsible.

Staphylococcal pneumonia has become clearly separated from the rest and viral infections are now more often recognized and identified.

Recurrent pneumonia suggests an underlying abnormality such as fibrocystic disease (p. 138), bronchiectasis (p. 256) or agammaglobulinæmia (p. 134).

In the temperate climates of the northern hemisphere, the great majority of cases of pneumonia are admitted to hospital from January to March.

Broncho-pneumonia

CLINICAL PICTURE

As a rule, low-grade infection and bronchitis have been present for a varying length of time, a few hours, days or possibly even weeks.

The extension of this infection to the terminal alveoli and through the walls of the bronchioles is determined by the nature of the organism and the general condition of the child. The temperature rises steadily to 101° F or higher. The cough, which has been previously present, becomes much more marked and may be almost continuous. There is an expiratory grunt, and the normal rhythm of breathing is reversed, the pause which usually takes place after expiration now taking place after inspiration. The pulse is rapid. The rate of the respirations increases from the normal 20 or 25 per minute to 40 or even 60 per minute and, instead of the normal ratio between respirations and pulse remaining as 1 : 4, it may be as 1 : 2. The face is flushed and cyanosed, the *alæ nasi* work with each respiration, and the diaphragm and intercostals overact. The child is restless, rolling his head from side to side on the pillow. The mouth is dry and the tongue furred. The lips are parched and the child is drowsy.

VIRUS PNEUMONIA

The viral pneumonias present a varying picture. Many cases show a persistent low fever, dry racking cough, moderate toxæmia and x-ray evidence of consolidation much in excess of that which would be expected from clinical examination. Meningismus is commonly found and may precede the development of pulmonary signs. In other cases, dyspnœa and cyanosis are marked, and the clinical findings bear more resemblance to those of a severe bacterial broncho-pneumonia.

In the highly virulent epidemics of influenzal-virus pneumonia that have occurred, particularly that of 1918, the clinical picture showed a typical heliotrope cyanosis, severe toxæmia and prostration, high initial fever (105–106° F), and a rapid course associated with a very high mortality.

STAPHYLOCOCCAL PNEUMONIA OF INFANCY

Staph. pyogenes, particularly the varieties resistant to standard antibiotics, present a particular problem in infants. Such infections may develop in an unexpanded lung in the newborn (p. 79) or may complicate a broncho-pneumonia of other bacterial or virus origin. Not infrequently, the infection is blood-borne and is in fact a part of a staphylococcal septicæmia arising from umbilical infection, paronychia, purulent conjunctivitis or other local staphylococcal infection.

Thus, apart from the pulmonary signs, the infant may show evidence of the local infection and possibly of other metastatic lesions, such as an osteomyelitis (p. 486). The infant is listless, reluctant to feed, vomits and fails to gain weight. The conventional clinical signs of pneumonia may be minimal, but on x-ray multiple abscesses are visible in both lungs. This tendency to cause rapid focal necrosis with multiple abscess formation is the especial feature of staphylococcal

9

pneumonia. If such an abscess occurs in the periphery of the lung, rupture into the pleural cavity, leading to empyema, is not unlikely.

In the lung, tension cysts, which may reach a considerable size, are not uncommon.

Staphylococcal pneumonia in infancy remains one of the most dangerous hazards of early childhood and still carries a high mortality rate.

DIAGNOSIS OF BRONCHO-PNEUMONIA

An examination of the chest at the very outset may show the signs of bronchitis only, that is, harsh breathing, inspiratory rhonchi, and occasional low-pitched moist sounds. In broncho-pneumonia, as a rule, both lungs are affected. Once the disease is established, the child's breath-sounds remain harsh, but they are higher in note. Where small areas of broncho-pneumonia have become confluent, there may be bronchial breathing. Accompanying the breath-sounds are many fine moist crepitations, which are high-pitched and crackling, indicating areas of consolidation. The percussion note may be resonant or even hyper-resonant (due to compensatory emphysema) or may be impaired. The vocal resonance and vocal fremitus may be increased. During the course of the disease it is common for a number of the pneumonic patches to coalesce, so that larger areas, varying from the size of a shilling to a whole lobe, may give the physical signs of consolidation. In such circumstances it is difficult to differentiate clinically between broncho- and lobar-pneumonia. In virus pneumonia, the pulmonary signs may sometimes be surprisingly slight.

In all types of broncho-pneumonia, the symptoms may precede the development of classical signs in the chest. In such circumstances, diagnosis and the institution of full treatment should not be delayed on this account.

X-rays. The physician may be surprised at the contrast between the physical signs as found by himself by percussion and auscultation and the picture revealed by a good x-ray. The stethoscope even in clever hands may be totally misleading, and an x-ray may show widespread disseminated infection in the lungs or patchy consolidation where none had been previously suspected. This is found particularly in the atypical pneumonias of virus origin.

It is well, therefore, not to believe that pneumonia is excluded by physical examination alone and, where there is ground for suspecting it, an x-ray of the chest should always be taken.

Generally speaking, x-rays will show whether the infection is of the broncho-pneumonic type, with the lesions widespread, or the lobar type, where the lesion is confined to one or more lobes. Very often in the latter, however, the clinical signs are widespread and the division is an x-ray classification rather than a clinical or pathological entity. The formation of multiple lung abscesses in staphylococcal pneumonia has already been described. These may progress in some cases to tension cysts which persist for many months but usually follow a benign course.

Laboratory Findings. Supporting evidence of the diagnosis is found in the polymorphonuclear leucocytosis which accompanies all bacterial pneumonias and in particular in pneumococcal lobar pneumonia, where the absolute polymorph count may sometimes rise as high as 50,000–60,000 per c.mm. In virus pneumonia, however, there may be leucopenia. The urine in pneumonia often contains a little albumin and a greatly reduced chloride content.

Confirmation of the diagnosis of virus pneumonia is obtained from samples of serum taken at the onset and again after a two-week interval; in this way active infection with adenovirus, Coxsackie, ECHO virus, psittacosis, ornithosis and Q fever may be identified.

COMPLICATIONS AND PROGNOSIS

Gastro-enteritis may be added to the clinical picture (parenteral diarrhœa, p. 198). Convulsions may occur in the early stages or cerebral thrombo-phlebitis (p. 454) may develop in a dehydrated infant. In virus pneumonia, encephalitis (p. 411) may be an added complication.

Empyema is a dangerous complication in infants (*see* p. 252). Small sterile pleural effusions, usually resolving without aspiration, are common in cases treated with chemotherapy. Delayed resolution of pneumonia or persistent collapse may follow the acute illness, and, in such cases, bronchiectasis may be a remote complication. Lung abscess, gangrene of the lung, and spontaneous pneumothorax are rare occurrences.

Septicæmia with metastatic pyæmic abscesses or meningitis is now rarely seen, except in staphylococcal infections.

The prognosis depends on several factors, but probably the most important is the age of the child. Children with cerebral palsy or with muscular dystrophy, in whom the chest movement is poor and who have difficulty in coughing up their secretions, tolerate broncho-pneumonia particularly poorly.

In otherwise healthy children the introduction of chemotherapy and antibiotics has not only greatly decreased the mortality from broncho-pneumonia but has reduced the frequency of complications. With few exceptions, fatal cases are confined now to infants and individuals already afflicted with a chronic debilitating illness such as fibrocystic disease.

TREATMENT

The patient should be kept in bed and nursed in a semi-recumbent position. Light, loose clothing should be worn and the bedclothes should be lightly held off the lower limbs with a cradle when the temperature is especially high or if the weather is warm.

Where cyanosis or marked dyspnœa is present, oxygen therapy should be begun early and is best administered in an oxygen tent. If the secretions are dry, " cold mist " can be given by means of a humidifier, for example, the Humidaire (Oxygenaire Ltd.) or Croupette (Air-Shields Ltd.).

Perfect quiet should be maintained and every effort made to get the child to sleep as much as possible. Taking the temperature, changing, and general attention should be arranged at intervals as long as possible, so as to ensure the maximum of sleep. During the hyperpyrexia, sponging the face and limbs with tepid water affords some relief. The diet should be similar to that given on p. 563. Breathing exercises and light percussion of the chest are started as soon as the patient is able to tolerate them.

In severe cases with intense toxæmia and peripheral circulatory failure, treatment with steroids and digitalis should be given, as for comparably severe cases of acute bronchiolitis (p. 243), until the general condition of the child is improved.

Specific Therapy. In all cases where a pneumonia is suspected and the temperature is raised, or where a pneumonia has been clinically or radiologically diagnosed, chemotherapy or antibiotic treatment is indicated. For routine use a sulphonamide or penicillin is to be advocated, at least until the sensitivity of the causal organism to the different antibiotics is known. Tetracyclines, erythromycin and methicillin should be reserved for those cases in which the symptoms are not responding to treatment or in which the organism is found to be insensitive to sulphonamide and penicillin (for dosages, *see* Appendix 1).

In infants in whom a staphylococcal pneumonia is suspected, it is justifiable to commence treatment immediately with an antibiotic to which the prevalent variety of *Staph. pyogenes* is known to be sensitive.

Although the viral infections are not susceptible to antibiotics, it is advisable, even where a virus pneumonia is suspected, to give treatment in view of the likelihood of a mixed infection or of secondary bacterial infection.

Lobar Pneumonia

ÆTIOLOGY

True pneumococcal lobar pneumonia is now uncommon, although the pneumococcus is still prevalent in the healthy population. Routine nose and throat swabbings of healthy children show that in cities in the United Kingdom from 30 to 50 per cent. of children may be expected to carry pneumococci, and typing with specific pneumococcal anti-sera shows that Types 3, 8, 14, 19 and 23 are most commonly found. In lobar pneumonia, however, pneumococcal Types 1, 2, 3, 8, and, in infants, Type 14, are most frequently isolated.

Young infants swallow their sputum and in such cases laryngeal swabs are taken to recover the organism.

PATHOLOGY

The four classical stages of pneumonic consolidation, namely, congestion, red hepatization, grey hepatization, and resolution, show no particular variation in children compared with adults.

CLINICAL PICTURE

(a) *Symptoms*. The disease starts abruptly, with vomiting and a rigor. The child is flushed, and the temperature and respirations rise rapidly; the usual pulse-respiration ratio of 4 : 1 becomes 3 : 1 or even 2 : 1. The pulse is full and bounding; the respirations are grunting, and the respiratory rhythm is reversed. The tongue is coated, and there is a disinclination for food. The cough is short and irritating, and is often accompanied by a stabbing pain on the affected side. If the diaphragmatic pleura is involved, the child may in the early stages complain only of abdominal pain, when the condition may need careful differentiation from an acute abdominal emergency. The child may be light-headed or delirious, and show some degree of cyanosis. There is often herpes about the mouth. Pneumonia may be ushered in by convulsions. Meningism, with delirium and a tendency to hold the neck stiffly, may be present, particularly with an apical pneumonia.

Physical Signs. Early in the disease there may be no local signs. Within 24 or 28 hours, however, the breath-sounds over the affected lobe will first be diminished, so that the air-entry is poor, and the normal harsh breath-sounds may appear exaggerated at the other base. As a rule, the base where the breath-sounds are damped down or diminished is the affected one. Accompanying this period of diminished air-entry and breath-sounds, there is slight impairment of the percussion note. A few hours later, bronchial breathing may be heard, unaccompanied by added sounds. Both the vocal fremitus and the vocal resonance are increased. The percussion note is grossly impaired and is dull, but not stony dull as when percussing over fluid. Very often, when listening at the opposite base, bronchial breathing, slightly less intense, may be heard. This is, as a rule, merely referred from the opposite side. At the time of resolution, the physical signs change; along with the bronchial breathing there are high, fine, crackling crepitations. A little later the accompanying sounds are larger, more bubbling, as if produced in the smaller bronchi, and lower in pitch, showing that there is less consolidated lung to convey them to the listener's ear (*redux* crepitations). Finally, bronchial breathing and the moist sounds clear up, leaving a normal, healthy lung.

X-RAY FINDINGS

The radiological findings are particularly important in cases of central pneumonia when clinical signs may be minimal or absent. A knowledge of the segmental arrangements of the individual lung lobes will also permit accurate localization of the extent of the consolidated area (*see* below).

For example, the confirmation of a clinical diagnosis of right middle-lobe pneumonia by x-rays may be important, especially if there is co-existing empyema in the interlobar fissure, either above or below the right middle lobe. It will be noted (*a*) that in an antero-posterior x-ray the right middle lobe occupies what might easily be assumed to be the position of the right lower lobe, and (*b*) that in the lateral view a portion of the right middle lobe abuts on both the diaphragm and

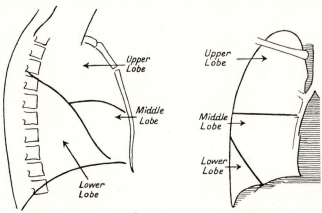

Fig. 21.—Diagram of right lung from the side and from the front.

sternum (*see* Fig. 21). A roughly comparable state of affairs exists in relation to the lingula segment of the left upper lobe, which in position corresponds to the right middle lobe.

LABORATORY FINDINGS

There is a marked polymorphonuclear leucocytosis sometimes reaching as high as 50,000–60,000 per c.mm. The blood culture may occasionally be positive for pneumococci and the organism can be recovered from sputum or by laryngeal swabbing and the pneumococcal type identified.

PROGNOSIS

Since the advent of chemotherapy and antibiotics the prognosis in lobar pneumonia is excellent. In no disease in childhood may the patient appear so ill, and yet so seldom die. When he seems as bad as possible he suddenly recovers in a dramatic fashion. Complications, such as empyema, fibroid lung, and pericarditis, affect both the immediate and the ultimate prognosis for the worse. A leucocyte count of 20,000–30,000 is of good prognostic value.   This should tend to fall along with the temperature.   If it does not do so, it suggests some complication.

TREATMENT

The most important aspects of treatment are careful nursing, oxygen (where respiratory difficulty is marked or where cyanosis is present) and early treatment with antibiotics.   The antibiotic of choice is usually penicillin or a tetracycline which should be started as soon as the diagnosis is made and should be continued for 7–10 days in an average case.   If secondary infection is present, other broad-spectrum antibiotics may subsequently be needed.   Physiotherapy with percussion and breathing exercises should be started early. Usually, the temperature falls by lysis over 48 to 72 hours, but the physical signs clear more slowly.   *Complications* are more likely to require treatment when chemotherapy is ineffective.   The commonest complication is otitis media.   Empyema (*see* p. 252) has become rare; a clear sterile effusion, requiring no treatment, is more common (*see* broncho-pneumonia, p. 247).   Pericarditis, meningitis and peritonitis are now very rare indeed.

Pulmonary Collapse

ÆTIOLOGY[1]

Following an attack of pneumonia, a lobe, or segment of a lobe, may remain unexpanded due to bronchial obstruction by retained secretion.   Segmental or lobar collapse will also occur from bronchial obstruction from many other causes: intraluminar obstruction may result from purulent or mucopurulent secretions in bronchitis and bronchiolitis as well as pneumonic infections, from tuberculous caseation when a hilar gland has ruptured into a bronchus, from an inhaled foreign body and following anæsthetics.   The bronchial wall itself may become constricted.   Thus, in bronchial asthma, as a result of spasm and œdema and from the sticky secretions, one or more bronchi may be obstructed giving rise to collapse of the relevant lung segments.   Bronchial stenosis with secondary pulmonary collapse may be the late result of childhood tuberculosis (*see* p. 580).   A bronchus may also be compressed from without by enlarged hilar glands in primary tuberculosis (p. 580) and pertussis (p. 546), and by the rare tumours and congenital malformations of the lung (p. 240) and mediastinum (p. 267) which are occasionally seen in childhood.

Pulmonary collapse also results from direct compression of the lung itself by pleural effusion, pneumothorax or by an enlarged heart.

CLINICAL PICTURE

Sudden pulmonary collapse may occur following an anæsthetic but more often the condition develops less dramatically.   The degree of

[1] James, Ursula, Brimblecombe, F. S. W., Wells, J. Weston (1956).   *Quart. J. Med.*, **25**, 121.

dyspnœa varies with the amount of lung that is collapsed and the extent to which the mediastinum is shifted to the affected side.   In addition to these signs, the chest movement is limited on the affected side, the percussion note impaired and the air-entry diminished.

TREATMENT

Where a sudden massive collapse has followed an anæsthetic or where the inhalation of a foreign body into a bronchus is suspected, immediately bronchoscopy is indicated.   In other cases of less acute onset but of a persistent nature, bronchoscopy is needed to discover or to confirm the cause of the bronchial obstruction.

Frequently, re-expansion occurs spontaneously, or follows a course of physiotherapy with postural drainage and breathing exercises, without recourse to bronchoscopy.   Secondary infection of the collapsed lung must be watched for and treated early with antibiotics in all cases.   In a small proportion of patients, re-expansion fails to occur and may be followed by the subsequent development of bronchiectasis (p. 256).

Empyema

This is a purulent effusion into the pleural cavity, as a rule accompanying or following pneumonia.

ÆTIOLOGY

The *Staph. pyogenes* has replaced the pneumococcus as the organism now most commonly found in empyemata in children.   The majority of cases are seen in infants.

The tendency in staphylococcal pneumonia to form multiple lung abscesses makes it particularly likely that a small sub-pleural abscess may rupture into the pleural cavity.   In pneumococcal infections, the pleura may be affected simultaneously with the lung, giving rise to a purulent pleurisy.   In some cases, however, it seems clear that there has been an extension of the infection from the lung to the pleura at an interval of some days after the actual onset of the pneumonia.

In the United Kingdom, a tuberculous empyema has become a great rarity, although tuberculous pleural effusions (p. 579) are still seen from time to time in childhood.

PATHOLOGY

The thin almost colourless effusion rapidly fills the pleural cavity. Quickly it becomes milky, opaque, and later purulent.   Within a few hours a thick layer of fibrin coats the parietal and visceral pleuræ. If this is opened and drained, large fibrin clots are evacuated.   There is a tendency for the pleura, whether drained or not, to be permanently thickened over the surface of the lung.   Usually the two thickened layers of pleura are bound together after an empyema, or strong adhesions are formed.

CLINICAL PICTURE

There are two main types of empyema; their clinical evolution is slightly different. In the first (*metapneumonic*), which is much the more common, the child has what appears to be an ordinary lobar pneumonia. The temperature settles and he appears to be doing quite well. Three or four days later the temperature rises slightly and he does not seem as well. Each day the temperature is slightly higher; ultimately it may reach 102° or even 103° F and is swinging in character. The other type (*synpneumonic*) is less common, and in this the temperature shows no inclination to settle down at the end of a week or 10 days, although an ordinary pneumonia has been diagnosed. A few days later the temperature begins to swing, the physical signs becoming more those of fluid than of pneumonia, and on aspiration of the chest pus is found.

Among the symptoms are pain in the affected part of the chest, with a short hacking, unproductive, painful cough, and dyspnœa getting progressively more marked. The breathing and pulse-rate are found to be rapid. Where the empyema is large, the child may be cyanosed, and the heart is displaced to the side opposite to that containing the empyema. On placing the hand over the two sides of the chest a definite thickening and œdema of the chest-wall is detected on the affected side. On percussion, the note is stony-dull, either over the whole lung or over the lower part where the fluid has collected. On auscultation, the breath-sounds are either absent or much reduced. At the upper level of the fluid there is ægophony. Vocal resonance and vocal fremitus are decreased. If heart failure is associated, the liver will be found enlarged. A marked polymorphonuclear leucocytosis is usually present. The blood culture may be positive. X-ray reveals evidence of fluid in the pleural cavity.

In the absence of treatment the fever continues for some weeks or months. The pus may gradually point at or somewhere about the nipple or in the axilla, becoming a so-called " empyema necessitatis." On the other hand, in pure pneumococcal infections, the pus may be gradually reabsorbed, leaving greatly thickened and adherent pleuræ. In this type there is a tendency for interstitial pneumonia to develop, giving rise finally to a fibroid lung with bronchiectasis. This type is, however, uncommon.

TREATMENT

Antibiotics should be employed in all cases as early as possible (*see* Appendix 1); they may arrest the process and avert the need for repeated aspiration or pleural drainage. The longer that treatment is delayed the more likely is it that pleural drainage will be required or that there will be thickening of the pleura and delayed re-expansion of the lung.

The diagnosis of empyema requires confirmation by pleural puncture, when as much of the purulent material as possible should be aspirated. Penicillin should always be injected and left in the pleural cavity; 10,000 units of soluble penicillin is advised for this. Subsequent treatment consists in aspiration and the introduction of penicillin as often as necessary. Where the pus thickens, continuous, air-tight, under-water drainage is advisable until the lung has re-expanded. In addition, systemic antibiotic treatment should be given until the temperature is normal.

In certain cases the treatment is less straightforward. For example, loculation of an empyema cavity may prevent satisfactory treatment and drainage, or there may be masses of fibrinous exudate obliterating the costophrenic sulcus and fixing the diaphragm. In such cases open operation is essential. Obliteration of the cavity and complete re-expansion of the lung are the aims of treatment. As soon as the general condition of the child allows, physiotherapy should be given by a trained therapist to aid expansion and prevent deformity. A period of convalescence should be the doctor's final recommendation.

PROGNOSIS

Before the days of chemotherapy, empyema had a high mortality in young children—up to 50 per cent. in the first year of life but falling to less than 5 per cent. by the age of four. Since the introduction of chemotherapy, empyema has become rare, and the outcome is favourable when an antibiotic to which the organism is sensitive is used. The greatest risk is in the neonatal period, particularly in staphylococcal empyema resistant to penicillin.

Aspiration Pneumonia

In a sense most cases of broncho-pneumonia are due to aspiration of material, including bacteria or viruses, from the upper respiratory passages or the mouth. The term is usually reserved for the introduction into the bronchial tree of gastric contents or foreign material, such as oil or milk. If more solid material is inhaled, a lung abscess (*see* p. 255) is usually the result.

Inhalation of stomach contents into the respiratory tree sets up an intense irritation and causes severe collapse. It is not infrequently the cause of death in patients, ill from other causes, in whom there is vomiting and a diminished cough reflex. Such patients should *always* be nursed well over on to their sides and with the foot of the bed raised. They should never be left unattended.

If inhalation of a vomit does occur, the child should immediately be held upside down and the chest firmly tapped. If the airway is not cleared by these means, bronchoscopy should be carried out as an immediate emergency measure.

The lipoid pneumonias, which are due to repeated inhalations of small quantities of oil or milk (oily nasal drops invariably find their way into the lungs and should never be used), set up a low-grade pneumonitis of patchy distribution which may take several months to resolve. Accidental poisoning with kerosene (p. 642) occurs in small children.

Lung Abscess

In the British Isles, lung abscess is comparatively rare. In America, the incidence appears to be much higher.

Lung abscess may develop after aspiration of any foreign material. The aspiration of pea-nuts is a not infrequent cause in the United States. Unless precautions are taken by the anæsthetist, the aspiration of small portions of adenoid tissue or infected blood may occur during an operation for removal of tonsils and adenoids. In staphylococcal infections in small children (p. 245), multiple lung abscesses may develop. In older children, a single abscess may form during the course of a pneumonia.

CLINICAL PICTURE

Some days after inhaling a foreign body, or after a tonsillectomy, or after pneumonia, a child develops a short cough and appears less well. The temperature rises. An examination of the chest reveals an area of poor air entry with many fine crepitations. An x-ray will show an opaque area at first and, later, a cavity with a fluid level.

After a varying time, usually between one and three weeks, the child, during a fit of coughing, may bring up some thick, foul-smelling material, and it will be found that the abscess has drained into a bronchus, with immediate relief and recovery. Rarely, an empyema forms.

TREATMENT

Antibiotics should be started at once and continued for at least 10 days. In many cases, as already mentioned, there is spontaneous drainage of an abscess, and provided adequate antibiotic cover is given no further treatment is necessary. Frequent x-rays are necessary to review progress.

If after a few days there is no sign of the abscess discharging itself, bronchoscopy should be performed and as much debris sucked out from the affected lobe as possible. Subsequent drainage may then occur. Physiotherapy with postural drainage is helpful if the patient's general condition is good enough to warrant its use.

Excision of a lobe of a lung is rarely necessary and should be carried out only after all other measures of treatment, including bronchoscopy, have been undertaken and when it has become clear that irreversible damage to the affected lobe has occurred. The prognosis of an isolated lung abscess in childhood is good, and few sequelæ occur as a rule. Bronchiectasis is the most common.

Bronchiectasis

ÆTIOLOGY AND PATHOLOGY[1]

The essential cause of bronchiectasis is bronchial or bronchiolar obstruction associated with damage to the bronchiolar walls peripheral to the obstruction from infection. The obstruction may be caused by a plug of mucus, or by a foreign body retained in the bronchus, or it may be due to the pressure of an enlarged lymphatic gland or tumour. The glandular component of a primary tuberculous complex may occlude by pressure from without, or it may erode the bronchial wall, more or less filling the lumen with caseous tissue.

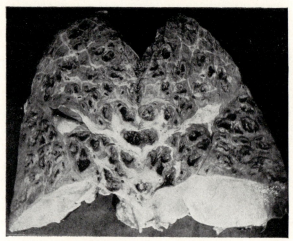

Fig. 22.—State of lung in bronchiectasis.

Whatever the cause, the result of obstruction to a bronchus, if complete, is always the same: absorption collapse of the distal alveoli· When massive collapse occurs, it seems probable that plugs of mucus are apt to be sucked piecemeal from larger bronchi into the smaller tubes. These changes are more likely to occur in broncho-pneumonia than in lobar pneumonia. A common sequence of events is for some of the bronchi to become obstructed during broncho-pneumonia and, these not being cleared, absorption collapse persists; the bronchial walls, softened by infection and having lost their supporting cushion of air, then dilate; obliteration of the alveoli is thought to precede this process.

Bronchiectasis may be saccular, fusiform, or cylindrical. The cavities may be clean and relatively dry, or they may be infected and retain pus or muco-pus; this is especially the case in saccular dilatations. The disease may be confined to a segment of a lobe, or it

[1] Lander, F. P. L., Davidson, M. (1938). *Brit. J. Radiol.*, **11**, 65.

may involve a whole lobe, or be widespread in most of the bronchial tree (*see* Fig. 22), depending upon the ætiology. Localized bronchial lesions, such as bronchial stenosis following primary tuberculosis or chronic localized obstruction by a foreign body, are more likely to cause segmental or lobar disease, while virus infections, such as measles or influenzal broncho-pneumonia, may be responsible for generalized basal bronchiectasis. There is a well-recognized association between bronchiectasis and para-nasal sinusitis. It has been

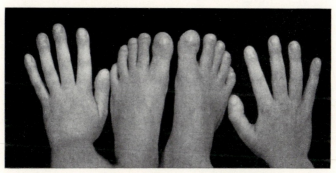

Fig. 23.—Clubbing of fingers and toes in bronchiectasis.

reported from Australia that bronchiectasis is not infrequently seen following pink disease. Occasionally persistent pulmonary collapse following asthma may lead to bronchiectasis.

SYMPTOMS AND DIAGNOSIS

There may be a complaint that, following broncho-pneumonia after measles or whooping-cough, the child has had a persistent cough. On the other hand the symptoms may develop insidiously after one of the causative illnesses already mentioned. In the great majority of cases, a persistent productive cough is a constant feature, the sputum being green and purulent or mucopurulent. In the rare cases of bronchiectasis limited to an upper lobe, where free dirainage is possible, sputum may be minimal but hæmoptysis may be the leading symptom. In most patients, the sputum is copious, amounting to an ounce or more in the day. The paroxysms of coughing are not frequent, perhaps three or four in 24 hours, but, as a rule, they are productive if the child is in a suitable position to ensure drainage of the cavities. In established cases there may be clubbing, oral fœtor and dyspnœa. The sputum must be examined to determine the nature of the infecting organism and to exclude pulmonary tuberculosis.

Examination of the chest often reveals definite flattening or retraction of the ribs on the affected side. On percussion the note is dull over the affected lobe. It may be so dull as to suggest fluid, but it

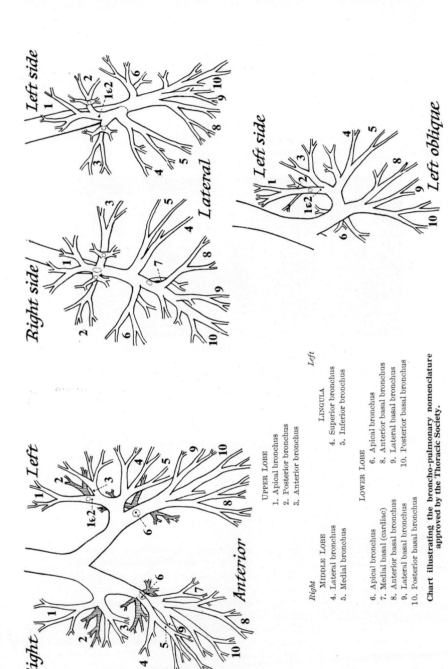

Right

Left

UPPER LOBE
1. Apical bronchus
2. Posterior bronchus
3. Anterior bronchus

LINGULA
4. Superior bronchus
5. Inferior bronchus

Right

MIDDLE LOBE
4. Lateral bronchus
5. Medial bronchus

LOWER LOBE
6. Apical bronchus
7. Medial basal (cardiac) bronchus
8. Anterior basal bronchus
9. Lateral basal bronchus
10. Posterior basal bronchus

LOWER LOBE
6. Apical bronchus
8. Anterior basal bronchus
9. Lateral basal bronchus
10. Posterior basal bronchus

Chart illustrating the broncho-pulmonary nomenclature approved by the Thoracic Society.

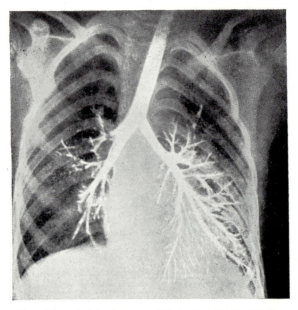

Normal bronchial tree in a case of slowly resolving pneumonia.

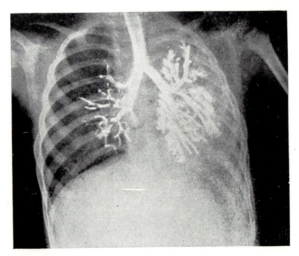

Bronchiectasis throughout left lung.

PLATE III. Bronchography.

is usually what may be termed apple dullness, not stony dullness. On auscultation the physical signs vary enormously, depending on whether or not the tubes contain fluid.   If they are well cleared out, the breath-sounds are bronchial or amphoric, suggesting cavity-formation.   In addition, the accompanying sounds are high-pitched, large and splashing.   If the bronchi are partially filled, the breath-sounds may be markedly diminished and distant, with a few accompanying moist sounds only.   If quite filled, as they are at certain times in the day, the breath-sounds may be absent and there may be no added sounds.   By inverting the child, so that the secretions tend to drain away, coughing is provoked and the cavities emptied, and in a few moments the auscultatory signs are completely changed. The question whether fluid is present in the pleura will often arise. It should be noted that in bronchiectasis the heart is drawn over to the affected side and not pushed away from it as with fluid in the pleural cavity.   The chest-wall is also definitely flattened on the affected side.

Bronchoscopy.   This is often of great value in ascertaining the reason why a lobe is collapsed and becoming bronchiectatic.   During bronchoscopy a foreign body may be removed, causing the re-expansion of the collapsed lobe, or a mediastinal gland occluding the lumen of a bronchus may be detected.

Bronchography.   The investigation of bronchiectasis by means of Lipiodol or Dionosil will throw light on the whole condition (Plate III).

The procedure is best carried out in children under general anæsthesia.   The technique varies in different centres.   In many, direct intubation is carried out and a rubber catheter passed into the appropriate main bronchus and the Lipiodol injected.   In others, a short rubber tube is passed to the back of the nose and with the head held back the Lipiodol runs into the trachea.   There is no place in pædiatric practice for bronchography by crico-thyroid injection under local anæsthesia, except in older children.

Whatever the method of introduction of the radio-opaque substance, the subsequent positioning of the patient to ensure that complete filling of all bronchial segments is obtained is the most important part of the technique.

Bronchography should not be undertaken until energetic physiotherapy, including postural drainage, has cleared the infected lung areas of as much as possible of their retained secretions.

TREATMENT

Experienced judgment is required to manage correctly the treatment of a bronchiectatic child.   Both medical and surgical treatment is available and a balance must be struck between them.

Medical Treatment. The following simple expectorant from the British National Formulary (1960) is useful.

> R Sodium Bicarbonate, 0·6 G. (10 grains)
> Sodium Chloride, 0·2 G. (3 grains)
> Emulsion of Chloroform, 0·3 ml. (5 minims)
> Anise Water to 15 ml. (½ ounce)

A five-year-old child to take 8 ml. (2 drachms) three times a day in hot water, a ten-year-old child 15 ml. (½ ounce) in the same manner.

The indications for antibiotic treatment have to be carefully considered. Short courses of treatment may be given when acute infections occur or as a preliminary to such procedures as bronchography. Some authorities advise prolonged courses of antibiotics lasting several years in an attempt to maintain the damaged areas of lung free from infection. To be set against this is the risk of encouraging the growth of *Staph. pyogenes* which are resistant to the usual antibiotics. Each patient must be judged as an individual, and it would seem advisable to restrict treatment of this kind to the more severely affected cases.

Physiotherapy is a vital aspect of treatment. Postural drainage carried out for periods up to a half to one hour twice daily, together with " frappage " of the chest-wall will do much to clear the infected lung segments. In addition, the question of the child sleeping on a tipping frame, so that the bronchial secretions are draining into the upper respiratory passages throughout the night, should be considered. Such treatment, however, carries the risk of repeatedly re-infecting the para-nasal sinuses which in turn contribute to the activity of the pulmonary lesion. Proper instruction in breathing exercises and insistence that they are carried out daily is essential.

After the diagnosis has been established, physiotherapy started and the teeth and sinuses attended to, long-term decisions about treatment must be made. Whether surgical intervention is eventually required or not, a prolonged period of medical treatment is usually a necessary preliminary. It is surprising to find that in that period a number of cases, which originally appeared to severe that lobectomy was considered to be necessary, improve so much that no operation is required. The prolonged period of medical treatment is best carried out in the country or at the seaside, and for this purpose residential open-air schools are provided. Physiotherapy, including postural drainage, regular medical supervision with immediate treatment with antibiotics for respiratory infections, nourishing diet, fresh air and exercise are the essentials of treatment. As most of the patients will be of school age, it is important that their education is continued during this period.

Every effort should be made to overcome para-nasal sinus infection in these cases. In no circumstances should surgical treatment be carried out for bronchiectasis until this has been done.

Surgical Treatment.   After six months to a year of medical observation it is possible to make an estimate of the progress of the disease and its rate of extension or regression.   In general terms, surgical intervention is required for those cases which fail to improve on medical treatment, and in which the disease is sufficiently localized to make surgical excision of all the lung segments affected by bronchiectasis a practical proposition.   Repeated review of individual patients is necessary. Surgery is contra-indicated in those cases in which widespread bronchiectasis is present, for, if attempted, there is frequently a deterioration in the state of the bronchiectatic segments which must necessarily be left *in situ*.   Localized bronchiectasis which shows a steady clinical and radiological improvement on medical treatment should be treated conservatively, but, if the improvement ceases, surgery should be considered.

PROGNOSIS

In properly selected surgical cases the prognosis is excellent and the mortality from operation not more than 1 per cent.   In cases which respond to medical treatment the prognosis is equally good.

In cases of widespread bronchiectasis which are unsuitable for surgery, the prognosis is very poor, cerebral abscess or death from corpulmonale and pneumonia being the likely outcome.

Spontaneous Pneumothorax

Spontaneous entry of air into the pleural cavity is an infrequent cause of symptoms in childhood.

In the newborn, a small pneumothorax may be detectable on x-ray but seldom gives rise to clinical abnormalities.   In older children, recurrent spontaneous pneumothoraces may very occasionally occur with asthma and emphysema, and a single episode may complicate the course of a lung abscess or tension cyst that has developed after a staphylococcal pneumonia.

TREATMENT

In severe cases, where there is evidence of considerable mediastinal shift and where dyspnœa is present, immediate aspiration of the air is essential.   Subsequently an underwater sealed drainage of the pleural cavity can be set up.   In milder cases, the air is slowly reabsorbed over several weeks, during which time the underlying cause of the pneumothorax is treated.

Pulmonary Tuberculosis

For tuberculosis of the respiratory system, *see* Chapter 25.

Fibrocystic Disease (Mucoviscidosis) (*see* p. 138).

Pulmonary Infiltrations from Other Causes

Symmetrical generalized pulmonary infiltrations, sometimes with calcification, are occasionally met with in children. They include *histiocytic reticulosis (Lettere-Siwe)* (p. 351), *tuberose sclerosis* (p. 447), *histoplasmosis and coccidiomycosis* (below), *idiopathic pulmonary hæmosiderosis* (below), *sarcoidosis, pulmonary eosinophilia* (below), *visceral larval migrans* (p. 630), and the *Hamman-Rich syndrome* (below).

Lettere-Siwe disease is usually fatal, the child showing rapidly increasing wasting and weakness apart from the other specific signs of the eosinophilic infiltration and xanthomatosis which may involve liver, spleen and reticulo-endothelial glands. Cutaneous eosinophilic granulomata may be present. The pulmonary infiltration in tuberose sclerosis is usually a chance finding on x-ray in a child who shows the classical neurological picture (p. 447). Cases of histoplasmosis and coccidiomycosis may be diagnosed by the intradermal skin tests which are highly specific.

Idiopathic pulmonary hæmosiderosis is a rare disease; the pulmonary deposition of iron is associated with increasing anæmia and hæmoptysis, and the prognosis is very poor. Sarcoidosis is rare in childhood compared with adult life. The infiltration spreads out from the hilum of each lung and is associated with a raised globulin in the serum proteins. The negative tuberculin reaction excludes tuberculosis. Pulmonary eosinophilia is usually seen in the tropics and, like visceral larval migrans, is associated with a massive eosinophilia in the peripheral blood. The Hamman-Rich syndrome, or diffuse progressive interstitial fibrosis of the lungs, has very rarely been encountered in childhood. Slowly progressive respiratory distress, cough, cyanosis and clubbing of the fingers develop with only minimal clinical signs in the chest. Pulmonary hypertension and cor pulmonale inevitably ensue with a fatal outcome. The x-ray shows diffuse mottling of both lungs and at autopsy gross destruction of lung tissue by interstitial fibrosis is found. The cause is unknown.

ASTHMA AND HAY FEVER

Asthma

ASTHMA may occur at any age, and sometimes appears to commence almost from birth. Two-thirds of the cases occurring before puberty start before the age of 3 years.

ÆTIOLOGY

In more than half the cases there is a family history of asthma, hay fever, eczema, or urticaria. This suggests a marked tendency for asthma to be inherited, or at least a constitutional tendency to this type of reaction under conditions of stress.

It is thought that asthma is (1) a spasm of the bronchial muscles, (2) an urticaria and swelling of the lining mucous membrane of the bronchioles, or (3) obstruction of the smallest bronchioles by plugs of mucus. It is possible that all three factors operate in some cases.

Various factors may precipitate an attack of asthma. Among the commonest are (1) infections, especially of the naso-pharynx, (2) hypersensitiveness to inhalants, (3) psychogenic; there is no doubt that excitement and nervousness without other influences can initiate attacks.

1. *Infections.* Naso-pharyngeal infections, together with the viruses of the common cold or influenza, appear to precipitate an attack of asthma in an allergic child. Frequently the lining membrane of the nose is swollen and more engorged than normal because of the presence of allergic rhinitis. Thus, the normal filtering mechanism of the nose against dust particles, pollens or bacteria may be less efficient than normal or indeed the nose may be so obstructed that nasal breathing is impossible.

2. *Allergy* (hypersensitiveness to pollens or other inhalants). Some children have severe asthma only during the pollen season. Other inhalants, such as feathers, horse-hair, house-dust, cat or dog fur, or orris root, are on occasion the exciting factors. They may account for nocturnal attacks, as when the child is in intimate contact with his feather pillow, eiderdown and horsehair mattress.

3. *Psychogenic.* There is no doubt that certain attacks are non-physical in their origin. Week-end asthma in schoolchildren is a not uncommon example, and emotional upsets at any time may precipitate an attack. *The importance of tensions and stress within the home in the causation of repeated asthma in the child can often be clearly seen when the child is sent to a convalescent home or some similar neutral environment. Although all the other causative agents of asthmatic attacks such as dusts, pollens and respiratory infections remain, away from home the asthmatic attacks cease.*

Given the basic allergic diathesis, a child tends to exhibit his underlying psychological difficulties in this way rather than by any of the other behavioural disorders seen in other children. The natural concern of the parents over the distressing nocturnal bronchospasm in their child and their own loss of sleep causes further anxiety and thus further bronchospasm in their offspring.

In the management of the asthmatic child psychogenic factors are thus of great importance and are more fully discussed in Chapter 18.

CLINICAL PICTURE

The child may be put to bed with what appears to be a slight cold, with or without a temperature, but wakes during the night, much distressed, coughing and wheezing and unable to get his breath. His difficult breathing worries him, and he looks anxious and care-worn and complains of tightness about the chest.　The attack may be over in a few hours or cease on waking in the morning; on the other hand, if accompanied by a fever, it may continue for some days, and manifest some degree of true bronchitis.

The term bronchial asthma may be reserved for cases starting very acutely and without signs of accompanying infection.　In other cases, bronchospasm is superimposed upon an upper respiratory infection and the term asthmatic bronchitis may be employed.　One child may suffer at various times from each type, although usually one variety will predominate.　The duration of the attacks will also vary, being sometimes short and sharp and sometimes long drawn out, lasting several days.

DIAGNOSIS

The percussion note is unchanged, or hyper-resonant due to an accompanying emphysema.　On auscultation, expiration is markedly prolonged, but both inspiratory and expiratory rhonchi are heard. The excursion of the chest is small and the air entry extremely poor. The chest may be barrel-shaped.　In asthma, the dyspnœa is primarily expiratory.

In every case, organic pulmonary disease must be carefully excluded as asthma may be simulated by such conditions as fibroid lung or bronchiectasis, especially cases of long standing.　An x-ray of the chest and a tuberculin test is of value as a routine.　Repeated attacks of bronchitis for no apparent cause in a child should always suggest asthma.　The blood-count may show an eosinophilia of from 4 per cent. to 10 per cent.　Asthma should also be suspected if the child has a previous history of well-marked eczema or urticaria.　The family history may be suggestive.

PREVENTIVE TREATMENT

Where repeated attacks commence with fever, it is reasonable to suspect an infection, and a careful examination of the tonsils and ears should be made; where necessary, infected tonsils and adenoids should be removed.　The sinuses may also require treatment.　In some cases, associated allergic rhinitis is troublesome and requires simultaneous treatment.　In a proportion of cases, pulmonary disease in the form of collapse, bronchiectasis, or even tuberculosis is found.

Physiotherapy.　Breathing exercises are a most vital aspect of treatment, both in the prevention and treatment of the emphysema and poor thoracic movement, and for use also in actual asthmatic attacks. By using proper diaphragmatic movement much of the distress and disablement during an attack may be overcome.

Allergy.　When the child is sensitive to feathers or horse-hair, both of which are commonly found in bedding, it is advisable to use a mattress and pillows made of kapok or rubber material, such as soft rubber latex foam. Exclusion of wool is only occasionally necessary, but no eiderdown should be used or other padded type of bedding.

Skin-Testing and Desensitization. Sensitivity to inhalants may be ascertained by a series of intra-cutaneous injections of group inhalants, such as feathers, hairs and pollens. A positive skin-reaction is revealed by a white wheal, surrounded by a reddened area, appearing within 5 or 10 minutes. In both scratch and intra-cutaneous testing, control tests are necessary.

Desensitization may be carried out against inhalants by means of a prolonged course of subcutaneous injections using an appropriate vaccine. It is occasionally helpful in cases where a clear-cut sensitivity such as a pollen allergy exists.

It is frequently found that a routine dose of a quarter of a grain of ephedrine (either in tablet form or as elixir) given at bed-time, and perhaps repeated once in the night, will prevent attacks of acute spasmodic asthma. If the child is troubled by attacks during the day, then ephedrine can be administered in the mornings in similar dosage.

General Management. The emotional aspect is often the most important and yet the most difficult one to treat. Incompatibility between the parents, broken homes and conflicts of similar kinds may all be contributory. Week-end asthma in schoolchildren can often be overcome most satisfactorily by giving ephedrine $\frac{1}{4}$ grain twice daily over the danger period. The subject of emotional stress is fully discussed in Chapter 18.

Open-air School. Many severely affected asthmatic children tend to miss a lot of school. The well-chosen use of residential and day open-air schools is often of great benefit both physically and educatively to such children.

The general approach of the physician is extremely important. Very often he will find that the life of an asthmatic child has become far too hedged in by restrictions. The child may have been forbidden such normal activities as swimming and games, and the eating of many foods in everyday use. Unless there is very clear evidence that any of these is a clear-cut causative agent of attacks, the purpose of the physician should be to inculcate an attitude of mind which can best be expressed as: " I went to school despite my asthma," rather than " I could not go to school because of my asthma."

Steroids. The place of long-term treatment with steroids as a preventive against asthma has to be considered. There is little doubt, if such treatment is given over a fairly prolonged period of three to six months, that in most of the patients the number and severity of the attacks will be greatly reduced.

On the other hand, the risks of long-term treatment with steroids are potentially so serious that they may either endanger the life of the patient or, if long continued, restrict the child's growth in height (*see* p. 661).

Herein lies a temptation to the physician who, taking a short-term view, can see at hand a quick advantage from successful treatment which may cause him to close his mind to the serious long-term dangers.

Before the physician decides on long-term steroid therapy, therefore, it should be clearly established that the risk to the child of continuing to undergo severe asthmatic attacks is greater than the known risks of long-term steroid therapy. It would seem to be a good working rule never to embark on such treatment without the benefit of a second opinion from a medical colleague. The techniques of steroid therapy are discussed in Appendix 2, p. 657.

TREATMENT OF THE ATTACK

In a bad attack of asthma, two to five minims of adrenaline are given subcutaneously, depending upon the age of the child; or inhalations of 1 in 100 solution of adrenaline, or isoprenaline may be given by means of a spray, and repeated if necessary. Alternatively, one quarter grain of ephedrine given in tablet form or as elixir of ephedrine will be found effective in the subacute case, and may be repeated once or twice in the night if necessary. Isoprenaline may also be given sublingually; ten milligrammes in a tablet to be dissolved under the tongue is a suitable dose for a seven-year-old child. Sublingual administration is not practicable in infants or toddlers. Aminophylline, given either as a suppository or by intravenous injection, is a valuable alternative. In all cases where the child is restless and wakeful, a suitable dose of phenobarbitonum (B.P.) should be given (*see* p. 664). ACTH or cortisone are indicated in cases of *status asthmaticus* which fail to respond to aminophylline. The dangers of steroid therapy on a long-term basis do not apply to the same extent to short-term treatment, and as a life-saving measure intravenous or intramuscular corticosteroid is indicated (*see* p. 660).

In many severe attacks, oxygen will be required; for small children, an oxygen tent with a humidifier attachment is the most convenient method (*see* p. 248).

PROGNOSIS

Often the prognosis is favourable and many children cease to have attacks as they grow older, this improvement being somewhat more consistent in the case of boys. On the other hand, when treatment does not succeed, frequent or prolonged attacks continuing to occur, a child may sometimes become a respiratory cripple. This is more likely to happen when asthma occurs almost daily for many weeks or months, and there is loss of thoracic movement with deformity which indicates chronic emphysema and the possibility of right heart strain. In a few such cases, death may occur during an attack of asthma; in others there is increasing enlargement of the right ventricle (*cor pulmonale*) and cardiac failure may ensue.

Hay Fever (Allergic Rhinitis)

Hay fever is the reaction of an individual to grass, plant and tree pollens, dust, and other irritating inhalants.

In the United Kingdom, about the middle of May, the sufferers experience an itching or burning sensation in the inner canthus of the eye, and in the naso-pharynx. Violent sneezing, with a profuse watery discharge, occurs; the eyes become congested, there is a tendency to cough, and there may be slight deafness. These symptoms are worse in the morning. Frequently, there is, in addition, a tendency to asthma. A family history of asthma, hay fever or eczema is common. Other patients have persistent symptoms throughout the year. The nasal mucosa is swollen and pink, and rhinorrhœa is profuse. Nasal obstruction is a constant feature. For such cases the more general term of allergic rhinitis is appropriate. Secondary nasal infection involving the paranasal sinuses is common. The constant inhalation of nasal secretions gives rise to a persistent cough, whilst the swallowing of the secretions sets up a secondary gastritis.

As in asthma (*see* p. 262), pollen sensitivity may be demonstrated by skin-tests, but specific desensitization is rather more valuable. This treatment is best given in the first quarter of the year—January to April.

Antihistamines are more effective in hay fever than in asthma. Diphenhydramine hydrochloride (Benadryl), chlorpheniramine (Piriton), and mepyramine maleate (Anthisan) are widely used. Often one particular preparation is found to be more effective than any other for a particular patient (for dosage, *see* p. 664).

DISEASES OF THE MEDIASTINUM

Infective Mediastinitis

THIS is an exceptionally rare condition which may occur as a part of an overwhelming staphylococcal septicæmia in association with pericarditis and empyema. It may occasionally follow chest injuries or chest surgery. *Mediastinal emphysema* has been described in whooping-cough and may be found after tracheostomy.

Mediastinal Tumours

Primary tumours of the mediastinum, if posterior in position, are likely to arise from nerve tissue as neurofibromata. Tumours arising centrally are found in the form of bronchial, pulmonary, pericardial or gastric cysts. The benign enlargement of the thymus and very rare thymic tumour (p. 167) account for most tumours arising in the anterior mediastinum. Dermoid tumours may sometimes be found in any part of the mediastinum. Retrosternal extension of a goitre is seldom seen in childhood.

Wherever the place of origin, mediastinal tumours may be symptomless and be discovered only at routine x-ray examination. They may, however, cause obstructive symptoms in any of the main intrathoracic structures. Thus, stridor and bronchial obstruction with increasing dyspnœa due to ball-valve emphysema of the affected lung, dysphagia due to œsophageal obstruction, or œdema and venous engorgement of the head and neck due to obstruction of the venous return *via* the superior vena cava may all be seen. Full investigation in a thoracic-surgery unit is then indicated to determine whether surgical treatment is possible.

Secondary tumours involving mediastinal glands, such as the neuroblastoma (p. 378), Wilms' tumour (p. 376), and lymphosarcoma, are seen in the malignant neoplasms of childhood. Hodgkin's disease (p. 351) and leukæmia (p. 347) may also involve the mediastinum. Tuberculous hilar adenitis (p. 585) can usually be differentiated from these conditions without difficulty.

CHAPTER 14

Cardiac and Circulatory Disorders

ALTHOUGH congenital and acquired heart disease are together major causes of morbidity and mortality in childhood, cardiac *symptoms* are often minimal in the young. The interpretation of cardiac *signs* is therefore of paramount importance.

SYMPTOMS OF HEART DISEASE IN CHILDHOOD

MANY children with congenital malformations of the heart have no symptoms of any kind, and in such cases care must be taken to ensure that symptoms are not suggested to the child by over-anxious parents. Where genuine symptoms occur, they may not at first sight suggest heart disease. Thus, in infancy, severe lesions can give rise to *reluctance to feed* and *inadequate weight gain*. In other cases, *tachypnœa* or *cyanosis* will immediately suggest a cardiac lesion. *Cardiac pain* is very rare in childhood but is found in the unusual condition of an aberrant left coronary artery arising from the pulmonary artery. Such infants appear to have true angina of effort, with *pallor and sweating*, and *cry as if in pain*, often during and after feeds. The symptoms of cardiac failure include *œdema*, which tends to be more generalized than the dependent œdema seen in adults, whilst in infants with left heart failure *repeated episodes of cough and dyspnœa* occur, which may be mistakenly attributed to uncomplicated respiratory infections. The full clinical picture of cardiac failure in infancy is described in detail on p. 283.

The principal symptoms of myocarditis (p. 309) are *listlessness* and *fatigue*, whilst in pericarditis (p. 301) *substernal discomfort and vomiting* should direct attention to the heart. In rheumatic carditis, the associated symptoms of rheumatism elsewhere will suggest the diagnosis.

GENERAL SIGNS OF HEART DISEASE IN CHILDHOOD

OFTEN is more learnt about the heart by general observation and by palpation than from the stethoscope.

In congenital heart lesions with a right to left intracardiac shunt (p. 282), *cyanosis* is either present at birth or develops later together with *clubbing of the fingers*.

Cardiac enlargement in infancy, from whatever cause, will give rise to *bulging of the praecordium* (which may be progressive during the first months of life). Such enlargement is associated with a *rapid respiratory rate* and with *indrawing of the lower intercostal spaces on inspiration (Naish's sign).* In older children, *tachypnœa* without cyanosis is a feature of the cases in which a large left to right intracardiac shunt is present (p. 282).

Examination should always include the palpation of both radial arteries and the femoral pulse (*see* coarctation of the aorta, p. 285). The blood pressure is recorded in one arm or in both, where the radial pulses feel unequal or where an abnormality of the ascending aorta is suspected. Where the *femoral pulses are absent or thin,* the blood pressure is recorded also in the legs. The normal values and techniques are described on p. 277.

Inspection and palpation of the præcordium gives valuable information in the majority of children with severe congenital lesions. Thus, *movement of the sternum* itself or of *the sixth rib close to the sternum* is indicative of *right ventricular hypertrophy;* this may be confirmed by placing two fingers below the xiphoid cartilage, upward palpation deep to the xiphoid then confirming the excessive pulsation. *Left ventricular hypertrophy* gives rise to *a forceful apex beat* and causes actual movement of the overlying rib, in contrast to the " tapping " impulse without rib movement (" all bark and no bite ") found in cases of right ventricular hypertrophy alone. The individual lesions which give rise to right-or left-sided hypertrophy are classified on pp. 281–282.

Heart failure during infancy is a not uncommon finding in congenital heart disease. Its early recognition and treatment is of great prognostic importance (pp. 283–284).

Finally congenital cardiac malformations may be associated with other specific congenital abnormalities, notably mongolism (p. 470), arachnodactyly (*see* Marfan's syndrome, p. 479), and the rubella syndrome (p. 540), but are also found in increased frequency wherever another congenital malformation of any kind exists.

The detailed signs of rheumatic myocarditis (p. 309) and of acute pericarditis (p. 301) are described in Chapter 15.

THE HEART SOUNDS

THE *first* sound is a mixed one produced by closure of the mitral and tricuspid valves, and possibly by the opening of the semilunar valves as well. Changes in the quality and duration of this sound are mainly due to the position of the valve cusps when the ventricles begin to contract, although the strength of ventricular contraction and the conduction of the sound to the stethoscope, through the lung and chest wall, also play their part.

The *second* sound is mainly caused by the closure of the aortic and pulmonary valves, and is best heard in the left and right second intercostal spaces. The closing of the semilunar valves is not exactly synchronous and when separately heard the result is referred to as *splitting* of the second sound (Fig. 24). The first component of the split " second " sound is usually aortic and the second component pulmonary. Splitting is most easily heard to the left of the sternum in the second and third interspaces, and in healthy children and young adults the gap widens slightly towards the end of inspiration. With advancing age the two components become indistinguishable, perhaps because closure of the aortic valve is delayed. *Pathological splitting* is a further widening of the interval between the aortic and the pulmonary components and indicates delay in closure of the pulmonary valve; in such cases there is a *fixed split*, the variation with respiration disappearing. In auricular septal defects, it is probably caused by the over-filling of the right ventricle.

The second heart sound is easily heard in all areas and in children is relatively louder in the second left interspace than in adults. The assumption that the aortic valve sound is best heard over the aortic area and the pulmonary valve sound over the pulmonary area is not always true. Accentuation of the second heart sound may be heard when the chest wall is thin or the lung retracted from the base of the heart. Hypertension, either systemic or pulmonary, also causes accentuation of the second sound and it may be possible to suspect which of its components is accentuated; in systemic hypertension it will be the first component, in pulmonary hypertension the second. Phonocardiography adds precision to this observation.

A *single second sound* may be heard where either aortic or pulmonary stenosis prevents proper closure of the particular valve.

THE PHYSIOLOGICAL THIRD HEART SOUND

The third heart sound is also a normal phenomenon. It is quite different from the splitting of the second heart sound. Soft and low-pitched, the third heart sound is *audible at the apex* and it is attributed to rapid filling of the left ventricle. With careful auscultation it can be heard in a majority of children after the period of infancy. It is also audible in adolescents and young adults; later in life it becomes less and less distinct. The differentiation between a normal third heart sound and a short diastolic mitral murmur can be difficult, especially as each of these sounds is brought into prominence by turning the patient towards his left side. Phonocardiography is helpful since a diastolic murmur is recorded just after the third sound (Fig. 32). An *abnormal* third heart sound may be prominent in certain forms of advanced disease especially when the auricles are fibrillating. Phonocardiography shows that the third heart sound tends to be accentuated in cases of mitral incompetence and diminished or absent in early mitral stenosis.

CARDIAC MURMURS

WHEN listening over the præcordium a systolic bruit is often heard in a child and the doctor has to make up his mind whether the systolic bruit is innocent (which is the more likely), or whether it means rheumatic carditis or a congenital cardiac lesion. Nearly all innocent murmurs are systolic in time. In contrast, the discovery of a diastolic murmur indicates, with few, if any, exceptions, an organic disorder of the heart.

EXTRACARDIAC MURMURS

These may be defined as audible vibrations caused by the action of the heart on surrounding structures. Only the friction rubs of inflamed serous surfaces have *pathological* significance. *Pericardial* friction sounds are superficial, systolic and diastolic in time, and often slightly out of step with the heart sounds. They may be fine, like the rubbing together of hairs, or coarse and somewhat leathery (*see* p. 301). *Pleuropericardial* friction waxes and wanes with respiration, and indicates pleurisy.

Innocent Murmurs. It is thought, although the explanation is uncertain, that the mechanism of production of a *cardiopulmonary* murmur is as follows: When the heart expands during diastole it may compress a portion of lung and drive air from the alveoli. During systole this portion of the lung is then decompressed and, as the air re-enters, a systolic vesicular murmur is heard. Such a murmur should be soft in character and should vary with respiration and change of posture. It may be heard at the apex although more often at the base. A cardiopulmonary murmur is recognized clinically by its disappearance with full inspiration, although a soft organic systolic murmur is usually lessened too by full inspiration.

Friction between smooth and healthy serous membranes can possibly cause a murmur almost indistinguishable in quality from the soft apical systolic bruit of early rheumatic endocarditis (*see* p. 311). A murmur caused in this way would be exaggerated by any increased action of the heart whether from exercise, anxiety or anæmia. Systolic murmurs which are innocent or " basal " in type often develop during a feverish illness when the heart is acting vigorously. The systolic murmur thus produced is likely to be transient. Phono-cardiography can be used to distinguish an innocent from an organic murmur (compare Fig. 24, p. 274, with Fig. 32, p. 311).

A *venous hum*, audible at the base of the neck as a continuous murmur, is to be regarded as a normal physical sign. It is abolished by jugular vein compression or sometimes by turning the head. It may be confused with the machinery murmur of patent ductus arteriosus, especially when it is heard beneath the manubrium sterni and below the inner end of the left clavicle. Such a humming type of murmur is heard in over 50 per cent. of children under three years old when the neck is extended. It is called the Eustace Smith murmur.

INNOCENT INTRACARDIAC MURMURS

Often short systolic murmurs produced within the heart are also *innocent*, and this should be considered when there is no accompanying enlargement of the heart or diastolic murmur. A possible mode of production is a pulmonary artery ejection murmur, especially when the cardiac output is increased. A murmur of this type is " basal " in character but may also be heard at the apex. Such a murmur occurs early in systole and does not continue up to the second sound (Fig. 24). Sometimes a harsh or musical systolic murmur may occur without discoverable explanation even including *post-mortem* study; possibly abnormal vibrations of the chordæ tendineæ are responsible.

Innocent murmurs generally show less intensity and conduction than organic ones; they are shorter in duration and more variable in behaviour.

The character of the second heart sound and the finding of *fixed splitting* (*see* below and also p. 271) also help to distinguish the organic from the innocent systolic murmur.

ORGANIC MURMURS

In contrast to the innocent systolic murmurs, the systolic murmur of ventricular septal defect and of mitral regurgitation may be pansystolic in continuing right up to the second heart sound. Atrial septal defects and mild pulmonary stenosis, on the other hand, may both give rise to pulmonary ejection murmurs identical with those heard in normal hearts. The associated physical signs distinguish the organic lesions; among these, the changes in the second heart sound are of some assistance. In healthy children, the splitting of the second sound is most marked on inspiration but is reduced on expiration. With atrial septal defects no such variation with respiration is noted. In pulmonary stenosis, the pulmonary component of the second sound is, in any case, greatly reduced in volume; in cases where it remains audible, the splitting may be most marked on expiration.

In the newborn infant, Burnard[1] has described a transient systolic murmur best heard in the second left interspace which is commoner in infants subjected to asphyxia neonatorum; it is thought to be due to persistent patency of the ductus arteriosus. In Bonham-Carter's[2] series, about one per cent. of all newborn infants had systolic murmurs and of these some forty per cent. were subsequently shown to have congenital heart disease.

SPURIOUS MURMURS

Spurious murmurs may be produced when the chest piece of the stethoscope is not applied firmly enough to the chest wall in the region of the apex; the first sound may then be blurred so that a

[1] Burnard, E. D. (1958). *Brit. med. J.*, 1, 806.
[2] Bonham-Carter, R. E., Benson, P. F., Smellie, Jean M. (1961). *Lancet*, 1, 627.

murmur is suspected. This is because too light a pressure accentuates low-pitched sounds. Such a spurious murmur is more likely to be heard when a child is examined in the standing position, because then he is apt to lean away from the stethoscope unless the doctor places a steadying hand upon his back.

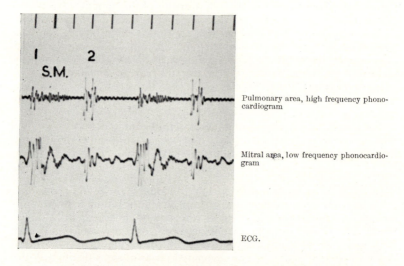

Pulmonary area, high frequency phonocardiogram

Mitral area, low frequency phonocardiogram

ECG.

Fig. 24.—Innocent " basal " type of systolic murmur (SM) and split second sound in a normal heart. The murmur occupies only the first part of systole.
1 = First heart sound, 2 = Second heart sound.

RATE AND RHYTHM OF THE HEART

RATE

In health the pulse rate varies with age, activity, and temperament. During the daytime it is 15 to 20 beats faster than when the child is asleep. Should the significance of a rapid pulse be in question, it is wise to count it at night when the child has been asleep for an hour or more, and this sleeping pulse may be taken as the true guide.

There is a wide range in the normal heart rate. The rate is sometimes noticeably slow in boys trained for athletics and it slows quickly after exercise.

Changes in the rate of the heart as growth proceeds are as follows: The fœtal heart rate is about 120–160. For a few minutes after birth the rate may go up, then, as vagal tone increases, the heart slows to about 120–140 within an hour or so. Occasionally, when this physiological slowing is delayed, there is sinus tachycardia for a few days or longer. In a young infant, activity such as crying causes a sudden acceleration to about 180. For some weeks after birth, the sleeping pulse is likely to be about 120 to 130 and the " alert " pulse (i.e. no crying, etc.) is often only a few beats faster. By six months of age the sleeping pulse will be around 110 to 115, with an alert pulse about ten beats faster. Between one and two years of age the sleeping pulse is perhaps 100 with the alert pulse 110. Afterwards the sleeping pulse gradually slows; by 10–14 years it will be about 80 with a difference between it and the alert pulse of 10 or more beats per minute.

TACHYCARDIA

By tachycardia, is meant a pulse rate faster than the upper limit of normality; that is, faster than what is known to be normal for a particular individual. A transient tachycardia will occur with most febrile conditions (enteric fever is usually an exception), and with recovery the rate subsides. When the sleeping pulse rate remains fast, myocardial damage may be suspected unless there is reason to think there is infection elsewhere. A sleeping pulse rate which keeps above 100 per minute, especially if it is within 10 beats of the waking pulse rate, suggests the possibility of carditis. In cases of rheumatic carditis (*see* p. 309), the erythrocyte sedimentation rate will usually be increased as well as the pulse and there will be other signs of carditis.

Nervous Tachycardia

Fear or excitement will increase the pulse rate. If tachycardia is being caused by the visits of the doctor or nurse, it will seem there is a constant elevation. However, the diagnosis can be easily established by taking the sleeping pulse rate, which will be normal.

Tachycardia from Illness

Most infections, however mild, tend to increase the rate of the heart, this tachycardia depending chiefly on the age of the child and the amount of fever. For example, in pneumonia and acute tonsillitis the temperature may be 103° F, the pulse rate 140, and there will be little or no slowing of the pulse during sleep. Again, in acute rheumatism the pulse may be increased even in the absence of fever. A rising pulse rate is one of the signs of shock. Tachycardia is also caused by a raised right auricular pressure which reflexly causes a reduction in vagal tone (Bainbridge reflex). This occurs in effort, anæmia, arterio-venous shunt (*see* p. 280) and congestive heart failure.

ARRHYTHMIA
Sinus Arrythmia

There is probably no such thing as an absolutely regular heart (Paul Wood). In childhood, acceleration of the pulse during inspiration and a corresponding slowing during expiration is physiological and this type of arrhythmia becomes more marked when the pulse is slow. It depends on alterations in vagal tone initiated by receptors in the lungs and its nature is shown by its disappearance when the patient holds his breath. A rarer form of sinus arrhythmia is independent of respiration and is abolished by exercise. In sinus arrhythmia the electrocardiogram shows variations in the cycle length but the complexes are normal. Because sinus arrhythmia is found in health, it is often said to be a sign of a healthy heart, yet it is sometimes found in heart disease if the heart rate is slow.

Ectopic Beats (Premature Systoles)

The next commonest disturbance of rhythm is due to *premature systoles*. These are caused by ectopic impulses discharged from excitatory foci in the auricles, the A–V node, or the ventricles. Their origin can be determined by the electrocardiogram. Ventricular ectopic beats are characterized by an early beat followed by a long compensatory pause. This is because the S–A node is not excited by the ectopic impulse and the sinus impulse which next follows, entering the ventricles during their refractory rate, is ineffective; thus there is a long pause until the next sinus impulse arrives. The beat that is premature is small or imperceptible, but the one succeeding the pause is fuller than normal and may be felt as a thump by the patient.

Extrasystoles are veritable heart beats, for they are ectopic beats (usually ventricular) in which the next succeeding sinus impulse manages to excite the ventricle. They can also be called interpolated ectopic beats.

Significance. Premature systoles, though not uncommon in the newborn, are rarer in children than in adults. In nearly all cases they can be regarded as benign since usually there is no evidence of structural disease (but *see* p. 310). They are more often heard when a heart is acting slowly, as in convalescence before the patient is getting up. They disappear when the rate is quickened. Sometimes the child is alarmed by the sensation of " pause and a thump ", and then reassurance is important.

Paroxysmal Tachycardia

The causation of paroxysmal tachycardia is the same as that of ectopic beats, the beats merely occurring in such rapid succession that the normal rhythm of the heart is obliterated. The ectopic foci of excitation may be auricular, nodal or ventricular. The condition may be associated with congenital malformations of the heart but more commonly it exists alone. The onset is always quite sudden and without any warning. A pulse rate of between 240–300 per minute can be attained from the very beginning of the attack and maintained until its end. The attack may last not more than a few seconds, a few minutes, or it may run into days. Older children are likely to complain initially of dyspnœa or chest pain. When attacks occur in infants there will be sudden dyspnœa and then a rapid onset of congestive heart failure, the tachycardia being discovered on examination. Most infants who have undergone an episode of paroxysmal tachycardia are subsequently found to have normal hearts and suffer no further attacks. Occasionally an attack in the neonatal period is found to be associated with a myocardial abnormality such as endocardial fibroelastosis (p. 283). Paroxysmal tachycardia usually responds well to digitalis (see p. 667).

Rare Cardiac Arrhythmias

All the other irregularities which occur in children are very rare. They comprise the various types of partial and complete heart block, which may be either congenital in origin or acquired (see p. 310), also flutter and fibrillation. The last mentioned occurs with severe mitral disease but is seldom seen before adolescence.

NORMAL BLOOD PRESSURE

It should be remembered in sphygmomanometry in childhood that considerable variations in apparent pressure can be obtained by the use of different sizes of pneumatic cuffs, the smaller the cuff the higher being the pressure. To achieve a comparable standard, a number of different sized cuffs should be kept, and the largest that will fit between axilla and cubital fossa is used for the particular child. The routine auscultatory method of taking blood-pressure is not easy in infants and small children, and often only a systolic reading can be obtained; moreover, a resting level may be difficult to achieve.

AVERAGE BLOOD-PRESSURES IN CHILDHOOD

Age	Blood-pressure (mm. Hg) Systolic	Diastolic
1 year	75	50
5 years	100	65
10 years	110	70

Where a satisfactory reading cannot be obtained on auscultation, the *flush method* is employed to obtain a systolic reading only. The limb is held above the level of the body to overcome congestion and a sphygmomanometer cuff is then inflated to well above the expected systolic level. The cuff is then gradually released and, once the systolic level is passed, the limb flushes and becomes rapidly congested.

Where coarctation of the aorta is suspected, the blood pressure in the lower limbs is estimated; the normal situation, in which the average femoral artery pressure is some 20–30 mm. of Hg higher than the brachial artery pressure, is found to be reversed with this malformation. Where there is an apparent difference in tension on palpation of the two radial pulses, the blood pressure should be taken in each arm.

CONGENITAL MALFORMATIONS OF THE HEART

THERE are many types of developmental lesion and they often co-exist. Common defects, such as ventricular septal defect, patent ductus arteriosus, and the tetralogy of Fallot, have received careful clinical study, whereas rare ones, mostly with a short period of survival, such as *cor biloculare*, are better known by their anatomical description.

FREQUENCY

It is useful to know the order of frequency in which the various lesions occur. The commonest is pure ventricular septal defect (35 per cent.), then patent ductus arteriosus (12 per cent.), then the tetralogy of Fallot (7 per cent.), then auricular septal defect; co-arctation of the aorta, isolated pulmonary stenosis, aortic stenosis, Eisenmenger's complex, anomalous venous drainage, transposition of great vessels, anomalies of aortic valve and ascending aorta, dextro-cardia, and others are more rare (Keith, 1953).[1]

In a significant proportion of cases, the exact diagnosis cannot be established except by special investigations, including cardiac catheterization, cine-angiocardiography, and dye-dilution studies, or by eventual *post-mortem* dissection. Those most readily diagnosed by ordinary clinical methods are single lesions, such as patent ductus arteriosus and coarctation of the aorta, which are accompanied by characteristic physical signs. The association of several lesions diminishes the chance of a completely accurate diagnosis unless the special investigations, such as cardiac catheterization (Plates IV and V) and angiocardiography, are employed.

In the " Atlas of Congenital Cardiac Disease " (Maud Abbott, 1936), there is an anatomical analysis of the various possibilities. Among a thousand specimens the following conditions occurred, either singly or associated with other cardiac defects: 377 examples of patent foramen ovale and auricular septal defect (a higher pro-portion than clinical experience suggests), 290 of ventricular septal defect, 277 of patent ductus arteriosus, 236 of transposition of arterial trunks, 178 of coarctation of the aorta, and 151 of pulmonary stenosis.

Pulmonary stenosis illustrates the way in which a developmental defect can occur alone or in association with other lesions. In pure pulmonary stenosis the septa are intact, there is no veno-arterial shunt between the two sides of the heart, and therefore no admixture of venous and arterial blood; thus there is no cyanosis until the hyper-trophied right ventricle begins to fail. In a small number of cases of

[1] In " Pædiatrics for the Practitioner ", Vol. I, chap. 43.   Ed. Gaisford and Lightwood.   London: Butterworth.

pulmonary stenosis, there is a patent foramen ovale which permits blood to be shunted from right to left when the pressure in the right auricle exceeds that in the left. Under these circumstances, un-oxygenated blood enters the systemic circulation and cyanosis occurs. In yet another type there is an associated ventricular septal defect and the aorta overrides a hypertrophied right ventricle (the tetralogy of Fallot); in this case, as well, there is usually cyanosis on account of a veno-arterial shunt.

AETIOLOGY

In the embryological development of the heart and circulation there occurs a remarkable change-over from the two entirely separate circulations characteristic of the higher vertebrates to the crossed systemic and pulmonary circulations of the mammalia, and this has to be effected by complicated structural changes *while the circulation is actually functioning*. The fact that various developmental errors should occur is not surprising; nevertheless we need to seek detailed explanations, those that Aristotle would have called the " efficient " causes, not merely the formal ones. How exactly do the various types of developmental defect take place? In most cases of congenital cardiac defect, there is no evidence of transmission by inheritance and a familial incidence is rare, yet it is common for other congenital defects to be found in association with cardiac ones: septal defects in mongolism; septal defects and abnormalities of the great vessels in arachnodactyly (as in Marfan's syndrome); and abnormalities of the aorta or pulmonary artery in Turner's syndrome (*see* p. 163).

Embryologically the heart is being rapidly fashioned between the third and the eighth weeks of fœtal development, and the majority of the cardiac malformations are believed to arise at about the fifth to the eighth weeks. Certain cases have indeed been traced to fœtal damage in this critical period of cardiac development, for example, the cardiac defects resulting from maternal rubella occurring within the first three months of pregnancy. In certain other cases, the developmental error consists in the persistence of some part of the fœtal circulation which should have become occluded soon after birth, such as the foramen ovale or the ductus arteriosus. Abnormal patency of the ductus is the commonest cardiac lesion to result from maternal rubella. Other environmental agents—toxic, infective and nutritional—are no doubt capable of acting on the fœtus, and for the present the exact cause of most lesions remains conjectural.

The parents of a child with congenital malformation of the heart may ask whether a child subsequently born to them is likely to be similarly affected and whether such lesions can be inherited. It is rare, in fact, for inheritance to play an obvious part. The malformations of Marfan's syndrome are determined by the presence of a single dominant gene but the heart is not affected in every individual carrying the gene; there are also a few recorded family pedigrees with more than one member showing an abnormality, such as atrial septal defect. The incidence of congenital heart disease in the siblings of affected patients lies between 1 and 2 per cent., a higher incidence than in control groups, but not high enough to suggest that inheritance is often concerned; thus, the responsible recessive genes are uncommon ones and appear to have a low penetrance, that is, they are only likely to produce lesions under the influence of unknown environmental factors. The physician can therefore give reassurance to parents who have one child with a cardiac malformation; if they are unrelated and there have been no other cases of congenital heart disease in the family, he can advise them that the chance of a second child being affected is less than one in fifty.

CLASSIFICATION AND DEFINITIONS

The term *shunt* is used to describe the short-circuiting of blood by means of an abnormal communication. Soon after birth the pressure on the left side of the heart becomes higher than that on the right, and if a communication exists a left-to-right shunt conveys arterial blood from the left side of the heart, or from the aorta, to the right side, or to the pulmonary artery; this is called an arterio-venous shunt. Sometimes this shunt may become reversed in direction. A reversed or veno-arterial shunt can only take place when the pressure on the right side exceeds that on the left; then venous blood mixes with arterial blood and cyanosis ensues, e.g. Fallot's tetralogy. A shunt can be intracardiac (ASD, VSD) or extracardiac (patent ductus arteriosus).

The frequency with which there are multiple defects renders a simple classification of developmental anomalies impossible, but it has long been the custom to divide the patients into two main categories—those with and without cyanosis. The clinical value of this distinction is that general cyanosis at rest usually indicates a right-to-left shunt, an exception being when cyanosis is due to a later developing right-sided failure. The cyanotic group needs to be further sub-divided into those with permanent cyanosis (*morbus cœruleus*, " blue babies ") and those with transient, deferred or terminal cyanosis (*cyanose tardive*).

THE SIGNIFICANCE OF THE PULMONARY BLOOD FLOW

The abnormalities can be further differentiated depending on the state of the pulmonary blood flow. Patients with increased pulmonary flow may be classified as *pleonæmic*, those with diminished flow as *oligæmic*. This difference can be recognized at fluoroscopic examination. Pleonæmic lungs have increased vascular markings and often their hilar shadows pulsate—the hilar " dance "—while oligæmic lungs have diminished vascular markings. Pleonæmic lungs indicate arterio-venous (left-to-right) shunt and so give an important clue towards a diagnosis.

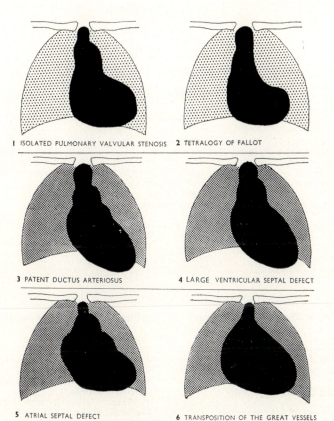

Pulmonary Oligæmia ∷∷∷∷   Pulmonary Pleonæmia ▓▓▓

Fig. 25.—The cardiac silhouette and pulmonary vasculature in some commoner types of congenital heart disease.

1. Isolated pulmonary valvular stenosis.

1. Small aortic arch.
2. Dilated main pulmonary artery.
3. Right ventricular hypertrophy.
4. Pulmonary oligæmia.

2. Tetralogy of Fallot.

1. Right aortic arch (present in 25 per cent. of cases).
2. Concavity of pulmonary artery impression.
3. Right ventricular hypertrophy.
4. Pulmonary oligæmia.
5. Little generalized enlargement of the heart.

3. Patent ductus arteriosus.

1. Large dilated aortic arch.
2. Dilated main pulmonary artery.
3. Left ventricular hypertrophy.
4. Pulmonary pleonæmia.

4. Large ventricular septal defect.

1. Normal aortic arch.
2. Dilated main pulmonary artery.
3. Left ventricular hypertrophy.
4. Pulmonary pleonæmia.

(This must be distinguished from the Maladie de Roger (i.e., a small ventricular septal defect) where the cardiac silhouette and pulmonary vascularity are normal.)

5. Atrial septal defect.

1. Small hypoplastic aortic arch.
2. Dilated main pulmonary artery.
3. Dilated right auricle.
4. Right ventricular hypertrophy.
5. Pulmonary pleonæmia.

6. Transposition of the great vessels.

1. Narrow upper mediastinal shadow.
2. Gross cardiac enlargement.
3. Pulmonary pleonæmia.

TABLE XVII
CLASSIFICATION OF CONGENITAL MALFORMATIONS AND DISORDERS OF THE HEART

(Derived from Wood's classification (1950)[1] and simplified)

Without Shunt: Acyanotic

General	Left-sided	Right-sided
Dextrocardia. Endocardial fibro-elastosis. Glycogen-storage disease. Other causes of infantile cardiomegaly. Gargoylism. Congenital heart block.	Coarctation of the aorta (adult type). Right-sided aortic arch. Complete or incomplete aortic vascular rings. Bicuspid aortic valve; supernumerary aortic cusps. Aortic and subaortic stenosis. Left coronary artery arising from pulmonary artery.	Simple pulmonary stenosis. Ebstein's malformation. Isolated pulmonary hypertension.

With Shunt

Left to Right Shunt: Acyanotic	Right to Left Shunt: Cyanotic
PLEONÆMIC LUNGS: *Enlargement of left ventricle:* Patent ductus arteriosus. Fenestration of the aortopulmonary septum. Ventricular septal defect. *Enlargement of right ventricle:* Atrial septal defect. Anomalous pulmonary veins joining superior vena cava or right auricle.	OLIGÆMIC LUNGS: *Reduced pressure in pulmonary artery:* Fallot's tetralogy and pulmonary atresia. Ebstein's malformation with ASD. Tricuspid atresia. Pulmonary stenosis with reversed interatrial shunt. *Raised pressure in pulmonary artery:* Pulmonary hypertension with reversed shunt (aorto-pulmonary, interventricular or interatrial).
	PLEONÆMIC LUNGS: Persistent truncus arteriosus. Transposition of great vessels with ASD and VSD or patent ductus arteriosus.

PRIMARY MYOCARDIAL DISEASE

UNDER this title are often included several different pathological conditions and the nomenclature will remain unsatisfactory until their causes are better known. Formerly glycogenic infiltration of the heart with cardiomegaly was included, but since the histology and

[1] Wood, P. (1950). Congenital heart disease, *Brit. med. J.*, 2, 693,

metabolic characteristics of *Von Gierke's glycogen storage disease* have become known this is no longer the case (*see* p. 133).

Endocardial Fibroelastosis

Formerly called fœtal endocarditis, hitherto seldom suspected during life, endocardial fibroelastosis is probably the commonest member of the group. It consists of a tough fibroelastic thickening of the subendocardial layer and myocardium, affecting the left auricle and atrium especially but extending in some patients to all parts of the heart. Its ætiology is obscure but occasionally developmental lesions co-exist, e.g. hypoplasia or coarctation of the aorta. The thickened endocardial layer results in a great increase in the work of the heart with consequent muscular hypertrophy, affecting especially the left side of the heart. Strands of fibrous and elastic tissue extend into the deeper layers of the myocardium. Three main clinical presentations are seen:

1. Cases of heart failure developing in infancy or early childhood (*see* below) and progressing to cardiac œdema and death.
2. Young children presenting without symptoms of failure but with grossly enlarged hearts for which no cause can be found.
3. Cases of mitral stenosis developing in infants or young children without evidence of rheumatic infection.

A diagnosis of fibroelastosis of the heart is largely a question of exclusion. The heart when screened will be enlarged and relatively inert; the lung fields will not be engorged unless there is left-sided failure or mitral stenosis. No shunt or other evidence of congenital heart disease is usually to be found. Pericardial thickening can be excluded by the physical signs, electrocardiography and cardiac catheterization.

PROGNOSIS

The prognosis is not easy to determine. Some infants appear perfectly well and are then found dead in their cots, heart disease not having been suspected during life. Other infants who may show variable degrees of heart failure or suffer attacks of paroxysmal tachycardia respond well to prolonged digitalization. Indeed, it seems to be of the highest importance to give digitalis therapy for several years. Although no statistical evidence is available, it seems possible that with such treatment some patients undergo spontaneous improvement. This by no means applies to all infants, and the majority deteriorate and die despite treatment.

HEART FAILURE IN INFANCY

A description of endocardial fibroelastosis provides an apt opportunity to consider the general clinical picture of cardiac failure in infancy. This may occur in many types of congenital heart disease including not only the myocardial diseases but many other malformations, and particularly patent ductus arteriosus, ventricular septal defect and the whole group of cyanotic congenital heart disease.

Before persistent heart failure is established, it may be noticed that an infant tolerates chest infections badly. In such cases a component of left heart failure has complicated an otherwise mild infection. Where repeated " chest infections " occur in infancy or where the breathing is more laboured than the severity of the infection would otherwise suggest, the possibility of congenital heart disease must be carefully investigated.

During the early months of infancy it may be noticed that although the infant is eager at the start of each feed, he quickly tires and the feed is left unfinished; inevitably there is failure to gain weight. Examination may show a tinge of cyanosis immediately after the feeds when the respiration is rapid. The characteristic indrawing of the lower intercostal spaces and pushing out of the upper abdomen with each inspiration (Naish's sign) become more pronounced. The soft chest wall of the infant becomes distorted by the progressive cardiac enlargement, with an increase in the precordial bulging. As the heart failure increases, œdema, which is generalized rather than confined to the ankles, becomes obvious and the liver enlargement more marked. Venous engorgement is not as easily measured as in the adult but can be detected in the neck and scalp veins.

TREATMENT

Whether or not the underlying condition is one for which surgery is contemplated, the infant with heart failure often responds well to general medical treatment. Digitalization (p. 667) remains the basic essential, but in addition supportive measures, including the use of a salt-free milk (Edosol), the giving of small frequent feeds, and where œdema is severe the careful use of chlorothiazide (for dosage, see p. 667), all have their place. Oxygen should be given as indicated by cyanosis. Respiratory infections are poorly tolerated; early and adequate antibiotic treatment is important.

DIFFERENTIAL DIAGNOSIS OF INFANTILE CARDIOMEGALY

A form of *myocarditis*, recognized by Fiedler in 1899, usually occurs in adult life but has been described in infants and children. It is characterized by infiltrations of the heart muscle with macrophages, plasma cells and lymphocytes, and sometimes giant cells and eosinophils as well. Patchy necrosis occurs and then fibroplastic repair. The disease lasts only a few months and causes general enlargement of the heart, disorders of rhythm and congestive failure. Its cause is not known.

In cases of familial cardiomegaly, *glycogen-storage disease* (p. 133) and *gargoylism* (p. 480) must be considered. Such patients sometimes develop congestive failure, others may die suddenly while young. *An anomalous origin of the left coronary artery from the pulmonary artery* is a rare cause of heart disease in infancy; attacks of acute left ventricular failure or attacks of dyspnœa, accompanied by what may well be acute chest pain resembling angina of effort of the adult, may occur; the electro-cardiogram shows the characteristic changes of ischæmic heart disease; the prognosis is extremely poor.

Finally, certain *virus infections* may involve the heart, especially in infancy—e.g. *Coxsackie* virus (but not polio virus) and perhaps SG virus (p. 99). In the acquired form of *generalized toxoplasmosis* (p. 413), myocarditis is a rare complication.

MALFORMATIONS PRIMARILY CAUSING OBSTRUCTION TO THE BLOOD FLOW

Coarctation of the Aorta

THIS is a developmental constriction of the aorta, the term being derived from *coarctatus* (tightened or contracted). It comprises not a single type but at least three anomalies. Two of these occur in a short segment of the aorta, opposite the ductus, which is called the " isthmus " because of the possibility of its being narrowed. (1) The first and commonest variety of coarctation consists of a constriction just below the attachment of the *ligamentum arteriosum* (obliterated ductus arteriosus); this is called the " adult type ", yet it can, by careful examination, be diagnosed even in early childhood although at this age the symptoms are not fully developed. These symptoms are caused by hypertension in the vessels of the neck and arms, and hypotension in the arteries supplying the lower part of the body, and eventually by gradual failure of the left ventricle; both signs and symptoms become more apparent in adolescence. (2) The second variety is called the " fœtal type " of coarctation because the fœtal pattern of circulation persists. In this the aorta is constricted below the origin of the left subclavian artery but above the ductus, which remains patent, and blood can therefore pass from the left pulmonary artery into the aorta below its site of constriction. This gives a right-to-left shunt and causes cyanosis of the lower part of the body, the upper being of normal colour. The condition is incompatible with life for more than a few years. (3) Still more rarely, there may be atresia of the ascending aorta whereby the whole of the systemic circulation has to be fed by the ductus arteriosus; the period of survival is very short.

The *adult type of coarctation* causes enlargement of the left ventricle since it has to overcome the obstruction below the obliterated ductus. Hypertension is found in the arteries arising above the obstruction and hypotension in those below. Thus, the systolic blood pressure in the arms is high and that in the legs low; indeed, the femoral arteries are usually impalpable. Boys are affected more often than girls; in some cases it may be associated with other defects, as in *Turner's Syndrome* (p. 163).

DIAGNOSIS

The " adult " type of coarctation is not very rare; the diagnosis is not difficult. In childhood, symptoms are usually absent but there may be epistaxis, throbbing and even intermittent claudication in the legs. Discovery of a systolic murmur down the left border of the sternum and through to the back draws attention to the possibility, and two very easily determined *signs* confirm the diagnosis; these are arterial pulsation in the suprasternal notch and weak or absent femoral pulses. Enlarged collateral arterial vessels will be present in older children. A mitral diastolic murmur is sometimes heard. An x-ray examination may show hypoplasia of the aortic knuckle and enlargement of the left ventricle. A sure sign is a double aortic knuckle; this is formed by the shadow of the aorta above and below the coarctation and an enlarged left subclavian artery. Notching of the inferior border of the ribs by enlarged intercostal arteries is often seen, though seldom before the age of eight years. If necessary, angiocardiography may help to confirm the diagnosis, but retrograde aortography is likely to provide more definite proof.

DIAGNOSIS IN INFANCY

There is a significant mortality from coarctation of the aorta in the first year of life. Thus, the routine examination of the newborn infant should always include palpation of the femoral pulse. Should this be absent or weak, the diagnosis must be strongly suspected. The infant may fail to thrive and the signs of cardiac failure (*see* p. 283) may develop.

TREATMENT

If coarctation is not relieved, hypertensive heart disease occurs and later on congestive heart failure develops in 40 per cent. of cases. There is also a risk of cerebral hæmorrhage and of bacterial endocarditis. The hypertension is said not to damage the kidneys because the aortic constriction protects them; nevertheless, renal ischæmia can itself be a factor contributing to hypertension. Operation provides a cure in most cases of coarctation and should, if possible, be done before hypertensive heart disease has occurred. It can be successfully performed in infancy and is indicated if any symptoms or electrocardiographic evidence of left ventricular strain are present. A number of infants have withstood surgical correction of the defect even in the first month of life.

Congenital Aortic Stenosis

The site of the stenosis may be aortic (valvular) or subaortic.

AORTIC STENOSIS

This is a rare congenital defect. The narrowing occurs at the aortic ring and causes left ventricular hypertrophy. On examination the results of this hypertrophy are evident and a systolic thrill will often be felt at the base of the heart, and in the carotid and subclavian arteries. At the base a rough systolic murmur, which is conducted into the arteries, is heard; it is also heard at the apex. There may be, in addition, a basal diastolic murmur due to associated aortic regurgitation. At the base the second sound may be diminished in intensity. The pulse is quite characteristic, being small and sustained (plateau pulse). The radial pulses may be unequal. When, very rarely, aortic regurgitation is also present, the pulse may show a double beat (pulsus bisferiens) due to premature systoles, which may be mistaken for coupling.

There is no cyanosis in these patients and sometimes they have a delicate pink complexion (" Dresden China " appearance). General growth may be retarded. Sometimes aortic stenosis is, like co-arctation, associated with gonadal deficiency and webbing of the neck (Turner's Syndrome, Fig. 12, p. 164).

TREATMENT

The first attempts at operative correction were not entirely satis-factory, although better results are now obtained using prostheses.

SUBAORTIC STENOSIS

Subaortic stenosis is a little commoner but more benign than aortic valvular stenosis. It is situated proximal to the aortic ring and is caused by a perforated membrane derived from the primitive *bulbus cordis*. Since it obstructs in the same way as valvular stenosis, the signs are similar, though the second sound is more likely to be clear. Sudden death may sometimes occur in these patients. It is not certain whether this is due to an occlusion of the stenosis with cerebral ischaemia or to a reduction in the coronary blood supply.

Surgical correction of subaortic stenosis is still unsatisfactory. It is reasonable to hope that in the next decade the technical difficulties of fashioning an effective aortic orifice will be overcome.

Aortic Vascular Rings

Persistence of the primitive double aortic arch, or part of it, is a rare defect and different kinds of vascular rings result from its variants. The condition deserves mention as a cause of dyspnœa or dysphagia in which exact diagnosis is possible by means of barium swallow.

Occasionally, in an x-ray it is noted that the aortic arch turns to the right and the aortic knob lies on the right instead of the left side. Such an aortic abnormality is seen in about 25 per cent. of cases of the tetralogy of Fallot but it may be associated with other defects.

When a right-sided aorta crosses over and descends on the left, a constricting ring may be formed by the participation of a patent ductus arteriosus or the fibrous remnant of a ductus which can exert pressure on the trachea and the œsophagus. This is an incomplete aortic ring. Alternatively, the condition may consist in an abnormal right subclavian artery arising as the first branch of the aorta, which passes behind the trachea and œsophagus to its destination. This abnormality is seen in association with a normal left-sided aortic arch. Symptoms of dyspnœa and wheezing may, like dysphagia, occur from birth. A complete double aortic arch is another form of vascular ring which produces comparable symptoms.

TREATMENT

Surgical treatment is possible as a result of the recent advances in anæsthesia and arterial grafting techniques.

Congenital Pulmonary Stenosis

Pulmonary stenosis can be (1) an isolated lesion, often called pure stenosis; (2) associated with patent foramen ovale or atrial septal defect; (3) associated with ventricular septal defect and an overriding aorta (*see* also Fallot's Tetralogy, p. 295).

ISOLATED PULMONARY STENOSIS

Pulmonary stenosis is not very rare, though not all cases are recognized; Gardiner and Keith (1948) placed it fifth in the frequency of congenital anomalies, saying that many of the affected children can lead fairly normal lives. The narrowing is either valvular (80 per cent.) or infundibular (20 per cent.), also called sub-valvular or sub-pulmonary. In valvular stenosis the cusps are fused. In the infundibular type there is an obstructive ring, derived from the *bulbus cordis*, which separates off a part of the conus arteriosus from the body of the right ventricle; this type is usually less incapacitating than valvular stenosis.

Diagnosis. Hypertrophy of the right ventricle, oligæmia of the lungs, and a hypoplasia of the left ventricle occur in both types (p. 281). In valvular, and perhaps in sub-valvular stenosis, the main pulmonary artery usually shows post-stenotic dilatation. Symptoms are entirely absent in mild cases of pulmonary stenosis, but in more severe ones there is increasing breathlessness on exertion, and failure of the right ventricle finally occurs. Cyanosis, which is late in appearing, is not *central* but *peripheral* in type, being caused by reduced cardiac output and compensatory peripheral vaso-constriction. This is not likely to occur until adult life has been reached, when the face may become bloated in appearance. The signs of valvular pulmonary stenosis consist of a systolic murmur and a thrill along the line of the pulmonary outflow track; this is maximal in the second and third left interspaces and in severe cases only a single second heart sound is audible; in cases of infundibular stenosis the murmur may be maximal a space or so lower and the second sound will be widely split. This is a *fixed split*, i.e. it does not alter, as in the normal heart, with respiration. The jugular pulse exhibits a conspicuous *a*-wave. The enlarged right ventricle becomes increasingly obvious on inspection and palpation of the præcordium close to the sternum. The electrocardiogram confirms right ventricular predominance. Catheterization shows a raised right ventricular pressure and a low pulmonary wedge pressure. In cases of extreme stenosis there is a risk of blocking the pulmonary artery with the catheter.

TREATMENT

Mild cases need no treatment and pulmonary valvotomy will only be considered in severe ones. Measures for the prevention of bacterial endocarditis should be advised.

PULMONARY STENOSIS WITH PATENT FORAMEN OVALE

In most cases of pulmonary stenosis, the foramen ovale, even when anatomically patent, is functionally closed. But with increasing age there is a gradual rise in the pressure in the right auricle which may be suddenly accentuated by exertion, perhaps causing a right-to-left shunt, and late *central* cyanosis (*cyanose tardive*) is then seen. Under similar circumstances reversed shunts may develop with auricular and ventricular septal defects. On the other hand, cyanosis may be seen early, even in infancy, and then valvotomy, though risky, gives the best chance of survival.

Isolated Pulmonary Hypertension

It has recently been appreciated that there is a rare condition in which the pulmonary arterioles become degenerate, even in childhood, giving rise to pulmonary hypertension, right ventricular hypertrophy and strain, and finally to right heart failure.

MALFORMATIONS LEADING PRIMARILY TO LEFT-TO-RIGHT CARDIAC SHUNTS

Patent Ductus Arteriosus

IN the fœtus, the ductus arteriosus carries blood from the pulmonary artery into the aorta, thus short-circuiting the pulmonary circulation. When the lungs become aerated at birth the flow changes, the blood passing from the aorta to the pulmonary artery. As the oxygen tension of the blood rises after birth, a mechanism comes into play which causes the ductus to constrict.[1] The blood flow through the

---

[1] Dawes, G. S. (1958). " Circulation." Oxford: Blackwell Scientific Publications.

narrowed ductus is thought to be responsible for the systolic murmur audible in the second left interspace of many newborn infants.   When the ductus closes completely the murmur disappears.   Under conditions of inadequate pulmonary expansion, the pulmonary artery pressure may remain high and the flow may remain in part from right to left.   Equally the stimulus of raised oxygen tension may be lacking and the ductus may fail to constrict.   A ductus arteriosus which has not closed within two or three months of birth can be regarded as being pathologically patent.   Probably many such cases had wide malformed ducti even before birth.

DIAGNOSIS

. This is the second commonest cardiac defect as well as being the most easily recognized.   Symptoms are usually absent and the characteristic murmur is discovered at routine medical examination; rarely, breathlessness on exertion draws attention to the heart.   A patent ductus is sometimes found as a component of a multiple set of defects.

Patency of the ductus results in a varying degree of left-to-right shunt and an increase in the pulse pressure.   In spite of the much increased output of the left ventricle, cardiac enlargement is not great. X-ray screening examination while barium is swallowed shows some enlargement of the left auricle.   The volume of blood shunted from the aorta to the pulmonary artery makes the lungs pleonæmic (p. 281); screening shows the pulmonary artery pulsating and dilated; the hilar shadows also pulsate though not so much as with atrial septal defect.   The ECG may be normal or it may show left ventricular preponderance.   Except in a child with a very wide ductus, cardiac function remains satisfactory until adult life when left ventricular failure may be expected.   Pulmonary hypertension is a dreaded complication in a few cases.   Bacterial endocarditis is another danger but a rare one during childhood.

A diagnosis of patent ductus is made when a *continuous murmur* is heard just below the left clavicle.   It is usually accompanied by a thrill and this highly characteristic bruit (Gibson murmur) has been nicknamed the " machinery " or " humming-top " murmur.   It increases towards the end of systole and wanes in late diastole.   A venous hum (*see* p. 272) should not be confused with a ductus murmur. A continuous murmur resembling that of a patent ductus is sometimes heard in the tetralogy of Fallot; this is caused by anastomotic communication between bronchial and pulmonary arteries.   Another and an early difficulty in diagnosis is due to the fact that the diastolic element of a ductus murmur may only develop after infancy.   Sometimes a " functional " apical diastolic murmur is present.   A collapsing pulse or a wide pulse pressure, e.g. 90/30, is an important observation in these cases.   The difference between the systolic and diastolic pressures increases on exercise.

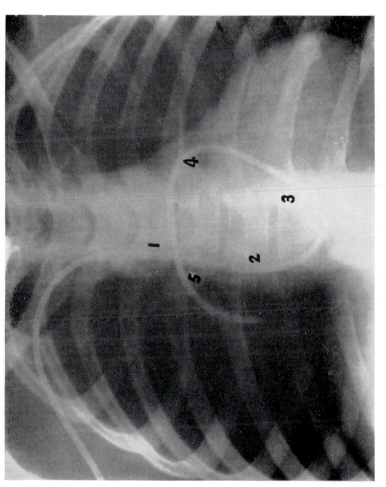

PLATE IV. Normal findings. Cardiac catheterization in a case of inactive rheumatic carditis. The catheter is seen lying in the superior vena cava (1), the right auricle (2), the right ventricle (3), main pulmonary artery (4), and in the right branch of the pulmonary artery (5).

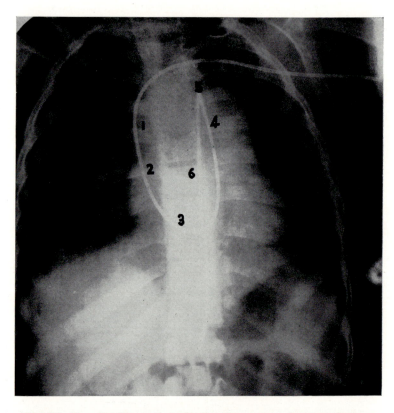

PLATE V.   Cardiac catheterization in a case of patent ductus
arteriosus.   The catheter is seen lying in the superior vena cava
(1), the right auricle (2), the right ventricle (3), the main pulmonary
artery (4); passing through the ductus arteriosus (5), it enters the
descending thoracic aorta (6).

The diagnosis should be considered in infancy whenever a systolic murmur is audible; particularly so when the murmur is high in position and when the pulse is collapsing in character. As a proportion of infants develop cardiac failure or pulmonary hypertension, it may be important to confirm the diagnosis and operate early.

In doubtful cases, the diagnosis of patent ductus may be proved by cardiac catheterization, the oxygen saturation of the pulmonary artery sample being greater than that of the right auricle and right ventricle, and the catheter may even traverse the ductus passing into the aorta (Plate V). Angio-cardiography and retrograde aortography are also available as aids in diagnosis. When *cyanosis* is present multiple defects are probable. Occasionally, however, cyanosis means a reversed shunt caused by pulmonary hypertension, in which case cyanosis will be most marked in the lower part of the body.

PROGNOSIS

The prognosis is very varied. A number of cases develop complications in infancy either from cardiac failure or from progressive pulmonary hypertension. There is a significant mortality in this group.

Many others remain asymptomatic, and the diagnosis is made at a routine examination. A number of these patients, nevertheless, are found to have pulmonary hypertension. Others develop complications only in adult life; among these bacterial endocarditis and heart failure are the most common.

TREATMENT

Operative treatment is now relatively safe and easy. The ductus should be tied or divided between ligatures and in expert hands the operative mortality is almost negligible. The operation can be undertaken with safety at any age, provided pulmonary hypertension has not progressed too far; therefore the diagnosis should be confirmed and operation performed forthwith on all suitable cases. Operation is strongly indicated in the case of infants with evidence of heart failure, breathlessness or of early pulmonary hypertension.

Ventricular Septal Defect

Clinically, patent septum ventriculorum is the commonest single cardiac defect and the one which is often found in mongols. When the septal opening is small, the condition is benign and symptoms are absent. During systole, blood shunts from the left ventricle into the right ventricle because the pressure in the former is about six times higher. Over the præcordium examination shows a harsh systolic murmur which is usually loudest in the third and fourth left interspaces near the sternum, although it may be better heard in the second interspace or nearer to the apex. Frequently there is a palpable thrill. It should be remembered that in cases of VSD the murmur is not present at birth but a few hours or days later when the pressure in the left ventricle comes to exceed that in the right. Sometimes a murmur disappears during childhood, not to return, and therefore it has been suggested that a small aperture may perhaps close spontaneously.

The majority of the children with VSD have little enlargement and good cardiac function. This was stated by Roger (1879), a physician on the staff of the Hôpital des Enfants in Paris, who from 1853 to 1874 examined many children's hearts and kept records of the localized systolic murmur and thrill with which we now associate his name. He was able to follow cases of ventricular septal defect for many years and he gave a lucid account of the normal-sized heart, normal function and good prognosis. But with a larger shunt symptoms may be marked, and Wood preferred to keep the term " Maladie de Roger " for asymptomatic cases. Taussig has stated that the position of the septal defect largely determines disability, a high one allowing the left ventricle to pump blood into the pulmonary artery, thus causing pulmonary overloading, and a low one causing only a trivial shunt; this view, however, does not appear to accord with the evidence.

DIAGNOSIS

The presence of a pansystolic murmur in the fourth left intercostal space suggests the diagnosis. Severe lesions cause considerable left ventricular enlargement and a functional mitral diastolic murmur may also be heard. The pulmonary blood flow is increased and on screening it is usual to see the pulmonary artery pulsating; thus, the x-ray appearances are almost identical with those of patent ductus arteriosus (Plate V) although enlargement of the left auricle is not present so commonly or so early as in patent ductus. The second heart sound shows a normal degree of splitting in contrast with the pathologically wide splitting of atrial septal defect (p. 271). Sometimes pulmonary hypertension supervenes; then the pulmonary component of the second heart sound is accentuated; moreover, as the hypertension progresses from increasing pulmonary arteriolar disease, there is danger of ultimate reversal of the shunt with persistent cyanosis (Eisenmenger's complex, p. 296).

TREATMENT

Surgical closure of ventricular septæ using the extra-corporeal circulation and deep hypothermia has become an established technique. It is indicated in patients who have progressive symptoms and in whom severe pulmonary hypertension has not yet become established.

In unoperated cases there is an ever present risk of subacute bacterial endocarditis.

In infancy, recurrent episodes of cardiac failure are not uncommon in patients with large defects. Such cases respond well to digitalization (p. 667), and to the general treatment of cardiac failure in infancy (p. 284). A proportion of these children lose their tendency to recurrent heart failure at about the age of twelve months, but in severe cases surgery has to be considered early[1] in view of the likely onset of irreversible pulmonary hypertension.

Abnormalities of the Atrial Septum

In its development the single auricle of the fœtus becomes separated into two cavities by the appearance of the *septum primum*; but this division is never fully completed by the septum primum itself, and the *septum secundum* grows on the right side of the septum primum covering it at all points except at the fossa ovalis where it forms a valve (the *foramen ovale*). In the fœtus the pressure in the right auricle is always higher than in the left auricle and this keeps the valve open; blood is shunted from right to left, side-stepping the pulmonary circulation. At birth the valve becomes functionally closed by increasing left auricular pressure. In 80 per cent. of cases the foramen ovale becomes closed by actual fusion of the septa (anatomical closure); in the remainder (anatomical *patency*) the foramen ovale can be rendered functionally patent by a sufficient rise in right auricular pressure, as for example in certain cases of pulmonary stenosis. It is important to differentiate between patients showing evidence of defects of the septum primum and septum secundum. The former have the more dangerous lesion and present a far more difficult technical problem to the surgeon for correction.

In *septum primum* defects there is a failure of fusion between the septum primum itself and the endocardial cushions. A defect remains immediately above the mitral and tricuspid valves, and in some patients extends to the upper part of the ventricular septum (atrio-ventriculare communis).

In patients having *septum secundum* defect, normal fusion has occurred between the septum primum and the endocardial cushions, but a defect remains above, either in the region of the foramen ovale or in some patients extending back to the orifice of the inferior vena cava.

Like other congenital anomalies, atrial septal defects are sometimes found in association with developmental faults elsewhere. Thus, the inherited condition called *arachnodactyly* (Figs. 26; 61, p. 479), or *Marfan's syndrome*, consists of spider digits, thin facies, hypotonia, high-arched palate, sometimes dislocation of the lenses, and various cardiac anomalies, of which atrial septal defect and defective aortic media are especially characteristic.

---

[1] Neill, C. A., Taussig, H. B. (1959). *J. Pediat.*, **55**, 374.

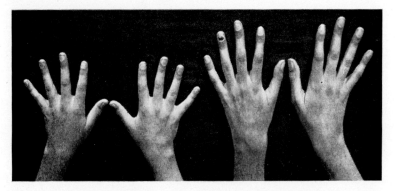

Fig. 26.—Hands in arachnodactyly (*right*), with control (*left*).

DIAGNOSIS

This condition ordinarily causes a left-to-right shunt. In consequence, the volume of the pulmonary blood flow may be two or three times the systemic flow, and the right ventricle therefore hypertrophies. The increased pulmonary flow is evidenced in an x-ray by dilatation of the pulmonary artery (*see also* p. 281). There is also pulsation of the artery and its branches (hilar dance) and increased vascularity of the lung fields. A systolic murmur, not loud, is usually heard in the pulmonary area; this is somewhat higher than is usual with VSD. There is no thrill. A basal diastolic murmur develops when a high pulmonary pressure causes stretching of the pulmonary ring (Graham-Steele murmur). Occasionally, mitral stenosis[1] co-existing with atrial septal defect causes a mitral presystolic murmur (Lutembacher's syndrome). Wide (i.e. pathological) splitting of the second heart sound is noted in cases of atrial septal defect, perhaps on account of interference of conduction (branch bundle block) but more probably from increasing over-filling of the right ventricle. The majority of the cases are reported to be associated with right bundle branch block in the ECG. As pulmonary hypertension increases, the pulmonary component of the second heart sound is accentuated. In such patients the Eisenmenger syndrome (p. 296) develops with increasing cyanosis.

The use of specialized techniques, such as dye, dilution curves, in addition to cardiac catheterization and angiocardiography, may be necessary in order to distinguish between the *septum primum* and *septum secundum* cases. The possibility of an anomalous form of pulmonary venous drainage must also be considered as a differential diagnosis or as an additional finding (*see* p. 295).

---

[1] The term *maladie de Durosiez* conveys the sense of mitral stenosis of developmental origin in contradistinction to *maladie de Vieussens*, mitral stenosis due to rheumatic infection.

Cardiac function usually remains good in most cases in childhood, but in the third and fourth decades progressive enlargement of the right ventricle leads to failure; the average length of life is therefore under 45 years. Finally, when the right ventricle fails, the pressure in the right auricle rises and the direction of the shunt may be reversed; in this way late central cyanosis and heart failure result.

TREATMENT

Children with major septal defects are limited in their capacity for exercise and are usually unable to take part in all school activities. Increasing breathlessness suggests a rise in pulmonary blood pressure. Candidates for operation are those with large shunts and large hearts, in whom pulmonary hypertension has not yet become irreversibly established. Patients with defects of the *septum primum* need the use of deep hypothermia and extra-corporeal circulation, whilst the closure of a *septum secundum* may be achieved with less elaborate techniques.

Anomalous Pulmonary Venous Drainage

The clinical picture of atrial septum defect may be produced in patients in whom one or more of the pulmonary veins drain either into the right atrium or into the superior or inferior venæ cavæ. The abnormal circulatory dynamics are similar to those in true atrial septal defects.

Such cases can now be diagnosed by the special techniques mentioned in describing the diagnosis of ASD, and correction has become a surgical possibility.

MALFORMATIONS LEADING PRIMARILY TO RIGHT-TO-LEFT SHUNTS

Fallot's Tetralogy

DEFINITION

THE tetralogy of Fallot accounts for about two-thirds of all cases of congenital heart disease with persistent cyanosis surviving beyond the first year of life. It is due to a faulty evolution of the *bulbus cordis* and consists of a combination of pulmonary or sub-pulmonary stenosis, ventricular septal defect, an " overriding " aorta, and hypertrophy of the right ventricle. The pulmonary obstruction is commonly infundibular (sub-pulmonary) and there may be no post-stenotic dilatation; indeed, the pulmonary artery is often small and thin-walled. The abnormality of the aorta is of great importance. Its root is displaced to the right so that it " overrides " the septum and receives about as much blood from the right as from the left ventricle. The aortic arch is right-sided in about a quarter of the cases.

DIAGNOSIS

Although breathlessness is present from infancy, there may be no cyanosis in the first months of life except with crying. For this reason it is helpful if, during part of the examination of a baby with a cardiac murmur, some crying should occur. The signs of dyspnœa should be noted as well (*see* p. 284). As the child grows, cyanosis becomes more constant; compensatory polycythæmia and clubbing of the digits is likely to develop; when he is breathless from walking the peculiar habit of squatting is sometimes adopted. Growth is likely to be stunted. The tetralogy is sometimes associated with mongolism but not so often as is septal defect.

Cardiac Signs. The size of the heart is often normal but the radiological outline is rendered characteristic by hypertrophy of the right ventricle and the reduced size of the pulmonary artery (p. 281). The cardiac shadow is rather upright and the apex, formed by the right ventricle, is raised. The left ventricle may be seen as a small prominence above it. This reminds one of the turned-up toe of a peasant's wooden shoe—the *cœur en sabot* (Plate VI). The shadow of the pulmonary artery is reduced so that the left cardiac border is either concave or straight. The lung fields are oligæmic although occasionally the opening up of compensatory broncho-pulmonary anastomoses gives them a somewhat reticular appearance. The electrocardiogram shows right ventricular hypertrophy and prominent peaked P-waves in leads 2 and 3. On auscultation a systolic murmur is heard over the præcordium; it is often rough in quality with its maximum intensity in the second and third interspaces near the left border of the sternum. A systolic thrill is present in about half the cases. The second heart sound is single owing to the absence of the pulmonary element. There is the possibility of cerebral embolism when cardiac catheterization is used to confirm the diagnosis, and rigid asepsis is essential to prevent the risk of cerebral abscess. Cineangiocardiography is often a more informative procedure (Plate VII).

TREATMENT

The palliative operations, Blalock-Taussig (anastomosis of subclavian artery to pulmonary artery), Potts (side-to-side anastomosis of aorta and pulmonary artery) and pulmonary valvotomy alone, are now being replaced by the total correction of all the defects under deep hypothermia. The palliative operations are still sometimes employed in infants and young children with severe symptoms as a preliminary to the major corrective operation at a later stage.

The operation still carries a high mortality which it is hoped will be reduced as further technical advances are developed.

Eisenmenger's Complex

Dr. Paul Wood recommended that this term should be used to refer to all patients in whom there is an abnormal communication

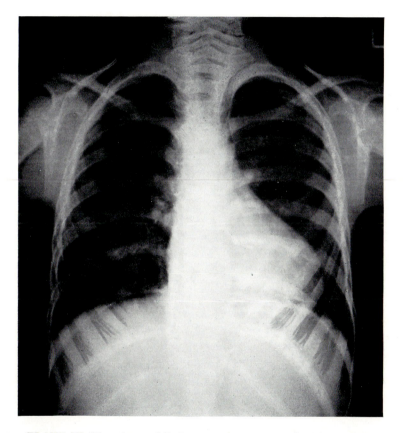

PLATE VI. Tetralogy of Fallot. The cardiac outline is upright and shaped like a French sabot. Note that the apex of the hypertrophied right ventricle is lifted above the diaphragm and the left upper border is convex. (From a girl of 12 years who was small for her age.)

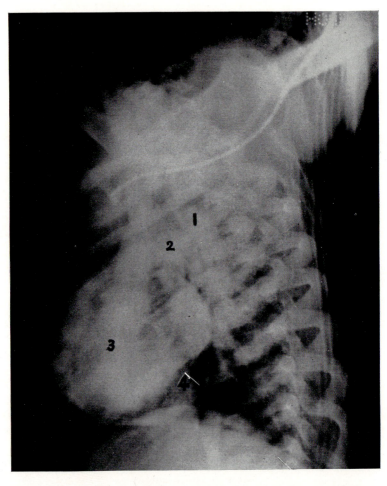

PLATE VII. Angiocardiogram in a case of Fallot's tetralogy.
Diodrast is seen entering the aorta (1) and pulmonary artery (2)
simultaneously from the right ventricle (3).   The left ventricle (4)
has not yet become opacified.

between the pulmonary and systemic circulations and in whom the onset of pulmonary hypertension has caused a reversal of the previous flow (i.e. from left to right) into a right-to-left shunt with the consequent development of cyanosis. Thus the Eisenmenger complex may be a consequence of atrial or ventricular septal defect or of patent ductus arteriosus where, as a secondary consequence, pulmonary hypertension has become established with reversal of blood flow through the defect.

In such cases, closure of the defect may be dangerous as the flow of blood from right to left through the defect has been acting as a safety valve in the relief of high pulmonary pressure.

Tricuspid Atresia

In tricuspid atresia the right ventricle is almost functionless. The blood passes from the right auricle through an atrial septal defect to the left auricle; the left ventricle maintains the systemic circulation through the aorta and also the pulmonary circulation through a ventricular septal defect and a vestigial right ventricle, or through a patent ductus arteriosus. Extreme cyanosis results from the right-to-left atrial shunt. In the diagnosis, angiocardiography gives conclusive proof, though it is hardly needed because the electrocardiogram shows left ventricular hypertrophy, and in a small infant this is an exceptional finding which, in the presence of severe cyanosis and an inactive right ventricle, points to tricuspid atresia. In the majority of such cases the period of survival is short.

Ebstein's Malformation

The tricuspid valve has a low position in relation to the right ventricle; the valve may be more like a net and the right ventricle is almost functionless. The right auricle is much enlarged and the jugular venous pressure is raised. A scratchy diastolic murmur, produced by blood-flow through the abnormal tricuspid valve, is heard. This murmur and the absence of right ventricular hypertrophy serves to distinguish Ebstein's malformation from pulmonary stenosis with ASD.

Cyanosis is not a feature of Ebstein's malformation, except when there is also an auricular septal defect.

Transposition of the Great Vessels

In this anomaly the pulmonary artery springs from the left ventricle and the aorta from the right one; if it were not for the presence of atrial and ventricular septal defects, on which life depends, there would be two independent circulations. Cyanosis is evident from the neonatal period and survival is brief. In many cases no murmur is audible. In an x-ray the lungs are pleonæmic and the cardiac shadow is shaped like an egg (p. 281 and Plate VIII). Angiocardiography gives a characteristic picture.

Persistent Truncus Arteriosus

When the aorto-pulmonary septum fails to develop, a common trunk arises from both ventricles. The severity of the condition depends on how the lungs are supplied with blood; if the pulmonary arteries spring from the truncus, cyanosis is moderate, but when the lungs are supplied by the bronchial arteries it is severe. Both ventricles are found to be enlarged, there is a loud systolic murmur and a thrill at the base. The second heart sound is single. Operative treatment, aimed at improving the pulmonary blood supply, has been attempted.

GENERAL PROGNOSIS OF CONGENITAL
HEART DISEASE

THE prognosis depends more on the nature of the lesions than on any other factor. Thus, anomalies such as simple dextrocardia carry no risk, small ventricular septal defects (maladie de Roger) have little effect on cardiac function, but more severe defects, such as Fallot's tetralogy, interfere drastically with hæmodynamics. The most serious lesions are those with persistent cyanosis dating from birth—transposition of the great vessels, common truncus arteriosus and tricuspid atresia—the infants rarely surviving for long. Campbell gives two general guides; the bigger the heart and the more multiple the lesions, the worse the prognosis.

The prognosis now depends on the feasibility of surgical treatment, and this has given an importance to exact diagnosis which it did not have before. The techniques of cardiac surgery are being improved; procedures at present relatively hazardous may soon become safer or quite new techniques may be introduced.

Any infant with severe congenital cardiac lesions starts life with a great handicap. He will probably gain weight slowly, and pulmonary infections will throw added strain on an already overworked heart. Before the days of cardiac surgery an infant with rapid breathing and cyanosis was unlikely to survive childhood. A young child who looks well but shows dyspnœa or cyanosis on exercise may survive for a considerable time, although there is likely to be progressive cardiac enlargement and heart failure. The prognosis is better when a lesion is found only on routine examination. It is to be remembered that other associated congenital defects, such as mongolism or skeletal deformities, may co-exist.

Certain forms of congenital heart disease, such as pulmonary stenosis and patent ductus, predispose to bacterial endocarditis but this is rare before adolescence.

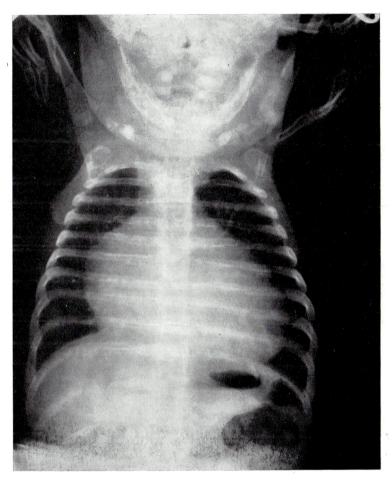

PLATE VIII. X-ray of a cyanosed infant, aged 4 months, with transposition of great vessels. The diagnosis was later confirmed at autopsy. There is transverse enlargement of the heart, which is somewhat egg-shaped; note the narrow upper mediastinal shadow.

GENERAL TREATMENT IN CONGENITAL HEART DISEASE

FEEDING

THE outlook is better for a breast-fed infant, but some dyspnœic infants cannot suck well; they tend to be underfed and thus the gain in weight is slow. It is often as well to give small feeds at shortened intervals, say 7 to 8 feeds in 24 hours; concentrated feeds of high caloric value are useful, or tube feeds may be given.

EXERCISE

In the case of an infant, the amount of exercise is not a problem but becomes so when he can walk or run. Up to school age it is usually best to let the child regulate his exertion himself, since breathlessness will stop him from living beyond his reserve; later on, competitive games and sports may be beyond the compass of children with congenital lesions, which limit the cardiac reserve. For example, in atrial septal defect the right heart output is increased leading to right ventricular hypertrophy, then to pulmonary hypertension and finally to right heart failure. *Each individual child should be studied before directions are given.* The full capacity of the heart should be ascertained by the test of exercise; thus can the patient be safely kept within his reserve yet allowed to do as much as is reasonable. For many patients a complete reassurance can be given that all normal activities may be undertaken. Excessive restrictions are pointless in conditions which are not curable. Insist on adequate rest and a long night in bed. The parents often needlessly fear that their child while exercising may have a sudden heart " attack " and die. Children with more severe lesions should attend " open-air " schools where physical handicaps can be especially catered for.

PREVENTION OF INFECTION

Routine procedures, such as dental extractions and tonsillectomy, should be covered by prophylactic penicillin; minor infections should be carefully observed and chemotherapy employed if extension of the infection to the lungs takes place.

ACQUIRED HEART DISEASE

Rheumatic Heart Disease (*see* Chapter 15)
Bacterial Endocarditis

INCIDENCE

IN childhood bacterial endocarditis is rare. The majority of infections occur either in association with developmental defects or after rheumatic endocarditis, and only a very occasional case arises *de novo*.

Pulmonary stenosis, bicuspid or supernumerary aortic valves, ventricular septal defect and patent ductus are the commonest predisposing lesions. In contrast, atrial septal defects are remarkably immune, and this is probably because it is the force of any abnormal jet of blood that causes local damage to the endocardium and so determines the site of infection with bacteria. Thus, in patent *septum ventriculorum* the vegetations are found on the wall of the right ventricle opposite to the patency as well as on the right side of the ventricular septum; again, in patent ductus they are found towards the pulmonary end of the ductus. Only a few infections are acute (the classical *malignant endocarditis*) and most of them, being caused by the *Streptococcus viridans*, are subacute (*endocarditis lenta*).

DIAGNOSIS

The most constant *symptoms* are fever, sweating and anæmia. Less constant ones are lassitude and embolic phenomena. Any unexplained pyrexia should, in a child with a developmental defect or rheumatic valvular disease, be a reason for suspicion; the urine and optic fundi should be repeatedly examined and blood cultures taken. It is essential that the cultures should be done before commencing penicillin or similar treatment. Positive bacterial cultures without signs are not sufficient proof of the diagnosis. The *signs* are splenomegaly and also those caused by emboli, including retinal exudates, petechiæ, and occult hæmaturia. Splinter hæmorrhages may also be detected in the nail beds. The location of embolic phenomena depends on the site of the cardiac lesion; in pulmonary valve and tricuspid disease, or when there is a left-to-right shunt, e.g. patent ductus, there are likely to be pulmonary infarcts; in mitral and aortic disease, emboli occur in the skin, kidneys, brain and fundi. Cardiac murmurs develop and often change. There may be clubbing of the digits or Osler's nodes. The latter consist of transient, tender, pink papules on the pads of the fingers, thumbs and toes, and the causative bacteria can often be cultured from them.

TREATMENT

Prevention may be attempted by adequate treatment of dental, cutaneous and pharyngeal infection. Dental extractions and removal of tonsils and adenoids should be covered with penicillin. Unexplained fever should be investigated. Patency of the ductus arteriosus should not go untreated beyond the age of twelve years.

Curative treatment is carried out with penicillin or other antibiotic to which the bacteria are most sensitive. Thus, it is a great advantage to obtain positive cultures before commencing treatment. It should be remembered that early treatment lessens the risk of permanent valvular scarring and mycotic aneurysms. The treatment must be adequate in dose and duration, that is, 1–2 million units of penicillin daily for 4 to 6 weeks, provided there is swift improvement, and longer if there is not. If there is a defect which can be surgically improved, operation should be planned to take place when the endocarditis has had time to heal and to consolidate, say, two months afterwards in the case of a patent ductus.

PERICARDITIS

INFLAMMATION of the pericardium may be *suppurative* (i.e. caused by septicæmic infection), *viral, tuberculous* or *uræmic* but is commonly due to the *rheumatic infections* or to *Still's disease.*

Pyogenic Pericarditis

Suppurative pericarditis causes much thickening of the pericardium and a rapid effusion of pus. The sac becomes distended and the heart sounds are faint. The pericardium is intensely inflamed with a shaggy surface and a purulent exudate; when opened it presents the so-called " bread and butter " appearance.

Clinical Picture. During a severe pneumonia or, say, an osteomyelitis, the child is found to be more ill than the condition warrants, though pericarditis is seldom suspected until a to-and-fro friction sound is heard. There is much fever and toxæmia; the pulse and respiration rates are rapid. Treatment with the appropriate antibiotic agent should be energetic and it may be advisable to aspirate the pus and to replace with penicillin. Occasionally surgical drainage is performed.

Tuberculous Pericarditis

Spread of disease from caseous lymph nodes in the mediastinum is the usual origin. It may take the form of a relatively benign non-suppurative effusion which reabsorbs, or there may be considerable pericardial thickening with *permanent pericardial constriction.* Occasionally the exudate is bloodstained or even purulent. If tubercle bacilli are recoverable the progress is poor unless streptomycin and Isoniazid are given early in the course of the condition. If tubercle bacilli are not recoverable, spontaneous cure is likely to occur, and even when the tuberculin reaction is positive the ætiology is uncertain.

Acute Benign Pericarditis

This is an acute form of pericarditis due to a virus, such as the *Coxsackie Group B,* and its course is self-limited. The onset is sudden with considerable fever, but fairly moderate symptoms. A pericardial rub is heard and the cardiac dullness rapidly increases. There is leucocytosis and a rise in the erythrocyte sedimentation rate. An effusion may also occur in the pleura. The condition resolves without treatment, and afterwards no signs of cardiac damage are discoverable. This, and the absence of rheumatic manifestations serve to distinguish the condition from rheumatic pericarditis.

Rheumatic Pericarditis

It is chiefly in the severe cases of rheumatic carditis that pericarditis occurs and along with it there are always changes in the endocardium and the myocardium (pancarditis). Often there is mediastinitis as well, and there may be pleurisy and pneumonia. The pericarditis is either *dry* with localized or widespread to-and-fro friction sounds, or it causes a sudden *effusion* which may be serous or serofibrinous. The effusion is sterile and rarely sufficient in amount to compress the heart. It is reabsorbed spontaneously. Adherence of the pericardium may follow one or more attacks of pericarditis, but chronic constrictive pericarditis is almost never rheumatic in origin.

Clinical Picture. The child has a pale and anxious face. Fever and tachycardia are present. Pain may be felt in the chest over the præcordium or it may be due to an associated pleurisy. When there is a large effusion, the heart sounds may be muffled, and on percussion dullness becomes evident in the second intercostal spaces close to the sternum. X-ray shows the heart shadow to be greatly enlarged and the left border is seen to be convex. An effusion similar to that in the pericardium appears at the base of the left pleura and this causes an area of dullness and bronchial breathing at the left base near the midline (Ewart's sign). A similar but smaller effusion may occur in the right pleura. Erythema marginatum (Fig. 31) and nodules (Fig. 30) may be present. In about two-thirds of the acute cases there are characteristic changes in the electrocardiogram (*see* p. 310).

Treatment is directed to the relief of pain and distress. Cardiac decompression is needed only in the rare cases of high-pressure effusion. Corticosteroids (p. 659) appear to have a beneficial effect in the acute phase.

Pericarditis in Still's Disease (*see* p. 317)

In some 10 per cent. of cases of Still's disease, electrocardiographic changes and sometimes friction sounds provide evidence of pericarditis, and pericardial adhesions are usually found at autopsy. The pericardial inflammation probably occurs in the acute phases of the disease but does not otherwise affect the prognosis. Endocardial and myocardial changes do not develop in these cases unless there happens to be co-existing acute rheumatic infection.

CHAPTER 15

Rheumatic Fever, Carditis, and Chorea

ACUTE rheumatism includes rheumatic fever, carditis, rheumatic nodules, erythema marginatum and chorea, occurring singly or in combination, but chorea more often occurs as a sole manifestation of the rheumatic process.

INCIDENCE

Acute rheumatism is notifiable in the United Kingdom in only a few areas. In these areas, the incidence of acute rheumatism among school children as judged by notifications was 45 per 100,000 school children during the year 1950. It is now considerably less than this. The incidence of acute rheumatism waxes and wanes with the attack rate of Group A β-hæmolytic streptococci, which are the main ætiological factor, but there are several *predisposing* factors which are imperfectly understood. The general incidence has shown a decline for at least half a century, and this decline has been accelerated where prophylaxis against rheumatism by means of penicillin is being used.

ÆTIOLOGY

The Group A (Lancefield) β-hæmolytic streptococcus acts as the trigger mechanism in acute rheumatism, but many children and young adults undergo such streptococcal infections without subsequently developing rheumatism; thus, there must be other factors which, in combination with a streptococcal infection, determine the onset and relapses of acute rheumatism.

Manifestations of acute rheumatism usually begin to develop about two weeks after the streptococcal infection, the order of events being (1) a streptococcal infection (usually a sore throat), (2) a silent (or latent) period, and (3) the attack of rheumatism, carditis or chorea.

Sex Incidence. Statistics show the disease to be rather more common in females than in males, and a difference in the manifestations in the two sexes; chorea is more common in girls than in boys, whereas arthritis is more common in boys than in girls; heart disease is equally common in the two sexes.

Heredity. A history of an increased incidence can be elicited in some families.

Age. Rheumatism is seldom seen below the age of three years, after which the incidence increases very slowly to the age of five. After five the increase is more rapid, reaching its maximum about seven years; from then to twelve years there is a steady fall. In both girls and boys, therefore, seven is the age at which rheumatism is most prevalent.

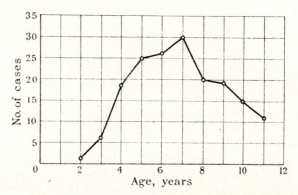

Fig. 27. — Age-incidence of initial attack in 172 cases of rheumatism (London area).

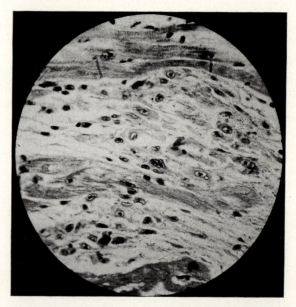

Fig. 28.—Large subendocardial Aschoff node in the left ventricle in a child, aged 7 years with rheumatic carditis. The muscle bundles are separated by a cellular infiltrate composed of Aschoff epithelioid cells, some multinucleate, and lymphocytes. This is an active lesion. (*Hæmatoxylin and eosin, medium power.*)

Social class. The class incidence of rheumatism should be noted. It is not the child of a well-to-do family who is likely to be affected. Rheumatism is a disease of the poorer class and the lower middle class.

It is probable that the fall in the incidence of the disease which has occurred in Britain[1] is due to improved nutrition, hygiene and social conditions.   But it would be unwise to assume that this decline will continue, and it is still necessary to guard against the risks, in particular by taking all possible measures to prevent streptococcal infections and by treating them promptly when they occur.

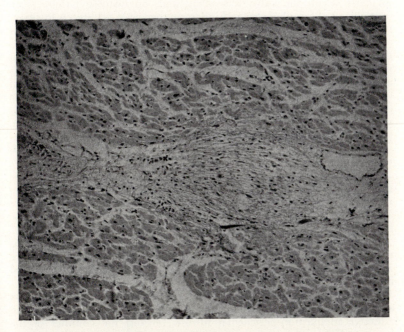

Fig. 29.—An Aschoff body in the interstitial tissues of the left ventricle. The lesion is spindle shaped. Fine collagen fibres run through the centre of the Aschoff body. The cellular component is mainly fibroblastic, this being an older lesion. From a case of rheumatic carditis, aged 7 years. (*Hæmatoxylin and eosin, low power.*)

PATHOLOGY

The essential lesion is a focal fibrinoid necrosis of collagen, usually situated close to a small vessel and surrounded by lymphocytes endothelial cells and fibroblasts; epithelioid cells, some multinucleate, are often seen as well. This is the *Aschoff* nodule or *Aschoff* body (Figs. 28, 29).   Such lesions are widespread in muscles and connective tissue, but their site of predilection is in the myocardium, valves and

[1] " The Health of the School Child, 1952–3."   London: H.M. Stationery Office

coverings of the heart, and also in subcutaneous tissues over the joints and tendon sheaths (*rheumatic nodules*). In its early and active stages an Aschoff nodule shows considerable cellular exudate but, as it becomes older, patchy necrosis and fibrosis occur; thus, a subcutaneous lesion may be felt at first as a soft and somewhat ill-defined pad and later as a small fibrous nodule.

ENDOCARDIAL CHANGES

The inflammatory reaction in a valve develops with the lesion. In an early lesion the valve is swollen, and, on histology, there is an outpouring of lymphocytes and inflammatory cells. Later, a fibrinous structureless exudate extrudes on the free surface of the valve. This stains badly, and the various circulating blood elements tend to deposit on the free surface of the exudate. Deep to the fibrinous material, however, endothelial cells, lymphocytes and early fibroblasts appear, so that the essential structure of a damaged valve is identical with that of the subcutaneous nodule or heart-nodule. Seldom is one portion of the heart alone affected; that is, rheumatic endocarditis is rarely, if ever, present without an affection of the myocardium. Certainly, rheumatic pericarditis does not exist apart from myocardial and endocardial changes. The term *rheumatic carditis* is therefore much to be preferred.

From the point of view of the functional efficiency of the heart, the outlook depends upon the ultimate state of the heart valves and the myocardium. Healing takes place by replacement fibrosis, the degree and site of which indicate the amount of damage to the cardiac muscle and interstitial tissue.

The endocardial valvular lesions heal by a process of slow fibrosis which may take several years to complete. Such fibrosis will give rise to the post-rheumatic endocardial lesions of valvular stenosis and incompetence.

The acute fibrinous pericarditis of acute rheumatism is followed by a fibrotic healing stage which may in rare instances give rise to an adhesive mediastino-pericardial fibrosis beyond the confines of the heart itself.

CLINICAL PICTURE

In the clinical syndrome of acute rheumatism, *rheumatic carditis, polyarthritis, the rheumatic rash* and *rheumatic nodule*, and *rheumatic chorea* may occur as isolated lesions or in combination.

The illness of rheumatic fever is usually preceded by a throat infection but this may be so mild as to escape attention. Then, after an interval of 10–21 days, the symptoms of the rheumatic attack develop. The commonest complaint is fever along with aching in the joints. The inflammation of the joints may cause no more than this, but in more severe cases there is tenderness, swelling, heat and, perhaps, synovial effusion (*see* under *Arthritis*, p. 308). In some cases the fever settles in about a week but in others it lasts longer. The *sedimentation rate is considerably raised and remains so as long as the*

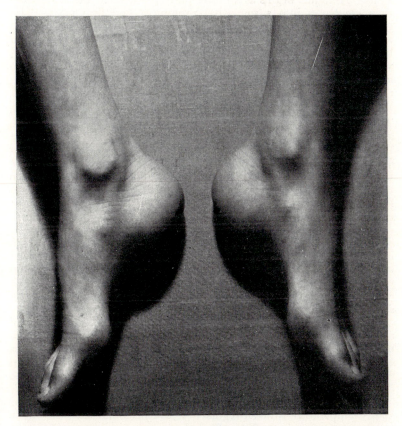

Fig. 30.—Nodules in the seventh week of acute rheumatism. The largest nodules are seen on the internal malleoli.

disease is active. The pulse is also increased and this too may persist. Treatment with aspirin, or with sodium salicylate, usually brings down the temperature and relieves the pain. An attack of rheumatism often leads to some degree of *anæmia*. In a child *acute leukæmia* may be misdiagnosed as acute rheumatism because it can cause fever, anæmia, a cardiac murmur and pain in the limbs (*see* p. 348).

Nodules. These are looked for at the subcutaneous bony surfaces over the elbows, occiput, vertebral prominences, knuckles and the ankles. On bending the knee, elbow, fist or ankle slightly, so as to draw the skin tensely over the bony prominences, the nodules stand out (Fig. 30). Pressed on slightly, they slide beneath the finger. Examination of an excised nodule shows a localized inflammatory focus. A nodule begins as a rather puffy pre-nodular thickening and then condenses into a somewhat prominent and firm mass. This gets harder and smaller, and in a few weeks disappears. Nodules are a sign of active rheumatic infection, and are generally accompanied by a cardiac lesion. They have occasionally been noted, however, without evidence of carditis. Rheumatic fever may occur either in an acute or subacute form. So long as rheumatic nodules persist, rheumatic activity remains, with the danger of further cardiac damage.

Arthritis. Rheumatic arthritis follows a streptococcal infection. There is a high swinging temperature up to 103° or 104° F at night, accompanied by sweating and anorexia. When the first joint has been affected for a varying period of hours, but seldom more than forty-eight, the pain shifts to another joint and flits in this manner from one joint to another. It is of the highest importance to realize that once the pain and tenderness have left a joint no residual deformity or abnormality of any kind remains; if it does, then the condition is not rheumatic fever.

One of the most important differential diagnoses in the early stages of acute rheumatism is *osteomyelitis*. Other evidence of rheumatism in addition to arthritis is often present, and as soon as the pain passes to another joint the true state of affairs becomes apparent. Abdominal pain, not uncommon at the onset of acute rheumatism, may cause confusion with *appendicitis*; again, other rheumatic manifestations should help to decide the diagnosis.

In a severe attack there may be involvement of the vertebral articulations in the neck and back. In such a case the patient is unable to move the head in any direction and a mistaken diagnosis of meningitis has been made. Arthritis is much commoner in boys than in girls, possibly two boys to one girl, and in this way the converse disproportion in the sexes seen in chorea is equalized.

In the less typical *subacute rheumatism*, the onset is more insidious. If the temperature is taken regularly it will be found that the night temperature may rise to 99° to 99·4° F, but rarely higher. The child remains pale, listless and anorexic, and loses some weight. It is to be noted that the pain not infrequently occurs in the mornings, as opposed to the muscle pain which results from fatigue or cramp; the latter commonly occurs at night and the child wakes from sleep because of the pain which by the morning has disappeared.

Multiple involvement of joints is usual in rheumatism, the pain disappearing from one joint and reappearing in another. Occasionally, however, *arthritis is non-articular* and the diagnosis is then difficult.

An example of this manner of presentation may be acute arthritis of one hip joint.

The Skin. Two types of rash have been described: (1) *erythema marginatum*, which appears over the trunk, thighs and arms and which may come and go for several weeks; the edge is characteristically

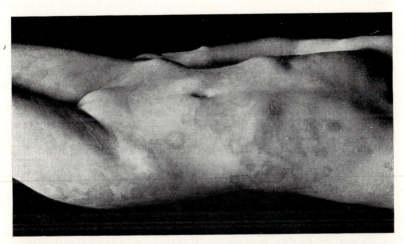

Fig. 31.—Erythema marginatum in a child with rheumatism. She had carditis and arthritis; the infection lasted several months. The erythema is more marked than is usually seen in cases of rheumatism. Note the raised œdematous edges of some of the lesions.

serpiginous or map-like, changing from hour to hour (Fig. 31); (2) *rheumatic purpura*, seen only in severe cases which are likely to be fatal.

Rheumatic Carditis

The significance of rheumatism depends upon the extent to which the heart is implicated. Rheumatic carditis usually involves the myocardium, the endocardium, and often the pericardium, simultaneously; for the purposes of description the clinical picture of each will be given separately.

Myocarditis

Some degree of cardiac enlargement takes place and the cardiac apex beat becomes prominent and more diffuse than normal. Thus, the apex beat in cardiac dilatation is diffuse and feeble, as opposed to the thrustful apex beat of left ventricular hypertrophy or the slapping impulse of right ventricular hypertrophy. As the acute condition heals, the apex returns to its normal position.

II

Tachycardia (*see* p. 275) which is out of proportion to the temperature is usually present and persists at rest and during sleep. The finding of a sleeping pulse rate which remains as high as the waking pulse is of the utmost importance, both as a diagnostic sign and as an index of progress during the subsequent weeks, for as improvement occurs, so the sleeping pulse rate drops to a level well below that of the waking pulse. Great care, however, is necessary to ensure that the sleeping pulse rate is properly taken, for the pulse rate of a healthy child when slightly disturbed from sleep will be raised often to the waking level (*see* p. 275).

Together with the acceleration of rate, *disturbances of rhythm* may be present. These are less commonly found than the other signs, but must always be sought for. In myocarditis, not only the muscle but also the conduction fibres may be involved in the inflammatory process. Thus, some degree of heart block may be present. This may be no more than a Grade I heart block, in which the rhythm is entirely normal but in which the electrocardiogram reveals an abnormal lengthening of the P–R interval. In healthy children the P–R interval is seldom more than 0·16 sec., but in myocarditis it may be prolonged to as much as 0·24 sec. without dropped beats occurring. Secondly, Grade II heart block may occur, in which the P–R interval is lengthened to such a degree that the ventricle does not respond to all auricular contractions. Thus 2 : 1, 3 : 1, 4 : 1 block may result. Finally, Grade III heart block may rarely occur; in this case conduction is so disturbed that the ventricle takes up a slow independent idioventricular rhythm unrelated to auricular contractions. Such a rate is usually between 40–50 per minute, and is little affected by exercise.

Other less common types of heart block may occur, such as the Wenckebach phenomenon, in which the P–R interval gradually lengthens in successive beats until a dropped beat occurs, after which normal rhythm is resumed with a normal P–R interval, which again gradually increases in duration.

In addition to heart block, multiple extrasystoles may sometimes be present in acute myocarditis. These may be distinguished from the dropped beats of heart block by the fact that they disappear on exertion.

As improvement occurs, all the signs of myocarditis may disappear, or some degree of residual dilatation may persist, together with a significant systolic apical murmur.

Endocarditis

In a first attack of rheumatic carditis no evidence of endocarditis may be detectable clinically. Its presence may only be revealed as fibrosis and shrinking of valves occurs and valvular lesions develop. This process takes months or years. The most constantly affected valve is the mitral, followed by the aortic and then the tricuspid.

Aortic lesions occasionally occur without disease of the mitral valve, but if the aortic or tricuspid valve is affected, it is usually in combination with a mitral lesion.

On auscultation, *the first sound may become muffled at the apex* and *a soft apical systolic murmur may be heard*: this murmur occupies the whole of systole (*see* Fig. 32), as opposed to an innocent murmur which is shorter in duration (*see* Fig. 24). In addition, transient *mid-diastolic*

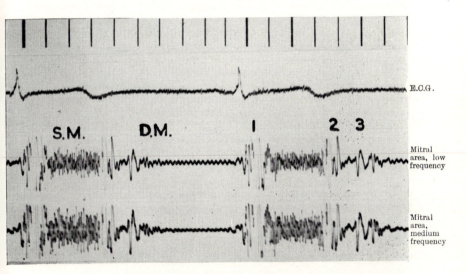

Fig. 32.—A case of rheumatic carditis with mitral incompetence. The recording of a mitral systolic murmur (SM) which occupies the whole of systole (compare with Fig. 33, p. 312). A mitral diastolic murmur (DM) follows the third heart sound.
1 = 1st heart sound; 2 = 2nd heart sound; 3 = 3rd heart sound.

apical murmurs may occur, which are very localized and variable; their significance lies in their appearance *de novo* in the course of an illness, and their tendency to alter.

As *mitral stenosis* develops, progressive enlargement of the left auricle occurs, followed later by hypertrophy of the right ventricle. The left auricular enlargement is not perceptible clinically, but may be demonstrated by a *barium swallow*, since a considerable backward indentation in the course of the œsophagus is produced by the enlarged auricle. The right ventricular hypertrophy may not be clinically evident until several years after the first attack of acute endocarditis, but eventually reveals itself by forceful pulsation which moves the sixth rib close to the sternum or even the lower end of the sternum itself; the apex beat also becomes slapping in character, but with no actual movement of the overlying rib.

On auscultation a localized diastolic murmur is heard at the apex with the patient lying on the left side. This murmur is usually presystolic in time with a crescendo element up to the first sound, but occasionally it is mid-diastolic in position. It may be associated with a palpable diastolic or presystolic thrill. Mitral diastolic murmurs are often sharply localized and can sometimes only be elicited with the patient on the left side or after exercise. They are often best heard just internal to the apex, and with a bell rather than the diaphragm chest-piece of the stethoscope. When a mitral diastolic murmur is present, the usual two-beat cardiac metre becomes a three-beat metre. In mitral stenosis the second sound is likely to be accentuated in the pulmonary area while at the apex it may show a characteristic " opening " snap of the mitral valve.

Mitral regurgitation may frequently be evident before mitral stenosis has progressed to a perceptible degree. This may be shown by the development of persistent cardiac enlargement, together with the appearance of an apical pan-systolic murmur (Fig. 32) which is conducted outwards to the axilla.

The development of *aortic regurgitation* is shown by the appearance of slowly progressive peripheral circulatory changes as well as cardiac signs. The blood pressure begins to show an increasing difference

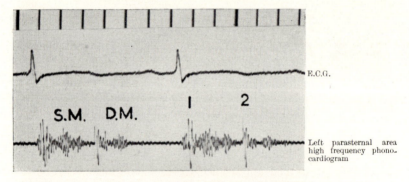

E.C.G.

Left parasternal area high frequency phono-cardiogram

Fig. 33.—From a child with rheumatic carditis (aortic incompetence), who had a " basal " type of systolic murmur occupying only the first part of systole (SM), and a soft aortic diastolic murmur (DM).
1 = 1st heart sound; 2 = 2nd heart sound.

between the systolic and diastolic levels, 130/50 mm. Hg being a typical final figure. Together with this, the pulse may take on a collapsing character, marked carotid pulsation becomes evident and capillary pulsation is visible in the nail beds.

As to the heart itself, aortic regurgitation gives rise to left ventricular hypertrophy, shown by displacement of the apex beat downwards and to the left and by the forceful character of the impulse which usually moves, with each beat, the rib which overlies it. This sign will not be evident in the early stages of the disease. A characteristic soft, high-pitched early diastolic murmur develops, which may be best heard at the base, or commonly to the left of the sternum in the third or fourth space (Fig. 33). The murmur is continuous with the second sound and, in contrast to a mitral diastolic murmur, the usual two-beat metre of the heart sounds is not altered. It may be accompanied by a diastolic thrill. An aortic diastolic murmur, being of high frequency, is best heard with a diaphragm chest-piece, and it is easier to hear it when the patient holds his breath in full expiration. The character of the murmur has been likened to a whispered " R."

Rheumatic aortic stenosis rarely develops to a clinically perceptible degree in childhood, but the physical signs are similar to those of congenital aortic stenosis (p. 286).

Tricuspid lesions are rarely detectable in childhood; it is to be noted, however, that tricuspid incompetence with a pulsating liver may complicate acute heart failure.

Rheumatic Pericarditis (*see also* p. 302)

Rheumatic pericarditis is remarkable in that it may give rise to a high temperature. Many rheumatic infections are not accompanied by much fever, especially if salicylates are being given. Despite salicylate therapy, however, pericarditis may cause fever for some days or even weeks, the child remaining distressed and ill. Vomiting and epigastric or substernal pain are warning signs. There is dyspnœa and often a short hacking cough reminiscent of pneumonia, together with a scattered bronchitis, and at the base of the left lung a patch of high-pitched tubular breathing. The cause of this is debatable, some regarding it as a rheumatic pneumonia and others attributing it to compression of the left bronchus by the enlarged heart and a consequent collapse of the left lower lobe.

When pericarditis develops, the pulse becomes rapid and the area of cardiac dullness increases. On auscultation, a harsh to-and-fro pericardial rub may be heard in varying areas in the early stages, but as fluid collects the murmur disappears and the heart sounds become faint. As healing with resorption of fluid occurs, the pericardial rub may temporarily return.

Additional evidence of pericardial effusion is given by the x-ray contour of the heart and the electrocardiogram, which shows elevation at first of the S–T segment in the standard leads followed by inversion of the T-wave at a later stage.

Adherent Pericardium

In an effort to compensate for this disability, the heart greatly hypertrophies, and in cases of rheumatic carditis the *cor bovinum* is seen *post mortem*. It seems probable, however, that " constrictive pericarditis " is seldom of rheumatic origin; instead, a condition of *adhesive mediastino-pericarditis* develops which can be detected by inspection of the intercostal spaces in the left axilla and at the angle of the scapula which occasionally shows a dragging in and out of the chest-wall with each cardiac impulse.

TREATMENT OF ACUTE RHEUMATISM

PREVENTIVE

IF infection by Group A β-hæmolytic streptococci could be prevented there would be no acute rheumatism; since nasal carriage of hæmolytic streptococci is found in ten per cent. of healthy school-children, this is not a practical possibility. The spread of hæmolytic streptococci is favoured by conditions of over-crowding and by carriers with chronic nasal discharges. Known cases of hæmolytic streptococcal infection in schools should receive prompt treatment. Where repeated infection is occurring in a particular school, a search for carriers should be made and treatment instituted. Penicillin should be used because the streptococcus is *never insensitive to penicillin* (*see* Appendix I).

Any child once having had an attack of rheumatism or chorea should have continuous penicillin prophylaxis in order to prevent future streptococcal infections. This is given as penicillin V 200,000 units (125 mg.) twice daily and a dose should never be missed. It should be continued for 5 years or until the child leaves school. Children known to be allergic to penicillin may have prophylactic sulphonamide or tetracycline as alternatives.

MANAGEMENT OF A CHILD WITH RHEUMATIC CARDITIS

In acute cases the child should be kept at rest, but pillows are allowed so that he can see what is happening around him without exertion. The pulse should be charted four-hourly and later twice daily, and a record of the sleeping pulse kept.

Penicillin should be given by intramuscular injection initially, followed by oral penicillin, which is afterwards continued as prophylaxis.

Salicylates are undoubtedly useful in relieving the pain of arthritis, and in stopping the fever; buffered aspirin, four-hourly, is well tolerated, but with high dosage tinnitus and vomiting can occur.

The place of cortisone and ACTH in the treatment of acute rheumatism is not yet settled, but in severe cases these drugs sometimes appear to be life-saving remedies (*see* Appendix 2). When they are used, the symptoms improve and the temperature, pulse and sedimentation rate are likely to fall more quickly, but this does not necessarily mean that hormone treatment yields better results in the long run. In a joint U.S.-U.K. study of rheumatic fever, comparisons between treatment with ACTH, cortisone, and salicylate were made, these comparisons being strictly based on a standard system of dosage used in courses lasting six weeks. Generally speaking, patients receiving the standard treatment prescribed in the three groups did not appear to show differences in the incidence of carditis in the final clinical state.

If the pulse rate drops rapidly with rest, there are no murmurs and the dilatation of the heart rights itself, more liberty of movement may be allowed; soon the child can sit up and feed himself, and finally may get up and slowly resume his ordinary life. The sleeping pulse rate, together with a declining sedimentation rate, are important observations in controlling this resumption. At any sign of a rise of pulse rate, or of the appearance of a murmur or fresh cardiac damage, more rest should be enjoined, this being maintained for many weeks if the cardiac damage is considerable. If an abnormal electro-cardiogram is found initially, repeat examinations may provide an index of progress. The weight and sedimentation rate also constitute helpful and reliable guides to the progress of the disease.

Occasionally, the course of rheumatic carditis is progressively downhill and the picture becomes complicated by acute cardiac failure. This is usually shown by œdema, which may not necessarily be dependent, as is seen in adults, and dyspnœa. Examination reveals engorgement of the neck veins and enlargement and tenderness of the liver. There is progressive cardiac dilatation. In some cases a tinge of cyanosis and signs of pulmonary œdema may develop. This is treated by digoxin (p. 667), diuretics, corticosteroids (p. 660) and oxygen, together with a restricted fluid and salt intake.

LONG-TERM CARE

The treatment of children with acute rheumatism including carditis has to be thought of in terms of months rather than weeks.

The special nursing and supervision can occasionally be provided at home, but this is becoming more and more exceptional, and for the majority of patients hospital care is indicated. The place of choice is a long-stay hospital where teachers are available to continue education and the gradual resumption of a normal active life can be supervised.

PROGNOSIS

With efficient care the immediate mortality is extremely low during the acute stage. The ultimate prognosis depends upon *whether the heart is irreversibly damaged in the first attack*, i.e. before prophylactic treatment can be instituted, and *whether further attacks can be prevented*; this largely depends on adequate and uninterrupted prophylaxis with penicillin (*see* treatment, p. 314). The greater the number of recurrences, the more certain it is that there will be permanent structural damage, and this is likely to shorten life.

Chorea (St. Vitus's Dance)

PATHOLOGY

The mortality is so low that very little material has been examined *post mortem*. Carefully investigated cases, however, have shown a characteristic cellular infiltration around the small capillaries, comparable up to a point with the picture of encephalitis. The brain is diffusely affected, especially the white matter, but particularly the corpus striatum and the red nucleus; minute emboli and blocking of the vessels by thrombi have been noted. In some cases extravasation of blood from the finest capillaries has been seen.

CLINICAL PICTURE

Chorea occurs mainly in children of school age. It is about twice as common in girls. The child is often of the bright, slim, rather nervous type; she may flag easily, become unduly emotional, laughing or crying too easily, and lose colour. The tendency to drop or spill things is common, the writing becomes less legible, the speech less articulate. Movements, in standing up or sitting down, are impetuous. The child tends to fall about, catching one foot behind the other, and on this account is often covered with bruises or abrasions, especially about the knees. As the disease develops, all the muscles in the body become involved. The involvement of the facial muscles causes grimacing whereby the child appears to smile or frown for no reason. Constant involuntary movements of the arms, hands, legs and feet are seen. The respiratory movements are also affected, resulting in grossly irregular breathing. The knee-jerks are active, giving rise to what is known as the " hung-up " knee-jerk; that is, after the jerk has occurred, the leg fails for a moment to drop back into its previous position. Sometimes the deep reflexes are diminished or absent (*paretic chorea*). Snorting noises and clucking with the tongue are characteristic. The movements continue throughout the waking period but always disappear during sleep. In a severe case even feeding is difficult. A pronounced case of chorea is a pitiful sight, and in some of the more severe cases the child may become almost maniacal. In some cases one side only may be affected (*hemi-chorea*).

The differential diagnosis from habit spasm is discussed on p. 387. Sometimes there is cardiac dilatation and carditis may occur in a first or subsequent attack. The disease is sometimes accompanied by rheumatic nodules but arthritis rarely coincides with the chorea. As many as eight recurrences of chorea may occur and this results in grave interruption of education.

PROGNOSIS

From the chorea there is very little to be feared; that is, there is no evidence of any permanent cerebral damage, and recovery appears to be complete. It is in possible accompanying heart disease that the danger lies.

TREATMENT

General Management. A child with chorea is confined to bed during the active stages. Choreiform movements mean that rheumatic infection is present and active, and the heart is therefore in danger.

The child should be placed in bed with two or three pillows. In severe cases the sides of the bed should be padded to prevent banging of the head and limbs. The sleeping pulse is much more important than the temperature in that it furnishes an indication of the cardiac condition. The ESR is not, however, raised in uncomplicated chorea.

Nursing. Much skill may be required in the management of chorea. The patients may need to drink from a special feeding-cup, and in the more severe cases are unable to feed themselves. They require much sympathy because of their emotional lability.

Drugs. A great variety of drugs has been employed. Aspirin or sodium salicylate do not appear to have any specific effect on the chorea. To understand the drug treatment of chorea it must be realized that there is an organic and a functional element. During the acute stages the disease is almost entirely organic. In six or eight weeks, however, provided the pulse has settled and the condition of the heart is satisfactory, it may be safely assumed that the movements are largely functional. Phenobarbitone, with or without aspirin (for dosage, *see* Appendix 3) may be given twice or three times daily. Cortisone and ACTH have no effect on chorea.

Re-education. During the later stages occupational therapy is valuable in re-educating the muscles.

RHEUMATOID ARTHRITIS (STILL'S DISEASE)

THIS condition in childhood was described by the late Sir Frederic Still in 1897.[1] His original description has been amplified[2] but not altered in any fundamental way.

ÆTIOLOGY

The affection is commoner in girls than in boys, and the majority of cases commence in the second, third or fourth year of life. Causation is obscure but is probably similar to that in adult cases. There is no evidence of direct infection of the joints or lymphatic tissues. It may be the result of an altered reaction of the tissues to stress and antigenic substances.

PATHOLOGY

The chief changes are periarticular, and the joints most commonly involved are the knees, ankles, wrists, elbows and interphalangeal joints. Every joint in the body, however, may be involved, including the vertebral joints, which are most frequently affected in the cervical

---

[1] Still, G. F. (1897). *Med.-chir. Trans.,* **80,** 47.
[2] Bywaters, E. C. L. in " Pædiatrics for the Practitioner." Vol. III.   Edited by Gaisford and Lightwood. London: Butterworth.

region. With disuse and the accompanying general ill-health, there is marked osteoporosis, revealed by x-ray examination. There is regional enlargment of the lymphatic glands, the epitrochlear nodes being often palpable, and the inguinal and axillary glands as well. The spleen is occasionally enlarged. In a case of long standing, the synovial membrane is thick and gelatinous, and the cartilage becomes more and more eroded until finally it shows gross destruction, with

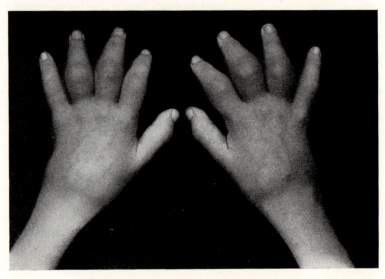

Fig. 34.—Still's disease. Characteristic wasting of the muscles and swelling of the dorsal tendon sheaths and fingers in a child of 3 years.

partial or complete ankylosis of the joint. Pericarditis with subsequent thickening of the pericardium may occur and adhesions within the sac (*see* p. 302) may develop.

CLINICAL PICTURE

A child aged two or more has a feverish illness, the joints becoming swollen and very painful. Fever is not always prominent, however, or may escape notice. Movement is limited by pain at the elbows, wrists, fingers, knees and ankles. The head is moved with difficulty, and chewing may be impeded because of pain or stiffness in the temporo-mandibular joints. The appearance of the various joints is typical: a fusiform swelling about the joint with wasting of the muscles above and below (Fig. 34). Although pain is often a feature at the onset, the joints gradually become less painful. At intervals, there is an acute fever for a day or two, with malaise and a return of pain in the joints; at the same time the glands become again enlarged, and then subside.   The spleen is sometimes palpable.   A fleeting macular rash may appear, particularly during the hours when the temperature is at its height; the macules are variable and a few have pale centres (Fig. 35).   The sedimentation rate is greatly raised in this condition, a rate of fall of 40–60 mm. in the hour being not uncommon.   It is likely to remain high for a long period.   In the early stages rheumatoid

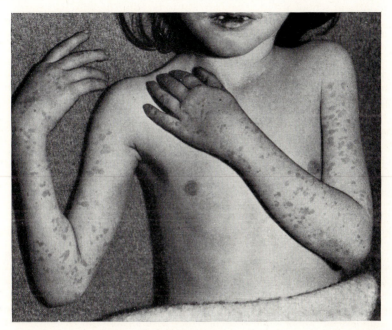

Fig. 35.—Still's disease.   Typical pale pink macular rash and swelling of dorsal tendon sheaths and of fingers.

arthritis can give rise to difficulties in diagnosis, for in some cases fever may be the outstanding feature and joint symptoms minimal or absent.

Rheumatoid arthritis may run a prolonged course.   Often there are remissions and exacerbations.   Gradually, in most cases, it subsides but may leave behind more or less permanent changes in the joints— limitation of movement, and ankylosis in a few cases.

DIFFERENTIAL DIAGNOSIS

The chronic joint involvement excludes acute rheumatism, and this is supported by the fact that carditis does not occur.   Brucellosis, tuberculosis, leukæmia and glandular fever may require exclusion in the early stages.   Biopsy of the affected synovial membrane may help in a doubtful diagnosis.

COMPLICATIONS

Anæmia and loss of weight usually occur. It must also be remembered that a child suffering from this chronic illness, perhaps in hospital for many months at a time, may suffer the effects of separation from the family. Lack of *joie de vivre* and lack of energy are seen in many such children and they become too reliant on others. If months at school are lost, they are apt to be educationally backward.

In severe cases there is often some interference with skeletal growth and the child ends up by being small in stature. Some bones are more affected than others, for example, the mandible.

In a small proportion of cases there are *ophthalmic* changes. Chronic and relapsing iridocyclitis may develop at any stage, even before the arthritis. Synechiæ are apt to bind the iris to the lens. Keratitis can occur. The child may end by being partially blind.

PROGNOSIS

The disease runs a long course, with relapses and remissions. There is complete recovery in some cases; in others there are residual disabilities. There is a small mortality in the acute stage, particularly in the younger age group.

TREATMENT

Until about 1950 rest was the underlying principle of treatment; these patients were kept in bed and the affected joints were immobilized for long periods. This was apt to result in much stiffness and great wasting of the muscles, even subluxation or ankylosis. It has now been shown that active movement, within reason, is beneficial; not only does it prevent fixation of the joints and maintain strength in the muscles, but there is no evidence that a small amount of movement increases the inflammatory changes around the joints. It is wise to institute physiotherapy at an early stage and as soon as the symptoms permit.

But in the acute stages the patient has to be made comfortable in bed; painful joints may need support and local heat; aspirin, codein and similar preparations should be used to relieve local pain. The child should be encouraged to eat. During periods of muscular wasting, protein is important in the diet. Vitamins, iron and calcium are advised.

In the acute stages, steroid treatment relieves the symptoms and makes increased activity possible. It helps physiotherapy and occupational therapy. Cortisone, however, *does not cure rheumatoid arthritis* and prolonged steroid treatment has important dangers; it causes osteoporosis, interferes with growth and makes the child more liable to infections. If steroids are required, it is wise to use the *smallest dose capable of relieving symptoms.* Prednisone or prednisolone are better than cortisone and, as soon as possible, the dose should be tailed-off. During the period of steroid treatment penicillin should be given by mouth.

As soon as the temperature is beginning to subside the patient should start getting up; there is no need to wait for a normal temperature and sedimentation rate. When the general condition allows, the child should start convalescence. The possibility of a relapse should be kept in mind and arrangements should be made for follow-up.

OTHER AUTO-IMMUNE DISORDERS OF THE MESENCHYME

In addition to rheumatoid arthritis, a number of other system disorders of mesenchymal tissue occur, many of which involve predominantly the walls of the small arteries and arterioles. These disorders include systemic lupus erythematosus, periarteritis nodosa, scleroderma (p. 519), dermatomyositis, Henoch-Schönlein purpura (p. 342) and acquired hæmolytic anæmia (p. 338). Other conditions, such as rheumatic fever itself and Bright's disease, have certain comparable features. Present knowledge suggests that in all these disorders, the normal immune tolerance is disturbed. Initiated by numerous factors, including infection, stress, drugs, and presumably many other endogenous causes at present not understood, an abnormal auto-immune reaction builds up within the patient; the abnormal antibody in some cases reacts against the DNA of the patients' own cell nuclei. (Recent observations suggest that the healthy thymus plays a part in regulating normal immune responses.) Certain individuals may well have a genetically-determined predisposition to auto-immune reactions.

Disseminated Lupus Erythematosus[1]

This rare disorder of childhood affects girls far more commonly than boys and almost always progresses to a fatal conclusion over a period of months or a few years.

PATHOLOGY

The characteristic lesion is the degeneration of collagen and the fibrinoid proliferation which involves all mesenchymal tissues and small arteries and arterioles throughout the body. Thus, the secondary effects are far reaching and involve many organs. Death is most often due to the renal damage.

CLINICAL PICTURE

The leading symptom is most commonly an erythematous rash of butterfly distribution on the cheeks and across the bridge of the nose.

[1] Cook, C. D., Wedgwood, R. J. P., Craig, J. M., Hartmann, J. R., Janeway, C. A. (1960). *Pediatrics*, **26**, 570.

Other early symptoms include fever and joint pains.   Later a general-ized rash, which may at times be petechial, develops together with enlargement of the liver and spleen and signs of renal involvement as shown by proteinuria and microscopic hæmaturia.   In fully established cases there may be progressive hypertension, cardiac enlargement or failure, hæmolytic anæmia (from the production of auto-immune antibodies), thrombocytopenia, convulsions (from involvement of the cerebral vasculature) and finally uræmia from the progressive renal involvement.

The finding of the typical cell (LE cell) in the peripheral blood helps to confirm the diagnosis.   Less specific laboratory tests show leu-copenia and reversed albumin-globulin ratio with a high level of gamma globulin (*see also* under plasma cell hepatitis, p. 217).   Other laboratory findings reflect the particular organs involved in the disease, such as the presence of hæmolytic anæmia, thrombocytopenia or renal damage.

TREATMENT

Corticosteroid therapy (for dosage, *see* Appendix 2, p. 660) may help to reduce the overt symptoms and may even slightly prolong life, but does not alter the bad ultimate prognosis.   Chloroquine is of value for the skin lesions (for dosage, *see* p. 664).   In most cases it is the pro-gressive renal damage which determines the downhill course of the disease.   The few cases that follow a more benign course are those in which no renal involvement has occurred.

Periarteritis Nodosa

Periarteritis nodosa in childhood is even more rare than dissemi-nated lupus erythematosus and, in contrast to that disorder, shows no difference in sex incidence.   The prognosis, however, is at least as bad.

PATHOLOGY

Medium-sized or small arteries throughout the body may be involved in a destructive process of nodal necrosis of their vessel wall, with aneurysmal dilatation and/or obliterative thrombosis and peri-arterial fibrinoid proliferation.

CLINICAL PICTURE

Almost any system of the body may thus be involved and indeed the diagnosis may often be suggested by bizarre combinations of symptoms involving different organs.   Fever and variable erythematous or petechial rashes are usually present.   Signs of renal involvement herald a fatal outcome.

The diagnosis is best confirmed by muscle biopsy which, when positive, reveals the characteristic vascular changes.

TREATMENT

Corticosteroids (for dosage, *see* Appendix 2, p. 660), as in disseminated lupus erythematosus, may diminish the clinical severity of the symptoms but probably have little influence on the ultimate prognosis.

Dermatomyositis

In this rare mesenchymal disorder, striated muscle is predominantly involved and other tissues to a lesser extent. Although fatal cases occur, the outlook is somewhat more favourable than that found in disseminated lupus erythematosus and periarteritis nodosa. Girls are slightly more frequently affected than boys.

PATHOLOGY

Except in cases which have progressed to extensive calcification of muscles and subcutaneous tissue (calcinosis universalis), the changes are seen on microscopy. The small arteries show medial thickening with perivascular round-cell infiltration, while the muscle bundles reveal degenerative changes and interstitial fibrosis.

CLINICAL PICTURE

There is usually an insidious onset of muscular weakness, together with pain on movement and muscle tenderness. All degrees of severity may be encountered, and the disease may be generalized or restricted, for example, to the lower limbs. The affected muscle feels indurated and actual swelling may be present.

Skin involvement may be shown by transient erythematous rashes, particularly on the face, and slight œdema may occur. In many cases the fingers have a typical appearance. The overlying skin becomes atrophic, red and shiny and is firmly attached to deeper tissues. Capillary microscopy of the nail beds show hypertrophied capillary loops and arcades. Where skin lesions are marked, the disease has to be distinguished from scleroderma (p. 519).

The diagnosis is confirmed by muscle biopsy of an affected area and in some advanced cases, x-ray reveals calcification in the soft tissues.

TREATMENT

With a disease which runs a prolonged but remittent course, it is not easy to determine the value of corticosteroid therapy. In severe cases, corticosteroids may help to re-establish mobility and thus prevent contractions, but where possible treatment should either be withdrawn completely or reduced to the absolute minimum once a remission has occurred (for dosage, *see* Appendix 2, p. 660), in view of the known dangers of prolonged treatment. Physiotherapy is helpful in severe cases.

The fatal cases occur when the muscles of respiration have become affected; in a proportion of cases the patient is left with severe fixed muscular and skeletal deformities.

CHAPTER 16

Blood Diseases

NORMAL BLOOD PICTURE IN INFANCY

BLOOD is formed during intrauterine life not only in the bone-marrow, but also (extramedullary) in such organs as the liver and spleen, and sometimes the kidneys, along with other portions of the reticulo-endothelial system.

During the latter months of pregnancy sufficient iron is transferred across the placenta to maintain the full-term infant's requirements for hæmoglobin production for the first months of extrauterine life. Studies using labelled iron have shown that this iron is used repeatedly in the formation of red cells, the iron liberated when a red cell is destroyed being utilized again for further red-cell production in preference to fresh iron absorbed from the gastro-intestinal tract. Thus, premature infants in whom this reserve of iron is deficient are at a disadvantage.

In fœtal life a large part of the hæmoglobin produced differs in chemical structural character from adult hæmoglobin. It is more resistant to denaturation by alkalis than adult hæmoglobin and is capable of combining at a given partial pressure with a slightly greater amount of oxygen. At the time of birth more than half the hæmoglobin is found to be of this fœtal type, but the proportion steadily diminishes thereafter. The significance of fœtal hæmoglobin persisting after the age of six months and the production of other abnormal hæmoglobins are discussed in detail in connection with hæmolytic anæmia (pp. 338–340).

NORMAL VALUES

Considerable variations are found in the blood volumes and hæmoglobin levels of normal newborn infants of similar weights. These wide ranges are partly explained by the varying extent to which the blood in the placenta (about 75 ml.) is allowed to enter the infant's circulation before the cord is clamped following delivery. Thus, if the cord is clamped early, a 3·0–4·0 Kg. infant may be deprived of virtually a quarter of the total fœtal circulating blood volume. Even so, the variation in extent of this autotransfusion cannot account entirely for the considerable differences in blood volume, which ranges from 70–120 ml. per Kg. body-weight in the newborn, and a complete explanation is at present not possible.

HÆMOGLOBIN

It is important to realize that samples of blood obtained by skin prick during the first hours after birth have on the average 2·0 G. per cent. more hæmoglobin than blood obtained simultaneously by venipuncture. The reason for this is not understood, but depends to some extent upon the temperature to which the infant is exposed. After the first day the differences between skin prick and venipuncture are less marked, being usually not more than 0·5 G. per cent.

Blood taken from the umbilical cord represents the true circulatory level before the infant's hæmoglobin has risen as a result of the " auto-transfusion " from the placenta which occurs immediately after birth. It has been found by Mollison and Cutbush that 95 per cent. of normal infants have cord hæmoglobin levels between 13·6 and 19·6 G. per cent., with a mean value of 16·6 G. per cent. It is a figure of the utmost importance in assessing the degree to which a particular infant may be affected by hæmolytic disease of the newborn (see p.110).

In the interpretation of hæmoglobin levels taken from the infant in the first day of life, either by skin prick or venipuncture, it must be realized that, as with the blood volume, wide variations exist. Differences in the extent of the autotransfusion from the placenta to the infant prior to the clamping of the cord again provide a partial explanation, but other, as yet unknown factors,[1] must also be involved. Thus, the finding of fœtal blood in the maternal circulation in considerable amounts, associated with severe anæmia in the newborn infant, has demonstrated the rare occurrence of a hæmorrhage from the fœtal circulation across the placenta into the maternal bloodstream.

The level of hæmoglobin at differing ages in childhood is shown on page 326. It seems probable that the low level reached at the age of three months starts to rise as soon as mixed feeding is begun. There is little difference in the hæmoglobin levels of artificially-fed and breast-fed infants under present-day conditions in Western Europe and North America. From the age of puberty onwards, girls have slightly lower levels than boys.

The premature infant usually shows a considerably greater fall in hæmoglobin between birth and three months than the full-term infant, the level at three months often being as low as 7·0 G. per cent.

RED BLOOD CELLS

Greater inaccuracies exist in the recordings of the red-cell count than in the determination of hæmoglobin by an accurate photoelectric

[1] O'Connor, W. J., Shields, G., Kohl, S., Sussman, M. (1957). *Amer. J. Obstet. Gynec.*, **73**, 768.

colorimeter. The changes in the red-cell count in infancy and childhood are similar to those found in the hæmoglobin level, and are summarized in Table XVIII.

NUCLEATED RED CELLS

Reticulocytes. Normal infants are found to have an average of 3·0 per cent. reticulocytes in umbilical cord blood. By the end of the first week the reticulocyte count is usually less than 1 per cent.

TABLE XVIII

CHANGES OF HÆMOGLOBIN LEVEL AND RED-CELL COUNT IN INFANCY

Age	Hæmoglobin (G.%)		Red-cell Count (in millions per c.mm.)
	Mean	Range	
Umbilical cord blood	16·6 (Mollison and Cutbush)[1]	13·6–19·6 (95 percentile) (Mollison and Cutbush)[1]	4·5–5·0
First day of life—venous	18·5 (Mollison and Cutbush)[1]	14·5–22·5 (Mollison and Cutbush)[1]	4·5–6·5
First day of life—skin prick ..	—	15·4–22·8 (Mollison and Cutbush)[1]	5·0–7·0
Fourteenth day—venous	17·5 (skin prick samples likely to be 0·59% higher) (Vahlquist)[1]	13·1–21·9 (Vahlquist)[1]	3·8–5·6 (Wintrobe)[4]
One to three months—skin prick ..	10·5 (Mackay)[2]	9–12	3·8–5·2 (Wintrobe)[4]
One year	11·5 (M.R.C. Special Report No. 252)[3]	10–13 (M.R.C. Special Report No. 252)[3]	4·0–5·0
Twelve years	13·8 girls 14·0 boys (M.R.C. Special Report No. 252)[3]	12·7–15·3 (M.R.C. Special Report No. 252)[3]	4·2–5·4

[1] Quoted in " Blood Transfusion in Clinical Medicine " by Mollison, P. L. (1961). Oxford: Blackwell Scientific Publications.
[2] Mackay, H. M. M. (1933). *Arch. Dis. Childh.*, **8**, 145.
[3] Medical Research Council Report No. 252 (1945). London: H.M. Stationery Office.
[4] Wintrobe, M. M. (1961). " Clinical Hæmatology." London: Henry Kimpton.

Normoblasts. A small number of normoblasts is usually found in the peripheral blood of normal newborn infants; these disappear by the end of the second day of life. Mollison[1] suggests that the presence of more than 10 nucleated red cells per 100 white cells in a full-term infant is usually pathological. Premature infants tend to have more circulating normoblasts at birth than full-term infants.

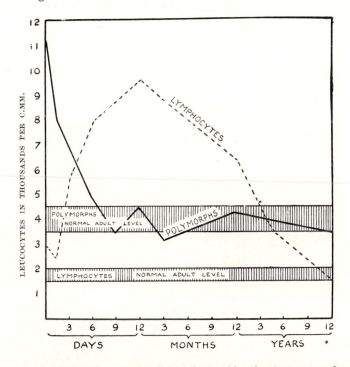

Fig 36.—**Absolute numbers of polymorphonuclears and lymphocytes per c.mm. from birth to 12 years of age.**
Reproduced from " Disorders of the Blood," 8th Ed. by L. E. H. Whitby and C. J. C. Britton.
London: Churchill.

Leucocytes (see Fig. 36). During the first 12 days of life, the total leucocyte count is approximately 18 thousand, but from this time on there is a steady fall, so that by the twelfth year the total leucocyte count is similar to that of an adult, i.e. 6 thousand per c.mm. However, the ratio of polymorphonuclear and lymphocyte cells, which at birth is that of the adult, rapidly reverses itself by the twelfth day. It is not until the sixth to ninth year that the higher polymorphonuclear and lower lymphocyte ratio of the adult is established.

[1] Mollison, P. L. (1961). " Blood Transfusion in Clinical Medicine." Oxford: Blackwell Scientific Publications.

Bone-marrow. At birth, all the bone-marrow including that of the long bones is of the red hæmopoietic type, and it is packed with nucleated erythroid and myeloid cells. By the tenth day the number of nucleated cells has markedly declined, rising again from the first to the third month, with a considerable increase in the number of lymphoid cells. During childhood the long bones begin to assume the adult type of yellow (fatty) marrow, and this is complete by the twentieth year. Red marrow remains in the adult only in the vertebræ and thorax girdle. In the young infant the bone-marrow is active at all times. If there is a fresh call for extra hæmopoiesis, extramedullary centres must partly answer it. Centres such as the liver, spleen and kidneys must consequently resume their hæmopoietic activity, and as a result many primitive cells are thrown out.

ANÆMIA

CLINICAL PICTURE AND DIAGNOSIS

THIS is sometimes difficult, as differentiation must be made between pallor of the skin and anæmia. Children with auburn hair or very fair children, often give a false impression; therefore examination of the palms of the hands is of particular help, as is that of the gums and conjunctivæ. The student should examine the sclerotics for jaundice and feel the abdomen carefully for enlargement of the liver or spleen. A hæmic murmur is usually present over the heart, especially in the basal region, if the anæmia is at all marked. Early symptoms include listlessness and undue tiredness. Anorexia, nausea and actual vomiting are frequently present. In more severe cases shortness of breath on exercise or evidence of heart failure may develop.

Classification of Anæmia of Childhood

1. DEFECTIVE BLOOD PRODUCTION

A. *Lack of Hæmopoietic Factors*

(i) Iron—Maternal iron deficiency during pregnancy. Prematurity. Dietary deficiencies. Malabsorption (cœliac disease, etc.).

(ii) Defective protein synthesis—Hypoproteinæmia and shortened protein life span.

(iii) Hæmopoietic factor—Cœliac disease (defective absorption). Zuelzer-Ogden anæmia (folic-acid deficiency, megaloblastic anæmia). Cirrhosis of liver (defective synthesis).

(iv) Vitamin c—Scurvy.

(v) Thyroxin—Cretinism.

(vi) Chronic renal disease.

B. Lack of Hæmopoietic Tissue

Primary

   (i) Primary aplasia of bone-marrow.

   (ii) Primary hypoplasia of bone-marrow.

   (iii) Fanconi's anæmia (familial).

Secondary

   (i) Infiltration of bone-marrow by neoplastic tissue (leuco-erythroblastic anæmia):

      (*a*) Leukæmia.
      (*b*) Secondary neoplastic deposits; e.g. neuroblastoma.

   (ii) Poisoning of bone-marrow:

      (*a*) Exogenous—Chemical (sulphonamides, benzol, etc.); physical (radiation).
      (*b*) Endogenous—Infections (pyogenic infections, syphilis, tuberculosis).

2. EXCESSIVE BLOOD LOSS

A. Hæmorrhage

   (i) Without blood disease:

      (*a*) Acute hæmorrhage from wounds.
      (*b*) Chronic hæmorrhage (hæmorrhoids, œsophageal varices, etc.).

   (ii) With bleeding disease:

      Hæmorrhagic disease of the newborn. Hæmophilia and related disorders of blood coagulation. Thrombocytopenic purpura. Other purpuras. Scurvy. Leukæmia.

B. Hæmolysis

   (i) Circulating incompatible agglutinins—Hæmolytic disease of the newborn (Rhesus incompatibility and A/B/O incompatibility). Acquired auto-immune hæmolytic anæmia.

   (ii) Acute infections (streptococcal, " Lederer's anæmia ").

   (iii) Poisons (lead, etc.).

   (iv) Congenital abnormality of erythrocytes (acholuric familial jaundice).

   (v) Abnormal hæmoglobin formation—Sickle-cell anæmia, Cooley's anæmia, thallasæmia minor, other abnormal hæmoglobins.

   (vi) Glucose-6-phosphate-dehydrogenase deficiency — Primaquine sensitivity. Favism.

DEFECTIVE BLOOD PRODUCTION

LACK OF HÆMOPOIETIC FACTORS

Nutritional Anæmia (Hypochromic Anæmia of Infancy)

THIS remains the commonest anæmia of infancy.

ÆTIOLOGY

Hypochromic anæmia does not usually develop until the fourth or fifth month of infancy or even later.   It is due to a diet deficient in minerals, particularly iron, and occasionally copper.   Infants who are fed exclusively on milk (either breast or artificially fed) develop this anæmia.   It may be seen at a rather earlier age in premature infants and twins who have been born before a proper store of iron has been given to them by their mother.

It is often seen in mental defectives who have refused solid food and who have been fed on milk only.   In underdeveloped countries iron deficiency anæmia is a measure of the poor nutritional state of the child population.   It is often associated with protein malnutrition.

In Western Europe and the United States the finding of iron-deficiency anæmia in an older child usually suggests an underlying illness such as a malabsorption state.   It may have to be differentiated from the anæmia of chronic hæmorrhage due to such conditions as œsophageal ulceration associated with a hiatus hernia, or the anæmia resulting from a chronic illness.

Poverty and poor diet still provide the explanation in a proportion of the children.

CLINICAL PICTURE

Infants with a pure iron-deficiency anæmia, although extremely pale, are often plump and well-grown.   If the condition has continued for any length of time the spleen is palpable, and there is a loud hæmic murmur over the heart.   This may be so marked that heart disease may be suspected.

From the work of Mackay[1] it appears that the average infant, whether breast or bottle fed, tends to develop some degree of nutritional anæmia unless mixed feeding is introduced at least before the age of six months or unless the milk feed is supplemented by iron. The present trend in Western Europe and the United States towards the early introduction of mixed feeding makes it unnecessary to add iron to the diet of the full-term infant, although this is still essential for premature infants.

BLOOD EXAMINATION

The red count is normal, or only slightly reduced; it is the hæmoglobin which is grossly depleted.   The cells are therefore pale, and

[1] Mackay, Helen M. M. (1933).   " Nutritional Anæmia in Infancy, With Special Reference to Iron Deficiency."   Medical Research Council Report.   London: H.M. Stationery Office.

contain very little hæmoglobin. The colour index varies between 0·7 and 0·3, the hæmoglobin being reduced to 50 to 20 per cent., with a corresponding reduction in the mean corpuscular hæmoglobin concentration (*see* end tables). Stained films show the cells to be hypochromic and microcytic. Poikilocytosis is usually present.

TREATMENT

Mixed feeding, with cereals, egg, green vegetables, particularly spinach, and broth, should be instituted at the earliest possible moment.
Iron may be given to infants in the following forms:

Mist. Ferr. Sulph. pro Inf. (B.N.F. 1960)

> ℞ Ferrous sulphate, 60 mg. (1 grain)
> Dilute hypophosphorous acid, 0·1 ml. (1½ minims)
> Dextrose monohydrate, 600 mg. (10 grains)
> Orange syrup, 0·6 ml. (10 minims)
> Water, to 4 ml. (60 minims)
> To be taken well diluted with water thrice daily

or:

Mist. Ferr. et Ammon. Cit pro Inf. (B.N.F. 1960)

> ℞ Iron and ammonium citrate, 0·4 G. (6 grains)
> Compound spirit of orange, 0·008 ml. (⅛ minim)
> Syrup, 0·6 ml. (10 minims)
> Chloroform water, to 4 ml. (60 minims)
> To be given thrice daily

Ferrous sulphate may be given to older children in tablet form: Tab. Ferri Sulphatis Co., B.N.F. 1960, contain exsiccated ferrous sulphate, copper sulphate, and manganese sulphate (for dosage at different ages, *see* p. 665).
Occasionally ferrous sulphate causes gastro-intestinal disturbances and in such cases organic compounds of iron may be used. These include ferrous gluconate, ferrous succinate and ferrous fumarate. A recent controlled trial[1] with ferrous sulphate and ferrous fumarate showed little to choose between the equally effective clinical responses obtained. Ferrous sulphate is, of course, considerably cheaper.
The place of intramuscular iron in treatment is at present *sub judice* because of the possible occurrence of neoplasms at the site of the injections in test animals.
Poisoning by iron (usually in the form of coloured tablets attractive to a young child) is not rare (*see* p. 644). Parents should be warned of this danger and adversed always to lock up ferrous sulphate and similar iron-containing tablets.
It has been shown that traces of certain metals, including cobalt, copper and manganese, are essential for normal hæmopoiesis. Copper sulphate is contained in Tab. Ferri Sulphatis Co. mentioned above.

[1] Gunn, C., Islip, M. C., Masters, P. L., Erskine-Murrary, H., Rigg, C. A., Stapleton, T. (1960). *Arch. Dis. Childh.*, **35**, 281.

Hypoproteinæmia and Microcytic Anæmia of Infancy

Recently a syndrome of severe iron-deficiency anæmia with œdema has been described in infants. These infants are found to have greatly reduced serum-protein concentrations and to be deficient also in serum iron and serum copper.

The basis of this syndrome appears to be both defective protein synthesis and also a shortened protein life span, despite a normal protein intake. It has also been suggested that there is loss of protein into the intestinal tract (*transient protein enteropathy*). Nevertheless, the condition responds rapidly to treatment with oral iron.

This syndrome is to be distinguished from kwashiorkor (p. 600), in which there is a gross deficiency of first-class protein in the diet.

Anæmia of Cœliac Disease

A minority of cases of cœliac disease shows a megalocytic hyperchromic type, with a palpable spleen. The bone-marrow is then found to be megaloblastic in character. Such patients respond rapidly to treatment with folic acid, which may be administered in doses of 5 mg. three times a day. In the majority of cases, however, the anæmia is of the iron-deficiency type. Such cases do extremely well on large doses of iron, once the gluten-free diet is established (p. 682).

Zuelzer-Ogden Anæmia

Very rarely a megaloblastic anæmia occurs in infancy. This is usually found either in infants who have developed gastro-intestinal disturbances, with a consequent failure to absorb folic acid, or in infants whose diet has been deficient, particularly as regards vitamin c. Treatment is with folic acid.

The Anæmias of Cretinism and Scurvy

These are orthochromic in type, with a comparable fall in the hæmoglobin and red-cell count, leaving the colour index at approximately 1·0. The missing factor in cretinism is thyroxine, and in scurvy it is vitamin c.

LACK OF HÆMOPOIETIC TISSUE

Primary Aplastic Anæmia

THIS type of anæmia is very rare in childhood. Without warning one or more of the bone-marrow functions (erythroid, myeloid or platelet formation) may fail. Soon pancytopenia is present. Thus the disease may commence with rapidly increasing anæmia, necrotic ulceration in the mouth due to agranulocytosis, or hæmorrhages and purpura from thrombocytopenia. Soon all the components are combined and the disease progresses rapidly to a fatal outcome.

The diagnosis is established by bone-marrow biopsy, when the marrow is found to be acellular and to contain chiefly reticulum cells. Whilst a number of causes for this disease are listed under secondary aplastic anæmia (*see* below), the origin of the primary type is unknown.

Whilst intensive treatment with full doses of steroids (p. 660), antibiotics to combat the secondary infection, and a transfusion of fresh blood should be given, the clinical state is only temporarily improved in most cases. It is possible, if the problem of immune reaction can be overcome, that transfusions of donor bone-marrow may offer hope in the future.

Congenital Hypoplastic Anæmia (Erythrogenesis Imperfecta)[1, 2]

This condition is also of rare occurrence. It differs from the aplastic type in that the depression of the bone-marrow is confined to the erythroid series, without disturbance of leucocyte or platelet formation. The anæmia is of the normocytic, normochromic type. It appears to be congenital in origin. A fault in normoblastic maturation has been suggested.

Hæmatinics and splenectomy are of no value in treatment, but patients have been kept alive for many years by repeated blood transfusions. However, such treatment leads to massive deposition of iron in vital organs, notably the myocardium, with eventual heart failure. Prolonged steroid therapy (Appendix 2) has been effective in a number of patients. In a few cases spontaneous recovery has occurred.

Fanconi's Anæmia

Fanconi[3] has described a congenital hypoplastic anæmia associated with other congenital defects, such as microcephaly, mental backwardness, pigmentation of the skin, squint, and abnormality of digits (Fig. 37). The condition is familial, probably of a recessive type. Repeated transfusions are the basic treatment, although splenectomy has improved the condition of a proportion of patients.

Secondary Aplastic Anæmia

This may be brought about by benzol, arsenic, radiation, and rarely sulphonamides, and may occur after severe infections, such as miliary tuberculosis, typhoid fever or diphtheria. The blood and bone-marrow picture resembles the primary aplastic type and the treatment is similar.

Leuco-erythroblastic Anæmia

When infiltration of normal bone-marrow by neoplastic deposits occurs, there is a considerable disturbance of normal marrow function,

[1] Ulstrom, R. A., Smith, N. J., Heimlich, E. M. (1956). *Amer. J. Dis. Child.*, **92**, 219.
[2] Cathie, I. A. B. (1950). *Arch. Dis. Childh.*, **25**, 124.
[3] Fanconi, G. (1927). *Z. Kinderheilk*, **117**, 257.

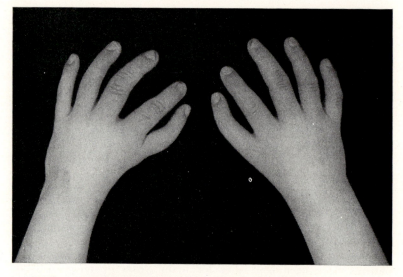

Fig. 37.—A congenital malformation of the hands seen in a boy with congenital hypoplastic anæmia of the Fanconi type. The commonest congenital abnormalities in this
condition are squint, smallness of the head, changes in the deep reflexes, pigmentation
and abnormalities in the development of the thumbs. In this case the thenar muscles
were imperfectly developed and the thumbs look like fingers.

with the appearance in the circulation of nucleated red cells and primitive white cells. The bone-marrow is hyperplastic in type. As
neoplastic infiltration extends, the anæmia becomes progressively more
severe. This type of anæmia may be seen with any neoplastic invasion
of bone-marrow, especially neuroblastoma (p. 378), and also in
leukæmia (p. 347).

Anæmia of Infection

Many chronic infections cause a general retardation in normal
hæmopoiesis. The anæmia is normocytic and normochromic in type,
and will often not respond to iron until the infection has been controlled.

THE ANÆMIA OF HÆMORRHAGE

THE blood changes produced by hæmorrhage depend upon the
severity and rate of the bleeding. An acute hæmorrhage from a
wound thus provides a picture different from that following repeated
small blood losses from hæmorrhoids or œsophageal ulceration or
varices.

In the former, the immediate findings may be of a normal hæmoglobin and red-cell count, because of the hæmoconcentration that

occurs; later, as hæmodilution ensues, a normocytic, normochromic anæmia is found. The bone-marrow responds rapidly to blood loss with an outpouring of cells, including many reticulocytes and even normoblasts, into the peripheral blood. If the anæmia is severe and the time of recovery prolonged, the newer cells formed in the marrow tend to be iron-deficient and hypochromic; thus, as recovery from hæmorrhage proceeds, a stage may be reached at which the red-cell count continues to increase but the hæmoglobin level remains stationary. This tendency to produce hypochromic cells can easily be overcome by the administration of iron.

In cases in which repeated small hæmorrhages are taking place, marked iron deficiency will become apparent sooner or later. A severe reduction in hæmoglobin (3–6 G. per 100 ml. of blood) may be associated with a red-cell count of 3,000,000 to 4,000,000 per c.mm. It is likely that the reticulocyte response of the marrow to small repeated hæmorrhages will be less marked than that seen following a single large hæmorrhage, and the reticulocyte count rarely rises above 5 per cent. Iron therapy will help to correct the hypochromic tendency, but the primary treatment is to control the source of the hæmorrhage.

Blood Transfusion

The usual requirements of compatibility of donor blood and the use of Rhesus negative blood for Rhesus negative female children are necessary, as in adult medicine. In cases of acute hæmorrhage severe enough to require a blood transfusion, account should be taken, whenever an accurate estimate is possible, of the volume of blood lost so that a comparable amount of donor blood may be replaced. Often, however, estimates of blood loss are highly inaccurate and unreliable or, as in cases of internal hæmorrhage, impracticable. In such cases the clinical condition of the patient, including particularly the degree of shock, fall in blood pressure and state of the pulse, must determine the volume of blood to be transfused. In infants and small children, there is a risk of overtransfusion which should be avoided if it is remembered that the normal total blood volume in infancy is approximately 85 ml. per Kg. body-weight. In patients with acute hæmorrhage whole blood is used for transfusion.

The total blood volume is also a basic consideration in deciding the volume of donor blood to be used in severe cases of chronic anæmia, whether caused by hæmorrhage or other conditions. Given the reduction in hæmoglobin and the total blood volume of the patient, a calculation can be made of the volume of blood necessary to restore the hæmoglobin to normal levels. In such cases, packed red cells rather than whole blood are usually given, and a calculated reduction is then made in the volume to be transfused to offset the amount of donor plasma removed (bearing in mind that in Britain 180 ml. of sodium citrate are included in each 540-ml. bottle of donor blood). In chronic anæmia, transfusions should always be given slowly—in general terms the rate should not exceed 30 ml. per hour. When dealing with small infants, it is of the first importance that an exact check be kept on the amount of blood transfused.

The insertion of a needle into a scalp vein is an elegant technique in small infants, whilst in older children the usual peripheral veins are utilized, either by percutaneous insertion of a needle when practicable or by the exposure of the vein and the introduction of a fine polyvinyl catheter.

HÆMOLYTIC ANÆMIA

ALTHOUGH intravascular destruction of red cells can arise from many causes, and some clinical variations exist which differentiate the various types, the basic features common to all hæmolytic anæmias can be summarized as follows:

1. The destruction of the red cells in the circulating blood, with some damage to the bone-marrow.
2. An increased level of indirect serum bilirubin, with or without clinical jaundice.
3. Urobilinogen in the urine in excess.
4. Anæmia of orthochromic type.
5. A marked reticulocytosis.
6. Splenomegaly.

Hæmolytic Disease of the Newborn (Icterus Gravis Neonatorum) (*see* p. 110)

Hæmolytic Anæmia caused by Infection

A hæmolytic anæmia may be caused by the streptococcus and staphylococcus. Such an event, however, is exceptional as the anæmia which accompanies infection is usually due to a general depression of hæmopoiesis. *Cl. welchii* (gas gangrene) may occasionally cause a severe hæmolytic anæmia.

In malaria, so severe a hæmolysis may occur that gross hæmoglobinuria is produced (blackwater fever). It seems probable that some cases may not be the direct result of infection but may be drug-induced, due to the individual being deficient of glucose-6-phosphate dehydrogenase (p. 136).

Acute Hæmolytic Anæmia : Type Lederer

This is a very rare condition which is usually seen between the age of 6 months and 3 years. The onset is sudden, and there is fever, jaundice, and sometimes blood in the urine. The blood shows a leucocytosis, with some myelocytes. There is a marked reduction of the red cells to one or two million. The cause of this condition is unknown; it appears probable that some cases may be due to G-6-P-D deficiency (p. 136).

A fresh blood transfusion is curative and recurrences of the anæmia are unusual.

Lead Poisoning (*see* p. 414)

Acholuric Family Jaundice (Congenital Spherocytosis)

This is a chronic disease characterized by crises of excessive blood destruction, sometimes associated with transient bone-marrow arrest, a constant high percentage of circulating reticulocytes, splenomegaly, spherocytosis, fragility of the red cells, a variable amount of jaundice, and an excess of urobilin but no bilirubin in the urine.

It is inherited as a dominant characteristic although the gene does not show complete penetrance. Family trees extending through four generations have been traced.

ÆTIOLOGY AND BLOOD CHANGES

The cause is unknown, but it is supposed that there is a congenital defect in the make-up of the erythron, probably related to carbohydrate metabolism. The red-cell envelopes are unduly fragile, and the cells themselves are spheroidal instead of the normal biconcave shape. Comparative tests of the fragility of the red cells as against normal corpuscles show destruction of the patient's red cells in concentrations of saline of the order of 0·6 per cent., whilst the normal red cells are not destroyed until more dilute solutions of saline (0·3–0·4 per cent.) are used. Unconjugated bilirubin is increased in the serum, and there is an excess of urobilin in the urine.

The reticulocytosis may be as high as 20 to 50 per cent. After splenectomy there is usually a clinical but not a biological cure.

PATHOLOGY

The spleen is much enlarged. The liver, spleen, kidneys and bone-marrow contain an excess of iron, and they give a strong Prussian blue reaction. Gall-stones are not uncommon; when they do occur, they complicate the clinical picture by exaggerating the jaundice, causing an associated rise in conjugated bilirubin.

SYMPTOMS

At extremely variable intervals crises occur in which the child (who may be of any age from infancy up) becomes anæmic and mildly jaundiced. The child is often feverish and ill, and there may be vomiting. Simultaneously with these episodes of acute hæmolysis, the bone-marrow may become temporarily aplastic. A crisis usually lasts for two to three weeks.

TREATMENT

Splenectomy is the treatment of this condition and operation should not be long postponed in cases showing much anæmia or if crises have occurred.

Idiopathic Acquired Hæmolytic Anæmia

Rare cases of hæmolytic anæmia, with a clinical picture comparable to acholuric familial jaundice, are seen in which there is no familial history and in which the characteristic hæmatological changes of spherocytosis and increased red-cell fragility are absent.

Hæmolysins may be found in the blood in some, and the Coombs' test may be positive. The spleen is enlarged. Such cases may be subacute or chronic but acute exacerbations occur and may cause jaundice. ACTH and cortisone are dramatically effective. Splenectomy is sometimes curative.

ABNORMAL HÆMOGLOBIN FORMATION

RECENT discoveries have helped to clarify our knowledge of a large number of diseases in which hæmolytic anæmia is the outstanding feature. It is now known that genetic differences linked with racial hereditary patterns are associated with the formation of abnormal types of hæmoglobin.[1] These different hæmoglobins, of which at least ten have already been identified, vary slightly from each other in the quality of their protein content and can be identified by means of electrophoresis. The presence of any one of these abnormal hæmoglobins may give rise to hæmolytic anæmia.

Normal adult hæmoglobin is designated A, fœtal hæmoglobin F, and the hæmoglobin in sickle-cell disease S. Other abnormal hæmoglobins which have assumed widespread clinical importance are types C, D and E. The other varieties so far described are less commonly found.

Racially, hæmoglobin S is found in a proportion of East and West African negroes; it is found in every country to which such negroes have been brought. It is also found in some of the descendants of the old populations of Arabia and India. As well as being of medical interest, it is thus a valuable indicator in ethnology. Hæmoglobin C is also carried by a high proportion of West African negroes and it is not surprising that negroes in this area are sometimes found with both S and C hæmoglobin in their blood. Like hæmoglobin S it has followed the exodus of West Africans to other countries, being found in the negro population of North America, South Africa and North Africa. Hæmoglobin D is found in India but in only a small percentage of the population, whilst hæmoglobin E is found farther east in countries of South-East Asia, such as Burma, Malaya and Indonesia.

[1] Jonxis, J. H. P., Delafresnaye, J. F. (1959). " Abnormal Hæmoglobins." Oxford: Blackwell Scientific Publications.

In all types of hæmolytic anæmia due to these abnormal formations of hæmoglobin, fœtal hæmoglobin is usually also present in varying proportions in the blood.

There remains one very important inherited hæmoglobinopathy, *thalassæmia*, which can occur in both a major form, Cooley's anæmia (when the individual is homozygous for the condition), or as *thalassæmia minor* (when the individual is heterozygous). In thalassæmia, the formation of adult hæmoglobin is partly suppressed and some fœtal hæmoglobin and an excess of hæmoglobin A_2 are present. Racially the disease is found in the populations around the Mediterranean Sea, and, as might be expected, individuals who carry the double traits of both thalassæmia and also of hæmoglobin S or C have been identified.

Sickle-cell Anæmia

Until the electrophoretic identification of the individual abnormal hæmoglobins was available, the clinical picture of sickle-cell anæmia was confused by the inclusion within the syndrome of diseases due to other hæmoglobinopathies.

Now the characteristics of pure sickle-cell anæmia due to the genetic inheritance of hæmoglobin S, in its homozygous and heterozygous forms, is well recognized. If the individual inherits hæmoglobin S from both parents and is thus homozygous for the characteristic, the anæmia starts in infancy with splenomegaly and, apart from the usual manifestations of hæmolytic anæmia, gives rise to recurrent swelling of the hands and feet due to associated bone involvement with characteristic radiological changes.[1] It appears that, if the patient survives childhood, the disease may become less severe, although during the early years mortality is high.

If the individual inherits hæmoglobin S from only one parent, then although the sickle-cell trait can be demonstrated electrophoretically, there are few or no clinical symptoms of disease.

An important observation led to the hypothesis that hæmoglobin S cannot be utilized by the malarial parasite to maintain the intracorpuscular phase of its life cycle. Thus, individuals whose blood contains hæmoglobin S are less liable to suffer from malaria. This may be one reason for the persistence of an inherited disease which might otherwise have been expected to become extinct.

The presence of hæmoglobin C, like hæmoglobin S, produces no clinical symptoms if the individual is only heterozygous for the disease; when present in the homozygous form or when found, as in West Africa, in combination with hæmoglobin S (hæmoglobin CS disease), a severe hæmolytic anæmia is manifest. In each of these clinical forms, as in pure sickle-cell anæmia, fœtal hæmoglobin is also found to be present.

[1] Trowell, H. C., Raper, A. B., Welbourn, H. F. (1957). *Quart. J. Med.*, **26**, 401.

Thalassæmia

As with hæmoglobin S, the inheritance of the thalassæmia trait is seen in both the homozygous (*thalassæmia major* or Cooley's anæmia) or heterozygous (*thalassæmia minor*) form. Its geographical distribution is described above.

The disease, *thalassæmia major*, starts in early childhood as a severe hæmolytic anæmia progressing to a fatal outcome. Up to 90 per cent. of the hæmoglobin is of the fœtal type and target cells are plentiful in the blood smear. X-rays of the skull and long bones show a characteristic trabeculation. Treatment is symptomatic, with repeated transfusions which only delay the inevitable outcome. The prevention of the disease is a problem in eugenics since it is now possible to detect the individuals who carry the trait (heterozygotes). Such individuals may have no clinical symptoms themselves or only a mild degree of hæmolytic anæmia (*thalassæmia minor*), but the offspring of two such individuals have a 1 in 4 chance of developing the major form of the disease. By examination of the hæmoglobin of all individuals prior to marriage in the geographical area affected, the risk of transmitting this fatal disease can at least be made clear to them.

Glucose-6-phosphate-dehydrogenase Deficiency, Primaquine Sensitivity, Favism (*see* pp. 136-137)

THE PURPURAS

THE term purpura refers to a purple eruption in the skin which can be shown to be of *hæmorrhagic origin*, as it does not fade when pressure is applied to the skin.

Although purpuric rashes occur in a large number of different diseases, there is a well-defined group generally known as *the purpuras*. This group may be divided into those in which there is a reduction in the number of circulating blood platelets, and those in which the platelet count is normal and the hæmorrhagic tendency can be ascribed to an increased permeability of the capillary wall. In the following classification, only the more common causes of purpura are mentioned:

A. Purpuras showing Quantitative Deficiency of Platelets.

1. Primary thrombocytopenic purpura (Werlhof's disease).
2. Secondary thrombocytopenic purpuras:
   (*a*) Aplastic anæmia (p. 332).
   (*b*) Neoplastic infiltration of bone-marrow (leukæmia, p. 347; neuroblastoma, p. 378; lymphosarcoma).
   (*c*) Poisoning of bone-marrow (p. 333) (benzol, x-rays, radium, etc.).

B. Purpuras with no Quantitative Deficiency of Platelets.

1. Anaphylactoid purpura (Henoch-Schönlein disease).
2. Secondary purpuras:
    (*a*) Acute fevers (platelets may be diminished in the early stages—pertussis, typhoid, measles).
    (*b*) Septicæmia (meningococcal meningitis, subacute bacterial endocarditis).
    (*c*) Toxic (snake venom, drugs such as Sedormid).
    (*d*) Mechanical (convulsions, asphyxia, violence).

C. Other Diseases in which Purpura may occur.

    (*a*) Scurvy (p. 117).
    (*b*) Vitamin-K deficiency (p. 109).
    (*c*) Hæmophilia and related disorders (p. 344).
    (*d*) Congenital afibrinogenæmia (p. 346).
    (*e*) Von Willebrand's syndrome (p. 346).

Primary Thrombocytopenic Purpura (Werlhof's Disease)

The disease is characterized by multiple hæmorrhages into the skin or from the mucous membranes, associated with a reduced platelet count, a prolonged bleeding time, a normal coagulation time, and a lack of proper clot retraction. It is most common in children and young adults.

ÆTIOLOGY AND PATHOLOGY

The reduction of the platelets is probably the basic factor. This may be due to a defective production of platelets by the bone-marrow, or an excessive destruction by the spleen. Another explanation is that the platelets are themselves defective.

CLINICAL PICTURE

Usually the disease is chronic, and there are frequent mild attacks of bleeding. In the acute form, purpuric patches appear over the surface of the body and the mucous membranes. Bleeding takes place from the nose, alimentary tract or urogenital tract (hæmaturia). The child bruises easily from slight knocks. The spleen is palpable in a proportion of cases. The capillary resistance test is positive. The platelets may be reduced below 40,000 per c.mm., which is the usual critical level at which purpura and hæmorrhage take place, but during remissions may approach a normal figure. The bleeding time is much prolonged. The clotting time is normal, but the clot is soft and poorly formed.

A proportion of patients appears to have only one episode of purpura and thrombocytopenia without later relapse, such cases being commonly associated with the acute specific fevers. Other patients have repeated episodes of hæmorrhage, with recurrent or persistent thrombocytopenia. The hæmorrhage may be so severe as to endanger life from blood loss or from damage to a vital structure such as the brain.

TREATMENT

A mild case, such as one associated with an acute specific fever, may require no special treatment. In a more severe case, treatment with steroids (Appendix 2) will stimulate a remission which is often permanent. Steroids are usually given for two to three weeks in gradually diminishing dosage. For any severe hæmorrhage, a blood transfusion should be given.

Where a second attack of purpura occurs, splenectomy is usually ndicated. This operation should not be carried out during an acute phase of the illness, but a remission should be first brought about by means of steroid therapy together with a blood transfusion if necessary.

After the operation the platelet count rises transiently, but although it may later fall to subnormal levels the clinical symptoms do not usually recur.

DIFFERENTIAL DIAGNOSIS

Henoch-Schönlein purpura may be excluded by the fact that pain in the abdomen and joints is not a feature; the reduced platelet count and the prolonged bleeding time are also not present. Aplastic anæmia may be excluded by the fact that in that disease all the blood elements are diminished, and there is no sign of regeneration, as shown by reticulocytosis. Bone-marrow examination confirms the diagnosis.

In hæmophilia the platelet count, capillary resistance test, and bleeding time are normal, but the coagulation time is prolonged.

Acute leukæmia, especially when there is an accompanying leuco-penia, may initially resemble thrombocytopenic purpura. The course of the disease and further blood counts will distinguish the two conditions. Bone-marrow examination is decisive.

Secondary Thrombocytopenia

Purpura as a result of aplastic anæmia has already been mentioned; rarely, bone-marrow poisoning by radiation or benzol has also been recorded. In addition to acute leukæmia, neoplasms such as neuro-blastoma and lymphosarcoma, which may invade the bone-marrow extensively, can give rise to thrombocytopenia and purpura. Gaucher's disease may act in the same manner.

PURPURA WITH NO QUANTITATIVE REDUCTION OF PLATELETS

Henoch-Schönlein Syndrome (Anaphylactoid Purpura)

THIS type of purpura, which may be associated with a variety of symptoms, such as urticaria, joint pains and swelling, abdominal pain and occasionally œdema, is of uncertain origin.

It is usually considered to be an auto-immune response, sometimes precipitated by a *Strept. pyogenes* infection. Histologically there is an acute inflammatory type of reaction in the corium of the skin, sometimes accompanied by an eosinophilic exudation.

In contradistinction to thrombocytopenic purpura there are no characteristic blood changes. The platelet count, bleeding and clotting time are normal, though there may be leucocytosis.

Relapses are common in this type of purpura, but the general prognosis is excellent except in cases complicated by nephritis.

SYMPTOMS

In some cases, there is a preliminary history of a sore throat two weeks before the start of the principal illness. The main symptoms

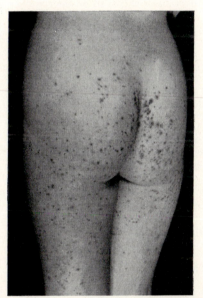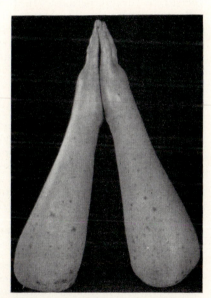

Fig. 38.—*Left:* **Typical skin lesions, maximal in the buttocks, in Henoch-Schönlein purpura.**
Right: **Upper limbs of same patient; note swelling in region of the dorsum of the hands in addition to the purpuric rash.**

may begin with abdominal pain or with painful swelling of the joints. If no purpura is present at this stage, the true diagnosis may be overlooked, appendicitis being suspected in the abdominal (*Henoch*) type and rheumatic fever in the joint-pain (*Schönlein*) variety. Sooner or later the purpuric rash appears, being frequently most extensive on the buttocks. In addition to the purpuric component, the rash may sometimes have papular or even vesicular elements. In the abdominal type, occult blood is present in the stools and because of this intussusception may be suspected. The symptoms may be prolonged for many weeks in severe cases with fluctuating episodes of acute abdominal colic, melæna, joint pains and recurrent purpura.

In thirty per cent. of the children, there is albuminuria and/or hæmaturia, indicating that an acute nephritis is present.

TREATMENT

The patient should remain in bed as long as fresh skin lesions are appearing or if there is nephritis.   Penicillin should be administered in full dosage (Appendix 1); steroid therapy is seldom helpful.

PROGNOSIS

In thirty per cent. of the patients, hæmaturia and proteinuria may persist for varying periods.   In a proportion of these, some degree of albuminuria persists long after the other symptoms have subsided. Some cases may progress to a latent nephritis comparable to that of patients who have had acute nephritis (p. 369) and in whom persistent albuminuria remains after the acute phase of the illness has passed. The place of long-term treatment with steroids in this group of cases is not yet evaluated.

Secondary Purpura without Platelet Deficiency

With acute fevers, such as scarlet or typhoid fever, and during treatment with drugs such as Sedormid, a purpuric rash sometimes occurs.   In debilitated children with poor resistance the rash of an exanthematous fever, such as measles, may be hæmorrhagic (black measles).

The purpuric rashes of subacute bacterial endocarditis and of meningococcal septicæmia are described under those diseases.

Hæmophilia and Allied Disorders

INHERITANCE

Hæmophilia is an inherited tendency to bleed.   It is transmitted by apparently normal females to their sons; thus, the inheritance is sex-linked, and in this and other ways it is unique among hæmorrhagic diseases.   But the responsible gene not infrequently arises by mutation, and sporadic cases are common; therefore, the absence of a family history does not exclude the diagnosis.   In advising parents, it must be appreciated that the daughters of hæmophilic fathers are able to transmit the tendency to their male children.

LABORATORY FINDINGS

The prothrombin and fibrinogen of the plasma, the platelet count, the bleeding time and the tourniquet test are normal, but in a typical case the coagulation time is prolonged although, between the attacks of bleeding, it tends to shorten.   In certain hæmophilic families the symptoms are relatively mild, hæmarthroses rare, and the coagulation time is only slightly prolonged and may even be normal.

In the clotting of normal plasma into serum most of its prothrombin is converted into thrombin. This disappearance of prothrombin can be measured in venous blood samples and the result expressed as a percentage loss (prothrombin consumption). In typical hæmophilia, the prothrombin consumption is very greatly reduced. Further, a special globulin fraction (antihæmophilic) is present in normal plasma which, on being added to hæmophilic blood, shortens its coagulation time and improves its defective prothrombin consumption; there is a diagnostic laboratory test by which to estimate the deficiency of antihæmophilic globin in hæmophilic blood. In the mild cases with a normal or almost normal coagulation time, the prothrombin consumption defect and the antihæmophilic globulin deficiency are only partial.

It is thought that the activation of prothrombin is brought about by " intrinsic " thromboplastin. The thromboplastin is formed by the interaction in the presence of ionized calcium of the various clotting factors of the plasma and the platelets:

1. Antihæmophilic globulin.
2. " Christmas " factor (or " plasma thromboplastin component ").
3. Factor V.
4. Factor VII.
5. Platelet factor.

Cases resembling classical hæmophilia but with the " Christmas " factor missing have been reported in England, " Christmas " being the name of the first patient described. Such cases can be distinguished from classical hæmophilia by the thromboplastin generation test. Rare cases with deficiencies of Factors V and VII have been reported.

SYMPTOMS

These usually appear at about two or three years of age, sometimes earlier. A steady slow bleeding takes place from a trivial cut, or after an operation for circumcision or dental extraction. Hæmorrhages occur from the skin and mucous membranes, especially the mouth and nose, or into the muscles and joints; these become swollen and tender, and the child is feverish. Repeated hæmarthroses lead to structural and radiological changes in the joints affected. On the first or second occasion the blood is absorbed, but subsequent bleeding tends to produce a partly ankylosed joint (see p. 493). The spleen is not enlarged.

DIAGNOSIS

Only males are affected and there is usually a family history. The blood coagulation time is much prolonged, except in mild cases. Thrombocytopenic purpura is excluded by the normal platelet count and the absence of purpura.

The recessively inherited *congenital afibrinogenæmia* affects both sexes and may cause bleeding in the neonatal period. Laboratory tests confirm the absence of fibrin in the plasma. *Von Willebrand's syndrome* is transmitted by a dominant gene. Bleeding occurs as a result of a capillary defect, revealed by capillary microscopy. In both these disorders, the bleeding is controlled by transfusion with fresh blood or fresh frozen plasma.

TREATMENT

(1) Firm pressure is applied to the bleeding site whenever possible, and other routine methods of controlling hæmorrhage are employed.

(2) Application of 1-in-10,000 solution of snake-venom to the area.

(3) Transfusion with normal blood or fresh frozen plasma; many such patients have had repeated transfusions before.

(4) Antihæmophilic globulin is of the greatest value in controlling hæmorrhage in cases of classical hæmophilia, but has to be given intravenously and repeatedly.

Many *prophylactic* measures have been advocated, but none seems definitely of value except antihæmophilic globulin. At present the technical difficulties of preparing and administering sufficient anti-hæmophilic factor to maintain long-term prophylaxis for all hæmophiliacs are too great; but a most useful part can be played by the selected administration of antihæmophilic factor, either in concentrated form or as fresh frozen plasma, before such procedures as dental extraction or general surgical procedures (*see also* p. 493).

DISORDERS OF LEUCOCYTES

Agranulocytic Angina

THIS is a severe disease characterized by marked leucopenia, due to extreme diminution or absence of cells of the myeloid series, and associated with necrotic ulceration, particularly of the mouth.

ÆTIOLOGY

In some instances the disease may be brought on by drugs, e.g. chloramphenicol, sulphonamide or amidopyrine series. Troxidone (Tridione) and the thiouracil compounds (very rarely used in childhood) are also potential causative agents. In other cases no cause can be ascertained.

BLOOD PICTURE

The leucocytes fall to fewer than 1,000 per c.mm., and the poly-morphonuclears are almost or entirely absent. The mouth and throat present a sloughing, ulcerated appearance. The cervical lymphatic glands become enlarged and œdematous.

In children the mortality in the acute fulminating type is high, probably 80 per cent. In the recurrent form the prognosis is very much better.

TREATMENT

Repeated blood transfusions offer the best hope in treatment, together with full doses of penicillin. There is no specific treatment. Corticosteroids are worth a trial (p. 660).

DIFFERENTIAL DIAGNOSIS

Clinical differentiation of cases of leukæmia with a marked leucopenia is not easy, and bone-marrow puncture is indicated. The benign form of cyclic neutropenia (*see* below) is distinguished by the non-progressive and intermittent nature of the symptoms. Glandular fever (p. 349) gives rise usually to additional symptoms and signs and is characterized by the presence in the peripheral blood of atypical lymphocytes and in most cases by a positive Paul Bunnell reaction.

Cyclic Neutropenia

This is a benign periodic condition in which the neutrophil count falls to below 1,000 cells per c.mm. during the active phases. The condition falls into the group of periodic diseases, including migraine and cyclic vomiting (described on p. 212), and may sometimes be found in association with them.

Acute Leukæmia

Leukæmia is a malignant hyperplasia of the reticulo-endothelial cells throughout the body, with differentiation towards one or other type of leucocyte. It is nearly always acute and very seldom chronic as compared with adult patients.

Cases are sometimes seen in the first two years of life, but the highest proportion is found between the third and fourth years. Thereafter the number of cases of acute leukæmia begins to decline.

The incidence of acute leukæmia is increasing at the present time. To what extent this can be attributed to the radiation hazards of modern life is not yet known; there is certainly sufficient evidence to make it inadvisable to x-ray the mother's abdomen or pelvis (entailing total body irradiation of the fœtus at the most critical stage of development) during the early months of pregnancy.

PATHOLOGY

The glands and all the other organs of the body are infiltrated with the cells corresponding to the type of response called up by the disease, i.e. lymphocytes, monocytes or myelocytes. The kidneys, liver, lungs, bone-marrow and spleen are infiltrated. Rarer sites are the retina and skin. Subperiosteal nodes have been described. The type of cellular metaplasia is shown by biopsy of the bone-marrow; although the reaction in some cases is of such a primitive type of blast cell as to make differentiation difficult.

The three types of leukæmia in their most active phases are *acute lymphatic, myelocytic,* and *monocytic*; since the clinical picture of all three is indistinguishable, they will be considered together.

CLINICAL PICTURE

The onset is extremely varied. It may be acute with *hæmorrhage, ulceration of the mouth, fever* or *pain in bones and joints*, or it may be insidious with *pallor* and *lassitude*. The following modes of onset may occur by themselves or in combination:

(1) Fever and pain in long bones and joints (resembles rheumatic fever).

(2) Hæmorrhage (gums, nose, tooth socket, purpura, bowel). Retinal hæmorrhages with a sudden onset of blindness may occur.

(3) Gingivitis (may resemble agranulocytic angina or glandular fever).

(4) Anæmia (progressive pallor, lassitude, anorexia and dyspnœa).

The disease is always fatal, the total course lasting only a few weeks or months, but it is possible to induce temporary remissions in most cases.

PHYSICAL SIGNS

As the blood platelets fall towards the critical level of about 40,000 per c.mm., hæmorrhage and purpura, with bruising, are common. Occasionally there is ulceration of the throat and bleeding from the gums.

Generalized lymphatic glandular enlargement may be present and the spleen is palpable in the majority of cases. Hepatic enlargement is progressive as the liver becomes more and more infiltrated with leukæmic tissue.

X-rays of the long bones show patchy absorption of the cancellous bone, or diminution or thickening of the compact bone, due to the proliferation in the bone-marrow. Occasionally the periosteum is raised, due to leukæmic deposits.

BLOOD CHANGES

(*a*) In the *lymphatic type* the cells are lymphocytes, or lymphoblasts, and it is rare to have less than 90 per cent. of this type of cell.

(*b*) In *monocytic leukæmia*, there may be monoblasts as well as monocytes. In addition, there are some lymphocytes and a number of other cells of the granular type. In a typical case, there would be perhaps 60 per cent. of the monocytic cells and their precursors.

(c) In *myelocytic leukæmia* there is a mixture of myeloblasts and mature neutrophils.

Leukæmic changes may not be evident from the peripheral blood count, particularly if the patient is in the aleukæmic phase. Even if numerous primitive white cells are present in the peripheral blood, it may only be possible to state with certainty that the diagnosis is acute leukæmia, the type of primitive cell remaining undetermined. Bone-marrow puncture is essential as a confirmatory investigation.

A progressive anæmia in which the red cells and hæmoglobin fall together, leaving the colour index at approximately 1·0 (orthochromic type), occurs along with the rest of the blood picture.

The platelets are reduced almost from the beginning of the disease.

TREATMENT

Although leukæmia is still a fatal disease, treatment with initial blood transfusions, followed by anti-folic acid substances such as Methotrexate, or with 6-mercaptopurin, combined with ACTH or steroids may produce good remissions, usually increasing well-being and postponing death for some weeks or months.

Occasionally a remission of up to two years' duration may be achieved by these means.

Acute Infectious Lymphocytosis

This is a very rare condition in which the lymphocyte count rises to 60,000–100,000 per c.mm. in association with a febrile illness. The lymphocytes are all of the mature type and the disease follows a benign course to complete recovery in two to three weeks. It is presumed to be of viral origin.

Glandular Fever (Infectious Mononucleosis)

Glandular fever is an acute infectious disease characterized by enlargement of the lymphatic glands and spleen, changes in the blood cells, especially mononucleosis, and the development of hetero-phil antibodies in the serum. The prognosis is favourable.

The condition is common in children of all ages and in young adults. Its cause is unknown and is probably a virus. It is not highly infectious and school epidemics are exceptional. The incubation period is 5 to 14 days but may be as long as six weeks. Isolation of cases is not usually considered necessary in view of the low degree of infectivity.

CLINICAL PICTURE

Few diseases are more variable in their mode of onset. Of particular difficulty are those cases which commence insidiously with a feeling of tiredness and irritability. Fever may be unsuspected until the temperature is taken and found to be 99°–99·6° F. There may be only minimal enlargement of the glands in the neck, axillæ and groins, and the spleen is palpable in only a proportion of these patients. In this form the disease may run a chronic course lasting several months.

In the more acute forms, the temperature rises rapidly to 103° or 104° remaining up for a week or longer; there is considerable malaise. The tonsils are enlarged and infected, and may be covered by a pale or white membrane which can be easily removed, but which may superficially resemble diphtheria. Conjunctivitis may be present. The spleen is usually palpable and enlarges with the glands. Very often these are not painful, but they may be slightly tender. The enlargement is chiefly of the neck glands, but also in the axilla and groin.

Rashes are said to occur in 15 per cent. of all cases and are of a morbilliform or macular type. Cases have been described showing well-marked jaundice with other symptoms suggesting hepatitis.

Meningeal Form. In a small proportion of patients the disease presents as a meningitis, without any of the usual signs of glandular fever. This type has to be distinguished from the other forms of benign viral (lymphocytic) meningitis (p. 409).

Occasionally, the other signs of glandular fever may be associated with the meningitis or may follow a week or more later.

Blood. The neutrophil count is reduced to 1,000–3,000 per c.mm., with an increase in lymphocytes of 7,000–15,000 per c.mm. The proportion of monocytes is increased and an atypical type of cell, variously described as a lymphocyte or monocyte, may be seen in the blood film.

Heterophil Antibody (Paul Bunnell) *Reaction.* This is the ability of a serum to agglutinate and hæmolyse sensitized sheep's cells. In glandular fever this ability rises rapidly, and by the fourth day has risen from the normal 1 in 8 to 1 in 64 or 1 in 250. The reaction is not positive in all patients presenting the clinical picture of glandular fever. This has given rise to the suggestion that a number of different viruses may be involved, of which only a proportion produce a positive Paul Bunnell reaction. The position will be clarified only when the causative agent or agents are finally identified.

The Wassermann test may be temporarily positive.

DIAGNOSIS

The enlarged glands must be differentiated from:

1. Tuberculous glands, mumps, septic glands, and Hodgkin's disease, by an examination of the blood for the mononucleosis and heterophil agglutination.

2. Monocytic leukæmia may be differentiated chiefly by the absence of the Paul Bunnell reaction, and the course of the disease. Bone-marrow puncture is decisive if any doubt remains.

3. Acquired toxoplasmosis (p. 413) may be distinguished by a positive dye and complement fixation test.

TREATMENT

This is symptomatic since no antibiotic treatment is applicable. Aspirin to relieve the headache, mouth-washes, gargles, and throat paints are indicated.

DISEASES OF THE RETICULO-ENDOTHELIAL SYSTEM

Histiocytic Reticulo-endotheliosis

THIS includes eosinophilic granuloma, Hand-Schüller-Christian disease and Letterer-Siwe disease, due to neoplasia of histiocytic cells originating in various parts of the reticulo-endothelial system.

EOSINOPHILIC GRANULOMA

The lesions may be solitary or multiple and can be situated in various parts of the bony skeleton. They may resolve slowly and the prognosis is much better in the case of single lesions; however, if other lesions appear, it is likely that a disseminated type of the disease will develop. The latter may conform to the classical type of Hand-Schüller-Christian disease or to that of Letterer-Siwe. These types rarely resolve.

HAND-SCHÜLLER-CHRISTIAN DISEASE

The classical triad of this disorder comprises: (1) Deposits in the skull bones (eosinophilic granulomata); (2) proptosis (orbital deposits); and (3) diabetes insipidus (involvement of the sella turcica or pituitary stalk). There may also be involvement of the skin, lungs, bone-marrow or liver; other parts of the skeleton may be affected including one or more vertebræ. Although a slow one, the process seldom becomes arrested.

LETTERER-SIWE DISEASE

This type is more acute. Fever, anæmia, pulmonary infiltration and involvement of the lymph nodes, spleen and liver are found, but various clinical pictures are encountered. The prognosis is bad, but some cases become chronic taking on the features of Hand-Schüller-Christian disease.

Hodgkin's Disease (Lymphadenoma)

Hodgkin's disease is a fatal disease characterized by a painless progressive enlargement of the lymphoid tissue of the body, in the glands, spleen, and other organs, associated with progressive anæmia.

The cause of the disease is not known but is probably a reticulo-endothelial new growth. It may be found at any age, but is rare below 10 years, and is commoner in males than females.

PATHOLOGY

The glands are enlarged and discrete, particularly the neck group. The glands of the mediastinum, abdomen, axilla and groin may also be enlarged. The spleen is greatly enlarged and is very hard; it has been termed a "hard-bake spleen." On section, patches of whitish lymphadenomatous tissue are seen scattered over the organ. Both the bone-marrow and the liver may show nodules of this tissue. The lungs, kidneys, and intestines may also be affected.

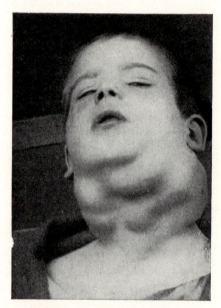

Fig. 39.—Lymphadenoma in a boy aged 10, showing massive glands in the neck.

Microscopically, the characteristic picture is an increase of the reticulo-endothelial cells, which replace the lymphoid tissue. There are multi-nucleated giant cells, the nuclei being centrally placed. Usually, there are many eosinophil cells. Towards the end, progressive fibrosis takes place, and little beyond fibrosis tissue is found in some of the lesions.

A progressive hypochromic anæmia is present. The leucocytes may be normal, increased, or decreased, but there is usually a leucopenia. Fifteen per cent. of the patients show an eosinophilia. The blood platelets are normal until the end, and the coagulation- and bleeding-time are also normal.

CLINICAL PICTURE

The onset is gradual, with enlargement of a group of glands, usually on one side or other of the neck. Wasting, pallor and weakness follow. The temperature may be high and continuous, remittent,

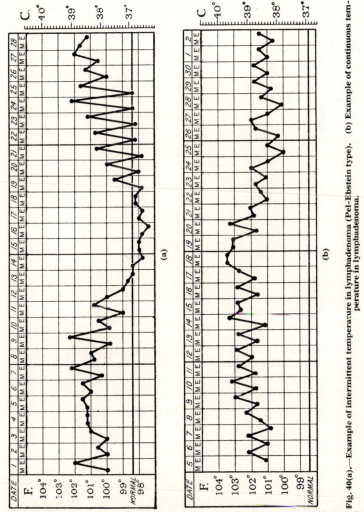

Fig. 40(a).—Example of intermittent temperature in lymphadenoma (Pel-Ebstein type). (b) Example of continuous temperature in lymphadenoma.

or of the Pel-Ebstein type (*see* Fig. 40(*a*) and (*b*)). X-ray of the chest may show considerable broadening of the mediastinum due to glandular enlargement. In other patients the glands are largely confined to the abdomen, with much splenic enlargement. The temperature slowly climbs for several days, then slowly subsides and remains down for approximately a week; it then once more repeats the rising undulations. With each rise in temperature the symptoms grow worse, but subside again along with the temperature. There may be pains in the bones, and pressure symptoms from the glands pressing on the trachea and bronchi. Collapse of the lung and pleural effusion may be present.

DIFFERENTIAL DIAGNOSIS

Tuberculosis must be excluded. Generally, enlarged tuberculous neck glands go on to abscess formation, but lymphadenomatous glands usually remain discrete. The temperature is irregular, and not characteristic of lymphadenoma. A Mantoux or tuberculin-jelly test should be done, and the removal of a gland makes differentiation easy.

Leukæmia is excluded by the blood picture. In chronic septicæmia, with generalized glandular and splenic enlargement, abscesses are formed. Infectious mononucleosis is distinguished by the course and positive Paul Bunnell reaction.

PROGNOSIS

All cases of lymphadenoma end in death; the duration of life may be prolonged by several years with treatment.

TREATMENT

X-ray treatment together with nitrogen mustard and other cytotoxic drugs may alleviate symptoms for the time being. Blood transfusion is definitely of value in correcting the accompanying anæmia. If the glands are greatly enlarged, causing pressure on the common bile-duct, with jaundice, or pressure on the bowel, or constriction of the trachea or bronchi, operative treatment may have to be considered. All such treatment is merely palliative and major surgery is rarely justifiable in childhood, particularly if the other forms of treatment have already been tried and have failed.

DISEASES OF LIPOID METABOLISM AFFECTING THE RETICULO-ENDOTHELIAL SYSTEM (LIPOIDOSES)

Gaucher's Disease

THIS is a rare disease which is familial, probably of a recessive type, characterized by an enlarged spleen and liver (both organs contain Gaucher's cells), leucopenia, and a hypochromic anæmia. It is found more often in the Jewish race, and is about as common in females as in males.

It may be recognized either in infancy or in older children or adults.

The disease is due to an inborn error of metabolism, and there is accumulation of abnormal cerebrosides in the reticulo-endothelial system. Pathologically, the spleen is enlarged and fibrotic and contains large Gaucher cells (20 by 40 μ). These have small round nuclei, and are distended with lipoid material. The cells are probably reticulo-endothelial cells, and are found in the liver, bones, bone-marrow, and lymphatic glands.

Infantile Form. There is mental and physical retardation in the first few weeks of life. Gross splenic and hepatic enlargement becomes evident, and is accompanied by neurological symptoms, including hypertonia, opisthotonus, with occasional lapses into hypotonia, dysphagia, laryngospasm, and, finally, clonic spasms. Death occurs several months from the onset.

At autopsy the brain shows sclerosis of the ganglion cells in addition to the reticulo-endothelial changes described below.

Older Children. Progressive enlargement of the spleen is followed sooner or later by hepatomegaly. The skin becomes dull brown or yellow, especially on exposed surfaces. Pinguecula (yellowish, wedge-like thickening of the conjunctiva) is occasionally seen.

Bone changes, including areas of rarefaction and sclerosis, and fractures, may occur.

There is anæmia, sometimes with lymphocytosis. If thrombo-cytopenia is present, purpura may occur as an additional symptom.

DIAGNOSIS

Typical Gaucher cells may be identified in the marrow specimens or biopsy specimens from glands or spleen.

TREATMENT

This is purely symptomatic. Splenectomy is advisable if purpura and thrombocytopenia occur. The disease is only slowly progressive.

Niemann-Pick's Disease

The disease is due to an inborn error of metabolism and results in widespread deposition of lecithin, causing splenomegaly and other manifestations. It occurs predominantly in Jews; both sexes are equally affected. It is a familial condition starting in infancy.

On microscopy reticulo-endothelial cells, distended with lipoid material, mainly lecithin, are found. The whole body is involved, including the nervous system. In the blood there is lipæmia with raised cholesterol and leucocytosis.

Clinically the spleen, liver, and glands become enlarged in infancy. After the first six months of life there is a considerable mental and physical deterioration. The skin is yellow, the child wastes and ascites develops. There is also anæmia. The nervous symptoms resemble those of Tay-Sachs disease (amaurotic family idiocy, *see* p. 444).

Bone-marrow puncture or bone or splenic biopsy will reveal the characteristic Niemann-Pick foam cells, which may reach 50 μ in diameter owing to their distension with lipoid material, mainly lecithin. Death takes place by two years of age.

Tay Sachs Disease (*see* p. 444)

Xanthomatosis

Two different conditions are given the name of cutaneous xanthoma.

In the infantile form, *xanthoma disseminatum*, multiple yellow nodules appear on the trunk and face. The serum cholesterol is normal. The condition is benign and the lesions disappear slowly but spontaneously; no treatment is necessary. The condition may be mistaken for the much more serious histiocytic reticulo-endotheliosis (p. 351).

By contast, *xanthoma tuberosa* are yellow-brown nodules, sometimes of considerable size, which usually appear on the limbs. The serum cholesterol is greatly raised. This hypercholesterolæmia may be either of the primary or familial type (cause unknown), or may be secondary to diseases such as diabetes mellitus or the nephrotic syndrome. The xanthomata are harmless although unsightly, but dietary treatment should be given for the hypercholesterolæmia in view of the danger of atherosclerosis.

CHAPTER 17

Diseases of the Genito-Urinary System

GENERAL EXAMINATION

In genito-urinary disease a careful general examination is essential. In all cases, signs of *hypertension* should be looked for by the estimation of the blood-pressure, the detection of left-sided cardiac hypertrophy and an examination of the optic fundi.

The presence should be sought of *œdema*, which may be generalized rather than dependent, and even in its absence a rapid, marked increase of weight may be suspicious.

The general appearance of the child should be taken into account; growth may be stunted, or definite *rachitic deformity* may be found (*see* p. 120); the skin is often sallow and anæmia may be present.

External genital abnormalities must be excluded and the presence of a normal urethral orifice confirmed. The *abdomen* is palpated to exclude dilatation of the bladder or ureters, or enlargement of the kidneys.

THE URINE

In normal conditions of hydration and humidity, a volume equal to about two-thirds of the fluid intake is passed per day as urine.

In the small infant the urine is passed about every half-hour. At 6 months of age, when picked up to be fed, he is often dry if he has been placed on the chamber after the previous feed. At one year the child may be able to retain urine for a period of 5 or 6 hours during the night, and 3 hours during the day. At three years the normal and properly trained child should pass urine only on waking, after breakfast, at dinner-time, after tea and at bed-time.

COLLECTION OF SPECIMENS IN INFANCY

(*a*) *Males.* The cleansed penis is attached with strapping to a sterile polythene tube, which is in turn connected with a sterile test tube or bottle.

(*b*) *Females.* From the female, when a sterile specimen is essential, catheterization is theoretically required. In practice, in infancy, to obtain a clean specimen, a special polythene collector is fastened with adhesive tape over the vulva and the urine collected; alternatively, the infant may be held over a clean utensil until the desired result is obtained.

TESTING THE URINE

A routine examination should be made in all cases for albumin, sugar, acetone, diacetic acid and bile, and microscopic examination made for pus cells, casts and red cells. The colour and reaction of the urine should be noted and, if sufficient quantity is available, the specific gravity measured.

RENAL-FUNCTION TESTS

Specific Gravity Test. Certainly the easiest and cheapest, and probably the most valuable, renal-function test is carried out by measuring the specific gravity of the urine. The patient is given nothing to drink after 6 p.m. and the early morning specimen of urine is collected and its specific gravity measured; it is normally over 1·020, and often over 1·025. The patient is then given a relatively large quantity of water to drink, e.g. 2 pints for an adult, 1 pint for a six-year-old child, and the specific gravity of the subsequent specimen estimated; it should certainly be below 1·010, and is often below 1·005. The less able a damaged kidney is to dilute or concentrate the urine, according to body requirements, the more fixed becomes the specific gravity of all specimens at 1·010.

Urea-concentration Test. In the normal individual the urinary output contains about 2–4 per cent. of urea.

Where the kidney is damaged, the concentration is reduced; it may be as low as 0·5 per cent. The technique of the test is as follows: 10 grammes of urea, dissolved and suitably flavoured, are given, say, at 6 a.m., the urine having been collected immediately before and no fluid taken since the previous evening. A specimen is obtained at hourly intervals for, say, four hours, and the urea content of the various specimens is ascertained by means of Doremus's ureometer, hypobromite solution being used. It is most important that the volumes of the specimens should be accurately recorded. This test is far less sensitive than the specific gravity test, and, if the specimens of urine are of large volume, is of no value.

Blood-urea Test. Normally the blood-urea should be between 15 and 40 mg. per cent. Higher values are also found, however, in the healthy newborn infant and in conditions of extrarenal disease, such as dehydration, as well as in kidney disorders.

Urea-clearance Test. This test is more applicable to older children and adults.

Proteinura (Albuminuria)

Albumin may be found in the urine in minor infections, as well as in serious renal disease. For instance, during infections such as diphtheria, whooping-cough and pneumonia, there is often a trace of albumin which disappears with the cessation of the disease. In infants with severe dehydration, as in diarrhœa and vomiting, transient albuminuria is common. It is sufficient to say that albuminuria may or may not be significant, but in all cases a thorough general examination of the patient should be made and its cause sought. The most common form of albuminuria is one which occurs quite apart from any apparent infection or organic disease, namely, *orthostatic albuminuria*.

This appears most often in children between the ages of 10 and 15, when the child is growing rapidly and approaching puberty, and is slightly more common in boys than girls. The specimen of urine obtained before rising in the morning is quite free from albumin. As the day goes on, each specimen contains a larger and larger quantity, until towards the evening an appreciable amount is found. When the patient goes to rest in the evening the urine once more becomes free. If the child remains in bed throughout the 24 hours, the urine remains free.

Hæmaturia

1. RENAL CAUSES OF HÆMATURIA

In *nephritis* there will be albumin apart from that accounted for by the blood, and granular casts will also be present in the urine. The blood-urea and blood-pressure may be raised.

Calculus is accompanied by pain, which radiates towards the bladder and even to the tip of the penis, or there may be aching in the groin. An x-ray of the renal tract and ureters will often show the stone. Such calculi are sometimes found in cases of spinal caries, where the child has been compelled to remain still in bed on his back for some time. They are often accompanied by a urinary infection.

Neoplasm. Hæmaturia may be the earliest symptom of Wilms' tumour (nephroblastoma, *see* p. 376). Such tumours are usually palpable and an intravenous or retrograde pyelogram will demonstrate the deformity of the kidney. Hæmangioma of the pelvis is a rare cause.

Scurvy. A general investigation will show the condition of the infant's gums, tenderness of the limbs on movement and a shortage of vitamin c in the diet.

Renal tuberculosis. Usually this condition is painless, and tuberculous infection may be found elsewhere in the body. An examination of the sediment from an early morning or twenty-four-hour specimen of the urine may show tubercle bacilli on microscopy or on culture, or when injected into a guinea-pig it may produce the disease. It is an extreme rarity in childhood.

Blood diseases. In leukæmia and the hæmorrhagic diseases an examination of the blood will confirm the diagnosis.

Oxaluria may produce slight bleeding. A careful examination for presence of crystals should be made.

Trauma is indicated by the history and often by some external bruising.

Sulphonamide administration may give rise to hæmaturia and oliguria, particularly if the fluid intake is inadequate or if dehydration is present.

Bacterial endocarditis may give rise to microscopic and occasionally macroscopic hæmaturia.

Red-coloured urine may be found after the eating of beetroot or dyed boiled sweets. This may be confused with hæmaturia unless the urine is examined under the microscope. *Hæmoglobinuria* is demonstrated by spectroscopy and may be due to blackwater fever, paroxysmal nocturnal hæmoglobinuria (the Marchiafava-Micheli syndrome), and incompatible blood transfusion.

In infancy the presence of urates gives rise to a pinkish stain on the napkin and may cause unnecessary alarm in the mother.

2. VESICAL AND URETHRAL CAUSES OF HÆMATURIA

Papilloma of the bladder. Bleeding will be profuse, and some of the papilloma may be seen microscopically, but a cystoscopy will be necessary to confirm the diagnosis.

Meatal ulcer. This is the commonest cause in boys under three years of age (*see* p. 381).

In *acute cystitis*, blood may be present as well as pus.

CONGENITAL ABNORMALITIES

THESE are comparatively common, being found in from 2 to 4 per cent. of all autopsies. Many are symptomless but since the introduction of intravenous and retrograde pyelography are more often discovered in life. X-ray cinematography using the image intensifier provides a dynamic as opposed to a static assessment of the state of the renal tract. The more frequent use of the cystoscope has made the detection of abnormalities of the bladder more common. The full investigation of the renal tract of a small child is thus a highly specialized procedure and is only undertaken in fully equipped centres. Similarly, surgery which should aim at conservation of the kidneys calls for a surgeon experienced in pædiatric urology.

ABNORMALITIES OF THE KIDNEY AND URETER

Congenital Cystic Kidney

Congenital cystic kidneys may be so large as to obstruct labour. Usually, they can be felt on palpation, but they may be unsuspected. The symptoms are those of chronic nephritis (*see* p. 373). The cysts are loculated, and the kidney substance almost destroyed. Death is due to renal failure, which may occur soon after birth or may be delayed until early adult life. In the latter case complications such as pyelonephritis, calculi and hypertension may sometimes be found.

Congenital Absence of One Kidney and Ureter, Fusion of the Kidneys (Horse-Shoe Kidney) or Double Kidney (Pyelon Duplex)

These abnormalities are discovered usually by chance. In pyelon duplex one half of the kidney may be hydronephrotic and non-functional. It may become infected and lead to pyelonephritis. In such cases an operation to remove the diseased portion of the kidney may be necessary.

Ectopic Kidney

This abnormality arises from an imperfect ascent of kidney in the intrauterine life. The kidney is commonly found in the pelvis or iliac fossa. Such ectopic kidneys produce no symptoms unless there is obstruction to the flow of urine when they will become infected or hydronephrotic.

Renal Agenesis

If the condition is bilateral it is incompatible with life. It is associated with a characteristic facial appearance (downward displacement of the ears and a frog-like face), absence of the anterior abdominal muscles and other congenital abnormalities.

Renal Hypoplasia

This condition is often difficult to distinguish from the end-result of renal infection, and for practical purposes the distinction is not important. Renal hypoplasia may be associated with renal dwarfism and rickets. There may be some dilatation of the ureter and a mild hydronephrosis.

Abnormalities of the Ureters

(*a*) A *duplication of the ureters* (with or without duplication of the associated kidney) will be discovered by pyelography or cystoscopy.

(*b*) *Aberrant renal vessels* may kink the ureters and be a cause of congenital hydronephrosis.

(*c*) *Megaureter*. Isolated dilatation of one ureter may be due to a stricture or a calculus (rare in childhood). When the most distal portion of the ureter, i.e. that within the vesical wall, becomes dilated it is described as a ureterocele.   In this situation a cystic enlargement may occur which protrudes into the lumen of the bladder and may further obstruct the ureteric outlet.   Chronic infection within the cyst quickly develops.

Bilateral dilatation of the ureter is frequently the result of urethral obstruction (*see* bladder neck obstruction, p. 363).   Occasionally, dilatation of one or both ureters occurs without evidence of any obstructive lesion and is thought to be the result of neuromuscular inco-ordination.

(*d*) *Ectopic Ureter.*   Occasionally, one ureter instead of draining into the bladder opens into the urethra.   As such an exit is beyond the internal sphincter, incontinence of urine is produced which is more pronounced when the child is up and about than when at rest in bed.

ABNORMALITIES OF THE BLADDER, URETHRA AND THE GENITAL ORGANS

Ectopic Bladder

This is due to a developmental failure of the ventral wall of the urogenital canal.   The anterior wall of the bladder and the corresponding midline portion of the abdominal wall are absent, and the symphysis pubis fails to fuse.   In males the penis is deformed, and epispadias results.   In the female the labia are separated, and the cleft urethra continues into the exposed bladder.   The bladder is seen as a red protrusion in the pubic region.   The urine runs away continually; eczema of the skin results.   When unrelieved the condition is not compatible with long survival.

Treatment.   Transplantation of the ureters into the colon is the usual procedure, after which renal function may remain surprisingly satisfactory, and, with training, a fair degree of continence can be obtained.   Recently, the isolation of a loop of ileum into which both ureters are drained, thus forming an ileal bladder, has been used as an alternative to transplantation of the ureters into the colon.

Subsequently, plastic operations on the ectopic bladder can be undertaken, combined with osteotomies to bring together the widely separated pubic bones.

Epispadias

The urethra opens on the dorsum of the penis.

Hypospadias

The urethra may open at the level of the glans, the body of the penis, or the junction of the penis and scrotum.

Undescended Testicle (Cryptorchidism) (*see* p. 162).

Phimosis

In a newly-born infant adherence of the prepuce to the glans penis is not of itself an indication for circumcision.   When there is sufficient room for the infant to pass urine there is no real need for operation. In phimosis a blunt probe may be passed down between the prepuce and the glans penis and adhesions broken down, the prepuce being stretched at the same time. In more severe cases a dorsal slit may sometimes be necessary. Generally, the prepuce becomes easily retractable by the age of five years. The commonly recommended grounds for circumcision, namely tight foreskin, balanitis (due usually to ammonia dermatitis in the small infant), or as a prophylactic against masturbation, venereal disease, nocturnal enuresis and carcinoma of the penis in old age, have little justification. There is no question but that meatal ulceration is more common in the circumcised infant.

In older boys, paraphimosis and recurrent balanitis present definite indications for circumcision, but these cases are very few in number.

Labial Adhesions

This condition is comparatively common. The labia minora are joined by a thin layer of adherent cells so that the urethra and vaginal opening are covered up. The treatment is to break down these adhesions with a probe and place in the opening a pledget of cotton-wool smeared with soft paraffin.

CONGENITAL URETHRAL AND BLADDER-NECK OBSTRUCTION

THERE is a group of congenital conditions found more commonly in males which give rise to urinary obstruction. These may be divided into those which are of organic origin, such as the presence of a posterior urethral valve, and those which are functional, due to a neuromuscular inco-ordination of the urinary sphincters. The clinical picture varies slightly in the different types, but broadly speaking they all give rise to vesical retention with overflow dribbling incontinence of urine and inability to pass a good stream, megaureter and hydronephrotic kidneys. A bladder that can always be felt raises a possibility of obstruction. The dilated ureters are also sometimes palpable. Pyelocystitis and later pyelonephritis invariably develop in those cases which survive the first month of life. In a small proportion of such cases there is an absence of the musculature of the anterior abdominal wall. Urinary obstruction, if untreated, and often despite treatment, always results in infection and renal failure. In children who survive infancy, renal rickets may develop.

Congenital Urethral Valves in Males

Valve-like mucosal flaps may be present below the verumontanum. Such valves present no obstruction to a catheter passed from below, but cause obstruction from above downwards. They are best demonstrated by contrast x-ray cinematography using an image intensifier during the act of micturition (voiding cysto-urethrogram), which reveals the marked dilatation of the posterior urethra above the obstruction.

Treatment of this condition, even when recognized in early life, may be of no avail, because the kidney substance may have been already destroyed in foetal life by constant back pressure. Nevertheless, relief by retropubic exploration of the posterior urethra and destruction of the valves should be tried.

Hypertrophy of the verumontanum without valvular formation may sometimes produce a similar condition to a urethral valve.

Marion's Disease

This condition is in many respects similar to achalasia of sphincters elsewhere. There is considerable hypertrophy of the internal urethral sphincter causing, in particular, an enlargement of the posterior bar of the bladder neck which pushes forward and occludes the internal urethral orifice. The condition is distinguished from urethral valvular obstruction by the voiding cysto-urethrogram.

Wedge-resection of the posterior lip of the internal urethral orifice, after exploration of the bladder, is indicated.

Bladder-neck Obstruction in Females

A lesion resembling Marion's disease is sometimes found, but it is difficult to obtain a surgical cure.

Other Congenital Causes of Urinary Obstruction

Urinary retention may arise from a *ureterocele* or from a *dilated ectopic ureter*, where either of these lesions presses upon the internal urethral orifice. *Congenital strictures* of the external urethral orifice are occasionally seen in males. Neurological lesions, such as *spina bifida with meningocele*, may give rise to a paralytic bladder with retention of urine.

INFECTIONS OF THE URINARY TRACT

Pyelitis, Pyelonephritis and Pyelocystitis

URINARY-TRACT infection is not infrequent, particularly in the neonatal period, and is quite as common in boys as in girls under one year. Among the causes of vomiting, lack of weight gain and general failure to thrive in infancy, remains one of the commonest and yet one of the most frequently overlooked explanations.

In older children, among whom girls are more frequently affected than boys, the patient is more likely to complain of specific symptoms which draw attention to the renal tract.

ÆTIOLOGY

It is known that pyelonephritis is common where there is malformation of the urinary tract which obstructs the free flow of urine. The various abnormalities which may be responsible have already been described (p. 363).

It follows that the finding of a persistent urinary infection, and particularly of recurrent urinary infection, should always lead to a full investigation of the renal tract from the point of view of congenital or acquired abnormality.

PATHOLOGY

Simple cystitis is seldom fatal. Cystoscopy in such cases reveals that the inflammatory process is usually localized to the area of the trigone of the bladder.

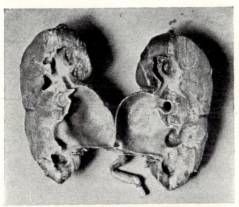

Fig. 41.—Pyelonephritis; note dilated calyces and pelvis and tortuous ureter. There are also inflammatory and fibrotic changes in the kidney.

The *post-mortem* appearances in pyelonephritis show that the whole kidney substance is involved. In long-continued cases the kidney is fibrotic and contracted. The capsule is stuck down to the underlying cortex. On the cut surface yellow, grey or white streaks of fibrosis are visible. Histologically there is interstitial fibrosis with progressive destruction of tubules, and later glomeruli, first producing capsular fibrosis and, finally, complete disappearance of the glomerulus. The renal pelvis and upper ureter may be dilated with a thickened wall, but if renal function has been completely destroyed the pelvis becomes shrunken and atrophic (*see* Fig. 41).

Esch. coli accounts for the majority of urinary tract infections; the remainder include *B. proteus, Ps. pyocyanea* and some mixed infections with *Strept. fæcalis* and *Staph. pyogenes.*

SYMPTOMS

In newborn and young infants there may only be failure to thrive with vomiting in the more acute cases. *There may be no symptoms to direct attention to the urinary tract.* It is therefore essential to examine the urine of all infants who fail to make normal nutritional progress,

In addition to the finding of an infected urine, investigation will show some elevation of the blood urea. Fever is not always present but in some cases the onset is marked by pyrexia of 103° or 104° F, and either drowsiness or irritability. The stools may be frequent, and with the vomiting there is refusal of food. The urine may be scanty and may stain the napkins. Sweating, rigors and meningismus or even convulsions may occur. In older children there will be a history of frequency and dysuria, often with pain at the end of micturition. Rigors, vomiting, headache and lumbar pain are common symptoms. The abdominal pain may be sufficiently severe as to suggest appendicitis. In pyelonephritis there will be lumbar tenderness, and in some cases the kidneys become palpable. In older children there is usually far less constitutional disturbance than in infants.

DIAGNOSIS

This can be made only by a careful *microscopical* examination of the urine. In males, the urine should be collected in a clean test-tube or bottle. In females, the method described on p. 357 should be used; catheterization is seldom required.

In the normal infant or child, not more than an occasional pus cell is to be seen in a microscopic examination of a shaken-up specimen of urine. In cases of pyelitis, however, there are, as a rule, from 5 to 100 or more pus cells per one sixth field in a shaken-up specimen, with marked clumping of the pus cells. Occasionally, at the commencement of the illness a specimen may be found with many organisms but few or no pus cells. There may be a varying amount of blood. A profuse growth of organisms will be found on culture. Albumin is often present, but there may only be a trace in some cases.

PROGNOSIS

Simple pyelitis responds rapidly to modern chemotherapy and antibiotics. Where a congenital malformation causes recurrent urinary infections, the prognosis depends upon the effectiveness of surgery or of long term prophylaxis against infection. Where chronic pyelonephritis is already established, the final result may be similar to that of chronic nephritis (*see* p. 373).

TREATMENT

The first requirement is to ensure that there is a good flow of urine. This necessitates a fluid intake higher than normal and, in cases in which urinary obstruction is present, treatment at the earliest possible stage, if practicable, to overcome the obstruction.

Specific Therapy. 1. Sulphonamides.—For the routine treatment of a urinary infection sulphonamides remain the initial drug of choice (for dosage, *see* Appendix 1).

Sulphonamide preparations are more soluble in alkaline urine than in acid, so the urine should be kept alkaline with a sodium citrate mixture while their administration continues. It is of the greatest importance to maintain treatment for an adequate period. Although the necessary daily dosage may be quite small, it should usually be maintained for at least three weeks in cases of urinary-tract infection.

2. Antibiotics.—The choice of antibiotic depends upon the sensitivity of the infecting organism; streptomycin and the tetracyclines are often appropriate (Appendix 1).

Other antibiotics, such as colomycin, and chemotherapeutic agents, such as nitrofurantoin, should be reserved for those cases in which the infecting organism is proved to be resistant to sulphonamides, and for pre- and post-operative use in operations on the genito-urinary tract (for dosage, *see* Appendixes 1 and 3).

PROPHYLAXIS

Where there is a predisposition to repeated urinary tract infection, long-term preventive treatment with Urolucosil or Gantrisin may be advisable (for dosage, *see* Appendix 1). It may be necessary to maintain such treatment for one to three years.

Mandelic acid is used in the prophylaxis of urinary infection in chronic cases as an alternative.

A full investigation of the urinary tract is carried out in all cases of recurrent urinary infection, followed by surgical treatment of malformations or calculi where this is indicated.

Renal Tuberculosis (*see* p. 586)

NEPHRITIS

THE terminology of nephritis has become confused by efforts to relate pathological variants to clinical types and to co-ordinate these with ætiology and prognosis. No attempt is here made to classify nephritis according to anatomical or pathological lesions. The classification of Addis is followed and its approximate correspondence with other classifications is shown, it being understood that widely differing ætiological agents may cause almost identical renal changes.

THE COURSE OF NEPHRITIS (After Addis)

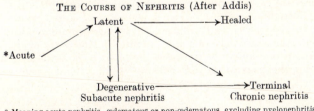

* Meaning acute nephritis, œdematous or non-œdematous, excluding pyelonephritis, and acute embolic nephritis.

The chief distinguishing clinical characteristics of these conditions may be summarized as follows:

1. Acute Glomerular Nephritis: Type I Nephritis

Both sexes are equally affected. The disease is very rare under the age of three years, becomes more frequent between five and ten years and has a small but persistent incidence among adolescents and young adults.

ÆTIOLOGY

In most cases, the symptoms follow a streptococcal throat infection. A Group A (Lancefield) Griffith type 12 organism is responsible, less often type 4. Thus, minor epidemics of acute nephritis restricted to a particular area or school may be seen when a " nephritogenic " streptococcus becomes prevalent. In some 25 per cent. of cases the initial infection is so slight that it escapes notice altogether. Occasionally a streptococcal infection in the skin is responsible, as in a case of nephritis occurring as a complication of a burn or a scald.

PATHOLOGY

Naked-eye examination shows the kidney to be swollen and engorged with blood. The cut surface bulges over the capsule and blood drips from the surface. Microscopically there is little doubt that the brunt of the infection falls on the glomeruli. The capillary loops of the tufts show necrosis in some instances. There is blood in the capsular spaces. Round cells may be seen near the affected glomeruli.

SYMPTOMATOLOGY

The onset of the disease is on an average 10 to 15 days after the infection, but it may start from 1 to 20 days after the initial illness. Much the commonest symptom is hæmaturia. The urine may suddenly become claret-coloured, or smoky brown, and there is marked oliguria. Slight œdema, especially of the face or about the eyes, appears. Occasionally, there is vomiting, abdominal pain, headache and backache. In the more severe cases there is drowsiness. The blood-pressure is often raised and examination of the optic fundi may show papillœdema or retinal hæmorrhages. Occasionally, the attack is ushered in with a convulsion. Hypertensive encephalopathy, with severe drowsiness, coma, repeated convulsions, and cranial or even limb palsies together with retinal hæmorrhages, exudates and papillœdema, is an extremely rare but potentially fatal form of the illness.

In about one-fourth of the cases the onset is so insidious that, were it not for the hæmaturia and perhaps slight œdema, little would be suspected.

COURSE

The illness is variable in duration. In mild cases, with only slight oliguria and without œdema, the hæmaturia will disappear in about a week. In less mild cases, a noticeable increase in the output of urine generally heralds improvement; hæmaturia and albuminuria then diminish, but in a few cases there is a persistent slight albuminuria, together with the excretion of a few red cells and granular casts. The sedimentation rate in the latter cases may remain raised. These are the patients who are likely to progress to chronic nephritis.

In a severe case, oliguria is more prolonged and there may be anuria, perhaps with hypertension and drowsiness.

In the majority of cases, a hypochromic anæmia develops during the course of the illness.

PROGNOSIS

The immediate mortality is less than 2 per cent. Signs which suggest danger are convulsions, broncho-pneumonia, gastro-enteritis and a rising blood-urea after the first week of the disease.

There is a complete recovery in about 90 per cent. of cases. The remainder may pass into the latent or second stage (*see* p. 370) and be symptomless. They are able to undertake sport and resume ordinary life, but a microscopical examination of the urine will show that the renal process has not healed. Such cases may develop hypertension and renal failure later.

TREATMENT

It is wise during the first week of the illness to administer a full course of penicillin, whether septic foci are evident or not, in order to eradicate any persistent hæmolytic streptococcal infection. Subsequently, maintenance therapy with a smaller dosage of an oral penicillin should be continued as a prophylactic. Apart from this there is no specific treatment.

The patient should be kept in bed until the œdema and oliguria have disappeared and until either the urine has returned to normal, or the steady diminution in albuminuria and number of casts in the urine have ceased and the position has become static.

During the acute stage a record of the fluid intake and the urine output should be kept. Until the diuresis occurs it is advisable to restrict the fluid intake to one pint daily. This should be given in the form of barley water or fruit juice. Until the hæmaturia has abated and the blood-urea fallen to normal, the protein intake should be small; then it should be increased only gradually. Milk should be restricted in the early stages and the basal caloric needs should be covered by giving carbohydrate. Iron is given, once the acute stage is passed.

FOLLOW-UP

The patient should be observed for the next few months at fortnightly, and later monthly, intervals, when a check can be kept on the urine and blood-pressure. During this stage, prophylactic oral penicillin 125 mg. twice daily should be continued. In cases of recurrent or chronic tonsillitis, evidenced by fibrotic distortion of the tonsils and enlargement of the tonsillar glands, tonsillectomy is indicated.

2. Latent-stage Nephritis

There are usually no symptoms; occasionally there may be acute headaches, with some vomiting, and at times slight puffiness about the eyes. The child may be listless and fail to gain weight. A slight hypochromic anæmia responding poorly to oral iron may persist.

Examination of the urine shows traces of albumin. Red cells are present in excess, together with granular casts.

Cases in this stage may recover completely, or may pass gradually in the course of 5–10 years into chronic nephritis and uræmia. Sometimes they pass into the subacute or nephrotic stage.

3. Nephrotic Syndrome : Type 2 Nephritis and Nephrosis

This syndrome is diagnosed in cases showing massive albuminuria, a reduction in the serum albumin, a reversal of the albumin/globulin ratio and a rise in serum cholesterol. Œdema is often present also because the osmotic power of the plasma is impaired by the loss of albumin. Among several possible causes, the nephrotic syndrome can be a sequel of latent nephritis which may, in severe cases, continue for many years until a nephrotic phase is reached. Such cases usually show gradual worsening of renal function and a bad prognosis. The majority of nephrotic cases occurring in childhood do not have a history of latent nephritis; moreover, their maximum age incidence (2–4 years) is earlier than that of acute nephritis which is seldom seen before school age. These are the cases which are called *childhood nephrosis* or *pure nephrosis*. In general they have a better prognosis than the cases of latent nephritis which have reached a nephrotic phase. This is because the lesion responsible for nephrosis is sometimes reversible. Rarely, acute nephrosis may be seen in infancy. In such cases the ætiology appears to be different; certain cases resemble cystinosis (p. 130), whilst others are a recessively inherited form of tubular dysfunction.

PATHOLOGY

In the terminal stage, the kidney is swollen and engorged; microscopically the tubules show cloudy swelling and fatty degeneration, and the epithelium tends to be shed into the lumen, forming casts. The Malpighian tufts show marked destruction, and crescent formation may occur.

However, renal biopsy carried out on patients during the acute nephrotic phase has shown a varying picture.[1] In some, the classical

[1] Squire, J. R., Blainey, J. D., Hardwicke, J. (1957). *Brit. med. Bull.*, **13**, 43.
Blainey, J. D., Brewer, D. B., Hardwicke, J., Soothill, J. F. (1960). *Quart. J. Med.*, **53**, 235.

picture just described is seen in the biopsy material; in others, the pathological changes are absent or minimal. Such changes as are present may involve the glomeruli, as shown by dilatation of the capillaries, whilst in other patients there is thickening of the basement membrane and some hyaline degeneration of the tubules. The changes in the basement membrane are the hall-mark of nephrosis; it is these changes which are reversible in some cases and thus permit recovery to occur.

SYMPTOMS

Nephrosis is usually ushered in by the gradual onset of massive œdema, and vomiting if there is nitrogen retention. At intervals there may be acute exacerbations of this subacute condition. At these times the urine is concentrated and diminished in quantity. The œdema involves the face, limbs and all dependent parts, including the scrotum, penis and labia. The eyes may be completely closed. The heart is rapid, and death may take place from dilatation and acute heart failure.

The characteristic feature is the large amount of albumin to be found in the urine. Red blood-corpuscles may sometimes be present, with some granular and hyaline casts.

Blood-cholesterol is raised to between 300 and 1,000 mg. per 100 ml. The plasma albumin is greatly reduced, often to 1–2 G. per cent. with a consequent inversion of the usual albumin-globulin ratio of 2 : 1. The blood-urea is somewhat raised or may be normal. The blood-pressure is usually normal or only slightly raised.

DIFFERENTIAL DIAGNOSIS AND PROGNOSIS

The presence of hypertension, together with red cells and granular casts in the urine and a raised blood-urea, distinguishes the group of patients in whom there is progressive nephritis and a poor prognosis.

In the majority, the blood pressure will be normal, the urine will reveal a massive albuminuria with no formed elements and the blood-urea will be within normal limits. Many such cases[1] will undergo a remission either of a spontaneous nature or following an acute illness such as measles. Treatment with steroids appears to have dramatic results in many patients. In all, it is estimated that between 50–60 per cent. of patients with nephrosis make a complete recovery from their illness. The effect of long-term treatment with steroids cannot as yet be fully evaluated, nor can the prognostic significance of the histological findings at renal biopsy during the acute stage.

Patients with nephrosis are highly susceptible to intercurrent infections, among which cellulitis, peritonitis and particularly broncho-pneumonia are to be numbered.

[1] Lawson, D., Moncrieff, A., Payne, W. W. (1960). *Arch. Dis. Childh.*, **35**, 115.

TREATMENT

The long-term objective of treatment is to minimize or correct the renal damage; for this purpose corticosteroids are believed by numerous authorities[1] to be of value in a proportion of the cases. Antibiotics also play a part by preventing intercurrent infections which exacerbate the kidney lesion.

On the short term, symptomatic treatment is required particularly

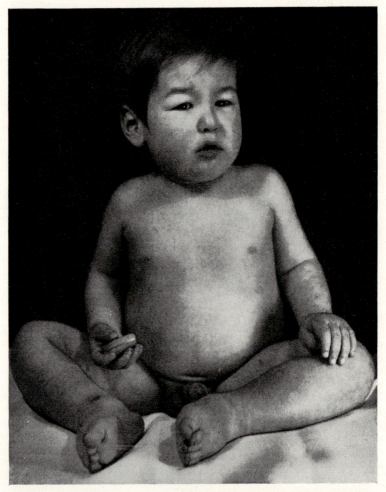

Fig. 42.—Nephrosis in a boy 16 months old. The puffy face and generalized œdema are characteristic.

[1] Recent Advances in Renal Disease (1960). *Proceedings of Royal College of Physicians Conference*, pp. 123–136. London: Pitman.

for the severe episodes of œdema; again, corticosteroids are considered by many authorities to be of direct value, but may need to be combined with other measures to overcome the negative nitrogen balance and to promote diuresis.

Management of Œdematous Phase.   The child is put to bed and given a high-protein, low-salt diet, with the fluid intake restricted to one pint daily.   Associated infections are treated with the appropriate antibiotic.

On such treatment, a proportion of the patients will lose their proteinuria and, following a brisk diuresis, their œdema and ascites. If the disappearance of the proteinuria and œdema is complete, the patient is followed up and regular urine examinations are carried out, but no additional treatment is given.

If, however, the proteinuria and œdema persist despite rest, dietary treatment and antibiotics, then corticosteroids should be given together with potassium replacement therapy (Appendix 2).   In cases of pure nephrosis there is usually a rapid improvement both in the proteinuria and œdema.   In a minority of cases, the corticosteroids are ineffective and other measures are added to the treatment.   These include diuretics, such as hydrochlorothiazide, used initially alone, but if ineffective in combination with spironolactone.   Attempts may be made to raise the serum-albumin level by the transfusion of specially prepared salt-free albumin, but this is unlikely to lead to more than transient benefit as long as massive proteinuria continues.   If all these measures fail, it is probable that the case is one with severe irreversible renal damage; but occasionally an unexpected remission may occur following an intercurrent illness, such as measles or malaria, in a child who has been unresponsive to ordinary treatment.

Long-Term Management.   The long-term treatment depends upon the initial response.   In children in whom there is rapid and complete clearance of proteinuria and œdema, long-term corticosteroid therapy with all its attendant dangers is hard to justify.   In the case of patients in whom proteinuria or œdema persists, or recurs after a transient remission, long-term steroid therapy (*see* p. 661) is given until complete clearance of the proteinuria has occurred.   In such circumstances potassium replacement therapy and prophylactic antibiotics (Appendix 1) form a part of the regime.   Such children need to be followed up for many years and further treatment is given if delayed relapses occur.

4. Chronic Nephritis (Chronic Bright's Disease with Uræmia and Hypertension)

In this stage, there may be no history of nephritis or there may have been a previous history of acute or subacute nephritis.   A precisely similar terminal picture may be seen as the end-result of chronic pyelonephritis or in severe congenital malformations of the renal tract, such as polycystic kidneys or severe bladder-neck obstruction. Chronic nephritis is more often seen in adolescence or adult life than in childhood.

Pathologically, all the elements of the kidney show destruction and fibrosis, and there is an increase of interstitial tissue, which tends to contract and produce the small granular or fibrotic kidney.

SYMPTOMS

There are symptoms of irreparable renal insufficiency—polyuria, thirst, headache, vomiting, retinal changes, hypertension, and dry skin. The urine shows albumin, epithelial cells and casts. The specific gravity of the urine becomes fixed at about 1·010 as the kidneys lose their ability to concentrate or dilute the urine.

Such cases frequently present with uræmia (*see* below) or occasionally with renal rickets (p. 375).

TREATMENT

A low-protein diet, with a low-urea production, is indicated, also bland fluid with fruit juice and carbohydrate, to make up the caloric intake. Often it is necessary to correct electrolyte disturbances, especially in the chronic case with renal rickets; but in most cases the outlook in this stage of the disease is practically hopeless.

Uræmia and Anuria

Uræmia occurs when renal failure is so marked that waste nitrogenous products accumulate in the blood and tissues. Other signs of renal failure include acidosis, phosphate retention and a fall in serum calcium.

Uræmia may be the result of a terminal nephritis, due either to chronic nephritis or irreversible renal damage from infection or severe congenital malformation of the renal tract. It may occur in severe cases of acute nephritis.

There is an additional group of patients in which there is sudden renal failure with anuria as a result of poisoning, anoxia, crush injury, incompatible blood transfusion, or an infection such as leptospirosis (*see* p. 615). In some of these patients the kidney damage may be reversible.

Finally, pre-renal uræmia may occur from such varied causes as repeated vomiting in intestinal obstruction, severe gastro-enteritis, liver disease, diabetic coma, acute adrenal insufficiency or in septicæmia, alkalosis and acute shock from any cause.

SYMPTOMS

The rapidity with which the symptoms develop will vary with the underlying condition. In the pre-renal uræmic cases especially, the clinical picture will be complicated by the symptoms of the associated condition and the attendant electrolyte disturbances.

Lassitude, muscular weakness, loss of appetite, coated tongue and sore mouth are some of the initial symptoms. Vomiting occurs, and sooner or later severe diarrhœa may be present. The temperature is, as a rule, subnormal, and coma appears at the end. Symptoms of tetany, with carpopedal spasm due to the low blood-calcium, occasionally occur. Finally, the overbreathing or hyperpnœa of acidosis is often seen as a terminal symptom.

Cerebral symptoms in company with hypertension may develop in both acute and in terminal nephritis, especially when uræmia is present. Major epileptiform convulsions, often known as " hypertensive encephalopathy, " occur; lesser degrees of these attacks are headaches, giddiness, amaurosis and mono- or hemiplegia; retinitis is a constant feature, and flame-shaped hæmorrhages are to be seen. There are no retinal changes or fits in uræmia until the blood-pressure rises.

TREATMENT

The palliative treatment of chronic nephritis has already been described (p. 374).

In cases of acute nephritis or of lower-nephron nephrosis (crush injury, incompatible blood transfusion, etc.) anuria should always be regarded as a medical emergency. All dietary protein should be forbidden and the calorie requirements given as hypertonic glucose. Fifty per cent. glucose may be given by stomach tube, or ten to twenty per cent. glucose intravenously. If the anuria persists for more than forty-eight hours, but yet the underlying condition is one which may be reversible, the patient should be transferred to a special centre where dialysis may be carried out (by artificial kidney).

In patients with extra-renal uræmia, the underlying cause must, if possible, be corrected. The adjustment of the disturbed electrolyte balance is discussed in Appendix 4.

Renal Rickets, Renal Dwarfism

ÆTIOLOGY AND PATHOLOGY

The renal lesion may be congenital, and be first noted when the infant is a few months old. The renal abnormality varies; it includes congenital hypoplastic kidneys and chronic urinary obstruction from congenital urethral valve. At necropsy, the kidney is often seen to be extremely small, weighing no more than one ounce. Microscopically, it is grossly fibrotic, and cysts are sometimes present.

Renal dwarfism is, however, more commonly seen in older children, of six to twelve years, brought to the orthopædic surgeon for knock-knee. Occasionally a history of chronic pyuria may be obtained, but usually there is no significant history of any previous renal symptoms. Undoubtedly some cases are secondary to pyelonephritis going on to chronic nephritis with osteodystrophy. In such cases, the brunt of the infection has fallen on both glomeruli and tubules.

SYMPTOMS

The infants are markedly rachitic.   Further examination will show polyuria, polydypsia, renal acidosis and high blood-urea.

Older children present for knock-knee or failure to grow.   They are anæmic, with a tendency to develop bouts of uræmia at intervals.   The blood-urea may be 100 mg. per 100 ml., or more.

DIAGNOSIS

The differential diagnosis includes the other causes of rickets (see pp. 119–123).

The urine is pale, excessive, with an extremely low specific gravity, say 1·004.   It contains a trace of albumin, some hyaline casts, and 1 or at most 2 per cent. of urea.

There is usually excessive thirst, with high blood-pressure, and retinal hæmorrhages appearing later.

The serum occasionally shows a low calcium, down to 5 mg. per 100 ml., instead of the normal 10 mg., and a phosphorus of, say, 10 mg. instead of the normal 5 mg.   The alkali reserve may be low.

PROGNOSIS AND TREATMENT

The infants survive only a few months, perhaps a year or two at most.   The older children rarely survive many years, and death takes place from uræmia.   Treatment with alkalis, such as Albright's solution (p. 141), will often prove helpful by correcting the associated renal acidosis.   High dosage of vitamin D 10,000 i.u. may be tried cautiously but should be abandoned if azotæmia increases.   The removal of the cause of the kidney lesion, such as a valve in the posterior urethra, should be undertaken if possible, but operations are badly tolerated.

A low-protein diet and iron should be given, and much care taken to prevent infections.

NEOPLASMS

By far the most common malignant tumour of the kidney in childhood is the *nephroblastoma* or *Wilms' embryoma*.   Very much less common are *renal sarcomata* or *carcinomata*.   The kidney may become secondarily invaded by the sympathetic nerve tumour, the *neuroblastoma* (*see* p. 378), which often originates in the suprarenal medulla.

Wilms' Embryoma

This is a malignant tumour arising within the substance of the kidney, partially encapsulated from it, and containing a variety of embryonic tissue, immature glomeruli, and fully-formed tubules, as well as muscle fibres and cartilage cells.

It is more common in males than in females: 90 per cent. of cases in the under-fives and 60 per cent. in the under-threes.

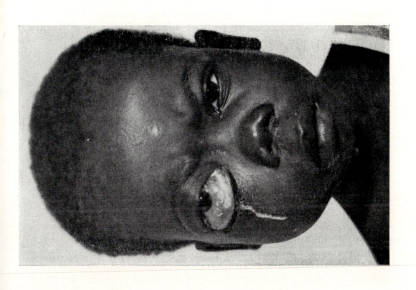

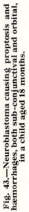

Fig. 43.—Neuroblastoma causing proptosis and haemorrhages, both sub-conjunctival and orbital, in a child aged 18 months.

Fig. 44. (*right*).—Malignant lymphoma, a neoplasm prevalent in the equatorial belt of Africa. Resembling lymphosarcoma, it usually presents in the jaw or retro-orbital region (*see* P. 621).

Symptoms usually commence insidiously, with enlarged abdomen, abdominal pain, hæmaturia (uncommon) and wasting, with pallor and debility, as the commonest, in that order. On palpation, a firm and painless mass can be felt in one loin, and bowel can be felt over it at times. The blood shows nothing but anæmia, and there is no characteristic fever. The tumour may be mistaken for a hydronephrosis, but a pyelogram excludes this. In a suprarenal neuroblastoma the growth is more central, and secondaries in the liver and bones, expecially the skull, are the rule. The tumour is encapsulated and easily removed, but recurrence is common in the operation bed. Metastases occur in the liver and lungs in 20 per cent. of cases. Early operation, combined with pre- and post-operative x-ray therapy, is carried out when practicable and is successful in perhaps a quarter of the cases.

Neuroblastoma of Adrenal Medulla

A tumour composed of nervous tissue is found in connection with the medulla of the suprarenal or of the sympathetic nerve ganglia in the thorax or abdomen. The tumour is found histologically to consist of relatively undifferentiated round cells often arranged in rosette fashion with a palisade network of the interstitial tissue. The tumour forms metastases by direct, lymphatic and bloodstream spread. Incidence in males is twice that in females. The age is usually between one and four years.

CLINICAL PICTURE

The symptoms that occur as a result of metastases are often the first indication of anything abnormal, although occasionally enlargement of the abdomen due to the presence of the tumour may be the first symptom. The bones are the usual site for metastases with progressive anæmia of a leuco-erythroblastic type (*see* p. 333) from interference with bone-marrow function, together with pain and local tenderness. Skull, ribs, spine and long bones can all be affected. The brain may also be involved and proptosis of the eye, together with local swellings of the skull due to bony metastases, may occur. Lung secondaries may develop. Local spread involves surrounding structures, particularly liver, kidney and pancreas. X-rays of the skull and long bones show mottling at the site of the metastases.

DIAGNOSIS

Wilms' embryoma does not show the early metastases which this tumour does. Osteomyelitis, scurvy, leukæmia and rheumatic fever may cause confusion in the early stages.

TREATMENT

Early operation with x-ray therapy may be tried but usually secondary deposits are already present. Recently, prolonged remissions have been claimed by giving vitamin B_{12} by intramuscular injection, in doses of 1,000 micrograms, on alternate days.   This large dose can be continued for two years without disadvantage.   It is still not possible to say if permanent cure is possible by this treatment.

Ganglioneuroma of Adrenal Medulla

This type of tumour is highly differentiated into ganglion cells and is usually of a non-malignant character.   It is discovered often as an incidental finding during abdominal palpation; it may occasionally reach a considerable size.

OTHER DISORDERS

Enuresis

IN the great majority of cases of nocturnal enuresis no physical abnormality can be found on examination.   In only 14 per cent. of his cases did Nash[1] find evidence of organic disease.

General metabolic diseases, such as diabetes insipidus, diabetes mellitus and chronic nephritis, must be excluded as well as neurological disorders such as meningo-myelocele and mental retardation.   Local urinary-tract abnormalities, such as urethral valvular obstruction (*see* p. 363) and urinary infections, must also be considered.   In this section will be considered the management of the great majority of enuretic children in whom no such organic abnormalities are present.

ÆTIOLOGY AND DIAGNOSIS

In general terms, the acquisition of urinary continence is a gradual process, with episodes of improvement followed by relapses which should be regarded as entirely normal.   Most children, however, have acquired permanent control by day by the age of two-and-a-half years, with lapses only during illness or extreme emotional upset. Night control should be permanent by the age of three to five years, and nocturnal enuresis should not be regarded as abnormal in any way until after that age.   These ages are the upper limits; many children acquire complete control at a considerably earlier age.

The cases of enuresis fall into three groups:

(1) Those in which enuresis has been persistent since birth without the normal phases of improvement and relapse.

(2) Those in which control is acquired by the fourth year and in which enuresis develops after a subsequent interval.

(3) Those in which control is normal by night but not by day. This group is almost always associated with local abnormality of the urinary tract and requires careful urological investigation.

In those cases in which organic disease plays no part, many factors may contribute to the ætiology.   The basic abnormality appears to be a persistence of, or a reversion to, an infantile type of bladder which to some extent is automatic, the normal relaxation of tone on distension and the higher cerebral control being absent.   In the

[1] Nash, D. F. E. (1951).   *Ann. roy. Coll. Surg. Engl.*, **8**, 193.

Group 1 cases, poor habit-training, unsatisfactory home life in general, and, perhaps, hereditary influence are important factors. In the Group 2 cases, emotional upsets, prolonged separation of the child from his home, severe illnesses, including transient urinary infections, and over-excitement may be responsible.

TREATMENT

A careful general examination should be carried out to make sure that the disease is not due to one of the organic diseases mentioned above.

The defects in management should be corrected so far as possible, proper habit-training instituted and in older children causes of over-excitement, such as evening visits to greyhound race-tracks or too much television, forbidden.

It should be fully explained to the parents and the child that enuresis is not a crime on the child's part and that as he grows older normal control will develop. In older children practice in holding their water for increasing periods during the day assists the development of cerebral control of the bladder and helps to give confidence.

One of the most important aspects of this disability is the child's outlook towards his complaint. In most cases, and certainly in the most difficult cases, a too serious view is taken by the mother. The child is cautioned and urged to try to be dry. He is commended when successful and reprimanded when unsuccessful. He is impressed with the importance of overcoming his failing, and with the fact that success or failure will make or mar his whole future. All this tends to place a conscious or subconscious strain on the child. An air of optimism about the whole matter must be carefully cultivated by those in charge; indifference should be shown when he fails and praise when he succeeds. He should occupy a room by himself, so that he alone knows when he has succeeded or failed. No discussion by the family or any outsiders should be allowed.

It is advisable to insist that the last drink of the day is given not later than 4 p.m., and that the child is wakened to pass his water when the parents retire to bed.

Drugs. It is doubtful whether any of the drugs in routine use for the treatment of enuresis has any more than placebo value. Indeed, some authorities deprecate their use altogether, suggesting that the giving of drugs tends to perpetuate the condition. Others are of the opinion that ephedrine hydrochloride and belladonna are of value in treatment.

Ephedrine hydrochloride may be given at bed-time, 15 mg. to a child of three to six years, and 30 mg. to an older child; this may not be a big enough dose, and more may be given if it is ineffective. It is often best to split the dose, giving one portion at bed-time and one when he is lifted at 10 p.m. If, after a week's trial, there is no improvement, the younger child's dose is increased by 15 mg. and that of the older by 30 mg. This can be repeated until 120 mg. are being taken by the older child, or until enuresis ceases. Dextroamphetamine 5–10 mg. is sometimes helpful for a child who sleeps very heavily.

Tincture of belladonna 0·3 ml. can be given three times daily to relax the wall of the bladder.

In children of ten years and older, the alarm blanket device may be found to be very effective. Two sheets incorporating metal strips and separated by an ordinary sheet are placed under the patient. When urine penetrates through the ordinary sheet an electric circuit is completed causing an alarm bell to ring. In this way a reflex inhibition of micturition during sleep may be established with permanent benefit.

PROGNOSIS

There is no doubt that our knowledge of the origin, and therefore our treatment, of enuresis remains very inadequate. The great majority of cases improve naturally, although treatment accelerates the process in many of them. Very few cases of enuresis persist after the age of puberty.

The place of psychiatric treatment in enuresis is discussed on p. 385. Child guidance is best reserved for those cases in which there is evidence of additional psychological disturbance apart from enuresis.

Meatal Ulcer

In circumcised male children who are still at the age when they cannot be kept dry both day and night, there is a tendency for an ulcer to form at the external meatus of the urethra. A crust forms and, when the urine is passed, this is torn off and remains bleeding, only to re-form before the next micturition. The condition is due to an ammonia dermatitis. (For treatment, *see* p. 502.)

Balanitis

In infancy this is probably due to the presence of napkin dermatitis, whilst in older boys poor hygiene is responsible. The preputial swelling may be great, and there is pain on micturition. In infants, the napkin area should be left exposed and the penis bathed with Roccal 1 in 80 every three hours. In older boys recurrent balanitis or paraphimosis may sometimes be corrected by training in proper cleanliness, but is often cured only by circumcision.

Hydrocele

There may be a hydrocele of the tunica vaginalis or of the cord. In all cases which persist for more than a few months, a hernia accompanying the hydrocele should be suspected. Spontaneous cure is common; therefore, unless great inconvenience is caused, nothing need be done until the child is continent, say at the age of two years, when an operation for both hernia and hydrocele is advisable.

Vulvo-vaginitis

The frequency of this condition varies with the climate and social class and is less commonly seen in cold countries and among the well-to-do. The proportion due to gonococci varies in different parts of the world; in the United Kingdom probably less than one per cent. is so caused at present. It occurs most commonly between the ages of two and five years, but may occur at any age. It is more prevalent in summer.

Among the non-gonorrhœal cases the chief source of infection is the *Staphylococcus aureus*, probably transmitted manually from nasal or skin infection. Another source is the fæces, the vulva being infected especially by *E. coli* and the intestinal streptococci. Occasionally, pneumococci are found or *monilia* (thrush). Threadworms, setting up an irritation about the anus and causing scratching of the anus and vulva, are often responsible for the spread of the organisms. The presence of a foreign body in the vagina should be suspected in cases resistant to ordinary treatment.

CLINICAL PICTURE

The vulva is red and swollen, and during the acute stage a thick purulent discharge can be seen appearing over the vaginal orifice and covering the labia. Pressure over the urethra may show a urethral discharge. There is pain on micturition in a proportion of cases. In the non-gonorrhœal type, the discharge tends to be less thick and watery and to have an offensive odour, and pain on micturition is less common.

TREATMENT

Bacteriological examination is indicated followed by treatment with the appropriate sulphonamide or antibiotic. Lotions can also be used, e.g. a 1 in 80 solution of Roccal. A search for threadworms (*see* p. 631) should be made. If a foreign body in the vagina is suspected, the child should be examined under a general anæsthetic and the foreign body removed.

CHAPTER 18

Emotional Disorders

OUR understanding of the nervous child or, as he is often called, the " problem child " (instead of the child with problems) has gained much from the psychoanalytic concept of personality development. Melanie Klein,[1] Anna Freud,[2, 3] and Winnicott,[4] to mention only three psychologists who have written about their work with children, have offered explanations of many psycho-pathological mechanisms. Not all their theories will be accepted by pædiatricians, and inevitably, in such a complex field as the inter-relation of mind, body and emotions, much will remain speculative. At least it cannot be said that this aspect of pædiatrics is stagnant. Far from being that, it is increasingly difficult to provide as much skilled help as is looked for, in pædiatric departments, for those children whose nervous ailments arise from psychological causes.

Hector Cameron[5] did much among pædiatricians to call attention to the unhappy state of so-called " nervous exhaustion " children. His description of such a child's response to stress, whether of an inter-current infection or arising from emotional conflict, remains a classic.

Usually these are only children, or the youngest by several years, and are too much thrown into the company of adults, thus being constantly on "mental tiptoes". Much benefit is derived from early kindergarten school, even at the age of three or four years. Here a child is taught to sit still, relax, and play along organized lines; mental and physical rest is obtained.

Emotional Maturation

No understanding of an individual child's difficulties can leave out the very important personal background of his family relationships. Inevitably, there are no tests of the quality of mother-child relationship, but no amount of good doctoring can take the place of good mothering. The helplessness of early infancy renders the human young vulnerable to every kind of neglect. On the other hand, successful breast-feeding means that a baby must be held warmly and closely during every feed, and if a good balance is established from the

---

[1] Klein, M. (1948). " Contributions to Psycho-analysis." London: Hogarth Press.
[2] Freud, A. (1946). " The Psycho-analytic Treatment of Children." (New Revised Edition). London: Imago.
[3] Freud, A. (1961). " Psychosomatic Aspects of Pædiatrics." Oxford: Pergamon Press.
[4] Winnicott, D. W. (1958). Collected Papers. " Through Pædiatrics to Psycho-analysis." London: Tavistock Publications.
[5] Cameron, H. (1945). " The Nervous Child." London: Oxford University Press.

383

start between what the baby needs and what the mother has to give, then this can become the foundation stone of a sense of trust in a good and giving environment.   Frustration has no stimulant effect on a baby's ability to learn adaptations, for the simple reason that he is not equipped with such capacities in his early weeks.   His few wants, all closely linked with biological needs and satisfactions, tend to be restricted in scope, and it is small wonder that his mother comes to be identified with the source of food and of all other good things.   Thus, human relationships become an essential part of a child's growth and development, a factor which gives him both a greater vulnerability and the capacity for a more complex development than is open to the young of non-human species, who can so soon depend on instinct and their own efforts to get what they want.

If the mother-figure is vital to the earliest phase of development, it follows that the father's role is complementary and in no sense secondary.   A father who is not there, or who chooses to contract out of his obligations, or who is a source of fear to either mother or child is likely to upset the balance of relationships within the family.   Similar tensions can be seen where grandparents, or even neighbours or school-teachers, become threatening figures within the child's imagination and so disturb his sense of belonging in a safe place.   Perhaps one of the greatest tests of his sense of security arises with the birth of a sibling. Nutritionally, he is not threatened as is his more primitive counterpart (*see* p. 592) but he commonly reacts by a regression and a temporary period of difficult and demanding behaviour.   Unless this is understood, advice to " ignore the tantrums " may only succeed in increasing the child's feeling that his loss will overwhelm him.   At these difficult phases in the development of a normal child, a mother often unconsciously does exactly the right thing by boosting his pride in new achievement or by allowing the father to take over more of the day-to-day care.   Here may be where an able and advanced child can take encouragement and stimulus from joining a nursery school or class. There is, however, real danger in supposing that merely sending him out of the home will get things right.

The stage at which the child is beginning to depend less absolutely on parental ties has been called by Susan Isaacs[1] the period of *normal negativism*, for in it he meets his first real frustrations.   By increasing his motor capacity, he has already learned to run more risks, and is inevitably more often restricted.   He is now expected to do simple things for himself in feeding, toilet and going to bed, which formerly were left easy or done for him.   It can now be seen why it is so important that he should be able to accept some authority without question, not because he has been drilled to do so but as part of a continuing experience of being able to trust himself to the hands of his particular authoritarians, his parents.   Their skill as parents will

---

[1] Isaacs, S. (1932). "The Nursery Years."   London: Routledge.

be greatly taxed by the child's need to test out both their endurance and their benevolence.

By the time school age is reached, the phase of conflict should have passed, enabling the child to emerge into some sort of independence and awareness of himself. Reiteration of these past conflicts will tend to recur, but his maturity, helped by his native endowment and good health, should at all times re-assert itself. It is usual, in what is called the latency period, for a real expansion in intellectual interests to take place, whereas often in adolescence there is a physiological slowing-up and even a throw back to some of the earlier emotional conflict. If these phases are seen as successive stages in developing independence, first as a child within the family and later as an individual within the world at large, the doctor and the nurse caring for a disturbed child can do much to avoid adding to his emotional difficulties.

Disorders of Habit

These are, of course, not confined to early childhood, but when bed-wetting or night fears are prolonged into later school age they can be seen as islands of unresolved infancy, and can often be related to the way in which early training was handled. Obviously, some training must be given, but each child has his own pace of development and it is not always easy to understand why one child, and not another, has so much difficulty in achieving maturity.

There can be little doubt that fantasy plays an enormous part in the lives of small children. At the same time that this is true, they are also living in daily close awareness of what goes on in their bodies. Feeding, sleeping and elimination can all in turn become linked with fantasy, a point shown in children's dreams and in their drawings. Battles over feeding, and potting, and sleep can thus be caught up and elaborated in fantasy, and can become threatening situations over which the child feels powerless. Or in reverse, they can become pleasurable in their own right and unconsciously exploited as means to an end. Thus, the jealous and deposed toddler, in his reversion to soiling, or his demand to be fed with his meals, may be demonstrating his need to be an infant for rather longer, while at the same time he lays claim to an infant's share of mother-dependence. He will not consciously work this out as a mechanism, so that exasperation with him can only increase his anxiety. Particularly at this stage hospitalization can easily fixate in him a feeling of defeat and despair, since by separation he seems to have lost his source of security by means of which he retains a relationship to those around him. The pendulum may have swung too far in the direction of awareness of danger in early separation; but persistent symptoms of habit disorder merit a careful study.

PSYCHOSOMATIC ILLNESS

JUST as every pattern of somatic behaviour, such as waking and sleeping, feeding and elimination, can be drawn on as a child's means of expressing conflict and maladjustment, so can almost any aspect of bodily illness be caught up and used as a manifestation of anxiety. Often there is an onset in physical disturbance, and, as Cameron showed, these anxious children tend to have a poor resistance to infection. Further than this, it is probably sound medicine to regard every childhood illness as likely to have a psychological repercussion. Put another way, the emotional care of the sick child cannot be separated from the physical care. The group of psychosomatic illnesses is therefore always increasing in range.

The Allergic Group

Elsewhere (p. 263 *et seq.*) the role of emotion in precipitating attacks of asthma has been stressed, and resistant cases of asthma should be given the benefit of psychiatric help whenever the patient and his parents are able to accept it, although the suggestion that a psychological factor may be at work often produces alarm and hostility. Nor is psychiatry by any means always able to achieve good results. A combined approach can sometimes offer more than either line taken separately, provided the pædiatrician and the child psychiatrist understand each other's language and realize that in some degree the approach of each is at variance with the other—a " double-crossing " situation which the patient or his parents may be ready to exploit!

Gastro-intestinal Disorders

Classifying in this way illustrates the difficulty of producing any clear-cut nosology in the concepts used by child psychiatrists.

Is constipation a disease or a habit disorder? Does it become the former only when it is associated with colonic inertia and a more or less permanently stretched bowel with great proneness to overflow incontinence? The same question could be asked of vomiting, or of Cameron's clinical picture of what is now called the periodic syndrome (p. 212), or of abdominal migraine (p. 214).

Abdominal pain can appear to be quite unrelated to physical causes, and if treatment uncovers an emotional problem, relief of which removes the attacks of pain, the situation then becomes comprehensible. Quite often it seems as if an initial disturbance of a physical kind undergoes a hysterical prolongation of symptoms associated with anxiety. As long as this is borne in mind, the pædiatrician can avoid subscribing actively to such prolongation by long courses of medical or surgical treatment (pp. 210–212).

Gastric and duodenal ulcer are not unknown in childhood and here, too, investigation of underlying personality difficulties, which might foster a chronic state of tension, may yield results.

Ulcerative colitis presents an unsolved problem where an association with strongly repressed emotional difficulty, even in very young patients, seems to offer at least part of the explanation for the onset of this disease (Higgins, 1954–5)[1].

Anorexia Nervosa

One of the rare complications of puberty, particularly in girls, is that of severe loss of appetite. Such children show no organic disease. Their mental outlook towards their surroundings, including parents, relations, food and life in general, is abnormal and psychopathic, with marked depression. They cannot be roused to take an interest in anything and, if left alone, may die. Fat children, in an effort to slim, may lapse into this condition, and it should be recognized that slimming carries this danger. In girls with anorexia whose periods have begun, amenorrhœa and some increase in hirsutes is the rule.

It must be recognized in all cases that this is a serious disorder, and it carries a high ultimate mortality. Even cases which improve for a time often relapse. From the psychiatric angle, the depression is in itself a risk and the whole illness may be an attempted suicide in the sense that it acts out a need, felt by the patient, to express her unworthiness to live. Some cases attempt a more direct kind of suicide and they therefore require psychiatric care rather than pædiatric nursing. While separation from home and parents may be needed, it should never be thought that removal from home is likely to effect a cure in itself. Good nursing, scrupulous attention to diet and even forcible feeding are all only adjuncts to a thorough investigation of the underlying emotional factors.

Motor Disorders, Tics and Habit Spasm

Tics seldom begin before the age of about three years, but probably six years is a commoner age, and the condition may continue into adult life.

Afflicted children are often the offspring of nervy parents, and they are thin, white-faced and over-active, both mentally and physically. Very often there has been some slight organic lesion, such as a mild conjunctivitis, or a tight collar, which has given rise to blinking or jerking of the head. The local irritation disappears, but the functional habit continues. Habit spasm is worse at the end of the day. It is primarily a sign of nervous tension.

There is often blinking of eyes, twitching of corners of the mouth, shrugging of shoulders, sudden rotation of the head, or hopping when walking. Sometimes audible tics, such as snorting, grunting, clearing the throat, short hacking coughs, or bleating noises are heard.

DIFFERENTIAL DIAGNOSIS

This lies chiefly between chorea and habit spasm. In chorea, the more attention paid to the child the worse the movements. In habit

[1] Higgins, R. (1954–55). *Gt Ormond Str. J.*, **8**, 99.

spasm, on the other hand, the movements may be more or less under voluntary control, the child being able to stop them temporarily himself. In chorea, the movement is never the same twice, different parts being continually involved. In habit spasm, the same movement is made over and over again. When one tic ceases, there is a tendency for a new tic to arise elsewhere.

It is interesting that some severe chronic instances of tic occur in adults who have in earlier life suffered from rheumatic chorea. This association suggests an underlying motor instability determining the choice of symptom. The hysterical tics, particularly those with vocal accompaniments, are often exceedingly difficult to cure, and even long and careful psychotherapy may fail to reveal the underlying anxiety; this is perhaps the more so since children who have this condition present a disturbing element at home or in the classroom. They are often told that they will grow out of it, but the motor habit has become a confirmed one by the time an attempt is made to understand it. Needless to say, the greatest care must be taken to exclude organic causes; for example, the rare condition of torsion spasm is in the first instance often incorrectly diagnosed as either a tic or an hysterical gait.

Fits and Faints

True unconsciousness in the form of a syncopal attack can be caused by emotional stress. Further, in an epileptic child, even where the EEG shows an epileptic diathesis, fits may occur more frequently when the child is distressed and under tension than in times of well-organized activity. Such convulsions can hardly, however, be labelled " psychosomatic " since this, or indeed any physical disorder, can be caught up in an existing anxiety situation. The differential diagnosis is, however, of great importance where very slight attacks of faintness are difficult to distinguish from *petit mal*, or where either is regarded as an hysterical manifestation. In children, the simulation of unconsciousness and the exploitation of any such attack is uncommon. Usually the quality of the onset and a careful investigation can establish the true diagnosis (*see* p. 453 *et seq.*).

Sleep Disorders

In the Infant. Nasal obstruction from a cold or catarrh is probably the commonest cause of broken sleep. A drop of 0·5-per cent. ephedrine solution into each nostril will help to clear the nasal passages. They may be cleared mechanically with pledgets of cotton-wool, or the infant may be made to sneeze. It is important to ensure that the infant does not sleep on his back.

Over-feeding, especially when the baby is not being held up afterwards to " break " or bring up the wind, tends to cause colic and indigestion, and with each bout of colic during the night the baby tends to cry out. Underfeeding, with consequent hunger-pains, will likewise disturb the infant. An adequate feed will cure this.

Although there is no scientific evidence to support the supposition, it is a remarkable fact that a great many children, who have seldom had a complete night's sleep during primary dentition, sleep soundly after cutting the last tooth.

" Hot " children require very little bed-clothing, and " cold " children may require bed-socks and hot-water bottles if they are to sleep the night through. Each child should be studied individually.

Older Children. Children living an indoor life may sleep badly because of a lack of fresh air and exercise. Late sleeping in the morning should be discouraged. Bed-wetting may wake a child, as he is cold and uncomfortable. As a result of bed-wetting, a meatal ulcer may develop; each time the urine is passed the child wakes because of painful micturition. Treatment is outlined on p. 501.

Some children are fanciful, and see in the shadows frightening objects. Such children should be encouraged to speak out, to reassure themselves, and should be given a night-light temporarily. The door of the bedroom should be left open, so that they can hear others passing by. Other children call out in the early part of the evening and will not settle off without several visits from the parents or nurse. Very often this form of exhibitionism follows the arrival of the new baby. If this be the case, the new infant should be placed asleep in the room with this child, and left in his charge. He must be told to be quiet, or he will wake the baby. He should be allowed to have his particular toy or plaything. Firmness and understanding will get round this short phase.

Some children go to sleep promptly, but wake either very early or during the night, quite refreshed and playful, and do not appear to require further sleep. It may be that they are having too much rest and insufficient exercise and fresh air. If necessary, they should be put to bed a little later. If awake in the night, they should be attended to, but if dry and warm they must be very firmly put down, and it must be made plain to them that this is not the time for play. Such children are sometimes better in a room by themselves, where slight noises will not wake them if they are light sleepers, and where, once awake, they can croon themselves to sleep again without disturbing others.

Yet other children are read to and played with during the last hour before bedtime. This may so " work them up " and stimulate them that it takes some time for them to become placid and quiescent enough to go to sleep. Such stimulation should be stopped.

It should be the aim to restrict the use of hypnotic drugs, in order to break a habit of wakefulness and to establish a normal sleep rhythm, to short courses (not more than two weeks). They should be used only when the simple measures described above have failed to achieve a normal sleeping habit.

Night Terrors

Repeated night terrors are less common than in the past. Such attacks must be carefully distinguished from epileptic seizures (p. 453), and the EEG findings are of value in this respect.

ANXIETY STATES

CHILDHOOD neurosis rarely takes the clear-cut forms of the adult disorders. An over-anxious child may appear truculent and aggressive, he may steal in an attempt to reinforce his confidence, he may wet his bed or vomit his food, or he may appear timid, shy, and withdrawn. He may show some or all of these facets of disturbed behaviour at different times.

Behind any anxiety manifestation is usually a deeper failure in relationships within the family. Some anxiety should be a normal part of growing up; it is met and adequately buffered by parental love and understanding. In some families, however, parents are unable to achieve this. They may themselves be anxious, or immature or may seek to compensate for a deeply rejecting attitude by an overlay of solicitude. Such attitudes are by no means consciously held, and for this reason it is often found that parents need help as much and as individually as their children. It is therefore better not to proffer good advice nor to attempt reassurance in such states, but to take time to try to understand what is really happening.

PSYCHOSES

NOWHERE is anxiety so clearly shown in every department of the child's organization of himself as in the psychotic states, where in fact disorganization and disintegration of the personality have taken place.

At one time, the psychoses of early childhood were regarded as excessively rare. Now a number of cases, which were formerly regarded as disturbed mental defectives, are seen as the end result of a failure to maintain an integrated development in the face of the threat of an overwhelming anxiety. Whether the particular vulnerability lies in the child's genetic endowment or in his nurture is still a matter for conjecture.

Grounds for the latter view are sometimes afforded by these children's parents, who are themselves rigid in their demands and emotionally arid. They may show an intellectual interest in precocious achievement while seeming to be unaware of how different their child is from his fellows. Sometimes they tolerate, perhaps because they have to, extremely odd behaviour. Such children on the other hand are often excessively disturbed by any small and apparently insignificant change in the environment. New foods are rejected and new toys are ignored; there seems to be an obsessional need to keep everything exactly the same and for the child to function montonously along one well-worn path. Thus, ritual behaviour and stereotyped mannerisms are very commonly seen. The psychotic child is often restless, his tense and anxious expression contrasting with this bird-like agility of movement. He may climb and poise himself without any fear, but scream uncontrollably at the bark of a dog or the sight of a fly, if these happen to be for him the objects which disturb him. His speech may be limited at first to a rather stilted diction, then to repetitive phrases and finally may be replaced by mutism. When this stage is reached there is often an associated regression, so that a previously clean child comes to be incontinent and to need feeding with his meals, and dressing and undressing. Parents often realize that it is a profound negativism rather than any real mental incapacity that makes him behave in this way. Nevertheless, it is at this stage that so often the condition can be mistaken for mental deficiency.

Perhaps the most striking feature is the extreme solitariness of such children. They pay little attention to what goes on around them and they withdraw from any attempt to interest them or to break into their self-absorption. Thus, they cease to learn, and administrative action, such as institutionalization or deeming the child ineducable, may be required. Even with intensive psychotherapy, the prognosis is doubtful and many seem doomed to irreversible disintegration, although no certain morbid anatomy has ever been established. It is interesting to note how some of these features, such as the solitariness, the restlessness and the tendency to stereotyped behaviour, occur for a time in the organic dementias, such as *tuberose sclerosis* (p. 447), only to be overtaken by the tide of advancing and increasing obvious mental failure. In the psychotic child, mental failure remains a failure of integration rather than a physical and mental reduction to helplessness.

BEHAVIOUR DISORDERS

THERE is no clear line between the anxiety states and the behaviour disorders, the distinction being based on the prominence of symptoms. The behaviour disorders are usually taken as those in which neurotic anxiety and unhappiness is less obvious; it must, however, not be assumed that these are absent.

Children whose behaviour is so disordered that they need treatment include those showing violent temper tantrums, stealing, aggressiveness towards others, and, in the psychopathic states, an apparent absence of concern regarding the harm that they cause.

A detailed discussion of juvenile delinquency and of the law in relation to juvenile offenders hardly comes within the scope of a pædiatric textbook, but one or two points deserve mention. Stott[1] and others have shown that there is a high correlation between broken homes and the more severe behaviour disorders. This is

---

[1] Stott, D. H. (1950). "Delinquency and Human Nature." Carnegie U.K. Trust.

understandable when the acceptance of good parental authority is seen as an essential part of normal development. Almost as important as this, is that parents and children should remain closely in contact whenever possible, and particularly during the formative years of early childhood.

Chronic or recurrent illness remains one of the commoner causes of separation in early childhood, and all is not well with the child who seems happier in hospital than he is at home. Every effort should be made to avoid long separations and to mitigate these by making parents' visits a real contact and a link between home and hospital. Bowlby's[1] work has underlined these points, but since the disordered behaviour does not occur in hospital but after the child goes home, there is still a risk of complacency.

EDUCATIONAL DIFFICULTIES

WHEN children fail to learn, they may do so from a variety of causes. Intelligence may be at fault and the child may be taxed beyond his capacities. (Intelligence testing is discussed on p. 23.) Bearing in mind that however skilfully it is devised and administered, an intelligence test remains a human estimate and therefore open to human error, it is still the most accurate method of estimating a child's ability. In skilled hands, a test should do rather more than this. The child's approach to a standard situation, his response to a need to work more quickly, his reactions to failure and to encouragement and the personal interest of the psychologist all provide situations which tell us not only of his ability but something of the kind of child he is.

No educational failure should be assessed without such a test, and further work may be needed to measure attainment in standard subjects such as reading and arithmetic.

Educational Retardation and Specific Disabilities

In some cases normal potential intelligence fails to function because a child is held back by sheer lack of learning. Through illness, he may have missed essential earlier stages, and a succession of quite minor illnesses can bring this about when it results in several broken terms early on in a child's school life. The moderately dull child is very apt to be adversely affected in this way and will seem to lack interest and incentive to catch up.

In others, a more specific difficulty in building up memory patterns, almost suggestive of an aphasic condition, results in a failure to learn to read (alexia) alongside evident abilities in dealing with non-verbal material. A similar severe degree of failure in number work (acalculia) is more rarely seen. For these conditions special remedial teaching and endless patience may be required. Difficulties clear-cut

[1] Bowlby, J. (1951). " Maternal Care and Mental Health." Geneva: W.H.O.

and of this degree are rare; very common is the general sense of defeat and discouragement in a child who seems to be academically "stuck." Every effort should be made to uncover underlying fears and inhibitions. Often jealousy of a brighter, younger sibling may be a source of intense discouragement; a really dull boy offered a bicycle if he " gets his scholarship " is another familiar problem. These need careful unravelling with the help of an educational psychologist and social worker, and it is important to be sure beyond all doubt that minor degrees of deafness or visual defect or motor weakness are not contributory factors.

CHILD GUIDANCE

IN psychiatric work with children, diagnosis and treatment often proceed together. The diagnosis may be in doubt until the child's point of view is better understood, or the patterns of his home and family are unravelled. Treatment is not specific in the sense of being different in a child with night fears or a maladjusted truant from school. Each must be understood in his own right and seen as part of a family situation.

A child does not usually seek treatment on his own account but he is brought, willy-nilly, with a series of complaints about him. It is, however, surprising how often quite young children realize that they want help. Even so, parental participation in the process is obviously essential and the help of the child's school is often sought. For these reasons it is usual to approach the problem with a team of workers; the psychiatric social worker will accept responsibility for work with the mother and for making home contacts, while the educational psychologist will do the same for the school and will be able to guide them from his knowledge of the child's response to tests. The psychiatrist cannot, of course, work in isolation with his patient, but he will need to give the child, in his interviews or play sessions, some sense of privacy and confidence. How quickly and easily a child will succeed in establishing *rapport* depends on many factors. It is a universal experience in psychotherapy that, while a patient may protest and over-react to interpretations which pain him, nevertheless, if through such work he comes to understand his own difficulties, he will experience relief and will be able to establish confidence in the therapist. The process is thus seen to be a lengthy one, for which adequate training is necessary. If interpretive work is undertaken, not only must the therapist recognize hints and indirect references but he will apprehend the situation through his own experience of working through to a deeper understanding of himself. A personal analysis will often have been part of his training.

It would be a mistake, however, to suggest that the pædiatrician has no share in dealing with emotional problems. His ear will generally be the first to hear the tale, and he will need to train himself to listen in order to recognize the overtones and the unconscious half-truths. Once he has got the story straight he will have to decide whether the parents can be helped by his advice or whether the patient must be referred to a children's psychiatrist. He can do a great deal to protect the child from further harm, and he will beware of unnecessary separations and unnecessary physical investigations and operations. Where the psychiatric team are at work in the pædiatric department each can learn from the other, but interpretive treatment which deals with material which has been repressed beyond the conscious level is best left to those whose special training enables them to deal with it.

MILDRED CREAK.

CHAPTER 19

Disorders of the Nervous System

PRACTICAL PROCEDURES

Lumbar Puncture

LUMBAR puncture in children is safe and simple if properly performed.

Dangers. (*a*) Sepsis. The needle and manometer should not be wet sterilized, but autoclaved. The physician should " scrub up " as for any surgical operation ; dry his hands on a sterile towel and not touch the child or the shaft of the needle. The child's skin is prepared as described on p. 396. Lumbar puncture must not be performed if there is local infection of the skin.

(*b*) Impaction of the medulla and cerebellum, in the form of a cone, in the foramen magnum, by withdrawing fluid below when there is increased pressure above (usually due to a cerebellar tumour). When an intracranial tumour is suspected, and especially if there is papilloedema, lumbar puncture should not be performed. If examination of the CSF is essential a lateral ventricle should be tapped.

(*c*) Breaking the needle. The risk is small; stainless steel needles are strong and flexible.

(*d*) After-effects. Where the child proves to have a normal fluid, the withdrawal of any considerable quantity may produce headache and vomiting. This is corrected by keeping the child lying flat or raising the foot of the bed. In meningitis, removal of fluid relieves the headache.

Indications for Lumbar Puncture. The chief indication for diagnostic lumbar puncture is the presence of signs of meningitis. Penicillin and streptomycin may be administered therapeutically by lumbar puncture, but intrathecal medication has its dangers and should be avoided unless the indications for it are very strong.

Pressure of Fluid. With the child lying on his side, the normal pressure is about 100 mm. of water as shown on the manometer. The pressure should be taken when possible, but if the child is crying it is often very difficult. Crying, coughing or holding the breath will cause the pressure to rise; with the child quiet an abnormally high pressure may indicate meningitis, encephalitis, brain tumour or abscess, hydrocephalus, etc. One can produce a temporary rise in intracranial pressure by compressing the jugular veins. This should cause the spinal fluid pressure to rise to over 300 mm. of water and to fall rapidly when the jugular compression is released (a positive Queckenstedt test). A negative result indicates obstruction to the CSF pathways at the base of the skull or in the spinal canal. A false negative may result from local obstruction to the end of the needle. This possibility should be eliminated by manual pressure on the abdomen, which will always produce a slight rise in pressure if the end of the needle is free.

Appearance of the Fluid. The CSF should be clear and colourless. Cloudiness is caused by the presence of excess cells; a turbid fluid will contain thousands of cells, and a very faint opalescence may be detected in fluid containing as few as 200 cells per c.mm. A clear yellow fluid is either an indication of old subarachnoid hæmorrhage or spinal block. A fresh subarachnoid hæmorrhage or a " bloody tap " will, of course, cause the fluid to be bloodstained. In the latter case, where a subdural vein has been accidentally punctured, the fluid as it emerges from the needle will be unevenly bloody and, if allowed to settle in a tube, the supernatant fluid will be clear. A few hours after a subarachnoid hæmorrhage the supernatant fluid will be yellow. Table XIX gives the cerebrospinal fluid findings in various diseases.

Equipment. The lumbar puncture needles should be No. 19 or 21 SWG, about 2 inches long, with a short, sharp bevel and a closely fitting stilet. A glass manometer, with connecting tube and adaptor, and dissecting forceps for holding swabs will also be required. Specimen bottles should be sterilized in order that they may be handled by the operator.

Anæsthesia. General anæsthesia may be necessary if the child is frightened, but as a rule lumbar puncture may easily be performed under local anæsthetic.

Preparation and Technique. The child is placed on his side, preferably on a table so that the spine does not curve laterally but is parallel with the floor. The knees are drawn up and the head, resting on a pillow, bent forwards towards the knees so that the back is well curved. The nurse or assistant grasps the patient behind the knees and at the nape of the neck, approximating the two hands. In this way the spines of the vertebræ are drawn as far apart as possible, allowing the needle to enter the spinal canal.

The whole lumbar and sacral region, including the upper iliac crest, is prepared with 2 per cent. iodine and spirit. The iliac crest is palpated through sterile gauze in order to indicate the elective level between the third and fourth lumbar vertebræ. A skin wheal is made with 2 per cent. novocain between the spines and the sub-cutaneous tissues infiltrated with about 1 ml. of the local anæsthetic for a short distance. The lumbar puncture needle is held with a sterile gauze swab and introduced at right angles to the back and

TABLE XIX

THE CEREBROSPINAL FLUID IN VARIOUS DISEASES

	Protein in mg. per 100 ml.	Sugar in mg. per 100 ml.	Chlorides in mg. per 100 ml.	Cells per c.mm.	Type of cell
Normal	15–25	55–80	About 725	0–5	Lymphocytes
Pyogenic meningitis	100–1,000	0–10	650–700	Thousands	Polymorphonuclears
Tuberculous meningitis	30–300	10–40	550–650	30–300	Lymphocytes
Aseptic meningitis	About 100	Normal	Normal	Hundreds or thousands	Lymphocytes, occasionally polymorphonuclears
Poliomyelitis	50 rising to 150	Normal	Normal	0–200	Mostly polymorphonuclears at first; later lymphocytes
Polyneuritis	50 to hundreds	Normal	Normal	0–5 (Rarely more)	Lymphocytes
Cerebral abscess	50–150	Normal	Normal	20–100	Lymphocytes predominate
Cerebral tumour	Normal to 200	Normal	Normal	Usually normal. Up to 200	Lymphocytes; rarely tumour cells

directed slightly towards the head. On entering from half to three-quarters of an inch, a click is felt as the needle pierces the stretched spinal theca. The stilet is withdrawn without inserting the needle farther and the fluid should flow freely. If the needle is pressed forwards through the spinal theca, striking the anterior surface of the spinal canal, a plexus of veins will be pierced, and the CSF will be mixed with blood.

How Much Fluid may be Safely Withdrawn? As soon as the flow is seen to be very slow, withdrawal should cease. In meningitis, where there has been increased pressure, it is well to run off as much as will flow freely, thus relieving pressure. The possible danger of lumbar puncture in cases of intracranial tumour is referred to on p. 450–1.

Cisternal Puncture

Preparation of the Patient. The back of the neck should be shaved well up to the external occipital protuberance. The child is placed on his side, and the head bent forwards, with the chin on the chest and firmly held there. It is well to give an anæsthetic to children who are quite conscious or normal mentally, but in meningitis, when the child is drowsy, this may not be necessary.

Technique. The patient's skin and the physician's hands are prepared as for lumbar puncture. The lumbar puncture needle, preferably one graduated in centimetres, is introduced in the midline, midway between the uppermost palpable spine of the neck (the axis) and the base of the skull. The needle is pushed forwards and upwards until it strikes the base of the skull behind the foramen magnum. It is then withdrawn slightly and redirected to point in the direction of the nasion. It is then pushed cautiously in and resistance will be felt as it penetrates the posterior occipito-atlantal ligament to enter the cistern at a depth of from 1·5 to 4 cm. from the skin, depending on the age of the child. (The depth is approximately one-eighth the circumference of the neck.)

Cisternal puncture can be a dangerous procedure in unskilled hands, as the cistern is only 0·5 to 1 cm. deep, and, if introduced too far, the needle may penetrate the medulla. Its chief indication is for obtaining a specimen of CSF when lumbar puncture has been unsuccessful.

Ventricular Puncture

The lateral ventricles may be tapped through the angle of the anterior fontanelle, if patent, or through drill holes in the skull; in the latter case the procedure should be carried out by a neurosurgeon.

The infant is given a teat stuffed with cotton wool soaked in sugar-water to suck. The scalp is shaved completely and the skin prepared. A lumbar puncture needle may be used, but there is a small danger of its sharp point piercing an intracerebral blood vessel. It is better to use a fine brain cannula into which can be fitted a sharp trochar or a blunt stilet. The trochar and cannula are introduced at the lateral angle of the fontanelle as far as possible from the midline to avoid the sagittal sinus. A resistance is felt as the dura is pierced. The trochar is then withdrawn and replaced by the blunt stilet and the instrument is pushed directly downwards. The stilet is removed as each centimetre is traversed; the ventricle should be reached at a distance of 3 to 5 cm. from the skin. (In cases of hydrocephalus it may be reached at a depth of only 1 cm.) If the first attempt is unsuccessful the cannula must be fully withdrawn from the brain before being redirected.

SUBDURAL TAP

The infant is prepared as for ventricular puncture. A fine lumbar puncture needle shortened to about 2 cm. and with a short bevel is introduced at right angles to the skull in the lateral corner of the anterior fontanelle. The needle is pushed in until the resistance of the dura is overcome. The stilet is then withdrawn. If no subdural collection of fluid is present, a few drops of clear CSF will exude from the end of the needle. As subdural fluid is often viscid it may be necessary to hold the needle in place for a minute or two to ensure that none is present. The procedure is repeated with a fresh needle on the other side.

MENINGITIS

Acute Pyogenic Meningitides

ÆTIOLOGY

PUS-FORMING micro-organisms may reach the meninges via the blood-stream or by direct spread from an adjacent site of infection, as, for example, in compound fracture of skull, osteomyelitis of skull or spine, cerebral abscess and so on.

Infecting organisms in children, in order of frequency, are: meningococcus, *Hæmophilus influenzæ*, pneumococcus, streptococcus, staphylococcus, *Esch. coli*, *Ps. pyocyanea* and others.

In the following sections features common to all types of purulent meningitis are outlined. In later sections the special characteristics of meningitis due to the several organisms will be described.

PATHOLOGY

At post-mortem examination the cortical veins are congested, and greenish-yellow pus is found throughout the subarachnoid space, in some cases thick enough to cover brain and spinal cord completely, in others confined to the cerebral sulci or to the basal cisterns. Here the foramina of the fourth ventricle may be blocked by inflammatory exudate with resultant internal hydrocephalus and flattening of cerebral convolutions. There may be microscopic evidence of inflammation within the brain substance.

GENERAL FEATURES

The onset is usually sudden, with vomiting, headache, high fever, dislike of the light and painful stiffness of the neck and spine. Fits may occur at the onset, or in the course of the illness, and are a bad sign. On examination, the child is drowsy, but results being disturbed. Meningeal irritation is shown by the limitation of passive flexion of the head and of straight leg raising. Kernig's sign is positive, and Brudzinski's sign may be present. The tendon reflexes may be exaggerated at first and then diminished, but they are not very helpful in diagnosis. The pupils may be small or unequal at the onset, and cranial nerve palsies (especially sixth nerve) occur occasionally. General hyperæsthesia is common.

Fulminating cases may present with the signs of septicæmia and shock overshadowing those of meningitis. This is commonest in meningococcal infections, in which there may be an extensive purpuric rash accompanied by signs of acute peripheral circulatory failure, restlessness preceding coma, cold, pale and clammy skin with distal cyanosis, rapid shallow respiration, rapid feeble pulse, and low blood-pressure.

Whenever a child is taken ill suddenly and presents with fever, drowsiness and signs of meningeal irritation, the diagnosis of meningitis should be confirmed as rapidly as possible by lumbar puncture. The cerebrospinal fluid is under raised pressure, and is cloudy with pus cells. The organisms are frequently seen on direct smear. The protein content is often raised, the chlorides normal or low and the sugar greatly diminished or absent. Blood count usually shows a polymorphonuclear leucocytosis.

The course varies with the infecting organisms. Untreated pyogenic meningitis is usually fatal, death being preceded by deepening coma, head retraction, dilated pupils and disappearance of tendon reflexes. Survivors may be deaf, blind, hydrocephalic, mentally defective, or hemiplegic. The younger the victim, the more likely is some neurological deficit to result, but sequels are very uncommon in older children who have received adequate treatment.

Meningitis in infants can occur in a much less acute and dramatic form, and is correspondingly more difficult to diagnose. Either convulsions or persistent, but not severe, vomiting, with gradual loss of weight, are nearly always the presenting symptoms. Fever and signs of meningeal irritation are often absent. Lack of interest in surroundings, staring eyes and a tense fontanelle in an ill baby should suggest the diagnosis. Even these signs may be absent and, if diagnosis is delayed, the head will begin to enlarge and become retracted, leading to the clinical picture of so-called post-basic meningitis. At this stage retinal hæmorrhages or papillœdema may be found.

DIFFERENTIAL DIAGNOSIS

Children presenting with fever and signs of meningeal irritation may be suffering from:

(1) Pyogenic meningitis,

(2) Tuberculous meningitis,

(3) " Meningism "—that is, meningeal irritation secondary to a disease such as upper lobar pneumonia, tonsillitis, otitis media or pyelitis,

(4) Aseptic or viral meningitis, as in anterior poliomyelitis, enterovirus meningitis, mumps meningitis, and so on, or rarely

(5) Meningitis caused by other organisms, e.g. spirochætes (congenital syphilis), leptospira (Weil's disease, canicola fever), protozoa (toxoplasmosis) or fungi (torulosis, histoplasmosis, coccidioidomycosis).

Posterior fossa brain tumours or abscess sometimes produce neck rigidity, and tetanus is sometimes mistaken for meningitis. A diagnostic lumbar puncture must always be performed, except when the history and examination strongly suggest that symptoms are due to a brain tumour and not to meningitis. However, the type of meningitis present can often be guessed correctly from the clues provided by history and examination, before examination of the cerebrospinal fluid. Thus the sudden onset in a previously healthy child will usually exclude tuberculous meningitis. *Drowsiness* is an important sign that distinguishes bacterial meningitis from most aseptic meningitides and meningism. The clinical features which may help to distinguish between the various infecting organisms are mentioned below, but again, a firm diagnosis can only be based on microscopic examination and culture of the cerebrospinal fluid.

TREATMENT[1]

1. *Specific Chemotherapy and Antibiotic Therapy.* The choice of drugs to be used will depend on the infecting organism, and, therefore, whenever possible a specimen of cerebrospinal fluid should be obtained before starting treatment. (In fulminating cases, however, sulphadiazine (0·1 G. per Kg. body-weight for infants) and crystalline penicillin (500,000 units) should be given intramuscularly without delay.) A lumbar puncture is performed, and 5 ml. of CSF collected in sterile test-tubes. If the specimen is cloudy, 10,000 units of crystalline penicillin (previously dissolved in 5 c.c. of saline solution) may be injected intrathecally. The CSF is then examined in the laboratory where it may be possible to identify the organism on staining a direct smear, in which case the appropriate specific therapy is prescribed. But if the organism is not seen, treatment must on no account await the results of culture.

Sulphadiazine, penicillin and chloramphenicol parenterally are a satisfactory combination of drugs, and administration should be begun

---

[1] For dosage, *see* Appendix 1.

promptly. The treatment may, if necessary, be altered when the results of CSF culture and sensitivity test are known. It is most important that dosage (*see* Appendix 1) should be optimal and treatment maintained until the temperature has been normal and the CSF sterile for at least four days, when the sugar content of the fluid should be normal and the protein and cells greatly diminished.

2. *Maintenance of Body Water and Electrolytes.* If the child is conscious and if vomiting is not severe, adequate amounts of fluid can be given by mouth. In other cases an intravenous drip infusion should be set up at once and a half-normal saline with 2·5 per cent. glucose solution administered in quantities sufficient to maintain normal daily fluid requirements, and to correct dehydration. Sulphadiazine and antibiotics may be administered in the transfusion fluid.

3. *Treatment of Acute Peripheral Circulatory Failure.* The most important measures are early and adequate chemo- and antibiotic-therapy and the administration of oxygen. An intravenous drip transfusion of plasma, followed by half-normal saline with $2\frac{1}{2}$ per cent. glucose, is started as soon as possible, but the total amount of fluid given should not be excessive for fear of causing cerebral œdema. In addition to antibiotics, soluble hydrocortisone should be added to the transfusion fluid, 50 mg. being given immediately and thereafter 25 to 50 mg. 6 hourly. Desoxycorticosterone 5 mg. is given intramuscularly. In cases of severe hypotension, noradrenaline may be added to the infusion fluid in the dosage of 4 microgrammes per ml. The rate of the infusion must then be carefully adjusted to keep the blood-pressure at the required level.

4. Sedatives are necessary in a restless patient and in any case of meningitis are advisable for the prevention of fits. Sodium amylobarbitone or phenobarbitone should be injected intramuscularly every six to eight hours for the first twenty-four hours, or longer if necessary. Actual convulsions are treated with intramuscular paraldehyde or phenytoin sodium.

5. Where a primary focus for the meningitis is found surgical eradication may be necessary. Subdural taps must be carried out if the persistence of symptoms suggests subdural effusion, which, although most commonly complicating influenzal meningitis, may occur in the course of any acute purulent meningitis, especially in infants.

SPECIAL FEATURES OF ACUTE MENINGITIDES

Meningococcal Meningitis (Spotted Fever)

Epidemics may occur, but sporadic cases are commoner. The disease may attack at any age, but half the children affected are under five years old. Invasion by the meningococcus takes place through the upper respiratory tract, where it is occasionally found on culture in healthy persons. Meningitis is secondary to septicæmia, which is frequently manifested by an extensive purpuric rash. (The association of fever, signs of meningeal irritation, and purpura is, with rare exceptions, diagnostic of meningococcal meningitis.) The spleen is usually palpable. The onset may be sudden and severe, the patient dying within a few hours of acute peripheral vascular failure. In such cases post-mortem examination sometimes reveals adrenal cortical hæmorrhages (Waterhouse-Friderichsen syndrome).

The CSF is usually purulent, and microscopic examination of a smear will show Gram-negative diplococci within polymorphonuclear leucocytes, or lying free. If examined early in the course of the illness the CSF is occasionally clear and acellular, and yet meningococci can be grown from it.

Sulphadiazine is the drug of choice, and, except in cases of fulminating septicæmia, the results of early treatment are excellent. In addition, penicillin is usually given parenterally, but intrathecal medication is unnecessary. Treatment should be continued for three days after the temperature has fallen to normal.

Influenzal Meningitis

Meningitis caused by the *Hæmophilus influenzæ* occurs in children under five years old, and is commonest in infancy. Unlike the other pyogenic meningitides it may have a subacute onset and be preceded by an obvious upper respiratory-tract infection. Blood culture is usually positive in the first few days of the illness, and very occasionally scattered purpuric spots may appear. Lumbar puncture reveals a cloudy fluid which on microscopy is seen to contain short pleomorphic Gram-negative rods. Even when correctly treated, the course is often long, and the temperature may not return to normal for many days. In some of these cases the persistence of fever is due to subdural effusions which may be revealed and removed by subdural tap. Rarely, the course is fulminant, the patient dying within a few hours of the onset of the symptoms.

Sulphadiazine, streptomycin and chloramphenicol should be administered parenterally in every case. In addition, 25–50 mg. of streptomycin should be given intrathecally once a day. Treatment may be altered when the sensitivities of the organism become known. Alternatively, sulphadiazine and chloramphenicol are used. Specific therapy should be continued for several days after the fever has subsided. Subdural taps should be performed if fever persists for more than four days, if vomiting or convulsions occur after the subsidence of the fever, or if any grossly abnormal neurological signs appear. Subdural effusions should be treated by daily tapping, not more than 10 ml. of fluid being removed on each occasion. In every case of subdural effusion the child should, following recovery from the acute illness, be referred to a neurosurgeon. Should burr holes reveal a membrane, craniotomy must be performed for its removal, to prevent reaccumulation of fluid.

Pneumococcal Meningitis

The meningitis usually results from direct or from blood-borne spread of infection elsewhere, e.g., otitis media, mastoiditis, sinusitis, pneumonia, or empyema. In infants, however, there may be no evidence of a primary focus. The purulent and fibrinous exudate is thickest over the convexity of the brain, rather than at the base as in other purulent meningitides. Moreover, the meningitis may for a time be circumscribed, and, with a normal CSF, cerebral abscess may be diagnosed in error. Difficulties in diagnosis may also arise when meningitis occurs secondary to pneumonia in an already ill and vomiting infant.

Once the meningitis has become generalized, the CSF becomes heavily purulent, and on microscopy Gram-positive lance-shaped diplococci are seen.

Penicillin is the drug of choice, and should be given both intramuscularly and by daily intrathecal injection. Sulphadiazine should also be administered by mouth. A primary focus, if present, will usually be dealt with effectively by the chemotherapy. Mastoidectomy or sinus drainage should be reserved for those cases in which the meningitis does not clear quickly with adequate drug treatment. The blood sedimentation rate is a useful guide to persistence of local infection.

Streptococcal Meningitis

In infants this is usually part of a generalized septicæmia; in older children, it is due to direct spread from a local infection (e.g. brain abscess, sinusitis, mastoiditis) or is occasionally secondary to bacteriæmia from a distant focus (e.g. tonsillitis). The treatment is the same as for pneumococcal meningitis.

Staphylococcal Meningitis

Meningitis due to this organism is always secondary to infection elsewhere—e.g. furunculosis, osteomyelitis. Penicillin, intramuscularly and intrathecally, is the first line of attack, but if the organisms prove to be resistant, one of the newer antibiotics must be administered by mouth or, if a soluble preparation is available, parenterally, but not intrathecally. It is important to make a careful search for signs of osteomyelitis of spine and skull, and for *congenital dermal sinus*. Staphylococcal meningitis from either source may not clear up until the primary focus has been dealt with surgically. (*See also* p. 438.)

Esch. Coli Meningitis

Meningitis due to *E. coli* seldom occurs after the newborn period. It usually follows bacteriæmia secondary to pyelitis (especially in infants with congenital renal-tract anomalies), or umbilical sepsis. Direct infection of meninges may take place through a meningocele.

Sulphadiazine and streptomycin, or chloramphenicol are the drugs of choice, and Colomycin is likely to improve the prognosis.

Colomycin is also used for *Ps. pyocanea* meningitis.

Tuberculous Meningitis

ÆTIOLOGY AND PATHOGENESIS

The disease develops as a complication of tuberculosis elsewhere in the body, usually following the primary infection. It is but seldom, however, that the primary infection is severe enough to be recognized, but when it is, it will be found to precede meningitis by one to three months. Tubercle bacilli are thought to reach the meninges through the bursting of an adjacent caseous focus that has developed in the brain following a blood-borne spread from the primary complex or other distant tuberculous lesion. In some cases this hæmatogenous spread is profuse enough to amount to miliary tuberculosis. The organism is usually the human bacillus and there is almost always a history of contact with an adult suffering from pulmonary tuberculosis. In recent years there has been a marked decrease in the incidence of and mortality from tuberculosis meningitis in children in England and Wales.

AGE INCIDENCE

The disease is commonest in the second, third and fourth years of life, but may occur at any age.

PATHOLOGY

Post-mortem the brain is pale, and the convolutions are flattened. On close inspection fine miliary tubercles may be seen on the meninges. A thin gelatinous exudate is found, chiefly at the base of the brain, but sometimes extending along the Sylvian fissures. This exudate commonly blocks the foramina of the fourth ventricle, and a varying degree of internal hydrocephalus is therefore present. Caseous tuberculous foci may often be found in the brain.

SYMPTOMS AND SIGNS

Three ill-defined stages may be recognized in the history, but symptoms may fluctuate markedly from day to day. The *onset* is usually insidious. The child, who was formerly active, wants to be nursed or carried about, and there may be lassitude, headache, drowsiness and irritability. Constipation is usually present, and all the early symptoms are often attributed by the parents to this fact. An occasional vomit, not necessarily in relation to food, may be noted. Symptoms in a young child may be attributed to teething. There is usually slight fever. This stage lasts from a few days to several weeks.

In the *second stage* the temperature rises, and signs of an increase in intracranial pressure, and sometimes of meningeal irritation, become more obvious. Vomiting, drowsiness and irritability increase.

The child lies curled up on his side, dislikes the light, and may pull the bedclothes over his head. He frowns continually, and may scream sharply at intervals, probably because of the headache. Teeth grinding is common. Hyperalgesia may cause him to cry when handled. Neck stiffness and limitation of straight leg raising are not invariably present. At the end of this stage, which lasts about one week, there is marked wasting, and the abdomen is scaphoid.

In the *third stage* the child sinks into stupor and finally coma. The temperature is high, but the pulse often slow. Breathing may be intermittent. Flushing, sweating, and " tâche cérébrale " become noticeable. Dilatation and inequality of the pupils, and squints may appear. Papillœdema may now be present. (Choroidal tubercles are seldom seen unless there is an associated miliary tuberculosis.) Generalized convulsions and localized muscle twitchings are common at this stage, and decerebrate rigidity may precede death, which in untreated cases takes place about one week after the onset of stupor. Occasionally the onset is *sudden* with vomiting, coma, convulsions or mono- or hemiplegia.

MANTOUX AND TUBERCULIN-JELLY TESTS

These are strongly positive in the first two stages, but may be negative in the stage of coma.

CEREBROSPINAL FLUID

The pressure is increased and the fluid clear or very faintly opalescent. On standing, a filmy clot suspended from the surface may develop. Cells are increased up to 200 or 300 per c.mm. and are mostly lymphocytes. The total protein is somewhat increased. Chlorides may be less than 700 mg. per 100 ml., and in the late stages fall below 650 mg. The CSF sugar is very occasionally normal at the first examination, but rapidly falls. It is the combination of a moderate pleocytosis and a low-sugar content which is so characteristic of the cerebrospinal fluid in tuberculous meningitis. If a satisfactory method is employed, tubercle bacilli may be found in most specimens. (*Method:* Ten ml. of CSF are centrifuged at 2,000 revs. per minute for 40 minutes. The fluid is then poured off and may be used for the chemical estimations. The centrifuge tube is left standing upside down to drain on blotting paper for exactly 10 minutes. Meanwhile a Pasteur pipette is heated and drawn out to a capillary tube, which is broken off squarely. The capillary tube is then scraped round the bottom of the centrifuge tube and will usually collect about one-eighth of an inch of sediment. This sediment is carefully blown out on to a clean slide, and *without being spread* is fixed in a flame and stained by the Ziehl-Neelsen method. Microscopic examination is made much easier by the use of a moving stage and should not take longer than half an hour.)

DIFFERENTIAL DIAGNOSIS

There are two problems. The first is to consider the possibility of the diagnosis in the early and more easily curative stage, when the symptoms are vague and commonplace. Variable irritability and listlessness lasting for more than a few days and accompanied by slight fever, constipation and occasional vomiting should suggest the diagnosis, and lead to lumbar puncture. A history of contact with an adult suffering from pulmonary tuberculosis will provide an important clue. The second problem arises in the differential diagnosis of cerebrospinal fluid abnormalities when the diagnosis has been suspected on clinical grounds. A rise in cell-count in the CSF in a child with active primary or miliary tuberculosis will usually indicate tuberculous meningitis, but may, of course, be due to another disease or to the rare " serous tuberculous meningitis." This is a self-limiting condition in which the CSF chemical findings remain normal, while the pleocytosis subsides in a week or two without treatment.

The finding of both tubercle bacilli in the CSF and a low-sugar content should precede the giving of specific therapy, which if begun while the diagnosis is still uncertain leads to complete confusion. In the writer's opinion it is permissible to wait for 24 hours, examining several specimens of CSF, before beginning treatment, and longer if there are few clinical signs to suggest meningitis.

PROGNOSIS

Before the introduction of streptomycin, the disease was always fatal. The prognosis to-day depends on the stage which the illness has reached when treatment is begun. With skilled treatment, about 90 per cent. of children who are conscious on admission should recover, the great majority with normal mental and physical health; relapse is very unusual. The prognosis in those unconscious on admission is bad; the majority die, and in those who recover, mental defect, hydrocephalus or hemiplegia are common.

TREATMENT AND COURSE[1]

Treatment should be begun as soon as possible after a firm diagnosis has been made, or within 24–48 hours of the presumptive diagnosis. (In these latter cases, positive culture or guineapig inoculation of the first specimens of CSF, or the subsequent course of the disease, may later confirm the diagnosis.)

Streptomycin is given intramuscularly every twelve hours in the dosage of 10 mg. per pound of body-weight per day and isonicotinic acid hydrazide orally six hourly in the dosage of 4 mg. per pound of body-weight per day. Unless it provokes severe vomiting, para-aminosalicylic acid is given by mouth in a dosage of 100 mg. per pound of body-weight per day in divided doses at meal times, a double

[1] Lorber, J. (1956). *Brit. med. J.*, 1, 1009

dose being given at night. This drug appears to reduce the risk of the tubercle bacillus becoming resistant to streptomycin or isonicotinic acid hydrazide.

Prolonged streptomycin treatment may result in permanent vestibular damage, although the child's ability to balance is not seriously affected, and it may occasionally produce permanent nerve deafness. Because of these toxic effects dosage should be reduced to 6 mg. per pound of body-weight per day, as soon as improvement in the child's condition is apparent. Isonicotinic acid hydrazide usually causes euphoria, excessive appetite and gain in weight. Other side-effects are rare—headache, acute mania, fits, peripheral neuritis and generalized drug reactions. It is possible that some of these side-effects may be checked by pyridoxine.

With the introduction of isonicotinic acid hydrazide the need for intrathecal medication has been reduced. However, intrathecal streptomycin should probably be administered daily to any child unconscious on admission, or to one whose general condition or cerebrospinal fluid abnormalities deteriorate while having the treatment outlined above. Fifty mg. dissolved in 5 ml. of pyrogen-free normal saline is injected slowly (and preferably warm) into the lumbar theca, after the removal of the same quantity of CSF, once a day. Nausea, vomiting and giddiness sometimes occur following the intrathecal injections, but may be relieved by antihistamine drugs. After one or two weeks of treatment it is usual to find a " meningitic reaction " on examination of the CSF. There are extreme fluctuations in the cell-count, which may rise to several hundreds (chiefly polymorphs) and fall to the previous level within a day or two, to be succeeded by a similar sudden increase. A rise in protein usually follows this pleocytosis. The " spikes " may recur for many days but gradually flatten out as the patient improves. This meningeal reaction is probably due to the release of tuberculin, and seems to represent a part of the recovery process. When the meningeal reaction does not occur and when the course is otherwise unsatisfactory, intrathecal tuberculin treatment may be considered.[1]

Tuberculin treatment may also be of value if the subarachnoid space has become blocked by exudate in the course of the illness. Signs of incipient spinal block are a decreased flow of the CSF on lumbar puncture, and a rising protein content. When such a block has developed, streptomycin must be administered by the cisternal or ventricular routes, 25 mg. only being given at each injection. Blocking at the free edge of the tentorium or in the basal cisterns will be accompanied by signs of rising intracranial pressure. Intrathecal streptomycin must be administered by the lumbar route.

Cortisone may be life-saving in cases presenting with acute intracranial hypertension due to cerebral œdema. Its value in cases of subarachnoid exudate is doubtful.

[1] Smith, H. V., Vollum, R. L. (1956). *Tubercle*, **37**, 301.

Treatment with oral isonicotinic acid hydrazide, para-aminosalicylic acid and intramuscular streptomycin should be maintained for at least six months, and not stopped until the patient is gaining weight and the CSF cells and protein have been steadily falling for at least two months. In cases in which intrathecal injections have been judged necessary, they should be continued daily for some time after the departure of the last clinical signs of active disease or the latest detection of tubercle bacilli on microscopy of the cerebrospinal fluid. (The only indication for abandoning treatment is the development of decerebrate rigidity.)

Following treatment, the child's return to a normal active life must be gradual.

ASEPTIC MENINGITIS[1]

This term is used to describe febrile illnesses characterized by signs of meningeal irritation, a benign course, and a sterile CSF containing excess cells, mostly lymphocytes. Most cases of aseptic meningitis are presumably caused by viruses, but as yet the virus cannot be identified in every case. The known causes of aseptic meningitis include the viruses of mumps, lymphocytic chroniomeningitis, herpes simplex and the entero viruses (poliomyelitis, Coxsackie and ECHO). The viruses of infectious mononucleosis and herpes zoster are other rare causes of aseptic meningitis. All these viruses may occasionally cause symptoms of encephalitis (disturbances of consciousness, focal neurological signs) as well as those of meningitis (headache, vomiting, neck stiffness).

IDENTIFICATION OF THE VIRUS

In most cases of aseptic meningitis the virus responsible is not identified, and this is in part due to the clinician's failure to realize that identification is possible in an increasingly high proportion of cases. There are so many antigenically different strains of the enteroviruses, for instance, that identification by serology becomes impracticable. It is therefore of the greatest importance to obtain specimens for virus culture *as early as possible* in the course of the illness.

Pharyngeal secretions should be obtained by using a throat swab on a wooden stick, the end of which is broken off into a sterile bijou bottle containing 1 ml. of a transport medium (usually 10 per cent. broth-saline with penicillin and streptomycin added). Stools (not obtained by enema) and CSF should also be collected. These specimens should be transported as soon as possible to a virus laboratory. If this cannot be done immediately, they should be kept in a refrigerator (4° C) and transported to the laboratory within 24 or 48 hours.

[1] " Virus Meningo-encephalitis." Ciba Foundation Study Group No. 7, 1961. London: Churchill.

The serum from at least 5 ml. of blood should also be obtained early in the illness and again 14 to 21 days later. The same precautions should be taken about cooling. The finding of a rise in titre of neutralizing antibodies will confirm that a virus previously isolated has in fact caused the disease.

Mumps Meningitis

There may be no associated parotitis, but if parotid swelling occurs it may precede or follow the central nervous symptoms by a few days. Fever, headache and occasionally coma are the presenting symptoms and, on examination, neck stiffness, limitation of straight leg raising and, rarely, ataxia and spasticity are found. A permanent nerve deafness sometimes results, but other cranial nerves are not involved. The CSF is under raised pressure and contains a few hundred cells, mostly lymphocytes. The disease is never fatal and, with the exception of deafness, symptoms disappear in a few days. Many weeks may elapse before the CSF is again normal.

The diagnosis may be suspected by a history of contact and confirmed by the presence of parotitis, or by the finding of a rising titre of mumps antibodies or a positive complement fixation test.

Enterovirus Meningitis

The enteroviruses (poliomyelitis, Coxsackie, ECHO) infect the gastro-intestinal tract of man and are excreted in the stools. Systemic invasion and viræmia may cause febrile illnesses and particularly aseptic meningitis. Poliomyelitis is discussed on p. 417. Sporadic cases and epidemics of Coxsackie and ECHO virus meningitis may occur throughout the year, but are slightly commoner in summer and autumn. The Coxsackie viruses are pathogenic to infant mice and hamsters; two groups, A and B, are distinguished by the histological damage produced. The ECHO viruses are not pathogenic to laboratory animals. There are many antigenically distinct types of each virus. It is not yet possible to distinguish the enteroviruses on clinical grounds. They usually cause fairly sudden and brief illnesses with high fever (sometimes diphasic), symptoms and signs of meningitis and sometimes rubella-like rashes, lymph-gland enlargement and muscle pains. The CSF shows a moderate pleocytosis usually lymphocytic, but, in some epidemics, mainly polymorphonuclear. Recovery is the rule.

Lymphocytic Choriomeningitis

This uncommon disease occurs sporadically, usually in persons living in houses infested by mice, which can harbour the virus. An influenza-like illness may precede the onset of headache, vomiting and signs of meningitis. There is usually a slight polymorphonuclear leucocytosis. The cerebrospinal fluid pressure is raised and a pleocytosis of from one hundred to several thousand lymphocytes is found. The headache may persist for several weeks, but complete recovery is the rule.

ENCEPHALITIS

INFLAMMATION of the brain may result from infection with bacteria, viruses and many other agents. Bacteria tend to produce localized lesions (*see* Brain Abscess, p. 415). Viruses cause more diffuse encephalitis, frequently accompanied by myelitis and aseptic meningitis. The term encephalopathy is sometimes used interchangeably with encephalitis; at other times it is used to describe acute degenerative disorders of the brain in which there is no evidence of inflammation. Various types of encephalitis are considered briefly under the following headings, but it must be admitted that many cases of encephalitis in children defy classification. Viruses known to cause encephalitis include those mentioned in the section on aseptic meningitis and the arbor viruses (arthropod-borne virus—ticks and mosquitoes). In addition encephalitis may occur secondarily to other virus illnesses.

ENCEPHALITIS OF KNOWN OR SUSPECTED VIRAL ÆTIOLOGY
Mosquito-borne Encephalitis

The viruses responsible for *Equine, St. Louis, Japanese B., Murray Valley* and *Australian X encephalitides* have been isolated. Epidemics of the first two named have taken place in America, of the third in Japan, and of the fourth and fifth, which are probably the same disease, in Australia. The viruses of the first three are known to be transmitted to man by mosquitoes.

Pathology. There is widespread involvement of brain and spinal cord, with œdema, congestion, cellular infiltration and neuronal degeneration.

Clinical Features. No age is immune and each disease causes a high mortality. The onset is sudden with high fever, vomiting, headache and various degrees of impairment of consciousness. Twitchings and convulsions are common, but focal signs are rare. The CSF contains several hundred cells per cubic millimetre— mostly lymphocytes. In survivors, the fever subsides gradually after a few days but permanent brain damage may result.

Tick-borne Encephalitis

The only type to occur in Great Britain is louping-ill, a disease of sheep, which is occasionally transmitted to man and usually produces a mild illness. European and Far Eastern tick-borne encephalitis are more serious illnesses with a higher mortality and higher incidence of residual symptoms.

Encephalitis Lethargica (Von Economo's Disease)

Epidemics occurred in England and other countries in the early 1920's and a few sporadic cases have occurred since. The virus has not been isolated.

Pathology. The inflammatory process is most marked in the basal ganglia and cranial nerve nuclei.

Clinical Features. The onset is usually gradual, influenza-like symptoms being followed in a few days by drowsiness and cranial nerve (especially oculomotor) palsies. Neither fever nor headache is usually severe. The CSF contains up to about 100 lymphocytes per cubic millimetre. About one-quarter of all cases die, one-quarter recover completely, while in the remainder permanent brain damage is manifested by paralysis agitans or emotional and behaviour disorders. Rarer sequels are oculogyric crises, myoclonus and intellectual deterioration.

Acute Demyelinating Encephalopathies associated with the Acute Infectious Fevers

This form of encephalitis complicates certain virus diseases, viz. measles, rubella, vaccinia, smallpox, chickenpox and influenza. There is no evidence of actual invasion of the brain by the virus concerned and the pathogenesis is thought to be that of an allergic response. Vaccinial encephalitis is rarest when primary vaccination is carried out between the ages of one and five years and seldom follows revaccination.

Pathology. There is generalized congestion and œdema, but, unlike the other encephalitides, little involvement of grey matter; instead there are patches of perivascular demyelination of the white matter of brain and spinal cord.

Clinical Features. The severity of the infectious illness seems to bear no relation to the chance of developing encephalitis. The onset is sudden and takes place from the fifth to twentieth day. The temperature rises again and the child may rapidly become comatose. Papillœdema may be present. Trismus is common and there may be convulsions. Occasionally a cerebellar ataxia is the main symptom. Myelitis may develop, producing flaccid paralysis of the limbs and retention or incontinence of urine. The cerebrospinal fluid may be normal or show a moderate increase in lymphocytes and protein. The illness is most severe when complicating measles and vaccination and least severe with chickenpox and rubella. Treatment with corticosteroids or specific immune gammaglobulins has been advocated, but the results are uncertain. When recovery takes place quickly it is usually complete. There may be an astonishing physical recovery after coma which has lasted for many weeks, but in such cases there is usually some selective mental defect which, without being obvious, causes difficulty in school learning.

ENCEPHALITIS OF UNKNOWN ÆTIOLOGY

Acute Toxic Encephalitis

This may complicate bacterial diseases, such as pneumonia, scarlet fever or pertussis, or may occur as a primary disease in small epidemics.

PATHOLOGY

There is generalized congestion and œdema of the brain, sometimes with scattered hæmorrhages. Miscroscopy shows neuronal degeneration and cellular infiltration.

CLINICAL FEATURES

The onset is acute with high fever, headache, vomiting and delirium or coma. Convulsions and cranial nerve and limb palsies may occur. The CSF is usually normal. There may be permanent brain damage in those who survive.

Subacute Inclusion Body Encephalitis

This is a rare disease of children from about five to ten years of age, lasting many weeks and invariably fatal.

PATHOLOGY

There is subacute inflammatory reaction in the grey matter with degeneration of nerve cells, which contain nuclear and cytoplasmic inclusion bodies.

CLINICAL FEATURES

There is an insidious onset of mental deterioration with, later, frequent generalized myoclonic jerkings. Death is preceded by a state of decerebrate rigidity. The CSF shows a paretic type of Lange curve, but is otherwise normal. The electro-encephalogram shows peculiar changes and may help in making the diagnosis.

ENCEPHALITIS CAUSED BY MICRO-ORGANISMS OTHER THAN BACTERIA OR VIRUSES

Encephalitis may be caused by yeasts (e.g. torulosis), fungi (e.g. actinomycosis), protozoa (e.g. malignant tertian malaria, toxoplasmosis) and rickettsia (e.g. typhus).

Toxoplasmosis [1]

This is caused by infection with the *Toxoplasma gondii*. As the sera of most adults contain antibodies to the organism, it is presumably a common infection of childhood which rarely causes clinical symptoms, although fever, lymphadenopathy, pneumonia or encephalitis are known to occur. Toxoplasmosis most frequently causes obvious disease when infection takes place *in utero*.

PATHOLOGY

The protozoon is found within cells of the brain and retina and less commonly in other organs. Granulomatous masses are formed, which soon become calcified.

[1] Wyllie, W. G., Fisher, H. J. W. (1950). *Quart. J. Med.*, **19, n.** ., 57,

CLINICAL ASPECTS

Symptoms are usually present at birth or shortly after. The infants do not thrive well and fever, jaundice, purpura and other rashes, convulsions and opisthotonos are among the commonest symptoms. On ophthalmoscopy a striking chorioretinitis is seen and x-ray usually reveals patches of calcification in the brain. The CSF is xanthochromic and contains excess protein and cells. Many infants develop progressive hydrocephalus and die within the first few months of life. Others survive to be blind, subject to fits and frequently mentally defective. The diagnosis can be confirmed by demonstrating the parasites in the CSF or by serological tests.

Treatment with sulphonamides and pyrimethamine may be beneficial, but usually irreversible damage has already occurred.

Lead Encephalitis

ÆTIOLOGY

Lead poisoning most commonly results from the chewing of repainted toys, cots, verandah railings, and so on. The serious dangers of lead paint are not realized by most parents. Nervous complications are not invariable, but in children usually take the form of encephalitis rather than peripheral neuritis.

PATHOLOGY

Post mortem the brain is greatly swollen, with serous exudate. There are capillary hæmorrhages and scattered areas of necrosis. Cerebral atrophy is found in long-standing cases.

CLINICAL FEATURES

A period of chronic ill-health, the symptoms of which are anorexia or pica, irritability, headache, abdominal pain and increasing pallor, usually precedes the encephalitis, the onset of which may be precipitated by an acute infection. Severe cerebral œdema causes convulsions, vomiting, papillœdema, enlargement of the head in young children, delirium, coma, and frequently death. In those who recover, even from milder poisoning, mental deficiency is common, while convulsions, blindness and spastic paralysis are rarer sequels. In older children, peripheral neuritis may produce widespread flaccid paralysis.

DIAGNOSIS

The diagnosis can be confirmed by the following examinations. X-rays of the skeleton may show dense transverse bands at the growing ends of the long bones (Plate IX). Examination of the blood reveals anæmia, reticulocytosis, and punctate basophilia of the red cells. The cerebrospinal fluid contains excess protein and sometimes a slight pleocytosis. A greatly raised pressure accompanies the encephalitis.

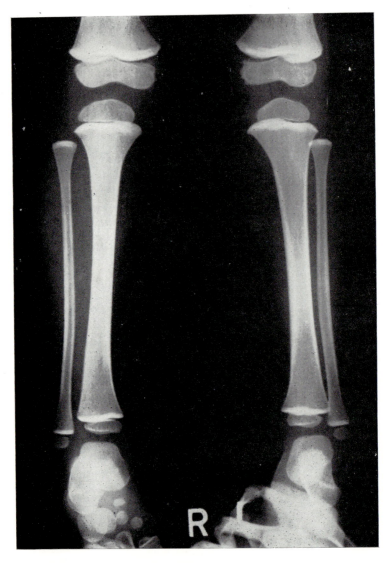

PLATE IX. Lead poisoning. The dense lines at the growing ends of
the long bones in a 2½-year-old girl are due to deposits of lead.

The estimation of the lead content of the urine is possible by spectro-graphic analysis and other methods, but is technically difficult; up to 50 microgrammes per 24 hours may be found in normal children; the amount detected in children with lead poisoning varies considerably, but greatly increased quantities may be excreted. Porphyrinuria is commonly found and is easy to detect. (*Method:* A test-tube is half filled with urine, which is acidified with acetic acid and then shaken with half its volume of ether. The tube is next held under a Wood's light, and if porphyrins are present the supernatant ether will show a cherry-red fluorescence. The test is not, of course, specific for lead poisoning.) Transient glycosuria and aminoaciduria are commonly found in lead poisoning. Estimation of the blood lead has to be undertaken in special conditions; the normal level is up to 40 microgrammes per 100 ml.

TREATMENT

Convulsions must be controlled by sedatives, and cerebral œdema reduced by the intramuscular injection of 25 per cent. magnesium sulphate solution (0·5 ml. per Kg. of body-weight given every four hours). Extensive surgical decompression may be needed. Acidosis is common and should be corrected by administration of sodium citrate. Treatment with the calcium complex of ethylene diamine-tetra-acetic acid (Calcium Disodium Versenate) should be carried out if there is no lead demonstrable by x-ray in the intestines and if a test dose of 0·2 G. intravenously produces no untoward symptoms. This agent is capable of binding lead ions in such a way as to render them chemically inert and so allow their safe excretion in the urine. Blood-lead levels can thus be reduced rapidly and the symptoms of acute and chronic lead poisoning relieved. The drug is usually given by slow intravenous infusion, the dosage being 1 G. per 30 Kg. of body-weight per day for a period of about 5 days. Several such courses may be needed with intervals of one week between them. Penicillamine (*see* p. 446) now provides an alternative method of treatment.

Brain Abscess

ÆTIOLOGY

The streptococcus, pneumococcus, staphylococcus, or *Esch. coli* are the usual infecting organisms, which enter the brain from a local or distant septic focus. The middle-ear or mastoid air cells are by far the commonest sites of the primary infection in children. Other sources are sinusitis, head wounds, empyema or bronchiectasis. In children with congenital heart lesions involving a " right to left shunt," cerebral abscess may be secondary to trivial local infections.

PATHOLOGY

Post mortem the appearance of the brain varies with the age of the lesion, i.e. between widespread, ill-defined areas of necrosis and a well-localized tumour surrounded by a thick capsule of connective tissue. The site depends on the source of infection. When secondary to otitis media or mastoiditis, the abscess is found in the temporal lobe, or, less commonly, in the cerebellum.

CLINICAL FEATURES

Characteristically there are two stages in the development of a cerebral abscess, but either may occur without the other. In the first stage there is fever, drowsiness, headache and vomiting, which may be followed by coma and death (often preceded by rupture of the abscess and purulent meningitis), or which may lead, immediately or after a latent period of days or weeks, into the second stage in which signs and symptoms of an expanding intracranial lesion appear.

In the second stage the general signs of a rise in intracranial pressure are commoner than localizing signs. It is noteworthy, however, that the headache is sometimes localized over the site of the abscess.

At this stage there is often no fever, no tachycardia and no leucocytosis. In either stage the cerebrospinal fluid may be normal, or, while sterile, may contain up to several hundred cells per cubic millimetre, a varying proportion of which are polymorphs, increased protein, but normal concentrations of sugar and chloride.

THE TREATMENT is surgical, with suitable antibiotics and chemotherapy.

SYPHILIS OF THE NERVOUS SYSTEM

OWING to routine Wassermann tests in pregnancy and antenatal treatment, congenital syphilis is now a rare disease in Great Britain, and syphilitic involvement of the nervous system in children is seldom seen. It is probable that the nervous system is involved early in a high proportion of congenital syphilitics, but there may be no clinical manifestations until late in childhood. As in adult syphilis, the manifestations of central nervous involvement are extremely variable.

Syphilitic Meningitis (*see also* p. 564)

When this occurs, symptoms usually develop in the first year of life and give rise to the usual signs of meningitis in infancy (*see* p. 400). There may be no fever. The spinal fluid usually contains about 100 lymphocytes per cubic millimetre, has increased protein and a positive Wassermann reaction. Ophthalmoscopy may reveal the characteristic chorioretinitis. Even if treatment with penicillin is begun early the prognosis is poor, and, if the child survives, residual defects such as cranial nerve palsies, blindness, hydrocephalus, hemiplegia, fits and mental deficiency are likely.

Vascular Syphilis

Thrombosis of vessels in the brain or spinal cord may occur independently of meningitis at any age, and give rise to disorders such as hemiplegia or paraplegia.

Juvenile General Paresis

This is the commonest form of late juvenile central nervous syphilis. Symptoms do not usually develop until the child is over the age of ten years, but occasionally they begin earlier. A previously normal child, often without physical stigmata of the disease, begins to deteriorate intellectually and becomes irritable, forgetful and dirty. His speech becomes slow and slurred. Fits may occur. On examination, Argyll-Robertson pupils are often found, together with tremor of the lips and hands, and an ataxic or spastic gait. The CSF contains a slight excess of lymphocytes and protein, the Wassermann reaction is positive, and the Lange gold curve is of the paretic type. Treatment is usually ineffective, and death occurs in a few years. Fortunately it is an extremely rare condition.

Juvenile Tabes Dorsalis

This is another rare manifestation of congenital syphilis. The age of onset is the same as in juvenile general paresis, and the first symptoms are optic atrophy leading to blindness, incontinence of urine, or an ataxic gait. The CSF may be normal apart from giving a positive Wassermann reaction. The course is slow, but the ultimate prognosis is poor.

ACUTE ANTERIOR POLIOMYELITIS
(Heine-Medin Disease)

A WIDELY prevalent virus infection is responsible. Usually, this causes a mild febrile illness, but in some cases produces flaccid paralysis of varying severity and distribution, due to central nervous involvement. The diagnosis is seldom made in the many cases in which there is no paralysis. In some countries the disease occurs in epidemic form.

ÆTIOLOGY

The disease is caused by one of a group of small viruses. Up to date three antigenically distinct types of poliomyelitis virus are known, the Brunhilde, the Lansing and the Leon strains, of which the first is thought to be responsible for most outbreaks of the disease. Infection with each type of virus is believed to produce a lasting, but specific, immunity. Second attacks of the paralytic disease are very rare and are probably due to infection with a second of the three types of virus.

EPIDEMIOLOGY

The mode of spread of the disease is not understood. Man is the only known living reservoir of the virus, which can be recovered from the fæces of individuals and from sewage during epidemics. It is likely that the virus is spread by healthy carriers. The cause of epidemics is not known; they occur in late summer and autumn, but whether the virus is fly-borne has not been proved. The reasons for the increasing frequency and severity of epidemics in certain countries in the past three-quarters of a century are thought to be related to the following facts: First, it is known that for every case of paralysis there are many of the mild illness and even more of the healthy carrier state. Secondly, the younger the individual when first exposed to the virus, the less likely is paralysis to ensue. Thirdly, epidemics have occurred in recent decades in countries with the highest social and economic standards. It is probable, therefore, that in less civilized countries to-day, as in all countries 100 years ago, exposure to the virus takes place in early life, producing a rare case of " infantile paralysis," but a lasting immunity in the population as a whole. But in countries with improved hygienic conditions and smaller families, exposures to the virus are likely to be postponed until an age at which paralysis is far more likely to result, and large-scale individual susceptibility results in epidemics. There are considerable fluctuations in the annual incidence of poliomyelitis, but it seems safe to say that there has been a significant decline in the numbers of victims in those countries in which large-scale vaccination has been introduced.

AGE INCIDENCE

The paralytic disease is most common between the ages of one and six years, but it may attack at any age and in recent years the proportion of all cases affecting both infants under one year and adults has increased.

INCUBATION PERIOD

This is variable, but is usually between one and three weeks.

PATHOGENESIS

The virus enters the body through the upper respiratory or gastro-intestinal tracts. Its route thence to the nervous system is via the blood stream (viræmia) or possibly along the axis cylinders of nerves. Some factors favouring damage to the central nervous system are known. The effect of age has been mentioned above. In the incubation period excessive muscular exertion, intramuscular injections (especially of diphtheria APT) and tonsillectomy are known to increase the risk of paralysis. Injections are usually associated with paralysis of the injected limb and tonsillectomy with brain stem poliomyelitis.

PATHOLOGY

Post mortem the spinal cord and medulla are œdematous and congested. There may also be cerebral œdema. Histological changes are widespread, but most marked in the anterior horns of the spinal cord and in the motor nuclei in the medulla, where there is vascular engorgement and perivascular infiltration with lymphocytes, plasma cells and microglia. The motor cells show changes varying from mild chromatolysis to necrosis and complete disappearance.

CLINICAL FEATURES

There are three stages in the illness of poliomyelitis, but one or more stages may not take place.

1. *The Initial Illness.* There is a sudden onset of fever, lassitude, and headache, frequently with sore throat and vomiting. Symptoms last from a few hours to two days. The initial illness is commonly the sole manifestation of poliomyelitis, but, unless followed by the second stage, is seldom recognized as such and usually called " summer 'flu."

2. *The Meningitic Illness* (preparalytic or nonparalytic illness). This may follow immediately on the initial illness, or after a latent period of two to four days, or may be the first sign of the disease. The temperature rises again to say 102° or 103° F and headache and vomiting may recur. The characteristic signs at this stage are stiffness and pain on flexion of the neck and spine. There may even be head retraction and opisthotonos. In contrast with the purulent and tuberculous meningitides, however, the child is usually not drowsy, but rational and alert. In older children there is often widespread muscle aching and tenderness. The pain may be severe and persist for several days. Transient hypertonus and increased tendon reflexes may be detected on examination. There is sometimes temporary retention of urine.

At this stage *cerebrospinal fluid changes* are usually, but not invariably, found. The cell count is increased up to a few hundreds, a variable proportion being polymorphonuclear cells. The protein level is slightly raised. The cell-count returns to normal in the course of a week or two, the polymorphonuclear cells disappearing first, while the protein gradually rises and returns to normal in four to ten weeks.

The meningitic illness may last from two to ten days. When paralysis occurs, it usually begins on the second to fourth day.

3. *The Paralytic Illness.* The fever of the meningitic illness may have begun to subside, but rises again shortly before the onset of paralysis. The paralysis is usually complete within 24 or 48 hours of its first appearance, but this is not always so and the danger of fresh paralysis is present for as long as the temperature remains raised. Paralysis results from damage to the cells of the lower motor neurones and is therefore of the flaccid type with loss of tendon reflexes and, eventually, wasting. There is no sensory loss. The main attack may fall on the muscles supplied from the spinal cord or the brain stem or both.

(a) Spinal type. The paralysis involves groups of muscles and is typically asymmetrical in distribution. It affects legs more than arms and arms more than trunk. In fatal cases death is nearly always due to paralysis of the intercostal muscles and diaphragm. Recovery of muscle power begins when the fever has subsided. Most of the ultimate recovery will have taken place within three to six months. The severity of the paralysis can vary from transient weakness and loss of reflexes in, say, one leg to a complete and permanent paralysis of all four limbs and trunk.

(b) Brain-stem type. It is fortunate that this type occurs much less frequently than the spinal paralysis, as the case mortality is high. Facial palsy is common and squints sometimes appear, but the main attack is on the motor cranial nerve nuclei and vital centres in the medulla—hence the term " bulbar poliomyelitis." Palatal, pharyngeal and laryngeal paralysis impair the mechanisms of swallowing and coughing, and suffocation may result from inhalation of secretions (a " nasal " speech is often the first sign). Frequently there is also involvement of the respiratory centre, producing shallow and irregular breathing, which may be followed by sudden respiratory failure. Other grave complications include peripheral circulatory failure and hyperpyrexia. Brain-stem poliomyelitis is frequently combined with the spinal type, and the co-existence of intercostal and diaphragmatic paralysis worsen the prognosis.

(c) A cerebral type of poliomyelitis producing delirium, drowsiness and stupor is rare. Convulsions in poliomyelitis are extremely rare.

(d) " Cerebellar " type. Ataxia occasionally occurs—usually in combination with signs of brain-stem involvement—but it is doubtful if the cerebellum is the site of the disorder.

DIAGNOSIS

In the initial illness a certain clinical diagnosis is not possible. It cannot be distinguished from influenza and other mild fevers, although a reasonable suspicion may be entertained if it occurs during an epidemic of poliomyelitis. The muscle tenderness may help to distinguish the meningitic stage from other types of aseptic meningitis, while the purulent and tuberculous meningitides are characterized by drowsiness and their CSF changes. In the paralytic illness the typical course, with fever, headache and neck stiffness followed by flaccid paralysis—usually asymmetrical—makes the diagnosis easy. Polyneuritis is distinguished by the distribution of the paralysis, by the CSF findings and the frequent occurrence of sensory abnormalities. " Pseudoparalysis " due to pain in scurvy, osteomyelitis and acute rheumatism may be confusing.

By modern methods of tissue culture, the virus can be isolated from stools and nasal washing, and a rising titre of neutralizing antibodies in the serum during convalescence makes a tentative diagnosis certain.

PROGNOSIS

In epidemics the mortality rate in paralytic cases is about 10 per cent. but various considerably. It is highest in the brain-stem type. Cranial nerve palsies usually recover completely if the patient survives. About half those patients with early recognizable limb palsies recover completely, the others being left with some degree of crippling. Little recovery can be expected in muscles in which no movement is detected after one month.

TREATMENT[1]

Meningitic and paralytic cases should be admitted to a hospital in which there are facilities for dealing with the various emergencies which may arise. The risk of cross infection is slight, but the child should be isolated until three weeks after the fever has subsided and excreta should be disposed of antiseptically. In the early stages complete bed rest and the minimum of disturbance are the rules. Analgesics may be necessary and frequently changed hot, wet packs help to relieve muscle pains. When paralysis has occurred each limb must be positioned to relax the paralysed muscle and stretch the antagonists in order to prevent faulty posture. Attention to the skin at pressure points and to bladder and bowels is important. A careful watch must be kept for the dyspnœa, restlessness and anxiety that mark the onset of respiratory paralysis. As paralysis of the intercostal muscles and diaphragm may take place rapidly, a mechanical respirator,[2] and someone who knows how to use it, must be quickly available. In cases of brain-stem poliomyelitis the most immediate danger lies in suffocation by aspiration of pharyngeal secretions. The foot of the bed (or stretcher, if the child is being taken to hospital) should be raised 12–18 inches and the child turned on his side or face to permit postural drainage. Repeated aspiration of the pharynx will be necessary. Tank respirators are usually ineffective in the treatment of the central respiratory failure which may result from brain-stem poliomyelitis. In these cases positive pressure respiration with the aid of an anæsthetic bag or automatic pump is the most effective method,[3, 4] combined with tracheostomy and a cuffed endotracheal tube to facilitate the artificial respiration and tracheal aspiration. Bronchoscopy will be necessary if pulmonary collapse takes place in spite of repeated aspiration. Barbiturates should be given to quieten an anxious and restless child. If the child is cyanosed oxygen must be administered, and antibiotics are usually given as a prophylaxis against inhalation pneumonia.

During convalescence from the acute illness, massage and carefully graded exercises are of value in helping the child to regain limb functions and in the prevention of contractures.

[1] Steigman, A. J. (1954). *Amer. J. Dis. Child.*, **87**, 343.
[2] Wilson, J. L. (1948). " Use of the Respirator in Poliomyelitis." New York: Publication of the National Foundation for Infantile Paralysis, No. 23.
[3] Lassen, H. C. A. (1953). *Lancet*, 1, 37.
[4] Russell, W. A., Schuster, E. (1953). *Ibid.*, 2, 707.

It should not be forgotten that throughout the illness everything should be done to sustain the child's courage and to occupy his interests.

Vaccination appears to afford considerable, but not complete protection. A killed virus vaccine (Salk) has been most generally used. One ml. is injected intramuscularly at intervals of one month, for three successive months, starting between 6 and 12 months of age. Extensive trials have also been made with a live attenuated vaccine given by mouth.

Contacts are usually excluded from school for three weeks. There are certain precautions which will lessen the chances of paralysis complicating an infection with the virus. If during a poliomyelitis epidemic a child is taken ill with symptoms which may be those of the initial illness, it is wise to limit muscular exertion as much as possible in the ensuing five or six days. Tonsillectomy and intramuscular injections, unless essential, should be avoided during poliomyelitis epidemics. Passive immunization with the gammaglobulin fraction of pooled human serum may provide a short lived and partial protection of contacts.

POLYNEURITIS

THIS term is used to describe a group of conditions of widely differing ætiology in which there is impairment of function of peripheral nerves producing symmetrical flaccid paresis and, usually, sensory loss. The cerebrospinal fluid characteristically shows no pleocytosis but instead a moderate to considerable increase in protein content. Death occasionally results from respiratory paralysis, but in the great majority recovery is complete and there is no residual weakness. There is usually no convincing explanation for acute polyneuritis in childhood, although its origin is thought to be infective. Pink disease and diphtheritic polyneuritis are rare to-day. Tetanus can be considered with the polyneuritides, but differs from them in the site of damage to the neuromuscular system. Rare forms of polyneuritis are associated with thiamine deficiency, lead and other heavy-metal poisoning and acute porphyria, and polyneuritis is a rare complication of almost all the acute specific fevers.

Acute Infective Polyneuritis (Infective Neuronitis, Polyradiculitis, Guillain-Barré Syndrome)

There is generally a history of a mild and short-lived febrile illness which precedes the onset of symptoms by one to three weeks. Pathological findings in the few patients who have died early in the course of the disease suggest that it is due to a sensitivity reaction of parts of the central nervous system rather than to an inflammatory disorder.

PATHOLOGY

The essential feature is an œdema of the spinal nerve roots followed by a mild inflammatory reaction, which may extend into the spinal cord, with in some cases neuronal degeneration.

CLINICAL FEATURES

The disease may occur at any age; the onset may be sudden and rapidly progressive, but it is more commonly gradual and increases over a period of one to four weeks. The legs are usually affected first, and the paralysis then ascends to involve the trunk and arms and in some cases the diaphragm and pharyngeal and laryngeal muscles. (A rapidly ascending paralysis is often called Landry's paralysis.) The paralysis is symmetrical and usually appears to involve the proximal more than the distal muscles. In many cases there is no sensory disturbance (" motor radiculitis "), but in others there is both pain and hyperæsthesia with objective signs of sensory loss, especially at the periphery of the limbs. Occasionally there are temporary signs of transverse myelitis with retention of urine and extensor plantar responses. The child is usually afebrile, but there is often a persistent tachycardia. The cerebrospinal fluid shows the characteristic changes mentioned above; in rare cases, in which the protein level is greatly raised, there may be an associated rise in intracranial pressure with headache, vomiting and papillœdema. Death may occur from respiratory paralysis, but most patients begin to improve after a few weeks and are perfectly well in about three months.

TREATMENT

There is no specific treatment. A mechanical respirator should always be available, and, if death from respiratory paralysis can be prevented, the eventual outcome, unlike poliomyelitis, is wholly favourable.

Diphtheritic Polyneuritis (see also p. 553)

ÆTIOLOGY

The neuritis is caused by toxin released by the diphtheria bacillus. It may follow a severe attack of diphtheria, a mild attack which has passed unrecognized or one in which antitoxin has been given late.

PATHOLOGY

The nerves show œdema, demyelination, and other degenerative signs, especially in their peripheral portions.

CLINICAL FEATURES

The first sign of neuritis usually appears in the second or third week when the child regurgitates fluids from the nose and acquires a nasal voice due to paralysis of the soft palate. In the third or fourth week paralysis of the ciliary muscle may lead to blurring of vision for close objects, although distant objects are seen clearly. Both palatal and ciliary paralysis recover in a few weeks, but from the fifth to twelfth weeks a generalized polyneuritis may develop. Loss of tendon reflexes is followed by symmetrical weakness—more marked in the legs than the arms. The limb paresis is rarely severe. Muscle tenderness and loss of sensation of a " glove and stocking " distribution may be present. Diaphragmatic paralysis may occur and will necessitate the use of a mechanical respirator. The greatest danger to life is the occurrence of a pharyngeal and laryngeal paralysis which may result in aspiration pneumonia or massive collapse of the lung. There may also be a recrudescence of an earlier diphtheritic myocarditis. If the child can be tided over these dangers, eventual recovery is complete.

Pink Disease (Erythrœdema Polyneuritis; Infantile Acrodynia)

This disease appears to be a form of polyneuritis with special involvement of the autonomic nervous system.

ÆTIOLOGY

The febrile illness which often preceded the onset of symptoms and the fact that the incidence seemed to vary with locality and season suggested an infective origin. It now seems certain, however, that the disease is the result of an exceptional sensitivity to mercury, and the incidence of the disease in England has markedly declined since calomel has been omitted from certain popular " teething powders."

AGE INCIDENCE

Incidence varies between 4 months and 7 years, but most cases occur between 9 and 18 months. Both sexes are equally affected.

Mental Upset. In perhaps no other disease is the child more wretched, and nothing will comfort him. A state of complete negativism develops; everything is refused. There is loss of appetite, all the good habits and training fail, and insomnia is most marked. The child with pink disease presents a picture of utter misery. The mind is not affected; he takes notice of his surroundings, and understands, but is markedly preoccupied with his own unhappiness.

There is usually insomnia, but the ordinary hypnotics have little or no effect. Wasting occurs, since there is obstinate refusal of food.

Rash. A pink macular rash may appear for a few days on the trunk early in the illness, and later there is often a profuse but mild folliculitis. The disease owes its name to the pink appearance of the nose and forehead, hands and feet. The latter show a diffuse redness in the glove-and-sock distribution, and have the appearance of having been dipped into very hot water. When touched, however, they are cold and slightly swollen, and do not pit on pressure. In time, these sodden hands and feet tend to peel, and the condition waxes and wanes, sometimes better and sometimes worse. The rash on the trunk, which is a typical sweat rash, also waxes and wanes and, because of the constant moisture of the skin, furunculosis is apt to develop. The

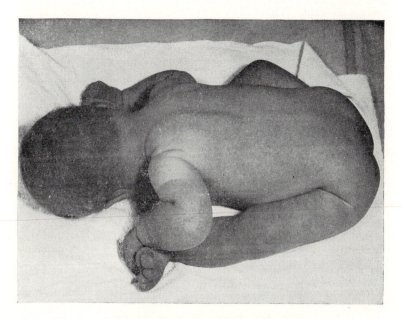

Fig. 45.—A characteristic posture in pink disease.

skin of the hands and feet irritates the child, so that they are constantly being rubbed one against the other. A much older child once told Dr. Paterson that his hands and feet " felt like fire."

Attitude in Bed. A typical attitude, except in very tiny infants, is that the child lies on his face, with the knees drawn up and the face buried in the pillow, in what might be termed the " kangaroo " or " knee-elbow " position. The head is slowly rolled from side to side in a burrowing motion into the pillow (Fig. 45), in an effort to allay the irritation of the forehead, cheeks, and tip of the nose, which look red from friction.

Photophobia. This is rather variable and where it exists is one of the reasons for the attitude in bed. At times it is the first and most marked symptom, and in some cases almost the *only* symptom of the disease.

Muscular Hypotonia. All the muscles are soft and flabby; the knee-jerks are very difficult to elicit, or absent. Rectal prolapse is not infrequent.

General. Small ulcers appear on the tongue and in the cheeks; these add to the difficulty of getting the child to take his food. Some of the teeth become loose, and may be swallowed and appear in the stools. The hair tends to fall out, and in severe cases large bald patches appear. The nails may fall off in more marked cases, although this is very rare. There is very definite dulling of sensation to pin-pricks over the feet, hands, and tip of the nose. Nothing characteristic is found in the fundi or in the respiratory system.

A prolonged tachycardia is one of the most characteristic features. The blood-pressure is almost invariably raised to 120–140 mm. of mercury. The clinical picture suggests that there is some disturbance of the autonomic nervous system, as shown by the sweating, rapid pulse, raised blood-pressure, vaso-motor paralysis at the extremities, salivation, rhinorrhœa, photophobia and trophic disturbances. The sedimentation rate is normal.

PROGNOSIS

The disease lasts from 4 to 6 months. This fact should be impressed on the parents so that they are not impatient. The mortality rate is very low; when a child with pink disease dies it is usually the result of emaciation and secondary infection. When recovery takes place, it is complete and the children are later normal in every way.

TREATMENT

Mercury intoxication may be treated by the administration of dimercaptopropanol (BAL) or Calcium Disodium Versenate, but it is not certain to what extent either treatment shortens the course of the illness.

An infant who suffers from insomnia, anorexia and irritability continually for weeks or months may well prove too exhausting to the mother unless she is helped by a nurse or relatives. The child may therefore have to be admitted to hospital. The additional danger of secondary infection is not to-day as serious a drawback to hospital treatment, especially if the child can be isolated.

An all-round, well-balanced diet should be maintained, together with a liberal supply of vitamins. Because of the ulcers in the mouth, spoon-feeding may be difficult, and when refusal of food is extreme, feeding by stomach tube is indicated. This, however, is rarely necessary.

Sedatives, barbiturates, chloral or paraldehyde may be necessary to combat insomnia and irritability.

For the sweating, frequent changes of clothing and much sponging and powdering are necessary, and the skin should be kept meticulously cleansed if boils and infections are to be avoided. The application of a methylated spirit rub to the body may be useful. The child should always be very lightly clad, and be on the cool side, rather than too warm.

Familial Dysautonomia

Dysautonomia[1] is a rare congenital condition sometimes seen in siblings. It may be due to a recessive gene. The manifestations are defective lacrimation, lability of blood pressure and instability of temperature control; also difficulty in swallowing which may interfere with feeding in early infancy, sometimes causing aspiration pneumonia and early death. Changes seen in the skin are transient blotching and excessive perspiration. Episodes of vomiting sometimes occur or diarrhœa. The corneal and deep reflexes are depressed. There is relative insensitivity to pain, as shown by diminution of response to pin-prick, and there may be emotional instability.

Tetanus (Lock Jaw) (see also p. 593)

This condition is caused by the exotoxin of the *Clostridium tetani* which is released when spores of this organism germinate in a septic wound. Local and general muscular rigidity results from a direct effect of the toxin on the muscles. Tonic convulsions are thought to result from a disturbance of the reflex arc caused by the toxin when it reaches the spinal cord, probably via the peripheral nerves.

CLINICAL FEATURES

Tetanus is most commonly seen following trivial wounds (abrasions, especially if covered with adhesive plaster, splinter and nail wounds, etc.) which have become septic and healed over. In some cases no wound can be found. Tetanus neonatorum is a rare complication of umbilical sepsis. The incubation period is usually between one and two weeks, but may be as short as three days or as long as several months. The symptoms can be divided into three stages, which consist of local rigidity, generalized rigidity and reflex tonic convulsions, and which appear in that order. The longer the delay in the appearance of each stage, the better the outlook. The first stage, consisting of aching and muscular rigidity near the site of the wound, may occur alone in mild cases or may precede the second and third stages. Most commonly, however, the first symptoms are those of the second stage of generalized tonic rigidity. The first muscles to be affected are usually the masseter and facial muscles, producing trismus and spasm of the face (risus sardonicus). The first sign is therefore difficulty in eating. A few hours later the trunk muscles become rigid. The more powerful spinal muscles produce opisthotonos, while the board-like rigidity of the abdominal wall might suggest acute peritonitis, except that there is no tenderness. This tonic rigidity remains unchanged for days or weeks and is not in itself dangerous to the child. The third stage, that of tonic convulsions,

[1] Riley, C. M. (1957). Familial dysautonomia. *Advanc. Pediat.*, **9**, 157.
Hutchison, J. H., Hamilton, N. (1962). *Lancet*, 1, 1216.

is superimposed on the second within one to seven days. Any sensory stimulus, such as handling the child, giving an injection, a loud noise or bright light, may precipitate a convulsion. The whole body is thrown into an extremely powerful spasm, the jaws clench, the back arches and respiration stops. A convulsion may last for several minutes and cause death from asphyxia. As the disease progresses, the convulsions become more frequent and severe, but in patients who survive cease after one to three weeks. Unless the illness is complicated by pneumonia, the child is usually afebrile throughout, but in some cases a sudden onset of hyperpyrexia proves fatal. Death may also be caused by central respiratory failure. There is no interference with the consciousness. The diagnosis is usually easy. In the early stages of trismus and dysphagia the condition must be distinguished from quinsy, impacted wisdom teeth, etc. There is no disease that can be easily confused with the stage of tonic rigidity. Certain forms of encephalitis may show trismus at the onset, but this is accompanied by drowsiness and fever. In the convulsive stage meningitis and epilepsy can easily be distinguished. Strychnine poisoning produces similar tonic convulsions, but there is no rigidity between paroxysms.

TREATMENT

The objectives are to neutralize any circulating toxin; to limit the frequency and severity of convulsions; to maintain the child's nutrition and general health, and to prevent infections. 100,000 i.u. of antitoxin should be given as soon as possible by intramuscular injection. (Intravenous, intrathecal and intracisternal injections are sometimes advocated, but there are dangers in these methods of administration which probably outweigh the advantages.) Before giving the injection, inquiry should be made about asthma or any allergic disease and about any previous injection of horse serum. With a positive history, 0·1 ml. of a 1/100 dilution should be given subcutaneously and tenfold doses repeated at two-hourly intervals for four or five doses before giving the full dose intramuscularly (Stanley Banks). 1/1,000 adrenaline should always be to hand in case of collapse. The wound should be excised and drained but not until the antitoxin has been given. It is of the greatest importance to limit the frequency and severity of the tonic convulsions. In some cases this can be achieved with the aid of hypnotic drugs and skilled nursing. The child should be put to bed in a darkened and quiet room. Quinalbarbitone (Seconal) is a particularly suitable drug; its dose (*see* Appendix 3) must be adjusted to control convulsions without depressing respiration. The combination of chlorpromazine or promazine with barbiturates is particularly effective in controlling spasms. The drugs should be administered every four hours as expeditiously as possible. Then one hour later, when the child is fully under the influence of the sedative, feeding, cleaning, change of position and other treatment should be carried out with as little disturbance as possible by two nurses. A nourishing fluid diet is best given in severe cases through a nasal tube. Alternatively bromethol (Avertin) may be given per rectum or paraldehyde intramuscularly (for dosage, *see* Appendix 3). These drugs are longer acting than quinalbarbitone and should be given eight to twelve hourly as required.

In cases in which these measures are unsuccessful in controlling spasms, muscle relaxant drugs (e.g. mephenesin or gallamine triethiodide) may help, but it is difficult to adjust the dose to produce adequate relief of spasms without impairing respiration. In the really severe case, it is probably best deliberately to paralyse all voluntary muscles, including the respiratory, with tubocurarine[1, 2] or succinylcholine[3], for several days if necessary, maintaining life by artificial respiration. In such cases tracheotomy is necessary to facilitate positive pressure respiration and tracheal aspiration and to overcome the danger of laryngeal spasm. In all cases antibiotics should be given as a prophylaxis against pneumonia. Artificial cooling has been recommended to prevent death from hyperpyrexia.[2]

The successful treatment of a severe case of tetanus[4] necessitates constant medical and nursing care, laboratory assistance and the co-operation of a physician or anæsthetist experienced in the use of the muscle relaxant drugs.

PROPHYLAXIS

Passive immunization may be obtained by the intramuscular injection of 3,000 units of antitoxin as soon as possible after the wound has occurred. Again an inquiry must be made about allergic tendencies or previous serum injections. If the wound suppurates, the dose should be repeated at weekly intervals. Active immunization may be achieved by three subcutaneous injections of 1 ml. of tetanus toxoid at intervals of one month to six weeks. This may be combined with diphtheria prophylaxis in infancy. The immunity lasts for probably a number of years, but if the child acquires a wound likely to be contaminated, immunity can be rapidly and safely increased by another injection of the toxoid.

Acute Porphyrinuria (*see also* p. 135)

This disease, inherited as a dominant characteristic, is an inborn error of metabolism which, however, does not usually manifest itself until late childhood or early adult life, and then in attacks. The illness begins with severe abdominal pain and vomiting and sometimes convulsions and delirium. These symptoms are followed in a few

[1] Honey, G. E., Dwyer, B. E., Smith, A. C., Spalding, J. M. K. (1954). *Brit. med. J.*, 2, 442.
[2] Rossi, E., Dodmer, A., Bettex, M., Graf, K. (1954). *Helv. pædiat. Acta*, **9**, 425.
[3] Forrester, A. T. T. (1954). *Brit. med. J.*, 2, 342.
[4] Powell, K. J., Brimblecombe, F. S, W., Stoneman, Margaret E, R. (1958). *Lancet*, 1, 713,

days by polyneuritis with pains in the limbs and muscular weakness. The urine becomes deeply red due to the excretion of porphyrins. The attacks, which may be precipitated by barbiturates, tend to recur and the ultimate prognosis is poor.

FACIAL PALSY

FACIAL palsy may be present at birth or acquired in later childhood. Congenital facial palsy is detected when it is noticed that the infant does not close one eye and that the same side of the mouth does not move. This condition is usually a complication of forceps delivery and is the result of pressure on the nerve; recovery almost always takes place in a few weeks. Rarely, damage to the facial nerve results from more serious birth injury with intracranial hæmorrhage or skull fracture. Developmental defects of the seventh nerve nucleus, usually bilateral and associated with other cranial nerve defects, are exceedingly rare. Unilateral dislocation of the jaw may be wrongly diagnosed as facial palsy. Supranuclear facial palsy, commonly part of a congenital hemiplegia, does not become apparent until the baby is several months old.

Facial palsy can be acquired in later childhood in several ways. A supranuclear lesion, usually a cerebral tumour, causes most obvious paralysis of the lower face and on voluntary rather than emotional movements. Nuclear lesions may result from poliomyelitis or pontine tumours. In the latter case, the palsy is often bilateral and associated with other cranial nerve palsies. Outside the brain, the nerve may be compressed by cerebello-pontine angle tumours, meningeal adhesions or skull fractures; it may be damaged in osteomyelitis of the facial canal secondary to otitis media, or in the stylomastoid foramen in the condition known as Bell's palsy. Acute infective and other forms of neuritis may involve the facial nerve. Bilateral facial palsy may also result from muscular diseases, e.g. myasthenia gravis, certain types of muscular dystrophy and dystrophia myotonica.

Bell's Palsy

ÆTIOLOGY AND PATHOLOGY

One facial nerve becomes œdematous and swollen within the stylomastoid foramen, possibly as a result of infection.

CLINICAL FEATURES

The palsy develops suddenly, sometimes after coryza or exposure to cold draughts. The first symptom is pain in the face, followed by inability to close one eye and to retract the corner of the mouth, which is drawn over to the normal side. The forehead cannot be wrinkled up. Recovery is the rule, although it may take weeks or months to be complete.

TREATMENT

Physiotherapy is of little avail. The angle of the mouth should be drawn back and up by a wire splint over the ear to prevent stretching of the paralysed muscles. Corticosteroids have been used in treatment but as recovery is usually spontaneous their efficacy is uncertain. In the rare cases in which there are no signs of recovery by six months, the hypoglossal nerve is sometimes transplanted into the degenerated facial nerve.

DEVELOPMENTAL DISORDERS

Hydrocephalus

HYDROCEPHALUS means an excess of cerebrospinal fluid within the skull. In external hydrocephalus the fluid lies outside the brain in the subarachnoid or subdural spaces. In internal hydrocephalus the main accumulation is within the ventricles. Excess fluid may simply replace diminished brain tissue (" hydrocephalus *ex vacuo* ") or it may result from obstruction to the escape routes for CSF. In practice the term hydrocephalus normally refers to *internal obstructive hydrocephalus*.

CSF is formed by the choroid plexuses of the ventricles and is absorbed into the dural sinuses. From the lateral ventricles it passes through the foramina of Monro into the third ventricle; through the aqueduct of Sylvius into the fourth ventricle, escaping into the subarachnoid space through the foramen of Magendie and the foramina of Lushka. Thence it passes forward through the basal cisterns or backward round the cerebellum and free edge of the tentorium to the surface of the cerebral hemispheres and along the sulci to the sinuses. (Some also passes downwards from the cisterna magna into the spinal subarachnoid space, but only a little can be absorbed into the spinal veins.) Hydrocephalus may result from obstruction at any point on the pathway. The obstruction may be due to a malformation, in which case hydrocephalus will be present at birth or begin in early infancy, or be acquired as the result of disease, although rarely before birth.

The terms " communicating " and " non-communicating " applied to hydrocephalus refer to the presence or absence of free communication between the ventricular system and the spinal subarachnoid space. This clearly depends on the site of the obstruction.

Very rarely hydrocephalus is caused by excess production of CSF due to hypertrophy of the choroid plexus.

ÆTIOLOGY [1]

The causes of hydrocephalus are many.

(1) Malformations: stenosis, " forking " or membranous obstruction of the aqueduct of Sylvius; absence of the foramina of the fourth

---

[1] Russell, Dorothy S. (1949). " Observations on the Pathology of Hydrocephalus." Medical Research Council, Special Report Series, No, 265, London: H,M, Stationery Office,

ventricle; myelomeningocele associated with the Arnold Chiari malformation (producing obstruction to the outlets of the fourth ventricle or to the basal subarachnoid space); similar obstruction due to deformities of the base of the skull (e.g. platybasia and achondroplasia); failure of development of the subarachnoid space.

(2) Acquired stenosis of the aqueduct of Sylvius, of unknown ætiology.

(3) Intracranial hæmorrhage (especially following birth injury) causing occlusion of the subarachnoid space by pressure (in subdural hæmorrhage) or by adhesions (in subarachnoid hæmorrhage).

(4) Meningitis, especially if treatment is delayed or inadequate, due to subarachnoid adhesions in the basal cisterns. (Some cases of " congenital " communicating hydrocephalus may be due to fœtal meningitis (e.g. toxoplasmosis) or to unrecognized meningitis in the neonatal period.)

(5) Brain tumours, by blocking, from within or without, the ventricles, aqueduct or subarachnoid space.

(6) Extensive dural sinus thrombosis.

CLINICAL FEATURES

Obstruction to CSF pathways produces enlargement of the ventricles and compression of the brain. If such obstruction begins in adult life there is a rapid increase in intracranial pressure, but in infants and young children the cranial sutures separate and the head enlarges.

In infantile cases the head may be large at birth, but more commonly the rapid growth first becomes obvious at two or three months of age. The head is uniformly enlarged in all diameters (Fig. 46). The forehead bulges forward, stretching the scalp and drawing up the eyelids, while pressure above the orbits pushes the eyes downwards, so that a rim of sclera shows above the iris. The fontanelles are large; the suture lines are wide and the bones thin, so that they may yield slightly on pressure. The scalp veins are prominent. The baby tends to be lethargic, and vomiting is a common symptom. Primary optic atrophy occurs more commonly than papillœdema, which is rare in infancy simply because the skull can expand in response to a rise in intracranial pressure.

If the head continues to enlarge the infant dies within a few months of infection or malnutrition. But sometimes a balance seems to be reached between CSF production and absorption. The head ceases to expand, and the small body " catches up " in growth, so that ultimately little enlargement of the head is noted. This is particularly the case in " communicating " hydrocephalus caused by subarachnoid adhesions (Lawrence[1]). There may be gross mental deficiency, although in many cases intelligence is but moderately retarded, even when air ventriculograms show the cerebral cortex to be markedly

[1] Lawrence, K. M. (1958). *Lancet*, 2, 1152.

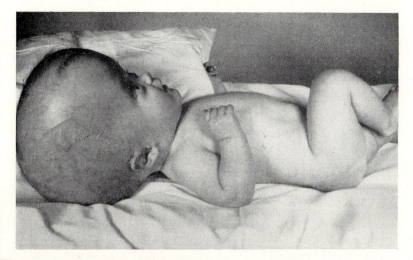

Fig. 46.—Hydrocephalus in a 3-month-old baby.

thinned. Other neurological sequelæ include spasticity, cerebellar ataxia, strabismus and convulsions.

DIFFERENTIAL DIAGNOSIS

The finding of large fontanelles and wide spaces between the vault bones of the skull may result from a disorder of bone (rickets, osteogenesis imperfecta or more commonly a simple delay in membrane bone growth not associated with any disease process), rather than from expansion of the head. When the skull bones are widely separated, the skull circumference should be measured; hydrocephalus should be suspected if the circumference exceeds the average for the infant's age by more than one inch.[1] If the enlargement is doubtful, measurements should be repeated at weekly intervals. Pathological enlargement of the head is usually due to hydrocephalus, but subdural hæmatoma and, rarely, enlargement of the brain (primary macrocephaly or secondary enlargement due to lipoidosis or other degenerative disease) must be distinguished. The diagnosis may be confirmed by ventriculography.

TREATMENT

The removal of a subdural hæmatoma or cerebral tumour may lead to permanent cure. With other causes of obstruction, however, treatment is directed to making alternative escape routes for the CSF, and although many ingenious operations have been devised, the results are not very satisfactory.

[1] Average head circumferences for male infants are as follows: Birth 14 inches; 3 months, 16 inches; 6 months, 17½ inches; 9 months, 18 inches; 12 months, 18½ inches; 18 months, 19 inches; 2 years, 19½ inches; 3 years, 20 inches; 5 years, 20½ inches (see also Appendix 5). Average for females is ½ inch less.

It must first be determined if the hydrocephalus is of the communicating or non-communicating type. This is best achieved by air studies. Alternatively, a dye (neutral phenol-sulphone-phthalein) is injected into the lumbar theca and a ventricular tap is made in half an hour, by which time the dye should have diffused to the ventricular CSF if there is no intervening block.

In non-communicating hydrocephalus a plastic tube may be inserted between a lateral ventricular and the basal cistern (Torkildsen's operation). In communicating hydrocephalus the tube is passed from the lumbar theca into the peritoneal cavity or ureter. Recently hydrocephalus has been successfully treated by the draining of the CSF directly into the venous system. One end of a plastic tube is placed in the right lateral ventricle and the other into the superior vena cava via the external jugular; a Spitz-Holter valve is interposed to prevent reflux of blood into the ventricle.

Hydrancephaly

In this condition the head is at first of normal size, but the skull is almost entirely filled with CSF so that on applying a powerful torchlight to the scalp the entire head transilluminates. The pathology is that of gross porencephaly rather than agenesis of the cerebral hemispheres. The condition presents with fits or failure of development, although the baby may behave normally in the neonatal period. Later the head enlarges. There is, of course, gross mental defect.

Craniostenosis

The bones of the vault of the skull are normally separated from each other by thin membranous strips. At birth the edges of the bones are straight and, after the first month, the gaps between them should not exceed 1 mm. From about the sixth month the bones begin to interdigitate, so that it is no longer possible to insert a needle between them. By about the tenth year they are so firmly interlocked that a rise of intracranial pressure no longer causes enlargement of the head. Bony union does not occur until late middle age.

In the condition of craniostenosis, however, bony fusion across one or more suture lines takes place before birth or in early childhood, and its effect is to prevent further growth of the skull in the direction at right angles to the line of the obliterated suture. Compensatory growth will take place across the line of the normal sutures, producing a distorted head.

Type	Sutures Involved	Shape of Skull
I	One coronal or one lambdoid.	Plagiocephaly—an asymmetrical head.
II	Both coronals (with rarely both lambdoids).	Acrobrachycephaly—a short, wide and tall head (Fig. 48).
III	The sagittal suture.	Scaphocephaly—a long, narrow head (Fig. 47).
IV	All sutures.	Oxycephaly—a small head, pointed in the region of the anterior fontanelle.

These malformations are probably determined genetically, as familial cases have been reported.

Craniostenosis is usually present at birth, but Type IV may not develop until the child is a few years old. Types II and IV may be associated with deformities of the base of the skull and with syndactylism of hands and feet (Fig. 48).

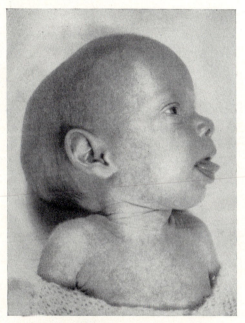

Fig. 47.—Scaphocephaly in a 2-month-old infant due to premature closure of the sagittal suture.

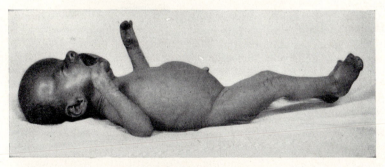

Fig. 48.—Acrobrachycephaly (turricephaly) due to premature closure of the coronal and lambdoid sutures in a month-old infant. Note the syndactyly of hands and feet.

The brain is usually normal in craniostenosis, and in growing within the small skull may press on surrounding structures, producing, for instance, a narrowed nasopharynx (and upper respiratory tract obstruction), exophthalmus and papillœdema and even blindness. Mental retardation occurs later, if the restriction to the growth of the brain is not relieved. These secondary pressure defects are common in Types IV and II, but not in Types I or III.

DIAGNOSIS

It is important to distinguish Type IV from the more common microcephaly, in which the head is small because the brain is small and the cranial sutures are all present. In craniostenosis the obliterated suture line is frequently marked by a palpable ridge, and the absence of a suture line may be confirmed by x-ray. (The metopic suture is normally closed before birth, and a central vertical ridge on the forehead is of no significance.)

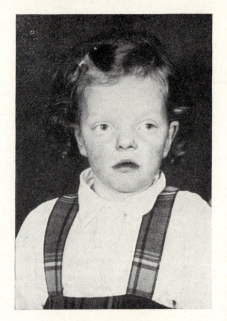

TREATMENT

Intracranial pressure signs may be relieved and normal brain growth permitted by the creation of artificial suture lines;[1] this operation should be performed early. The final cosmetic result is, however, not always satisfactory, because of associated malformation of the base of the skull.

Fig. 49.—Hypertelorism.

Hypertelorism

This is a rare malformation of the sphenoid bone, the greater wings being small and the lesser wings large. As a result, the eyes are widely set apart and the bridge of the nose broadened (Fig. 49). The head is often brachycephalic. Unilateral hypertelorism has been reported. Children with hypertelorism are usually mentally defective.

Sturge-Weber Syndrome

This is a sporadically occurring malformation in which a capillary nævus (" port wine stain ") in the area of distribution of one trigeminal

[1] Ingram, F. D., Alexander, E., Matson, D. D. (1948). *Surgery*, **24**, 518.

nerve is associated with angiomata of the cerebral cortex. X-rays usually show wavy lines of subcortical calcification. Hemiparesis, focal fits and mental deficiency are frequent associations (Fig. 50).

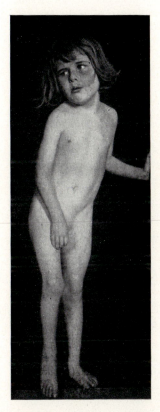

Fig. 50.—A child of 5 years with the Sturge-Weber syndrome. Note the left facial nævus and the hemiplegic posture of the right arm and leg.

CONGENITAL MALFORMATIONS OF THE SPINAL CORD

Spina Bifida

SPINA BIFIDA is a defect in the spinal column. It usually takes the form of a failure of the laminæ to unite, producing a posterior defect, commonly in the lumbar or sacral regions, less commonly in the upper cervical region or elsewhere. (Rarely, a vertebral body may be defective, leading to anterior defect and thoracic' abdominal or pelvic tumours.)

Spina Bifida Occulta

This is a common condition, a simple bony defect which can only be detected on x-ray examination, but the presence of which may be suspected from the finding of a (mid-line), dimple, tuft of hair, lipoma or skin sinus overlying the spine, usually in the lumbar region. In itself it is harmless, but it is occasionally associated with fibrous adhesions to the cord, or congenital defects of the cord, resulting in weakness of the legs and lack of sphincter control. In such cases operation is indicated. Enuresis can rarely be attributed to spina bifida occulta, and when related, incontinence is found by day as well as at night.

Spina Bifida Cystica

The bony defect is large and the meninges protruding through it are adherent to subcutaneous tissue and skin, producing a globular tumour (Fig. 51). This is fluctuant and translucent. When it contains CSF only (meningocele) it may be repaired surgically. Unfortunately parts of the cauda equina or cord are usually also adherent to the wall of the sac (meningomyelocele) and may be visible on transillumination. In such cases there are varying degrees of paralysis of the legs and sphincters, with sensory and trophic disturbances. This is invariably the case in meningomyelocele, presenting at birth with a raw area, which is in fact exposed spinal cord.

Hydrocephalus frequently develops in association with meningo-myelocele. In most cases this is due to the presence of the *Arnold Chiari malformation*, in which the medulla and cerebellar tonsils are misplaced within the upper cervical spinal canal. In other cases there are developmental defects in the aqueduct of Sylvius or else-where.

Myelo-meningocele is often not amenable to surgical treatment, and, although these infants may live for many months, death eventually

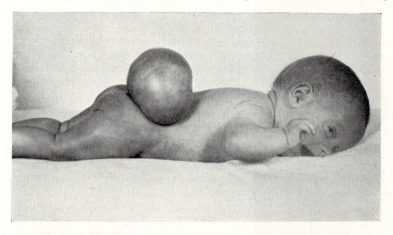

Fig. 51.—Spina bifida cystica myelo-meningocele in a 2-month-old infant.

results from infection of the sac and meningitis. If they escape this fate, they may survive with paraplegia only to die ultimately of chronic pyelonephritis, unless an ileal conduit operation (p. 362) is done.

Congenital Dermal Sinus

Local failure of closure of the neurenteric canal in embryonic life results in midline sinuses overlying the skull or vertebral column. Whenever such a sinus, which is usually of only pinpoint diameter, is located above the level of the second sacral vertebra, it may be assumed that it is connected to the dura. It frequently terminates in a subdural dermoid cyst. Eventually the cyst becomes infected through the sinus, and unfortunately it is seldom that a diagnosis is made before meningitis has developed. Even then, however, the sinus track and cyst may sometimes be removed, with a satisfactory outcome.

Diastematomyelia

The cord is pierced in the lower thoracic or lumbar regions round a central bony spine projecting from a vertebral body. As the spinal column grows more rapidly than the cord, the latter is slowly split; weakness of the legs and enuresis develop and become progressively worse. X-ray usually shows spina bifida, widening of the spinal canal and a bony septum. Removal of the bony septum often prevents the symptoms worsening.

CEREBRAL PALSY [1]

CEREBRAL palsy includes a number of conditions in which paresis and other derangements of movement result from non-progressive disorders of the brain originating before birth, at birth or in the first few years of life.

There are several fairly well-defined types of cerebral palsy, but various combinations and variations may be recognized.

ÆTIOLOGY

It is seldom that one can be certain of the cause of the original brain damage in a child with cerebral palsy. In cerebral palsied children as a whole certain significant associations are known. Histories of toxæmia of pregnancy in the mother, prematurity, perinatal anoxia or traumatic delivery are commoner than in normal children. But most babies who survive these hazards eventually prove to be normal and the limits of tolerance of the brain of a newborn baby to anoxia, for instance, are not known. Some cases of cerebral palsy appear to be caused by an arrest of development of the brain (agenesis cerebri) in prenatal life. With certain exceptions, attempts to correlate particular types of cerebral palsy with particular events in early life have hitherto been unsuccessful.

Spastic Quadriplegia and Paraplegia (Spastic Diplegia, Little's Disease)

ÆTIOLOGY

Of the factors mentioned above prematurity is particularly common. Very rarely, spastic quadriplegia or paraplegia appears to be genetically determined.

PATHOLOGY

The brain is usually small. In the cases of agenesis the external appearance of the brain may be that which is normal for early fœtal life with a greatly simplified convolutional pattern. In other cases there are numerous small gyri, and in yet others the brain may appear macroscopically normal. The cortex appears immature on microscopic examination, showing fewer than the normal number of cell layers, a reduction in ganglion cells and defects of myelinization.

[1] Recommended for further reading:
Crothers, B., Paine, R. S. (1959). " The Natural History of Cerebral Palsy." London: Oxford University Press.
Woods, G. E. (1957). " Cerebral Palsy in Childhood." Bristol: Wright.

In other cases the pathological picture of " atrophic lobar sclerosis " is found, with minute scarring on the surface of the shrunken brain and, on microscopic examination, evidence of neuronal degeneration and neuroglial overgrowth, especially in the deeper layers of the cortex.

SYMPTOMS

In many cases there are abnormalities in the neonatal period, such as prematurity, with attacks of cyanosis, convulsions, muscular hyper-tonia or hypotonia, feeding difficulty, vomiting, etc. The child may then be thought to be normal until he is several months old, when he is noticed to be backward in learning to sit up or stand. Examination at this time reveals a symmetrical weak-ness of the limbs, with increased resistance to passive movements, which is of the " clasp knife" variety. In infancy the spasticity is most noticeable in the adductors of the thigh, so that when the child is lifted the legs tend to cross (" scissors deformity", Fig. 52). Involvement of other muscle groups including the arms becomes more obvious in the second or third year of life, but paresis is always more severe in the legs than the arms and in some cases may be confined to the legs (spastic paraplegia). The spasticity is worse on attempted movement and disappears in deep sleep. The ten-don reflexes are usually brisk, but may be limited in range by the spasticity; the plantar responses may be extensor, but the abdominal reflexes are usually present. Ankle clonus may be elicitable, and tonic neck reflexes, normal only in early infancy, may be retained.

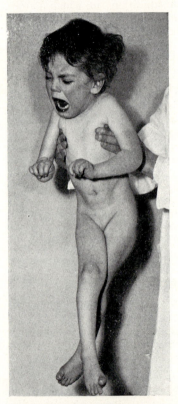

Fig. 52.—A spastic quadriplegic show-ing marked adductor spasm of the thighs. Note the characteristic posture of the hands.

The severity of the condition varies considerably. In some cases, there may be but mild paresis of the legs with spasticity, chiefly in the ca.f muscles, producing an equinus deformity of the feet, so that the child tends to walk on his toes. In the severest cases there is gross spasticity and paresis of all four limbs, and the child may be per-manently bedridden.

ASSOCIATED FEATURES

There is frequently some degree of mental deficiency—commonly in children with the most extensive limb involvement—and these children usually have small heads. There may be visual defects or even optic atrophy. Delay in talking, usually attributable to mental defect, may also result from deafness or apraxia of the tongue and lips. Dribbling from the mouth may occur for the last reason. In the most severely affected children dyspagia may be present, and vitamin deficiencies (especially scurvy) and anæmia may result from dietary limitations. Many cases are complicated by epilepsy. Paralytic dislocation of the hip is not uncommon.

Double Hemiplegia

This is sometimes distinguished from spastic quadriplegia; the degree of paralysis is asymmetrical and the arms are more affected than the legs.

Hemiplegia

One side of the body is affected as a result of a defect in the opposite cerebral hemisphere.

ÆTIOLOGY

In about three-fifths of all cases the disorder of the hemisphere originates at or before birth. There is frequently a history of difficult labour or of other abnormalities in the neonatal period. In the remaining two-fifths of cases the child has been normal at birth, the hemiplegia developing usually suddenly in infancy or early childhood. This may occur in the course of a febrile illness, but not infrequently a perfectly healthy child has suddenly been struck with unilateral convulsions and on recovery is found to have a hemiplegia. Some of such cases result from obstruction to the middle cerebral artery, whilst others are possibly caused by cerebral venous thromboses. Hemiplegia may also result from subdural hæmatoma, cerebral tumour, or lead poisoning.

PATHOLOGY

A common finding is a large " pseudoporencephalic " cyst within the affected hemisphere, usually in the area of distribution of the middle cerebral artery. This probably represents the end result of a vascular lesion. In other cases the hemisphere is atrophied, and on microscopy shows loss of nerve cells and gliosis. There may be evidence of old subdural hæmatoma. Rarely, there may be a unilateral cerebral agenesis. The skull covering the affected hemisphere is smaller, and the bone is thicker than on the opposite side.

SYMPTOMS

Even in cases undoubtedly originating from birth, the paralysis is seldom detected by the parents until the child is several months old. From that time, defective use of one arm and leg gradually becomes more obvious. (A distinct preference for one hand is unusual in normal children in the first year of life.) Examination shows a spastic paresis which is always more marked in the arm than the leg. In older children the arm becomes adducted, the forearm flexed and pronated, the wrist flexed, the thumb adducted and the fingers, usually, extended. All movements are weak and the arm is generally of little use. In contrast, the paresis of the leg is slight. The hemiplegic child always learns to walk, but may limp, or slap down the affected foot. There is usually a mild facial palsy on the same side. In about half the cases of hemiplegia the affected arm, and less frequently the leg, fail to grow normally. In such cases examination will show loss of stereognosis and other sensory defects. The sensory defects usually include a homonymous hemianopia, which, however, does not seem to inconvenience the child. Athetoid movements of the affected arm sometimes appear in later childhood.

Major convulsions, often beginning with clonic movements of the affected arm and leg, occur in more than half the cases of hemiplegia; not infrequently, convulsions first appears everal years after onset of the palsy. Temper tantrums and outbursts of violent behaviour are particularly common in those who have fits. Mental deficiency is also common, but many hemiplegic children are of normal intelligence.

Congenital Athetosis

ÆTIOLOGY

This condition results from disorders of the brain originating before birth or at the time of birth. There is frequently a history of birth injury and neonatal asphyxia. Some cases of athetosis follow "kernicterus" due to erythroblastosis fœtalis or other cause of neonatal jaundice (see p. 95).

PATHOLOGY

The usual finding is disorganization, loss of cells and gliosis in parts of the caudate and lenticular nuclei.

SYMPTOMS

Like spastic cerebral palsy, this condition is often not recognized in the first half of infancy, and medical advice is usually sought when it becomes obvious that the child is slow in learning to sit up. At that time examination may disclose symmetrical weakness of arms and legs with some rigidity or flaccidity. In the second year, however, the abnormal and involuntary movements become distinguishable from the normal incoordinate movements of infancy. Athetoid movements are slow and writhing, and are most obviously seen in the hands, forearms and face, but can affect all voluntary muscles. Irregular diaphragmatic and laryngeal actions, for instance, lead to explosive, distorted speech and uncouth noises. The involuntary movements are made worse by any attempted muscular action but are distinctly less if the child is relaxed; they disappear during sleep. Especially as a result of kernicterus, athetosis may be combined with quicker and jerkier movements like those of Sydenham's chorea (choreo-athetosis). Together with the athetosis, there is sometimes a symmetrical extrapyramidal rigidity (" lead pipe " rigidity) which may also disappear if the child is mentally relaxed. The tendon reflexes and plantar responses are usually normal.

ASSOCIATED FEATURES

Mentality is often normal in these children, in spite of appearances to the contrary. There is sometimes an associated nerve deafness, especially in cases resulting from kernicterus. Swallowing is often impaired.

Quadriplegic Rigidity

Rarely, a symmetrical extrapyramidal type of rigidity is found in older children without athetosis. These children usually have severe mental defect.

Flaccid Quadriplegia

Many mentally defective children have hypotonia of voluntary muscles (e.g. mongols). In rare cases of cerebral palsy there is marked flaccidity and weakness. These children may be thought to be suffering from amyotonia congenita, but the condition is distinguished by the mental defect and the presence of tendon reflexes.

Ataxic Quadriplegia

This is another rare condition, in which the child's motor development is delayed and intention tremor of the hands is noticed early. Later there is a staggering gait. Muscle tone is usually good. There is a tendency to spontaneous improvement. The anatomical basis for this disfunction is unknown, but agenesis of the cerebellar hemispheres has been described.

Treatment of Cerebral Palsy[1,2]

It is of the first importance to try to obtain an estimate of intelligence in children suffering from cerebral palsy, but this may be extremely difficult to do, particularly in those children who are severely handicapped physically. Special methods and experience are necessary in

[1] " Notes for Parents on the Home Care of Children Handicapped by Cerebral Palsy." 4th Ed., 1952. London: British Council for the Welfare of Spastics.
[2] Lucas, H. Keith. " The Cerebral Palsies of Childhood." 2nd Ed., 1952. London: British Council for the Welfare of Spastics.

doubtful cases. It is clearly useless to attempt to train the child who has gross mental defect. Next, it is important to realize that as the cerebral palsied child is relatively immobile, he is deprived of much sensory experience which is needed for intellectual growth in early life. Such experience—and the companionship of children—must be brought to the child, and this can probably be best accomplished in a nursery day school for the physically handicapped.

PHYSIOTHERAPY

Passive exercises may be of value in the prevention of contractures in the spastic types, and splints may be necessary. The value of muscle training is controversial, and the improvement which indubitably takes place in some cerebral palsied children treated at special centres may not be the direct result of physical therapy.[1] Special equipment may be of value in enabling the child to learn to walk and feed himself, but the aim should be for him to use everyday articles. Speech therapy has its advocates, but the dangers of over-tiring the child with " training " of various types should be remembered.

SURGERY

Tendon lengthening and other orthopædic operations have a place in the treatment of spastic paresis, but are of no value in athetosis.

Hemispherectomy has been successful in abolishing severe fits and behaviour disorders in selected cases of infantile hemiplegia. Chemo-pallidectomy may prove to be of value in incapacitating cases of athetosis.

DRUGS

Apart from the control of epilepsy, drugs have little place in the treatment of cerebral palsy.

Weaning the child from dependence on his parents, arranging his schooling, and providing him with work in adult life remain the greatest problems in handling cerebral palsy.

DEGENERATIVE DISORDERS

CEREBROMACULAR DEGENERATION

SEVERAL rare familial degenerative disorders are characterized by deposits of lipoid substances in the ganglion cells of the entire central nervous system, including the retina. Each disease is inherited as a Mendelian recessive.

Tay-Sachs' Disease (infantile amaurotic family idiocy) occurs most commonly in Jews. The child is normal at birth, but when about six months old becomes apathetic and loses interest in his surroundings. Blindness, progressive muscular weakness and mental deterioration soon become obvious. There is the unusual combination of marked muscular hypotonia with brisk tendon reflexes. Tonic

---

[1] Tizard, J. P. M. (1955). In " Pædiatrics for the Practitioner." Vol. 3, chap. 93. Ed. Gaisford and Lightwood. London: Butterworth.

neck reflexes can be elicited. Tonic fits occur in the later stages. On opththalmoscopy the normal fovea stands out as a cherry-red spot surrounded by pale retina, in which the ganglion cells are loaded with lipoid. Death occurs at about two years of age. - *3 yrs in Kathleen.*

Batten's Disease (early juvenile cerebromacular degeneration, Bielchowski's disease) begins between three and four years of age, usually with mental deterioration followed by blindness, tremors, paralysis and fits. A dull red spot (or pigmentary changes) may be seen at the macula. Death takes place in a few years.

Spielmeyer-Vogt's Disease (late juvenile cerebromacular degeneration) begins between five and ten years of age. Macular vision is first affected, so that when the child looks at an object his gaze appears to be directed elsewhere. Later, mental deterioration and convulsions appear and finally extrapyramidal rigidity and paralysis. The cherry-red spot is seldom seen, but instead atrophy and fine brown pigmentation. The average age at death is eleven years.

Neither of the latter two varieties shows any racial predilection.

DEMYELINATING DISORDERS

Schilder's Disease (Encephalitis Periaxialis Diffusa)

Pathology. Within the white matter of the cerebral hemispheres there are large translucent areas sharply demarcated from normal tissue. Histological examination shows destruction of myelin sheaths and microglial infiltration as the earliest stages, followed by degeneration of both axis cylinders and glial tissue and, finally, complete disappearance of tissues and cavitation. There is little or no evidence of inflammation.

Clinical Features. The disease occurs sporadically, and may begin at any age. The symptoms include mental deterioration, emotional instability, blindness, deafness and spastic paresis, but the order in which these appear varies with the part of the subcortical white matter first to be affected. As the blindness is caused by destruction of the optic radiations, the fundus oculi appears normal and the pupillary reactions are preserved. Rarely, however, the intracranial pressure rises, producing papilloedema, headache and vomiting. Convulsions may occur. The CSF is usually normal but may show a slight rise in cells.

Pelizæus-Merzbacher's Disease is a similar condition, which is usually transmitted as a sex-linked recessive character, afflicting chiefly male infants or young children. It differs from Schilder's disease pathologically in that the white matter of the cerebellum and spinal cord is affected as well as that of the cerebral hemispheres. Clinically it is characterized by rotary nystagmus, ataxia, spasticity and mental deterioration. The course is slower than that of Schilder's disease.

Krabbe's Disease is an acute form of cerebral sclerosis which occurs in infants.

Late Infantile Metachromatic Leucodystrophy (Greenfield)

This rare disease, which appears to be inherited as a recessive character, probably represents an error of inborn metabolism. Pathologically the disease is characterized by evidence of destruction of myelin sheaths and axons, absence of oligendroglia and presence of metachromatic[1] granules. These granules are also found in the wall of the gall bladder and the renal tubules and may occasionally be detected in urinary deposit. The disease is first manifest at the age of about 18 months with ataxia and hypotonia of limbs. Tremor, nystagmus, fits and mental deterioration follow. The CSF protein is raised. Death occurs in two or three years.

Kinnier-Wilson's Disease (Hepato-lenticular Degeneration)

Ætiology. This rare disease is known to be inherited as a recessive character. The essential metabolic defect is the innate inability to form cæruloplasmin, a serum protein which contains copper. As a result of this deficiency, excess copper is absorbed from the intestine and is subsequently deposited in abnormal amounts in the brain, liver, kidneys and cornea.

Pathology. Neuronal degeneration and gliosis is found in the putamen and other basal ganglia. The liver shows a nodular cirrhosis.

Symptoms. Signs generally appear in late childhood. The first symptom is usually loss of emotional control; this is followed by tremor and an extrapyramidal type of rigidity. Among the first manifestations are a fixed foolish grin, unclear speech and difficulty in writing. Rigidity and abnormal movements increase. The cirrhosis usually gives rise to no symptoms, but occasionally there are attacks of jaundice or signs of portal obstruction. A common and pathognomonic finding is the *Kayser-Fleischer* ring. This is a ring of brownish-yellow pigmentation near the edge of the cornea. Aminoaciduria, due to renal damage, occurs early. The diagnosis is confirmed by the finding of an abnormally low level of serum cæruloplasmin (normal 27–38 mg. per 100 ml.) and a high urinary excretion of copper (normal—less than 50 microgrammes per 24 hours).

Course and Treatment. Courses of BAL or penicillamine produce a marked rise in urinary excretion of copper, and temporary remissions of symptoms. The dose of penicillamine, when used as a chelating agent, varies with the individual. A daily dosage of between 1·0–2·0 G. should be tried initially, the maintenance dose being that which continues to promote urinary excretion of copper and prevents clinical relapses. It may need to be continued for months or years.

The disease has a naturally fluctuant course, but without treatment

---

[1] The term metachromasia was introduced by Paul Ehrlich to describe situations in which a dye changes colour on staining a tissue. In Greenfield's disease the granules stain golden brown with methylene blue.

death occurs in a few years. The effect of long-term treatment with penicillamine, if started early in the disease, appears promising but cannot as yet be fully evaluated.

Friedreich's Ataxia

This disease is usually inherited as a Mendelian recessive character, occasionally as a dominant.

PATHOLOGY

The spinal cord and sometimes the cerebellum are atrophied. Histology shows demyelination and gliosis in the posterior column of the spinal cord and, to a lesser extent, in the spinocerebellar and pyramidal tracts.

CLINICAL FEATURES

Symptoms usually appear insidiously, but become obvious between the fifth and tenth years of life. The child is found to have a staggering gait and, later, clumsiness of the hands and arms. The ataxia is in part due to loss of postural sense, and in part to cerebellar dysfunction. Muscle tone is diminished and tendon reflexes are reduced or absent. The plantar responses are extensor, due to the pyramidal tract degeneration. Later, nystagmus may be elicited, and speech becomes slurred and swallowing difficult, due to bulbar involvement. A bilateral pes cavus usually develops, and spinal scoliosis or kyphosis are quite common. Electrocardiograms show evidence of myocardial damage, and patients may die of cardiac failure. The course is usually steadily progressive, but death may not occur for many years. Rarely, the disease is spontaneously arrested.

Neurofibromatosis (von Recklinghausen's Disease)

This rare and complex disease, seen in children and adults, is inherited as a Mendelian dominant, but is expressed in an individual in widely differing degrees. It may be manifested by:

(1) spots or large areas of light-brown pigmentation on the skin; (2) small, frequently pedunculated, subcutaneous tumours (fibromata), chiefly on the trunk; (3) multiple tumours of varying size on peripheral nerves and spinal nerve roots (neurofibromata); (4) various congenital skeletal defects. Thus, the clinical picture may vary from a child showing only a few harmless pigmented patches to one with widespread existence of all four types of lesion. The neurofibromata do not usually interfere with the function of the nerve, except by compression within a bony canal; in this way the function of the auditory nerve and spinal roots may be interfered with. Pressure by an acoustic neuroma may also produce signs of cerebellar dysfunction and a rise in intracranial pressure. Symptoms may commence at any age.

Tuberose Sclerosis (Epiloia)

This somewhat similar disease is probably inherited as a Mendelian dominant, but in varying degrees of completeness (" expressivity "). It is characterized by: (1) sebaceous adenomata—small plaque-like

tumours producing a " butterfly " rash round the nose and cheeks—
and rough, dark skin in the lumbar region; (2) multiple small gliomata
of the brain; and (3) tumours of the heart (rhabdomyomata), of the

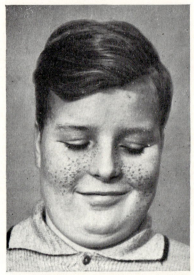

kidney (fibroadenomata) and of
the retina (phakomata). The
latter appear as grey plaques on
ophthalmoscopy. Pulmonary
infiltrations sometimes giving a
" honeycomb " appearance (*see* p.
262). Fits, major or minor, often
occurring in infancy, are the first
signs of the disease. Mental
deficiency usually follows.

Fig. 53.—Adenoma sebaceum in a butterfly
distribution in a boy with tuberose sclerosis.

Progressive Spinal Muscular (Werdnig-Hoffmann's Disease)[1]

This rare condition is genetically determined, almost invariably
by a recessive gene. Thus, when
one affected child is born, there
is a one-in-four risk of a subsequent
child having the disease.

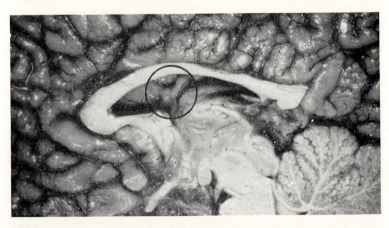

Fig. 54.—The brain of a child who had tuberose sclerosis, showing " candle-guttering "
tumour masses in the wall of the lateral ventricle, and enlargement of the third ventricle
due to obstruction by other tumour masses.

[1] Brandt, S. (1950). " Werdnig-Hoffmann's Infantile Progressive Muscular Atrophy." *Opera
ex Domo Biologiæ Hereditariæ Humanæ Universitates Hafniensis*, Vol. 22. Copenhagen.
Paterson, Donald (1929). *Westminster Hosp. Rep.*, **20**, 43.

PATHOLOGY

The defect lies in the ganglion cells of the anterior horns of the spinal cord and of the lower motor cranial nerve nuclei, the changes varying from swelling and chromatolysis to atrophy and "ghost cells." There is no inflammatory reaction. The voluntary muscles are very small and on microscopy show a patchy atrophy, but no specific changes.

CLINICAL FEATURES

Weakness may be present from birth or may even be detected before birth by feeble intra-uterine movements, but more commonly the infant is normal for the first few months of life. Progressive

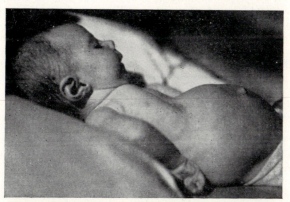

Fig. 55.—Werdnig-Hoffmann's disease. The chest wall is pulled in, due to paralysis of the intercostal muscles, and respiration is entirely diaphragmatic. The arms hang in a lifeless position, owing to their almost complete paralysis.

muscular weakness and atrophy then begin and involve trunk and limb muscles symmetrically, the weakness being most obvious around the shoulder and pelvic girdles. Later, intercostal muscles, palate and tongue become involved. Fibrillation may be seen in the limbs and tongue. There is marked muscular hypotonia and excessive range of passive movement at the joints. The tendon reflexes disappear early. There are no sensory changes. The infant's cry becomes feeble, as does his ability to cough, and death is usually caused by pneumonia within the first three years of life. The alert mentality is an important point of distinction from other causes of flaccid weakness in infancy. There is no treatment.

Amyotonia Congenita (Oppenheim's Disease)

This condition, similar pathologically and clinically to Werdnig-Hoffmann's disease, has been differentiated on the grounds that there is no evidence, either clinical or pathological, of active degeneration.

The paralysis is present at birth and remains unaltered. Also, familial cases are less frequent. The prognosis of this extremely rare disorder is less grave than in Werdnig-Hoffmann's disease, but few patients reach adult life.

The diagnosis is often made erroneously in children with Werdnig-Hoffmann's disease, atonic types of cerebral palsy, mental defect and the many rarer causes of flaccid weakness.

BRAIN TUMOURS [1]

TUMOURS of the brain occur almost as commonly in children as they do in adults, but differ in pathology, localization and symptoms. In general, the types of tumour that are common in childhood are rare in adult life, and vice versa. Then, in contrast with adults, about two-thirds of all intracranial tumours in children arise from below the tentorium, from the cerebellum or pons, while supra-tentorial tumours are found more frequently in midline structures than in the cerebral hemispheres. As in adults, symptoms are caused both by local damage to the brain and by the rise in intracranial pressure, due to blocking of cerebrospinal fluid pathways, but the effects of increased intracranial pressure are modified in children, and especially infants.

SYMPTOMS AND SIGNS OF RAISED INTRACRANIAL PRESSURE

The well-known triad of headache, vomiting, and papilloedema may occur early in older children. The younger the child, however, the less closely are the cranial bones interlocked (see Craniostenosis, p. 434), with the result that a rise in intracranial pressure will produce expansion of the head and a more gradual onset of symptoms. Vomiting is the commonest symptom, often occurring in the early morning, and frequently not preceded by nausea. Headache is intermittent at first in older children, while in infants and young children it may be absent or at least not recognized. Papilloedema is often a late sign, and in infants retinal haemorrhages are commoner. The scalp veins may be dilated and, in infants, the anterior fontanelle may be tense. Raised pressure may stretch the sixth cranial nerves and produce an internal squint. There is often little disturbance of general health. X-ray of the skull may show separation of the sutures and, in late cases, decalcification of the posterior clinoid process. Some tumours calcify (see p. 452). Moderate convolutional markings of the inner table of the skull are common in normal children.

DANGER SIGNS

Increasing intracranial pressure may force the medulla and cerebellar tonsils through the foramen magnum and cause death through compression of vital centres. This is especially liable to

[1] Bodian, M., Lawson, D. (1952). Intracranial neoplastic disease in childhood. *Brit. J. Surg.*, **40** 368.

happen following lumbar puncture, which should not be carried out in cases suspected of brain tumour. Signs which suggest that this herniation is taking place are impairment of consciousness, severe pain in the neck, and slowing of pulse and respiration rates. An enema of four ounces of 50 per cent. magnesium sulphate solution, or an intravenous injection of 25 ml. of 50 per cent. glucose solution may produce temporary relief, but a ventricular tap must be carried out as soon as possible to relieve pressure from above.

THE COMMONER VARIETIES OF BRAIN TUMOUR IN CHILDREN

1. Cerebellar Medulloblastoma

The medulloblastoma is a soft, rapidly growing and invasive glioma. It arises from undifferentiated neural cells. It grows most commonly from the vermis of the cerebellum spreading into one or both cerebellar hemispheres. It may occur at any age in childhood, and is commoner in boys.

Clinical Features. The first symptoms are those of a rise in intracranial pressure and a staggering gait. Formal tests for ataxia are usually negative, however, and nystagmus is unusual. With surgical excision and radiotherapy almost half the victims survive for five years, but unfortunately late recurrences are common. Metastases spread into the subarachnoid space and invade the spinal nerve roots and cord.

2. Cerebellar Astrocytoma

This is a slow-growing, relatively acellular glioma, which also arises from the vermis of the cerebellum and spreads into one cerebellar hemisphere. It frequently gives rise to large cysts and is, as a rule, easily separable from surrounding tissues.

Clinical Features. Symptoms of increased intracranial pressure appear slowly, and are combined with unilateral cerebellar signs. There are ataxia, flaccidity and diminished tendon reflexes in the arm and leg on the side of the lesion; the child may stagger towards the affected side when he walks, and use the affected arm clumsily. Nystagmus is present, and is slower and coarser when the child looks towards the side of the tumour.

In contrast to other intracranial tumours in childhood, the prognosis following surgical excision is good.

3. Pontine Astrocytoma

This is a diffuse, infiltrative glioma that grows in the pons and extends slowly into the medulla and midbrain. It occurs in the middle years of childhood.

Clinical Features. There is a slow onset of cranial nerve palsies and involvement of nerve tracks. Paralysis of the external rectus muscle on one or both sides, producing a convergent squint, is often the earliest sign, and is slowly followed by facial palsy and other cranial nerve lesions, together with ataxia, due to involvement of cerebellar connections, and weakness, of an upper motor neurone type, in the limbs. Vomiting is common, but headache, enlargement of the head and papillœdema occur late or not at all.

Radiotherapy may produce temporary improvement, but death is inevitable.

(Diffuse astrocytomata may also arise from the basal ganglia, hypothalamus, midbrain, cerebral peduncles or optic nerves.)

4. Ependymoma

This is a slow-growing, uninvasive glioma, which arises beneath the ependymal lining of the ventricles, usually the fourth. In this situation it produces, early, signs of increased intracranial pressure and also various symptoms due to local pressure on pons, medulla, cerebral peduncles or cerebellum. Calcification within the tumour may be seen on x-ray. The prognosis, following attempted surgical excision, varies with the site of the tumour; viz. those in relation to a lateral ventricle may be removed entirely, while ependymomata of the fourth ventricle are inoperable.

5. Craniopharyngioma (Adamantinoma, Rathke's Pouch Tumour)

This tumour arises from ectopic buccal mucosa in the pars tuberalis of the pituitary. It usually forms a large cyst, the fluid in which contains cholesterol crystals. The cyst walls become patchily calcified.

Clinical Features. The cyst grows slowly, so that symptoms are unusual before middle childhood, and may be delayed until adult life. The cyst compresses (1) the optic chiasma and nerves, producing visual field defects or optic atrophy, (2) the hypothalamus, producing obesity, (3) the pituitary, producing delayed skeletal growth and sexual maturation, and (4) the third ventricle, producing hydrocephalus and signs of raised intracranial pressure.

The calcification may often be seen on x-ray, and there is sometimes widening or erosion of the pituitary fossa. Surgical removal is extremely difficult, but symptoms may be relieved for years by repeated tapping of the cyst.

6. Tumours of the Cerebral Hemispheres (ependymomata, medulloblastomata and astrocytomata) may occur, but are rare in children. They produce pressure signs, upper motor neurone palsies and local or generalized convulsions. (Plate X.)

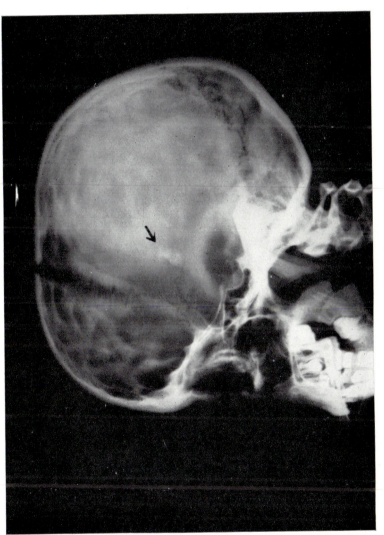

PLATE X. A partly calcified, right temporal lobe glioma in an 8-year-old girl. The x-ray shows characteristic changes, namely, greatly increased intracranial pressure, separation of the sutures, decalcification of the posterior clinoid process, widening of the sella turcica and excessive convolutional markings.

TREATMENT

Once an intracranial tumour is suspected it must be localized accurately by means of air ventriculograms and sometimes arteriograms. In every case a craniotomy must be performed, because only direct inspection will reveal whether or not the tumour is removable.

EPILEPSY
(Fits, Convulsions, Seizures)

EPILEPSY may be loosely defined as a condition in which there is a sudden cerebral disturbance, nearly always associated with loss of consciousness and usually with involuntary movements, which ceases spontaneously but shows a strong tendency to recur. The term epilepsy may be applied correctly to any form of convulsion, but is usually reserved for cases of recurrent fits without an obvious organic basis.

ELECTROENCEPHALOGRAPHY

If a pair of electrodes is placed on the scalp and connected to an amplifier, it can be shown that between them there is an electrical potential difference which tends to fluctuate rhythmically. These potential changes may be recorded on moving paper, to appear as waves. In practice, many electrodes are spaced evenly over the scalp, and the potential differences between four, six or eight pairs are recorded simultaneously. At birth, recordings are irregular and there is little rhythmical activity, but by four months waves of a frequency of $\frac{1}{2}$ to 4 per second (δ rhythm) can be recorded. As the child grows older the recordings become simpler and the rhythm faster. At five years the dominant rhythm is 4 to 8 cycles per second (θ rhythm), and by the age of ten years the adult rate of 8 to 13 cycles per second (usually 10 cycles per second—α rhythm) is reached. There is, however, considerable individual variation in the age at which electrical " maturity " is reached.

Abnormal electroencephalograms (EEG) are characterized by alteration in rate, amplitude, waveform or symmetry. During a fit, abnormal electrical discharges appear; in a grand mal attack, for instance, the dominant rhythm quickens and is followed by a series of tall spikes; while in petit mal a slow wave of large amplitude is followed by a sharp spike, each complex occurring three times per second. Seizure discharges may also be recorded in between fits, but the clinical value of this is mitigated by the fact that some individuals who have never had clinical fits show " abnormal " EEGs, while a small proportion of epileptics show normal EEGs. Brain damage may result in the production of slow waves and, if these can be shown to arise from a constant focus, they may help in the localization of tumours, etc. In various behaviour disorders, the EEG tends to be immature for the child's age, but the significance of this finding is not clear.   Some of the clinical applications of electro-encephalography are mentioned in the section on diagnosis.

ÆTIOLOGY

There are three separate factors to be considered in the causation of fits: (1) Inherent predisposition; (2) added predisposition in the form of disease of the brain; and (3) the immediate exciting factors.

(1) A history of fits is found five times as frequently in the families of epileptic children as in the families of those who have not had fits.   The incidence of " abnormal " EEGs is much higher in the relatives of epileptics.   This and other evidence suggests that there is an hereditary predisposition to fits.

(2) Almost any disorder of the brain, and especially of the cerebral cortex, predisposes to fits.   Minor injuries to the brain at birth may cause fits in later childhood.   Developmental anomalies, such as in spastic cerebral palsy and hydrocephalus, degenerative disease, such as cerebromacular degeneration and Shilder's disease, in-flammatory conditions, such as meningitis and encephalitis, and neoplastic disease may all be accompanied by convulsions.   Mentally defective children are more liable to have fits than are the normal.

(3) In children with an inborn predisposition to fits, or with acquired brain disorders, fits may be precipitated by quite minor upsets, such as constipation, a dental eruption, emotional excitement and so on, while in many cases no immediate exciting factors are apparent. Thus in idiopathic epilepsy fits take place most frequently when the child is at rest physically and mentally—most commonly when asleep.

More serious disturbances of body equilibrium may also precipitate fits in children who have no obvious inherent or acquired tendency to epilepsy.   Amongst these conditions are:

(a) High fever at the onset of illnesses such as otitis media, lobar pneumonia or pyelitis.

(b) Poisoning, with lead, ether or chloroform.

(c) Metabolic upsets, such as tetany (in rickets or hypopara-thyroidism), hypoglycæmia (idiopathic or due to insulin therapy or to pancreatic islet tumour), uræmia, alkalosis.

(d) Cerebral anoxæmia in nitrous oxide anæsthesia, pertussis with laryngospasm, breath holding attacks, etc.

VARIETIES OF SEIZURE

Only the commoner of the many clinical varieties will be described.

Grand Mal

Major epilepsy typically has four components: the aura, the tonic phase, the clonic phase, and the post-ictal phase.   The aura consists of a variety of usually unpleasant sensations, generally in the head or the belly, which warn of the onset of a fit. The child may be seen to appear frightened or bewildered, and may have time to run to his mother and clasp her. At the onset of the tonic phase the child loses consciousness and falls. A single cry is often emitted, due to tonic spasm of the larynx, before respiration ceases. Every voluntary muscle then contracts, the most powerful muscles arching the back and extending the limbs. The child may bite his tongue, and the bladder or bowel may be emptied. The tonic phase lasts not more than one minute, during which the child becomes cyanotic. This is then followed by the clonic stage, consisting of jerkings of the limbs, irregular respiration with frothing at the mouth, and partial return of the normal colour. This phase may last several minutes. The movements then cease and the body relaxes. At this stage the tendon reflexes are usually absent and the plantar responses extensor. The temperature is often raised. The child sleeps heavily for up to an hour or so, and usually wakes with a headache. The post-ictal phase is sometimes accompanied by " automatism "—irrational acts for which the patient has no subsequent memory.

A fit may be represented by a fragment of the major convulsion, one or more of the phases being omitted. Thus, the aura may occur alone, or the fit may not be preceded by any aura. The tonic phase may occur alone, as in breath-holding attacks, and rarely a state of post-ictal automatism may take place without there having been a previous recognizable fit. Again, especially in infants, a fit may take the form of a few clonic jerks, and in these cases it is perfectly correct to speak of a " minor grand mal " attack.

Petit Mal

This is characterized by brief, and usually frequent, attacks of loss of consciousness, with little or no convulsive element. The child will pause, turn pale, the eyes will momentarily turn upward, and the arms sometimes twitch. The child does not fall, but is occasionally incontinent of urine. The attack is usually so brief that it may escape notice. A petit mal attack can often be precipitated by overbreathing. Rarely, similar attacks are associated with loss of postural tone, and the child falls to the ground (akinetic fits).

Focal Epilepsy

The symptoms of focal epilepsy depend on the site in the brain from which the abnormal discharges arise. The most easily recognized are those which begin with clonic movements confined to one part of the body. The commonest sites of onset are the thumb and index finger, the great toe and one angle of the mouth. From these sites the clonic movements may spread in a gradual and orderly progression to involve adjacent muscle groups (Jacksonian epilepsy), consciousness being lost when the opposite half of the body becomes involved.

Lightning Attacks (Infantile Spasms)

This form of epilepsy is confined to infancy and early childhood and carries a bad prognosis in terms of mental development. There is a sudden flexion of the head; the arms jerk forward and the legs stiffen. The fit is over in a second, but is frequently repeated, perhaps every few seconds. Variants are " nodding " and " salaam " fits, in which there is a brief flexion of the head or trunk. The electro-encephalogram shows gross dysrhythmia with large amplitude irregular slow waves and spikes. It has recently been shown that corticosteroids will often control the fits and occasionally, if treatment is started early, restore normal mental development. The relationship of pyridoxine dependency to a rare variety of convulsions in the newborn is discussed on p. 143.

Myoclonic Epilepsy

A sudden local muscular jerking without loss of consciousness.

Status Epilepticus

Rarely, one major fit succeeds another so rapidly that there is no recovery of consciousness and, unless arrested, the condition may lead to peripheral circulatory failure, hyperpyrexia and death.

Abdominal Epilepsy

Fits in children may rarely take the form of sudden, brief attacks of abdominal pain and pallor.

Psychomotor Epilepsy

These are rare forms of epilepsy in which organized and apparently purposive movements take place. Or they may take the form of complicated sensory or emotional experiences, and the latter may lead to violent acts. Obviously the clinical diagnosis is extremely difficult, but the EEG often shows an epileptogenic focus in the anterior temporal lobe.

Breath-holding Attacks

These may cause tonic fits but should be considered separately from epilepsy, because the prognosis with respect to fits in later childhood is uniformly favourable. The attacks occur in " highly-strung " children from late infancy until the third or fourth year. They are precipitated by an emotional upset, especially if the child is thwarted or scolded. He begins to cry loudly and continues to do so, with a series of expiratory efforts, until he becomes blue and falls to the ground unconscious with generalized tonic rigidity of limbs and trunk. The child remains unconscious for from a few seconds to a minute or two.

DIFFERENTIAL DIAGNOSIS

The first problem is to decide if a given incident has in fact been a fit. The parents' diagnosis of a fit is usually correct, although masturbation in young infants is occasionally mistaken for a convulsion. On the other hand, fits may masquerade under a number of disguises. The commonest is perhaps fainting. Syncope is unusual in young children, and occurs only when the child is standing up. Petit mal may take the form of a behaviour disorder, temper tantrums, aggressiveness and the like, the short lapses of consciousness being unnoticed. Bed-wetting, especially when it develops in a child who has previously been dry at night, may be the sole manifestation of epilepsy to be noticed by the parents. The possibility of epilepsy causing recurrent abdominal colic must also be remembered. The lightning attacks of infancy are seldom thought to be fits and are often attributed to " wind " or colic.

The second problem concerns the origin of the fits—are they due to " idiopathic " epilepsy or are they symptomatic of some other disease? The type of fit is of importance in this connection. True petit mal is always indicative of idiopathic epilepsy. Major convulsions, both complete and incomplete, may be a symptom of idiopathic epilepsy, or of some organic disease of the brain, of poisoning, of a metabolic disorder, and so on (see p. 454). Focal attacks may occur in idiopathic epilepsy, but the site usually changes, and a persistent local focus of onset should always suggest the probability of a tumour or other local brain lesion. Fits in the newborn are usually indicative of anoxic or traumatic brain damage, but may be due to metabolic disorders or infections. In children between the ages of six and thirteen months the possibility of latent tetany must be considered. In all cases associated with fever, it is important to know if the temperature was raised before the onset of the fit (see Prognosis), and whenever the suspicion of meningitis arises a lumbar puncture must be performed. Hypoglycæmic attacks both in the newborn and as a cause of major convulsion in young children are discussed on p. 172.

The EEG may help in the differential diagnosis. A symmetrical three-per-second spike and wave tracing is found only in idiopathic epilepsy, with either grand mal or petit mal attacks. A *persistent* focus of abnormal waves in focal epilepsy or grand mal may point to the presence of a local lesion (e.g. tumour) before neurological signs appear.

PROGNOSIS

The prognosis of fits associated with an organic lesion of the brain clearly depends on the nature of the lesion, but it must be remembered that fits may continue even if a tumour or superficial scar has been completely removed. The prognosis for fits unassociated with organic brain disease varies with the nature of the precipitating factors, if any, or the frequency of the attacks. For instance, a single fit occurring at the onset of a high fever in childhood, does not seem to increase the risk of fits in later life. On the other hand, frequently repeated convulsions without obvious cause usually mean that the child will continue to have idiopathic epilepsy, although if such children are treated adequately about one-quarter may later be entirely free from fits. Mental deterioration rarely occurs, and is probably due to underlying degenerative conditions rather than to the fits themselves. A small proportion of patients with petit mal will recover completely, but the majority later develop major convulsions. Lightning attacks typically begin at six months of age, and are associated with severe mental deficiency and a poor prognosis.

TREATMENT OF ATTACKS

An attack nearly always ends spontaneously, and no treatment is necessary other than to ensure that the child does not injure or smother himself. Prolonged attacks can usually be cut short by an intramuscular injection of paraldehyde or phenytoin (for dosage, see *p.* 665). In status epilepticus, once the convulsions have been controlled by these means, repeated injections of phenobarbitone may be necessary.

The question of when to give prophylactic drug treatment is difficult, but the physician has to be guided by the probability of future attacks (*see* Prognosis). Prophylactic treatment, once started, should continue for at least two years after the last fit. Phenobarbitone should probably be tried first in any type of convulsion, except true petit mal. If this is ineffective in controlling major convulsions epanutin should be added. Primidone may be of value in otherwise uncontrollable grand mal. Tridione is often markedly successful in suppressing petit mal attacks, but there is a danger of its producing agranulocytosis. Acetazolamide (Diamox) is also sometimes effective in cases of petit mal. It must be emphasized that the choice of drugs, their combination and dosage vary with individual children, and can only be decided on the basis of trial and error.

Finally, the child who is subject to fits must lead as nearly normal a life as possible. Parents and doctors must, in the child's best interests, be prepared to take some risks in not restricting his activities unless they endanger the lives of other people.

DISORDERS OF MUSCLES

MUSCULAR DYSTROPHY (MYOPATHY)[1]

This term covers a group of genetically determined diseases in which a degeneration of muscle fibres leads to progressive weakness and wasting. The central nervous system is not affected.

Most children with muscular dystrophy have normal intelligence, but mental defect is more than a chance association.

[1] Walton, J. N., Nattrass, F. J. (1954). *Brain*, **77**, 169.

PATHOLOGY

The muscles are usually small, but may be large and firm due to excess deposition of fat in between the muscle fibres.   In a microscopic section fibres of normal size can be seen next to both enormously swollen and abnormally small muscle fibres.   The degenerated fibres are replaced by connective tissue and fat.   The histological appearance of the muscles is not always characteristic enough to permit a firm differentiation from muscular atrophy of central nervous origin.   As in other diseases involving loss of muscle tissue, there is an increase in urinary creatine and a diminution in creatinine.

ELECTROMYOGRAPHY [1]

The EMG may be of use in differentiating the dystrophies from spinal muscular atrophy and other conditions.

VARIETIES OF MUSCULAR DYSTROPHY

There are a few well-recognized types of muscular dystrophy, but intermediate forms exist.

Duchenne's Muscular Dystrophy

This is the commonest and the most clearly defined type of muscular dystrophy.   It is inherited as a sex-linked recessive character, but the disease does very rarely occur in girls which can probably be explained on the basis of a fresh mutation.

The onset is insidious, but the child is usually brought to the doctor at about five years of age with the complaint that he tires easily, runs slowly, and has difficulty in getting upstairs.   Inquiry then will often reveal that he learned to walk late, and occasionally there may even be a history of muscular weakness in infancy.

On examination, muscle weakness is symmetrical and most marked in the proximal groups of limb muscles.   Thus, weakness of the muscles round the shoulders may make it impossible for the child to raise his arms above his head, while, if an attempt is made to lift him under the arms, he tends to slip through the examiner's hands. Weakness of the muscles attached to the pelvis results in an exaggerated lumbar lordosis and pot belly, a waddling gait and inability to get up from a lying position, without the following complicated manoeuvre. The child rolls over on to his front and raises himself awkwardly on to his hands and feet.   He then places first one hand and then the other above each knee, and by shifting his hands up his thighs, pushes his trunk into the upright position.   This manoeuvre is not, of course, diagnostic of muscular dystrophy, but of any condition in which there is weakness of muscles fixing the pelvis.

At first, little muscular wasting is detectable; instead, certain muscles, especially the gastrocnemii, triceps and infraspinali, are enlarged and have a characteristically firm, inelastic consistency.

[1] Luder, J. (1952).   The value of electromyography in pædiatrics.   *Gt Ormond Str. J.*, **3**, 1–8,

The enlargement is due to deposition of fat—hence the term pseudo-hypertrophic (pseudohypertrophy is not invariably a feature of Duchenne's muscular dystrophy). Later, however, there is obvious muscular wasting, first round the buttocks and shoulders, later in the arms and thighs, forearms and legs. The tendon reflexes are at first present, but later disappear. Contractures may develop.

The weakness and wasting become progressively worse and the child seldom lives into adult life, dying usually of pneumonia, but sometimes of heart failure due to myocardial degeneration.

Facio-scapular-humeral Muscular Dystrophy (Laudouzy-Dejerine).

This type of dystrophy is inherited as a dominant or occasionally a recessive character. The weakness first involves the facial muscles, so that the face is somewhat expressionless or even mask-like. The eyes are not closed during sleep, and the child cannot blow or whistle. The onset is usually in childhood and sometimes even in infancy, so that there may be difficulty in sucking breast or bottle. The course is very slowly progressive and is not usually incapacitating in childhood. The muscles of the shoulder girdle are next involved, and later those of the pelvic girdle. Patients may survive until 30 or 40 years of age.

Limb-girdle Form of Muscular Dystrophy.

This form is usually inherited as an autosomal recessive, occasionally as a dominant characteristic. It involves first either the shoulder girdle or pelvic girdle muscles and slowly spreads from one to the other. In most cases the onset of weakness and wasting is deferred until adolescence or early adult life, but it occasionally begins in childhood. The course is very slowly progressive.

TREATMENT

There is no specific treatment. Massage and exercises are of some help in maintaining residual muscle function and preventing contractures. As disuse often results in a rapid progression of the weakness, children with muscular dystrophy should be confined to bed during illness for as short a time as possible.

Myotonia Congenita (Thomsen's Disease)

This is a rare disease characterized by sustained muscular contraction and muscular hypertrophy. The defect is thought to lie in the muscles themselves or in the myoneural junctions; the central nervous system is normal. It is inherited usually as a dominant characteristic, occasionally as a recessive.

CLINICAL FEATURES

The onset is usually in early childhood. Following any voluntary movement, muscular relaxation is slow and a new movement cannot be initiated quickly. School teachers may complain that the child is slow to obey. The more a movement is repeated, however, the easier it becomes, so that the child may be able to run quite fast, after a slow start. The myotonia is best demonstrated by asking the child to let go after gripping the examiner's hand, or to open the eyes after shutting them tightly. Percussion over a muscle produces a prolonged tonic contraction. The reflexes are normal.

TREATMENT

Quinine by mouth will relieve the myotonia for a few hours, and the child may be greatly improved by taking this drug several times a day.

Dystrophia Myotonica (Myotonia Atrophica)

This is a very rare hereditary disease characterized by progressive myotonia with muscular atrophy, and by developing cataract, premature baldness and gonadal atrophy. The onset of symptoms is generally in early adult life, but may occur in childhood.

Myasthenia Gravis[1]

Myasthenia gravis is a disease characterized by excessive fatigue of muscle due to some defect, the nature of which is unknown, in transmission at the myoneural junction.

PATHOLOGY

There are no constant pathological changes in the muscles or in the nervous system. In many cases collections of lymphocytes (lymphorrhages) are found scattered through the voluntary muscles. In about half the cases of myasthenia gravis the thymus is enlarged, or, rarely, contains a benign tumour (thymoma).

CLINICAL FEATURES

The onset of the disease is usually in adult life, but it sometimes begins in childhood, and in rare instances has been present at birth. Most of the congenital cases have been in infants of mothers suffering from myasthenia gravis, the symptoms being generalized weakness, difficulty in sucking and swallowing, drooping eyelids, and little facial movement. If untreated, death is likely, but if treated, signs of the disease disappear in a few weeks. In the majority of cases, however, there is no family history of the disease, and the myasthenia, although fluctuating in severity, is permanent.

The onset is usually gradual, and the first muscles to be affected are those supplied by the cranial nerves. Ptosis, limitation of ocular movement, diplopia (due to extraocular muscular weakness), dysphagia and dysarthria are early signs. Early fatigue can be seen following repeated movement of any group of the muscles involved. Thus the child may chew and swallow normally at the beginning of a meal, but be unable to complete it. When he begins to talk his

[1] Wyllie, W. G., Bodian, M., Burrows, N. F. E. (1951). Myasthenia gravis in children. *Arch. Dis. Childh.*, **26**, 457.
Mackay, R. I. (1951). Congenital myasthenia gravis. *Ibid.*, 291.

speech is clear, but it becomes nasal, hoarse and weak after a few sentences. Moreover, weakness is always worse in the evening than in the morning.

Muscles of the neck, arms, legs and trunk later become involved, usually in that order, and show the characteristic fatigability.

Rarely the disease has an abrupt onset, and in these cases death may occur in a few days from respiratory paralysis.

DIAGNOSIS

The diagnosis may be confirmed by a therapeutic test. Depending on the age of the child, 0·1 to 0·5 mg. of prostigmine with 0·1–0·3 mg. of atropine is injected subcutaneously. In myasthenia gravis but in no other disease a marked increase in muscle power is observed in about 15 minutes.

COURSE AND TREATMENT

Prostigmine will usually abolish weakness for about four hours, and must therefore be given three or four times a day, either in the form of subcutaneous injections of 0·1 to 0·5 mg., or by mouth in 5 to 15 mg. doses. In about half the cases of myasthenia gravis removal of the thymus results in improvement, but in most it is still necessary to continue to administer prostigmine. The disease undergoes spontaneous fluctuations and the child may live for many years, but on the whole the course is unfavourable. Prostigmine becomes less effective and sudden relapses occur, often precipitated by infectious illnesses. Death usually results from respiratory failure.

Polymyositis[1]

This syndrome of unknown ætiology may occur with dermatomyositis but sometimes without skin changes, in which case the signs may be thought to be due to muscular dystrophy. Muscular weakness is disproportionate to atrophy and muscle pain and tenderness may also help to distinguish the syndrome from myopathy. The progress of the disease is more rapid than is the case with the dystrophies, but spontaneous recovery may take place.

Muscle biopsy is of value in the differential diagnosis. The corticosteroids are of therapeutic benefit.

J. P. M. Tizard

[1] Walton, J. N., Adams, R. D. (1958). " Polymyositis." Edinburgh: Livingstone.

CHAPTER 20

Mental Subnormality

Mental Defect (Oligophrenia)

THIS may be defined from a social standpoint as " a state of incomplete mental development of such a kind and degree that the individual is incapable of adapting himself to the normal environment of his fellows in such a way as to maintain existence independently of supervision, control, or external support " (Tredgold, 1937).[1]

The legal definitions (Mental Health Act, 1959) are as follows: " Severe subnormality " means a state of arrested or incomplete development of mind which includes subnormality of intelligence and is of such a nature or degree that the patient is incapable of living an independent life or of guarding against serious exploitation or will be so incapable when of an age to do so. " Subnormality " means a state of arrested or incomplete development of mind (not amounting to severe subnormality) which includes subnormality of intelligence and is of such a nature or degree which requires or is susceptible to medical treatment or other special care or training of the patient (*see* Appendix 7).

These two categories now replace the three classes of mentally defective persons recognized by the Mental Deficiency Act, 1927: idiots, imbeciles, and feeble-minded persons. The writer believes that the modern euphemistic substitutions have not removed the usefulness of the older classification.

Idiots are persons in whom there exists mental defectiveness of such a degree that they are unable to guard themselves against common physical dangers.

Idiots cannot speak well, have a very limited understanding, cannot find their way about in the house or in the street, are incapable of work of any kind, and have to be washed and cared for, and even fed, like children.

Imbeciles are persons in whom there exists mental defectiveness which, though not amounting to idiocy, yet renders them incapable of managing themselves or their affairs, or, in the case of children, of being taught to do so.

Imbeciles can be taught to understand and to do simple tasks, though they need to be watched over in washing and dressing. They can manage to find their way about the house or school, but not usually in the streets.

[1] Tredgold, A. F. (1937). " A Text-book of Mental Deficiency." 6th Edn. London: Baillière, Tindall & Cox.

Feeble-minded persons are persons in whom there exists mental defectiveness which, though not amounting to imbecility, is yet so pronounced that they require care, supervision and control for their own protection or for the protection of others, or, in the case of children, that they appear to be permanently incapable by reason of such defectiveness of receiving proper benefit from instruction in ordinary schools.

Feeble-minded persons can be taught to do a varied range of simple or repetitive work, and sometimes can learn to do a single thing in a more expert manner. They can be taught a little reading and arithmetic, but are incapable of planning things out for themselves, or of managing their own earnings.

A distinction should be made between amentia, in which mental defect is present from birth and is non-progressive, and dementia, in which the defect develops in a child of previously normal mentality and in which progressive intellectual deterioration takes place. The distinction is clear as, for instance, between mongolism and juvenile general paresis, but it is not as easy to define other conditions (e.g. Tay-Sachs' disease, post-natal brain injury) in these terms.

INCIDENCE

About 1·2 per cent. of children need special education on account of mental defect and about 3·5 per thousand are ineducable.

ÆTIOLOGY AND CLASSIFICATION [1, 2]

Mental deficiency may result from both hereditary and environmental causes; that is, it may be determined by single abnormal genes, or combinations of genes, by unfavourable external influences (such as disease or injury) acting on the brain of the embryo, fœtus or child or by combination of hereditary and environmental factors.

It has been suggested that there are two different types of mental deficiency. The individuals in any population vary greatly in intelligence, and those whose intelligence is of the highest degree should be balanced by an equal number whose intelligence is correspondingly below the average. The latter may be said to have " physiological " or " subcultural " mental deficiency. In practice, however, when the " mental age " of a large number of individuals is measured and plotted on a graph, it is found that instead of a distribution curve which is symmetrical about the mean, there is a preponderance of those with low-grade intelligence. This preponderance results from the addition of individuals who are defective as the result of malformation, disease or injury, and who may be said to have " pathological " mental defect.

The ætiology of the physiological type lies in a combination of numerous genetic and environmental factors, each of which has by

[1] Penrose, L. S. (1949). " The Biology of Mental Defect." London: Sigwick & Jackson.
[2] Fraser Roberts, J. A. (1952). The genetics of mental deficiency. *Eugen. Rev.*, **44**, 71–83.

itself little effect, but which summate to produce a condition of low mental development. The ætiology of the pathological group is to be found in simple genetic factors, or in single external incidents producing disease or malformation.

Certain points of distinction may be made between the two groups. Firstly, the great majority of physiological mental defectives will belong to the feeble-minded group, while most of the pathological type will be imbeciles or idiots. Secondly, the average intelligence of the parents of physiological mental defectives is below that of the general population, while the parents of the pathological types will be found to have high, medium or low intelligence in the same proportions as in the general population. Thirdly, the size of families of the physiological group is larger, and their economic status lower than the average, while in neither respect is there any deviation from the normal range in the families of the pathological defectives.

It will be noted that these points of distinction apply to groups, and are not necessarily applicable in individual cases. Moreover, there is neither in theory nor in practice, a clear demarcation between the two groups. Obvious pathological processes may cause minor as well as major degrees of mental defect and may indeed be a factor in producing biological variation.

CAUSES OF SEVERE MENTAL SUBNORMALITY

Certain disorders are known to be determined *genetically*. These include malformations, such as hypertelorism, some cases of microcephaly, Sturge-Weber syndrome, tuberose sclerosis, Laurence-Moon-Biedl syndrome; and degenerative diseases (more correctly causes of dementia), such as amaurotic family idiocy, Schilder's disease, Friedreich's ataxia, late infantile metachromatic leucodystrophy and metabolic disorders such as phenylketonuria, galactosæmia, gargoylism, Niemann-Pick disease, maple-syrup disease, glycogen-storage disease of the central nervous system, hereditary fructose intolerance, cretinism with goitre, pyridoxine dependency, idiopathic infantile hypoglycæmia, arginosuccinic-aciduria, etc. (*see* Chapter 10).

It has recently been discovered that certain forms of congenital abnormality, which may include mental defect, owe their origin to anomalies of *whole chromosomes* rather than genes. The cells of these patients contain more or fewer than the normal number of 46 chromosomes. In mongolism there is usually an additional *autosome* (No. 21), or a translocation defect may occur (p. 18). Other autosomal abnormalities are known to be associated with multiple congenital malformations including mental retardation (p. 20).

Environmental factors may operate in *intrauterine life, at the time of birth,* or *in infancy* or *childhood.* Maternal rubella occurring in the first three months of pregnancy may result in the birth of a mentally defective child, although certain physical defects are commoner.

Later in pregnancy, fœtal infection with the *Toxoplasma gondii* may cause mental defects, usually in association with hydrocephalus. X-irradiation of the pelvis in pregnancy is a known cause of microcephaly in the infant. In districts where cretinism is endemic, it is probably related to iodine deficiency in the diet of pregnant women. Fœtal hypoxia may be a cause of mental deficiency, but it is difficult to obtain definite evidence that this is so.

At the time of birth, prolonged anoxia or cerebral injury (e.g. subdural hæmatoma) may be followed by mental deficiency, as may brain damage secondary to erythroblastosis (kernicterus). There is a higher incidence of mental defect in children born prematurely than in those born at term.

In infancy or childhood, permanent intellectual impairment may result from brain damage secondary to head injury, anoxia (suffocation, carbon monoxide poisoning), encephalitis, meningitis (especially in infancy), lead poisoning, hydrocephalus from any cause, untreated craniostenosis, hypothyroidism, prolonged or repeated hypoglycæmia and severe dehydration.

DIAGNOSIS

Physical abnormalities, such as are seen in mongolism, gargoylism, microcephaly, etc., will imply the existence, but not necessarily the degree of mental deficiency. However, the majority of defective children show no gross physical abnormalities. In most cases, therefore, it is clearly impossible to arrive at a diagnosis at birth, but mental defect will first be suspected either by recognition of a paucity of accomplishments, compared with other children of the same age, or by reason of certain characteristic disorders of behaviour or because the physician detects certain physical symptoms or signs or biochemical abnormalities which are indicative of disease known to lead to or to be associated with mental defect.

BACKWARDNESS IN ACCOMPLISHMENTS

The existence of mental deficiency will begin to be noticed at the time when the infant's behaviour ceases to depend largely on spinal cord and brain-stem reflexes, and when the cerebral cortex should begin to play its part in enabling the infant to acquire proper control of the muscles and special senses that are necessary for voluntary activity.

Thus, backwardness may be suspected when the infant is seen to take little notice of his surroundings after the first six weeks of life, or when he is unable to remain sitting at six months, or to walk unaided at eighteen months. In minor degrees of feeble-mindedness there may be no great delay in reaching the various stages of psychical and motor development, and the child may be thought to be normal until he goes to school and is found to be behind his fellows in his capacity to learn.

Delay in *speech development* is an important symptom of mental defect. All degrees of language impairment are found. Idiots may be speechless, while in children with the highest grades of feeble-mindedness conversational powers, at least, are not obviously inadequate. The use of words may be deceptive. The parents of a young mentally defective child may truthfully claim that he has a large vocabulary. On inquiry, however, this may be found to consist of nouns, which are used reflexly or parrot-wise, but not to convey an idea. Thus, if shown a spoon, the child may say " spoon," but he cannot ask for one. Such children may have astonishing powers of memory—the " idiot savant " is the extreme example—and be able to repeat by rote many nursery rhymes, which an intellectually active child would not bother to learn. Then powers of language may also be misleading in a child who has sustained brain damage after learning to talk. as he may retain good verbal abilities but have difficulties in abstract reasoning and in appreciation of symbols on which school learning depends.

ABNORMALITIES OF BEHAVIOUR

The behaviour of a mental defective may simply be like that of a younger child, but may also show certain characteristic abnormalities, viz. underactivity, overactivity, peculiar habits. Thus the defective infant may appear entirely apathetic, may cry little, show no interest in his surroundings, have little muscular activity and slow reaction to stimuli. Alternatively, he may be of a restless type and cry almost unceasingly, although the significance of this is seldom realized except in retrospect.

After infancy, behaviour may vary between that of the child who sits placidly drooling at the mouth and indulging in some repetitive movement, such as rolling the eyes, shaking the hands or rocking the trunk, to that of the hyperactive type of defective, who displays ceaseless activity and who is irritable and distractable. An object is no sooner picked up than it is thrown down again, and nothing can claim the child's attention for more than a few seconds. Such children are often destructive and difficult to manage.

Finally, mentally defective children do not develop adequate powers of moral judgment, consideration for others and capacity to anticipate. Amongst juvenile delinquents the incidence of mental deficiency is high.

PHYSICAL STIGMATA

Mentally defective children are often short in stature, and tend to have heads smaller than the average. Minor physical peculiarities, such as abnormal pinnæ or irregular teeth, are found more frequently than in children of normal intelligence. These physical abnormalities are not reliable evidence of mental defect. Many defective children are subject to fits.

DIFFICULTIES IN DIAGNOSIS

Hasty judgments must be avoided in the diagnosis of mental deficiency, but even in cases in which there is only a suspicion of backwardness, every effort must be made to exclude treatable disease such as cretinism, phenylketonuria or deafness.[1] In doubtful cases in which no specific diagnosis can be made, many periods of observation and repeated mental tests may be necessary. Special difficulties are encountered when the child suffers from severe physical defects or from emotional maladjustment. Deafness, blindness and cerebral palsy may all be accompanied by mental defect, either through co-existent disease of the brain or through lengthy deprivation of those normal sensory experiences which are necessary for full intellectual development. On the other hand, these defects may give a wrong impression of mental deficiency in a child who, if taught early by special methods may be found to be of normal or even high intelligence. The greatest difficulties in diagnosis are met in children deprived of normal emotional stimuli, for instance the motherless child for whom no adequate " mother substitute " has been provided. Here again there may be the appearance of mental retardation, which becomes permanent if the abnormal emotional environment persists. The very rare instances of juvenile psychosis may also provide difficulties in diagnosis.

PROGNOSIS

Except in those rare cases in which a specific and treatable disorder is diagnosed, the prognosis is hopeless in the sense that no treatment or training will change a mentally defective child into a normal one. The feeble-minded and imbeciles will, of course, learn, but the rate of learning is slower than that of a normal child. The idiot, if he reaches adult life, will seldom have a mental age exceeding that of a two-year-old child; the mental age of the adult imbecile will not be greater than six years and that of the feeble-minded not greater than ten years.

The expectation of life is lower than that of normal children, both because of the defective's greater liability to accidents and of his lowered resistance to disease.

MANAGEMENT

The question of whether a mentally defective child should be cared for at home or in an institution is one that has to be faced sooner or later by the parents and doctor. It is a problem that must be influenced by numerous factors, including the degree of mental defect, the existence of brothers and sisters, social and economic circumstances and so on. In general it may be said that, if the child is capable of

[1] Tizard, J. P. M. (1960). " The Role of the Family Doctor in the Prevention of Mental Defect." Suppl. to " Pædiatrics for the Practitioner." Ed. Gaisford and Lightwood. London: Butterworth.

making a distinction between home and institution, he should if possible be kept at home. Idiots and many imbeciles are best cared for in institutions, especially if there are other children at home who may be neglected because of the demands made by the defective.

The type of mental defect is of some importance. Mongols, for instance, are usually placid and easy to manage at home, while true microcephalics are often just the reverse.

If a mentally defective child is to be reared at home, his parents will have to teach him diligently and patiently things which the normal child learns for himself.[1] At the same time they must not expect too much from him, nor attempt to train him, before he is ready to learn. " Pushing " the child readily causes confusion and irritability, and leads to temper tantrums and destructive behaviour. As the child grows, he should be encouraged to carry out simple tasks for which he shows an aptitude. Many high-grade defectives may become skilled in manipulative work of a simple nature. The high-grade mental defective will also benefit greatly from training in an ESN school, where, surrounded by others of his kind, he feels no sense of inferiority, and where the education is limited to that which he is capable of receiving.

TALKING TO THE PARENTS OF A DEFECTIVE CHILD [2]

To learn that their child is mentally defective is the most cruel blow that can befall any parents. The physician must learn the difficult task of presenting the facts and giving advice in a manner that leaves no feeling of resentment and does not increase their distress.

No two situations involving a defective child and his parents are quite the same and the right approach in one case may be unsuitable in another. When the existence of mental defect in early infancy is obvious to the doctor, but not to the parents, as for instance in cases of mongolism, it is usually best to warn the parents that all may not be well; and the policy of the truth and nothing but the truth, but not, at first, the whole truth is to be commended. When the doctor suspects mental deficiency, but is not certain, extreme caution must be exercised in what is said to the parents, and investigations may have to be arranged without revealing their true purpose.

In some cases it is the parents themselves who are the first to suspect that their child is backward. Again, the doctor should be cautious in expressing a definite opinion. Repeated examinations and, in most cases, hospital investigation are desirable and in the case of older children intelligence tests should be carried out. When the existence of mental defect is certain, the parents may be asked in what manner the child's behaviour differs from that of his brothers and sisters or of other children they know of the same age. In discussing the

---

[1] " Opening Doors " by Dr. John Thomson (Oliver & Boyd) is a helpful book for parents.
[2] Brennemann, Joseph. The approach to the parents of a subnormal child. Brennemann's "Practice of Pædiatrics," Vol. 4, Chap. XIII, Section 2. W. F. Prior & Co. Inc.

matter in this way, most parents will admit that the child is " backward," and it is never necessary to introduce other expressions such as mental defective, imbecile or idiot unless first mentioned by the parents. It is useful to point out that the child's behaviour is similar to that of a younger child, and the physician and parents will usually come to an agreement about the degree of retardation, deciding, for instance, that a three-year-old child acts more like one of eighteen months. Too often parents are left with the impression that no further development can be expected, but the physician should explain that the child will learn, albeit slowly, and may, if asked, give a rough estimate of the degree of future mental development that can be anticipated.

Then, although the question is seldom asked, parents are frequently obsessed with the thought that the child's condition is due to their fault, through the unsuccessful use of contraceptives, venereal disease, and so on. The physician should make it clear that they are not responsible, and that mental defect may occur by mischance in the child of perfectly healthy and highly intelligent parents.

Finally, there is the question of future children, and here the physician can usually be reassuring. Where the mental defect is known to be due to a simple genetic factor, the risks must be admitted. Thus, the parents of a child with phenylketonuria—inherited as a recessive character—must be told that there is a one in four chance of a subsequent child being similarly affected. In other cases, even where there is a statistically increased risk of repetition, the risk is so slight that for the parents' peace of mind the physician had better not mention it.

Mongolism

This makes up 5 per cent. of the total of mental defectives in institutions, but 50 per cent. of those mental defectives noted during the first year of life. About 1 in 600 children born are mongols.

ÆTIOLOGY

It is now known that mongol children have chromosomal abnormalities which may be detected by means of tissue culture of their leucocytes. In most cases so far studied there are 47 chromosomes, the extra chromosome (No. 21) having arisen by nondisjunction during germ cell formation (*see* p. 18). Nondisjunction seems to occur more frequently in the ova of older mothers. The following table shows the incidence of mongolism in children born to mothers at different ages.

Maternal age	14–19	20–24	25–29	30–34	35–39	40–44	45 +
Incidence per thousand births	0·0	0·3	0·3	1·7	3·5	14·2	26·3

In a small proportion of mongols the total number of chromosomes is 46, but one chromosome is abnormally large. In these cases the cells of one parent may be found to contain only 45 chromosomes, one large chromosome representing the fusion of (or " translocation " of parts of) two chromosomes.[1] This necessarily results in imbalance of chromosomal material during germ-cell formation and may explain the rare instances of familial incidence of mongolism, especially where the mother is relatively young. In the future, tissue culture of the child's and parents' blood will be a necessary part of the investigation of mongolism in assessing the risk of recurrence in future children.

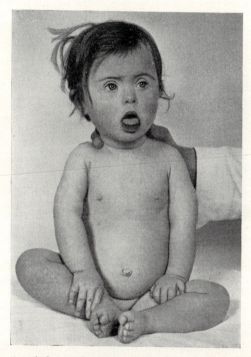

Fig. 56.—A typical mongol aged 11 months. Note the open mouth and visible tongue, the curved little finger and the characteristic slant of the eyes. There was cyanosis due to Fallot's tetralogy.

PATHOLOGY

The brain is unduly small, with simple convolutions, and the cortex is thin. Microscopically, there is defective neuronic development. The endocrine system is not involved. Congenital heart disease is present in 15 per cent. of all cases. The commonest defects are atrial or ventricular septal defects and atrio-ventricularis communis. Duodenal atresia not uncommonly coexists.

[1] Polani, P. E., et al. (1960). Lancet, 1, 721.

CLINICAL PICTURE

The appearance is so characteristic that once one mongol has been seen another is recognized at once (Fig. 56). It is seldom that there is any difficulty in diagnosis except sometimes in the first few weeks of life. The most striking features are the eyes, which slant upwards and outwards and which frequently have large epicanthic folds. Squints, white spots on the iris (Brushfield's spots), myopia and blepharitis are common. The face is rather flat; the nose short and squat; the lower lip protuberant and the corners of the mouth turn down.

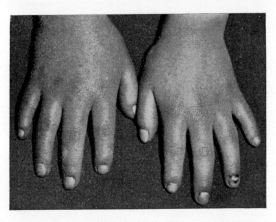

Fig. 57.—The hands in mongolism ; note short, incurved, little finger.

The child is given to sucking the tongue, which tends to protrude from the mouth and is included to be slim and pointed at its tip, and in time shows furrows on the dorsum. The teeth are late to erupt and irregular.

The head is small and nearly always brachycephalic, being flattened at the occiput. The posterior fontanelle and the central part of the sagittal suture often remain patent for several months and the anterior fontanelle also closes late.

The whole muscular system tends to poor tone. This hypotonia is best seen in the arms and legs, especially the hands. A nurse holding the child will remark that he lies in her arms like a bag of jelly, instead of having the firm live feel of the normal infant. There is a tendency to umbilical hernia. Mongols are always somewhat dwarfed, both trunk and limbs being short. The hands are small, the fingers tapering, and the little finger especially is shortened and inclined to curve in (Fig. 57). There is often one instead of the normal two transverse palmar creases. The proximal triradius (where three sets of fine lines meet) is frequently displaced towards the centre of the palm (Fig. 58). The skin is smooth, but tends to roughness in parts

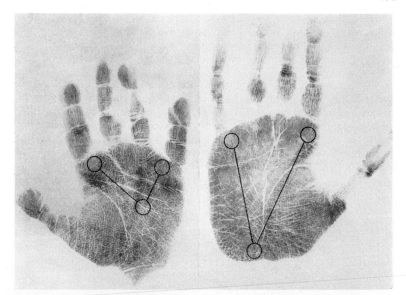

Fig. 58.—*Above:* The palm print from a mongol child on the left shows (1) a short second phalanx of the little finger; (2) a transverse alignment of the distal palmar creases which have not, in this case, fused to give a simian crease; (3) a centrally situated palmar triradius, giving an angle of over 66° (in this case 79°) with the triradii at the base of the index and little fingers. The palm print on the right is from a normal child. *Below:* Human chromosomes. Normal male karyotype arranged according to the Denver system of classification; the chromosomes of a male mongol are identical with these except for the 21-22 group, which is shown in the rectangular inset.

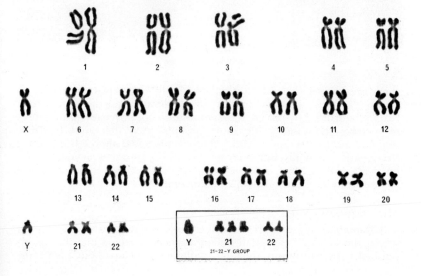

which are exposed to the weather. The colour of the cheeks is high. With the exception perhaps of the slanting eyes, there is not one of these physical abnormalities that may not be absent in an individual mongol, nor one that cannot exist as a single physical peculiarity in a normal person.

The mentality may be very deceptive, as he seems bright, takes a great interest in his surroundings, smiles up into the face of his mother and is most affectionate. But in fact most mongols are imbeciles (many are idiots) and the I.Q. rarely exceeds 50. The average mongol learns to sit alone at 2 years, to walk at 3 years, to be toilet trained at 4 years, to say words at 5 years and sentences at 7 years. As a rule, mongols are fond of music and are affectionate and gentle; occasionally,

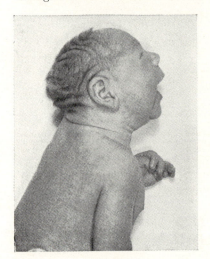 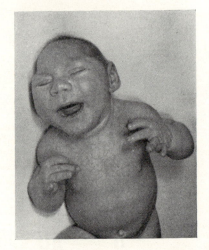

Fig. 59.—True microcephaly in a boy aged 2 months.

they are destructive. Imitation is highly developed, initiative is lacking. They can be taught to be moderately obedient, but they cannot be trusted to any great extent and do not prove useful members of society. Because of the short nasopharynx, the child tends to make a snorting noise as with enlarged adenoids, almost from birth. Frequently, adenoids and enlarged tonsils do appear later and should be dealt with. Most mongols who survive develop cataracts in the second decade of life. Epilepsy is uncommon.

Microcephalia Vera

Although many mental defectives have small heads, a group in which the head is very small and of a peculiar shape may be distinguished. In institutions, the microcephalics make up about 5 per cent.

of defective children below ten years of age, and 0·5 per cent. of all defectives.

ÆTIOLOGY

In most cases the cause is unknown, but in some the defect is known to be inherited as a recessive character. Microcephaly may result from x-ray therapy to the pelvis of a pregnant woman.

PATHOLOGY

The brain is much smaller than normal, and often has a convolutional pattern similar to that of a three-month fœtus. On microscopy, the nerve-cells are few in number. There is no evidence of inflammation or degeneration.

CLINICAL PICTURE

The head appears small at birth, and the disproportion in size between the head and the normal face and trunk becomes more obvious as the child grows (Fig. 59). The fontanelles close early, but normal suture lines are visible on x-ray. The head circumference never exceeds 17 inches, and may be smaller. The vertical measurement is greatly diminished, so that the skull slopes sharply on all sides to the vertex. The scalp is often wrinkled. Limb and trunk musculature may be well developed. These children are nearly always idiots or imbeciles. At home they are inclined to be aggressive and difficult to manage, but they may be happy and docile in institutions. Epilepsy is common, and in some cases there is spasticity of the limbs.

J. P. M. Tizard

CHAPTER 21

Diseases of the Bones and Joints

THIS chapter is primarily concerned with diagnosis; details of orthopædic treatment are not described, but will be found in standard text-books of orthopædic surgery.

For detailed information about the less common diseases of the skeleton the reader is referred to the work of the late Sir Thomas Fairbank,[1] which will, in the authors' opinion, remain the standard reference work for many years to come.

CONGENITAL DISORDERS

Congenital Skeletal Limb Deficiencies

INFANTS may be born with complete deficiency of one or more limbs (amelia) or with a variety of partial skeletal deficiencies. For the latter, a considerable nomenclature exists including such terms as phocomelia, hemimelia, ectromelia and so on. For clinical purposes, it seems more helpful with a particular patient to describe the extent of the defect in simple language, that is " absent radii " or in another case " absent humerus, radius and ulna with carpus attached direct to shoulder girdle." Infants with skeletal limb deficiencies have an increased chance of other congenital malformations involving one or more different systems: central nervous; cardiovascular; alimentary; genito-urinary.

Major symmetrical skeletal deficiencies used to be among the rarer congenital malformations, although minor unilateral deficiencies involving usually only the hand or phalanges were seen somewhat more frequently. From 1958, coinciding with the first administration of thalidomide to women during the early months of pregnancy, there was a marked increase in the number of infants born with major symmetrical deformities, although the number with unilateral abnormalities did not alter significantly.

THALIDOMIDE BABIES [2, 3, 4, 5]

It is established that the administration of thalidomide in the first trimester of pregnancy carries the risk of major congenital deformities

---

[1] Fairbank, Sir Thomas (1951). " An Atlas of General Affections of the Skeleton." Edinburgh: Livingstone.
[2] Lenz, W. (1962). *Lancet*, 1, 45.
[3] Spiers, A. L. (1962). *Ibid*, 1, 323.
[4] Smithells, R. W. (1962). *Ibid*, 1, 1270.
[5] British Pædiatric Association Memorandum (1962). *Brit. med. J.*, 2, 522,

in the infant. These deformities predominantly involve the limbs; almost all the infants have major symmetrical deficiencies of their upper limbs and in about one-third of the cases there are deficiencies of the legs also. A rather smaller proportion have imperfectly developed external ears although the hearing may not be affected. A nævus extending from the forehead over the nose to the upper lip is seen in many of the children. Malformations of the heart and alimentary tract are associated in a small but significant proportion. The intellect is not impaired.

PREVENTION

The risk of further cases, now that the dangers have been so widely publicized and since thalidomide has been withdrawn from general use, comes from the residuum of the tablets of thalidomide prescribed in the past and retained in medicine cupboards in containers with such anonymous labels as "The Tablets. Two to be taken at night." Arising from the thalidomide tragedy, the attention of both the medical profession and the general public must be drawn to the potential dangers of drugs in the early months of pregnancy. Whilst no additional drugs have as yet been incriminated with certainty, evidence suggests that the adverse effect of thalidomide on the fœtus may occur as a result of its action as a riboflavine antagonist. Other drugs with similar actions must thus fall under suspicion. There is no doubt that in a number of the children with major symmetrical limb deficiencies there is no history of thalidomide administration to the mother during the pregnancy.

TREATMENT

Expert help is required both for the family who have to care for the patient as well as for the child. The physician needs to work in co-operation with the social services in order that the child may receive all the necessary medical care and still retain his place within the family circle.

Medical treatment in the early years involves the conservation and use of every piece of limb tissue present. Expert physiotherapy is required to help such children obtain mobility and a sense of balance and to utilize their rudimentary limbs with the object of obtaining the maximum degree of independence for themselves. Prosthesis plays an important part as the child grows older. Such children present a special problem in education and later in training for employment as disabled persons.

OTHER SKELETAL DEFICIENCIES

The various degrees of partial limb deficiencies are too numerous to enumerate individually. The basic principles of treatment, already mentioned, apply.

Congenital absence of the radii has been noted for many years in association with purpura and thrombocytopenia and constitutes a special syndrome. Fanconi's anæmia (p. 333) may also be present.

Hereditary Cleidocranial Dysostosis

In this rare condition there is a failure of development of membranous bone, thus giving rise to a congenital absence of the whole or part of the clavicles with imperfect ossification in the skull in the

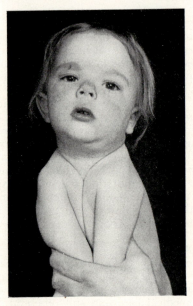

Fig. 60.—Cleidocranial dysotosis in a girl of 2 years.

region of the fontanelle. The teeth and the centres of ossification in the hands, feet, and elsewhere are delayed. Such children can approximate the shoulders in front of the chest. The condition is inherited as a dominant characteristic.

Cranio-facial Dysostosis (Crouzon's Disease)

This disease is inherited as a dominant characteristic. The patient presents a striking and characteristic appearance. The skull is oxycephalic, with atrophic maxillæ. There is exophthalmos and a beak-shaped nose. The eyes may show malformations, including coloboma; optic atrophy, due to compression of the optic nerve in the deformed middle cranial fossa, may occur in some cases.

Acrocephaly Syndactyly (Apert's Disease)

Congenital fusion of the cranial sutures giving rise to a brachy-cephalic skull is associated with webbed fingers and toes. Exophthalmos and nasal obstruction occur as a result of the foreshortened skull. Surgical separation of the cranial sutures is essential to allow the brain to develop (p. 436). Plastic operations are necessary on the fingers.

Arachnodactyly (Spider Fingers)

In this rare condition the fingers and toes are unduly long and thin (*see* Fig. 26, p. 294). X-rays show that all the bones are likewise elongated and thin. Abnormalities of the iris frequently accompany this condition. The association of dislocation of the lens, congenital heart disease and arachnodactyly make up Marfan's syndrome (*see* p. 293). Often these patients are hypotonic and their ligaments lax (Fig. 61).

Congenital Elevation of the Scapula (Sprengel's Deformity)

The condition is rare. It is commoner in girls than boys. The scapula on one side is small, and fixed high up, with the inferior angle nearer to the spine. Movement of the arm is restricted.

Klippel-Feil Syndrome (Webbed Neck)

Such children have congenital abnormalities, including fusion or absence of some of the cervical vertebræ, causing the neck to be extremely short. The head is therefore set between the shoulders and there is a fold of skin running from below the ear almost to the tip of the shoulder. It may be associated with a Sprengel deformity of the scapula.

Marble Bones (Albers-Schönberg's Disease)

The bones are unduly dense, due to the deposit of much lime; x-rays confirm this. The skull is involved, and optic atrophy may result from encroachment on the optic nerves. Anæmia is present because of the involvement of the bone-marrow. Death takes place from intercurrent disease, before

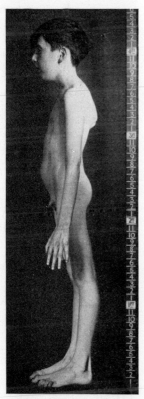

Fig. 61.—Marfan's syndrome. A boy aged 7 years with arachnodactyly, lordotic stance with round shoulders, muscular hypotonia and lax ligaments. He is tall for his age.

puberty as a rule. This condition is rare. It is sometimes familial, sometimes of a dominant and sometimes of a recessive genetic type.

Punctate Epiphyseal Dysplasia

In this condition the infant is born with considerable foreshortening of some of the long bones, the humeri and femora being particularly affected. In addition, the epiphyses are fragmented, giving a stippled appearance on x-ray. The child may also show congenital cataracts or a congenital cardiac malformation. Such patients as survive are dwarfed but may be of normal intelligence.

The radiological appearance of the epiphyses is to be distinguished from the epiphyseal dysplasia seen in some cases of cretinism (Plate II).

Osteochondrodystrophy

Morquio-Brailsford Type. This hereditary condition consists of dwarfism, kyphosis, and abnormalities of the femoral head and acetabulum in a child of normal intelligence. Other parts of the skeleton in addition to the spine and hips may be affected to a varying degree.

Clinically, no abnormality may be recognized until the age of four years, when progressive kyphosis and stunting of growth are noted (Fig. 62), together with a characteristic posture whereby the child stands in a crouching position with the head thrust forward. Varying degrees of limitation of movement may be noted in the joints, depending upon the extent of the disease.

Radiologically, there is found to be flattening of the vertebral bodies, particularly in the dorsal region. In the lateral view they have a characteristic shape, since the upper and lower surfaces are irregular and ill-defined, with a tendency to approximate anteriorly which gives rise to a wedge-shaped appearance, accentuated further by a central prolongation in front. In the region of the hip joint the acetabulum is found to be enlarged and irregular, with flattening and fragmentation of the femoral head.

The disease is progressive and crippling, becoming more and more marked until unassisted walking may become impossible.

Gargoylism (Hurler's Disease). This condition differs from the Morquio-Brailsford type in that changes are not confined to the skeleton but include a typical gross facies, mental deficiency (*see* p. 464), corneal opacity and marked enlargement of the liver and spleen. It is often familial. The name *dysostosis multiplex* has been employed as well as *gargoylism*. The latter term was given as an affectionate nickname by the late Dr. F. J. Poynton to a patient who was in fact the first case of Hurler's disease to be described in England.

Formerly classified as a disorder of lipoid metabolism, and sometimes called *lipochondrodystrophy*, it now seems that the material which is found deposited in the cytoplasm of the cells is probably a mucopoly-

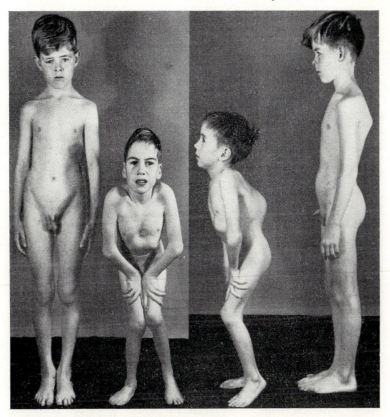

Fig. 62.—Morquio's disease. A patient, aged 10 years, showing severe dorsal kyphosis and dolichocephaly; he is standing beside a normal boy of the same age. The standing attitude of flexion of the hips and knees and the support by the hands on the thighs is very pronounced. There is a marked knock-knee deformity.

saccharide. A simple test for Hurler's disease[1] is based on the excretion in the urine by these patients of excessive amounts of mucopolysaccharide by a colorimetric method.

CLINICAL PICTURE

Clinically, dwarfism is usually recognizable by the end of the first year; the head is seen to be large, with widely separated eyes and a depressed bridge to the nose. The facial appearance generally is characteristic, being ugly in the extreme, with the mouth often open and the tongue protruded. Mental deficiency and corneal opacity are present in most cases, with enlargement of the liver and spleen, often

[1] Fisher, O. D., Robinson, M. (1961). *Arch. Dis. Childh.*, **36**, 691.

associated with umbilical or inguinal herniæ. There is kyphosis in the dorso-lumbar region, with variable degrees of limitation of movement in other joints. Cardiac enlargement, with abnormalities evident on the electrocardiogram, is often present.

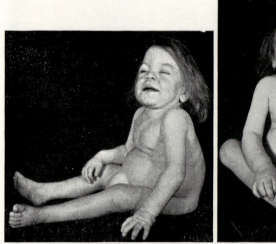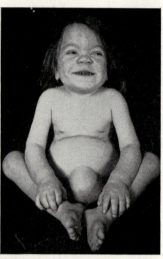

Fig. 63.—Gargoylism in a 3 year old; she was mentally defective. She had profuse nasal discharge, a large umbilical hernia, lumbar kyphosis and genu valgum. Note the broad flat face with mid-frontal bossing of the skull.

Radiologically, there is enlargement of the sella turcica, with or without hydrocephalus. The vertebral bodies are convex and the vertebral discs are biconcave and deeper than normal. The kyphosis often appears to be associated with one vertebra " slipping back " out of alignment. Such a vertebra will often show a concave upper margin with a beak-shaped anterior projection at the inferior margin. The most commonly affected vertebra is the second lumbar, but the first lumbar vertebra and occasionally several vertebræ may be affected (Plate XI). Kyphosis may sometimes be present without displacement of any vertebræ.

The condition is progressive, and few cases survive the age of ten years.

Infantile Cortical Hyperostosis: Caffey's Disease [1]

This condition makes its appearance during the first four months of life, and is characterized by *laminated* cortical thickenings of the aw, facial bones and elsewhere (Plate XII). The hyperostoses are

[1] Annotation (1961). *Lancet* 1, 394.

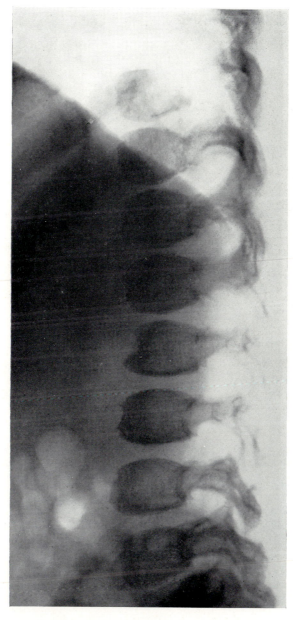

PLATE XI. Lumbar spine in an 8-year-old boy with
gargoylism.   Note   typical   anterior   " beak "   of
vertebral body.

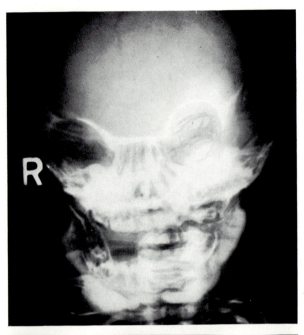

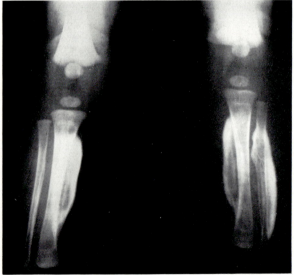

PLATE XII. Infantile cortical hyperostosis.

surmounted by somewhat tender, soft-tissue swellings. After varying periods, in which fever may occur, the swellings and the hyperostoses slowly resolve. The level of vitamin A in the blood is not raised in this disease (*see* diagnosis).

DIAGNOSIS

Caffey's disease may require to be distinguished from neoplasm, subperiosteal hæmatoma, scurvy and chronic vitamin-A poisoning. The latter may cause a picture of liver enlargement and tender cortical hyperostoses, but with only one layer of periosteal proliferation to be seen in the x-ray; the age of onset is later than in Caffey's disease. There is also a difference in the distribution of lesions: in vitamin-A poisoning the metatarsals and long bones, commonly the ulnæ, are affected but the jaw bones are not; moreover, there are general symptoms such as anorexia, irritability, pallor, a dry erythematous skin, scaling lips with bleeding cracks, as well as hepatomegaly. The level of vitamin A in the blood is raised and dramatic recovery takes place when the excessive intake of this vitamin is stopped.

Achondroplasia (Chondrodystrophia Fœtalis et Micromelia)

This is recognizable at birth. The long bones are shortened, but the trunk is normal. The head is large (Fig. 64). The hands are characteristic, as the digits are approximated in pairs, giving rise to the trident appearance. The elbows show some limitation of full extension.

The condition may be hereditary, of a dominant genetic type, but as labour is difficult among achondroplasic women the strains tend to die out, mutations accounting for the continuation of the disease. It is due to an interference with endochondral ossification, especially at the extremities of the long bones. Mentally these children are normal. They seldom exceed 4½ feet in height.

Osteogenesis Imperfecta (Fragilitas Ossium, Brittle Bones and Blue Sclerotics)

This is a familial and hereditary condition (dominant gene). In the more benign form, the disease may not be diagnosed before the third or fourth year, when fractures begin. At this time the sclerotics are noticed to be intensely blue, as opposed to the pale blue sclerotics of many normal babies, and the skull tends to bulge in the temporal region above the ears.

In the *mild form*, the fractures are infrequent and the children live a normal life; only a few progress to invalidism. Liability to fracture grows less with the years. In adult life, otosclerosis is a common complication. In the more *severe form*, fractures may be present at birth and gross deformities result (Fig. 65). The ætiology is unknown, but there is deficiency of the fibrous trabeculæ binding the osteoid tissues together.

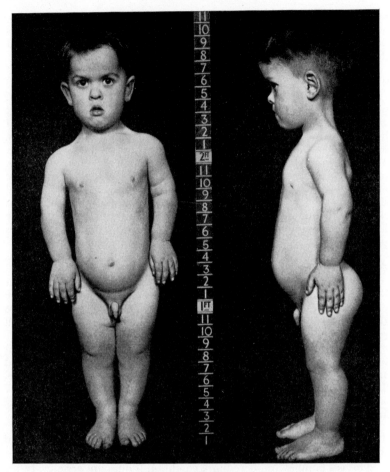

Fig. 64.—Achondroplasia.

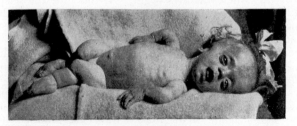

Fig. 65.—Osteogenesis imperfecta in an infant aged 18 months.

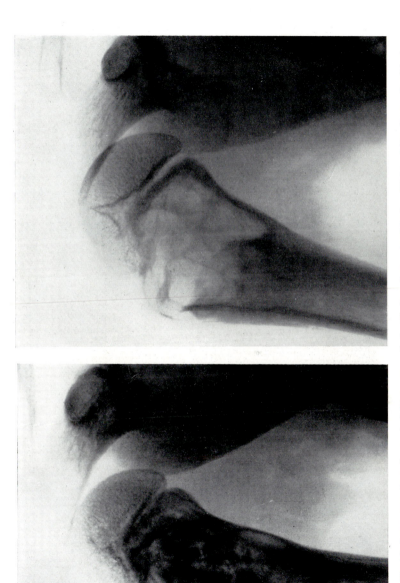

PLATE XIII. Single bone cyst in a boy aged 12 years. *Left*: Before bone grafting. *Right*: After bone grafting.

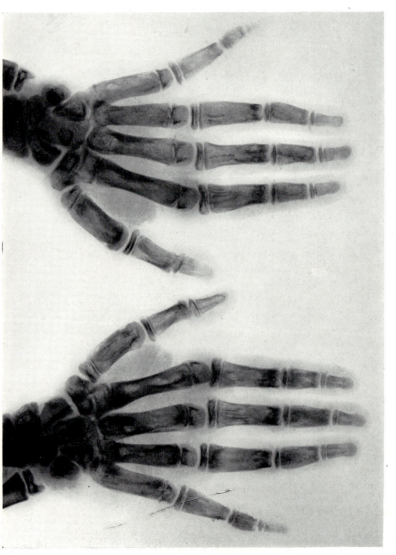

PLATE XIV. Polyostotic fibrous dysplasia. Translucent areas of bone absorption together with thinning of the cortex are visible in the metacarpals and some of the phalanges. Many of the other bones of the skeleton showed similar changes. Biopsy: osteitis fibrosa, residual bone trabeculæ embedded in dense fibrous tissue. An X-ray of the patient shown in Fig. 66.

The calcium and phosphorus levels in the blood are normal.
No treatment seems of use beyond general care to prevent fractures.

Generalized Osteitis Fibrosa

The majority of the patients in whom profound decalcification and osteoporosis of a generalized nature occurs are found to have hyperparathyroid tumours (p. 158). Such cases are very rare in childhood.

Localized Osteitis Fibrosa

Localized decalcified bone cysts, often single but sometimes multiple, may be found unassociated with any disturbance of calcium or phosphorus metabolism. The condition when multiple is to be distinguished from Albright's syndrome (*see* below) in view of the absence of pigmentation and sexual precocity. Pathological fractures may occur.

The condition responds well to cleaning out of the cyst and packing with bone fragments obtained from other sites (Plate XIII).

Polyostotic Fibrous Dysplasia of Bone (Albright's Syndrome)

This is a rare congenital disorder which is characterized by disseminated osteitis fibrosa, pigmentation of the skin and, in girls, precocious

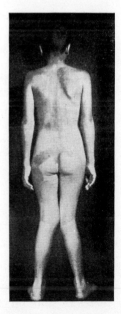 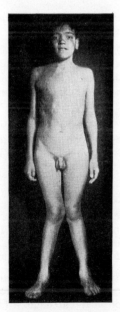

Fig. 66.—Authors' case of polyostotic fibrous dysplasia (Albright's syndrome) at the age of 13½ years. Note the genu valgum, which had been increasing for 7 years, and the pigmentation.

sexual development. There is no evidence of the condition being inherited. Albright postulated an endocrine cause.

Osseous deformities may occur, and in a male seen by the authors[1] there had been increasing genu valgum for some years. The patient, a Greek, presented at 13 years (Fig. 66) and the radiological diagnosis was made by Dr. L. G. Blair (Plate XIV). The condition does not get worse after the bones cease to grow. It is at this stage, therefore, that the question of corrective osteotomy should be considered and, if necessary, carried out.

INFECTIVE STATES

Acute Suppurative Arthritis

THIS disease may be primary, or secondary to some infective process elsewhere. The cause is most commonly the *Staph. pyogenes*, but the pneumococcus, gonococcus, *Salmonella byphosa* and *Esch. coli* have all been implicated.

The condition may occur at any age, but it is to be noted that staphylococcal arthritis or *Esch. coli* infections may occur in the newborn as a part of a septicæmia or pyæmia.

Site. Any joint may be infected, the knee, hip, shoulder and ankle being most common.

Clinical Picture. There is fever, pain on movement, and the child appears ill. Examination shows heat, swelling and marked local tenderness. Aspiration is needed to confirm the diagnosis and provide material for isolation of the infecting organism in the laboratory.

Prognosis and Treatment. Since the advent of antibiotics, the outlook has been much improved; these infections rapidly yield to them, together with rest and surgical treatment where necessary. Infections of the newborn, despite chemotherapy, however, still have a significant mortality.

Osteomyelitis

Ætiology and Pathology. Apart from injury, the infection is blood-borne from a skin lesion or from some other infected part of the body. It is usually the *Staph. pyogenes*, but may be the streptococcus or *Esch. coli*. Osteitis in the newborn is easily overlooked.

Site. The disease starts in the metaphysis, which is the most vascular part of the bone, and lies at the diaphyseal side of the epiphyseal cartilage. This diseased area is therefore shut off and gives rise to severe pain and toxæmia.

---

[1] Vines, R. H. (1952). Polyostotic fibrous dysplasia. *Arch. Dis. Childh.*, **27**, 351.

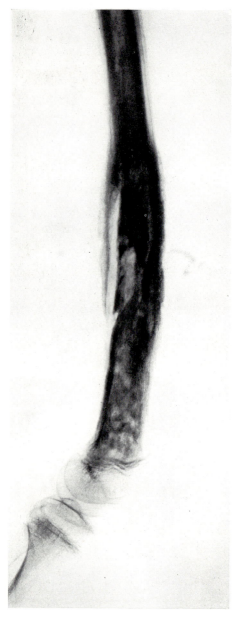

PLATE XV. Chronic osteomyelitis of the femur due to *Staphylococcus pyogenes* in a 14-year-old boy.

Clinical Picture. In older children, there is severe local pain followed later by swelling and heat. The child can appear gravely ill from the first, with a high fever, coated dry tongue and rapid pulse. In infants the signs may be less obvious.

Differential Diagnosis. This must be made from acute rheumatism (p. 306), which can cause confusion until the pain removes to another joint. A marked leucocytosis suggests osteitis. X-rays are of no value for diagnostic purposes in the first 7–10 days of the infection, but the characteristic changes (raising of the periosteum and bone destruction) appear later (Plate XV).

Treatment. Early treatment with antibiotics, in particular penicillin (for dosage, *see* Appendix I), has revolutionized the treatment and prognosis of this condition. Initial surgical drainage remains essential, but chronic sinus formation, with recurrent acute episodes, is now rarely seen.

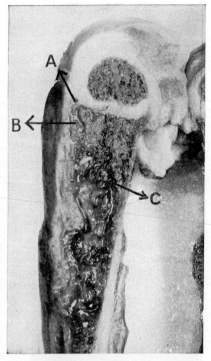

Fig. 67.—Femur from a case of osteomyelitis.
A, path taken by infection into knee-joint.
B, primary focus of infection.
C, path taken through necrosed bone to popliteal space.

TUBERCULOUS DISEASE OF BONES AND JOINTS

TUBERCULOUS osteitis is always secondary to some focus in another part of the body. Joints are affected secondarily to disease of the adjacent bone. (For a general description of tuberculosis, *see* Chapter 25.)

The organism is usually the human strain of tubercle bacillus in countries, such as the United Kingdom, where retailed milk is now virtually safe from contamination with bovine tubercle bacilli. One-third of the cases occur in the spine, one-third in the hip, and the remaining third are distributed in the knee, ankle, elbow and shoulder. The disease is most frequently found in the juxta-epiphyseal region, but does not give rise to formation of new bone beneath the periosteum, as shown by x-rays. (The exception to this is tuberculous dactylitis.)

Spinal Caries (Pott's Disease: Tuberculous Spondylitis)

The commonest site is the lower dorsal region, and the condition becomes increasingly rare up to the cervical region.

The bodies of the vertebræ are attacked in the central portion where there is cancellous tissue. Abscesses may form in the paravertebral region, or the bodies of the vertebræ may collapse, causing kyphosis and pressure symptoms on the cord.

Occasionally pain may be referred to the abdomen from a dorsal caries, or there may be pain in the limbs, if the appropriate region of the spine is involved. Usually there is rigidity of the spine, and the child complains of pain accompanying any violent movement. Local tenderness is present over the spines of the affected vertebræ. In the later stages deformity of the spine may be marked, but the diagnosis should be made before this stage is reached. Usually there is little temperature or constitutional disturbance.

DIAGNOSIS

There is marked limitation of movement of the spine in the affected region, thus differentiating the condition from one of postural scoliosis. There is acute tenderness on jarring of the spine from above or below or tapping the spines of the vertebræ in the affected area. A tuberculin test, x-rays and the sedimentation rate will confirm the diagnosis and indicate the activity of the lesion.

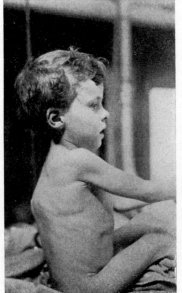

Fig. 68. – Spinal caries.

The combination of general anti-tuberculous therapy (p. 490) with local treatment to provide immobilization in the optimum position produces excellent results, although treatment remains a long and tiresome business. Paravertebral abscess has to be watched for and in cases in which the lesion affects the lowest dorsal vertebræ may track downwards to form a psoas abscess.

Tuberculous Dactylitis

The fingers and toes show a spindle-shaped tender enlargement. Usually more than one bone is affected. Caseous material may form, burrow to the surface, and evacuate through the skin.

Accompanying this process there is a subperiostitis, which produces new bone, as shown in the x-rays

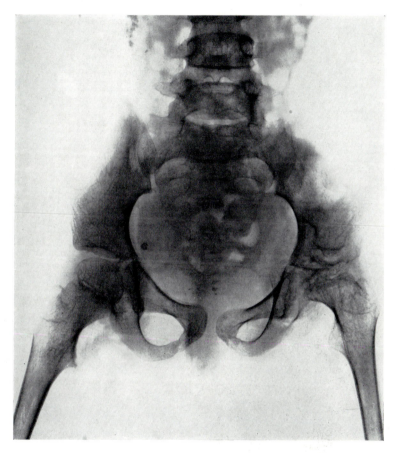

PLATE XVI. Tuberculous arthritis of the left hip in a girl aged 6 years.
Note complete disappearance of the head of the femur.

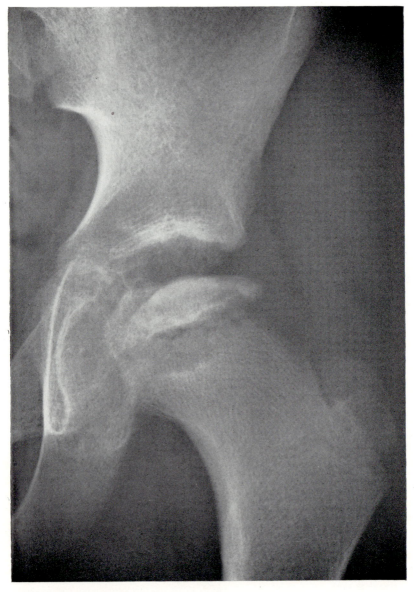

PLATE XVII.   Perthes' disease in a boy aged 9 years.   Note, in addition
to the sclerosis of the head of the femur, the rarefaction and widening of
the metaphysis.

Syphilitic dactylitis bears a close resemblance and may not be distinguishable except by a tuberculin test and the Wassermann reaction.

Tuberculosis of Long Bones and Joints (Tuberculous Hip)

Usually the infection occurs at the juxta-epiphyseal region, and extends into the joints secondarily.

PATHOLOGY

The synovial membrane of the joint becomes infected and is studded with miliary tubercles. Ulceration of the cartilage, and adhesions between the synovial membrane and surrounding parts occur. The joint may be come distended with fluid in which tubercle bacilli can be demonstrated.

CLINICAL PICTURE

The hip joint is the most commonly affected; the knee, ankle, and joints of the upper extremities are affected less frequently. Usually the child complains first of pain, particularly at night, and then he is seen to be limping. This contrasts with Perthes' disease, where the child is first seen to limp, and later complains of pain.

On examination, the joint, usually the hip, shows limitation of movement in all directions. The surrounding muscles are in spasm. As the process continues, " starting pains " are complained of at night. As the child dozes off to sleep the muscles relax, and the inflamed surfaces of the joints come together, causing pain. Muscular wasting always occurs in the vicinity of the affected joint.

X-rays in the early stage show no abnormality in the affected joints; a repeat x-ray, however, in a few weeks will show a fluffy appearance of the articular surfaces of the bones and progressive rarefaction of the epiphyses and approximate areas of the diaphyses (Plate XVI).

DIFFERENTIAL DIAGNOSIS

Rheumatism is seldom monarticular, but may occasionally be so. Usually, a few days on full doses of salicylates will cause the pains to disappear. In addition, the tuberculin skin-tests are negative, and no lesion is seen in an x-ray. The sedimentation rate is raised in both conditions.

In acute infective arthritis the differential diagnosis may be very difficult. The onset, however, is usually more acute, with high fever and a leucocytosis. A negative tuberculin test is helpful.

Congenital syphilis may be excluded by a negative Wassermann. In Clutton's joints (*see* p. 491), in which the knees are affected, the disease is bilateral and the swelling painless.

Trauma, or the so-called irritable hip syndrome, giving rise to a painful restriction of movement of the hip, with a limp, may cause difficulty in diagnosis, but the condition subsides in a few days.

Hæmophilia with hæmarthrosis may also cause confusion, but a history of a tendency to bleed and the finding of a prolonged coagulation time will settle the diagnosis.

TREATMENT

For cases of bone and joint tuberculosis the treatment must be considered in terms of months and years rather than days and weeks. The basic principles of treatment are chemotherapy and complete rest, achieved by adequate immobilization of the affected area, until active tuberculosis has ceased. As it is possible that a stiff joint will be the end-result, the joint must be immobilized in the position of maximum function. Chemotherapy is with INH and PAS or streptomycin (*see also* p. 578). The treatment is best carried out in special hospitals where facilities exist for occupational therapy and the continuation of education.

Osteochondritis Juvenilis

ÆTIOLOGY AND PATHOLOGY

This conditions appears to be a degenerative type of lesion of unknown origin affecting various skeletal sites, including the head of the femur (*Perthes' disease*), the tibial tuberosity (*Osgood-Schlatter disease*), the os calcis (*Sever's disease*), the tarsal scaphoid (*Koehler's disease*), the metatarsal heads (*Freiberg's disease*), and the vertebral bodies (*Scheuermann's disease*). There is first an erosion and irregularity of the affected bone, which later becomes fragmented and radiologically shows increased density. As recovery occurs, reconstitution of bone takes place with a return to an almost normal radiological picture.

For the purposes of description only Perthes' disease (pseudo-coxalgia), the most frequently encountered, will be mentioned in detail.

CLINICAL PICTURE OF PERTHES' DISEASE

The disease occurs most often between five and nine years of age; it starts with a limp and later gives rise to a pain in the hip. This is in contrast to tuberculous disease of the hip, where pain is the first symptom and limp comes on afterwards. There is limitation of movement of abduction and rotation.

X-ray examination in early cases reveals flattening of the head of the femur (Plate XVII); later there is fragmentation of the head of the femur, and thickening of its neck. In late cases the x-ray appears almost normal again, but the head is inclined to be mushroom shaped.

The majority of cases recover completely, though some are subject to osteoarthritis in this hip-joint later. The degree of recovery depends largely upon the extent to which adequate immobilization is carried out in the early stages.

Differential diagnosis is from tuberculous disease of the hip, *see* p. 489.

Treatment. Adequate immobilization in the position of maximum rest is the vital factor in treatment as long as signs of activity persist. Later a caliper may be worn.

Syphilis of Bones and Joints

EARLY CHANGES : SYPHILITIC EPIPHYSITIS (PARROT'S DISEASE, SYPHILITIC PSEUDO-PARALYSIS)

This condition occurs in the first three or four months of life.

Pathology. The syphilitic infection is at the metaphysis, where softening and separation of the epiphysis may occur. It is common at the upper end of the humerus, tibia and around the elbow-joint, and is often symmetrical. Periostitis is frequently present also, and may be seen in the x-rays.

Clinical Picture. The affected limb is held perfectly still and is quite flaccid, but not painful.

The joint may be swollen.

Diagnosis. The diagnosis is made certain by the positive Wassermann reaction and the x-rays, showing the separated epiphysis, the " bitten out " portion of adjacent bone, and periostitis in the shaft or other bones. Erosion of the upper end of the tibia is sometimes called Wimberger's sign.

Prognosis and Treatment. This is as for congenital syphilis (*see* p. 567), and provided treatment is instituted early the outlook is excellent.

Syphilitic dactylitis occurs in the first two years of life. The swelling of the proximal phalanges is painless and symmetrical, and yields to anti-syphilitic treatment.

LATE CHANGES

Syphilitic changes in the skull and tibiæ and synovitis of the knees are present in a few cases of congenital syphilis.

Tibiæ. These may be sabre-shaped and thickened, and the x-ray shows osteitis.

Syphilitic Arthritis. This occurs in older children, over the age of six years. There is a bilateral painless effusion in the knees, due to a syphilitic synovitis (*Clutton's joints*), often accompanied by a keratitis (*see* p. 566). This yields rapidly to anti-syphilitic treatment.

BENIGN TUMOURS OF BONE

Multiple Exostoses (Diaphyseal Aclasia)

THIS is more common in males, and is inherited as a sex-linked condition. It is transmitted through the females.

The exostoses arise from bones that are formed in cartilage and particularly from the diaphysis near the epiphysis of the long bones,

system. In the latter case, the tumour metastases are frequently found in the skull and may cause proptosis. In cases of leukæmia deposits may occur in the bones and under the periosteum, causing considerable pain.

MISCELLANEOUS DISORDERS

Hæmophilic Joints

CHILDREN with hæmophilia fall and bruise their knees and elbows. Bleeding takes place, and the joint becomes distended with blood (hæmarthrosis) and painful. If this is repeated on several occasions, adhesions and ankylosis occur.

Felt-lined leather pads can be worn over the knees and elbows, and rough games should be avoided (*see also* p. 344).

Clubbing of the Fingers

Ætiology. This may be found in bronchiectasis and other chronic infective conditions of the lungs, such as empyema, and in congenital heart disease. It is also seen in subacute bacterial endocarditis, cirrhosis of the liver, cœliac disease, and ulcerative colitis.

Clubbing of the fingers appears to be related to the more extensive condition of hypertrophic osteo-arthropathy, in which changes are found in the bones of the hands and feet; sometimes these changes are extensive, involving all the long bones and the scapula and patella. In such cases a layer of new bone is formed beneath the periosteum extending for a variable distance along the shaft.

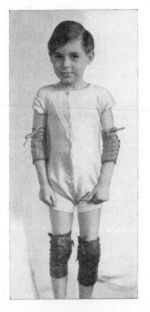

Fig. 69.—Use of pads in hæmophilia.

The cause of the condition is unknown, but appears to be related to an alteration in blood flow.

Clinical Picture. The clubbing appears gradually, and in congenital heart disease there is also swelling of the tip of the nose, and lobes of the ears.

In slight cases the nails of the fingers and toes appear to be " floating". There is a tendency for the nail to curve convexly in a longitudinal direction. The fingers may be said to be " bulbous," with filling in of the normal depression between the base of the nail

and the skin immediately proximal to the nail (Fig. 23, p. 257).   The
end of the finger is splayed out.   With the removal of the cause, the
fingers return to normal.

MECHANICAL DISTURBANCES

Congenital Dislocation of the Hip

SEVEN females are affected for each male, and the condition is bilateral
in 40 per cent. of cases.   A proportion of the cases are genetically
determined as a dominant characteristic.   Such inheritance is found
in Italy and in Jugoslavia.

The condition should be recognized at birth, but may not be noted
until the child begins to walk, at 12 to 14 months of age, when a
definite limp, with one hip higher than the other, is noted.

If the newborn infant is placed on the back, abduction and external
rotation of the hip are limited on the affected side; when the movement
of abduction of the hip is carried out passively, with the knee flexed, a
distinct click may be heard or felt (Ortolani's sign); this is produced
by the femoral head returning to the acetabular fossa in the reduced
position as abduction is completed.   In unilateral cases asymmetry of
the skin creases is often noted and there is disproportion in the length
of the legs.   In some cases the dislocated femoral head may be felt
posteriorly.   X-rays confirm the diagnosis.

In bilateral cases, overlooked in infancy, the child has a waddling
gait and shows marked lordosis.   Occasionally, cretinism and juvenile
myxœdema may be associated conditions.   Paralytic dislocation as
opposed to congenital dislocation may occur in cases of meningo-
myelocele and is also seen as a complication of spastic diplegia in
children with cerebral palsy.   In such instances, the adductor spasm
acting relatively unopposed against the weak voluntary power of the
other muscle groups is responsible for the dislocation.

The earlier the diagnosis is made, the easier will be the technical
problems of correction and the better the end result.   It is thus highly
desirable that the routine examination of all newborn infants should
include the simple clinical examination described above to exclude
the presence of this abnormality.   A patient in the authors' care,
who weighed 2 lb. 7 oz. when born, was diagnosed at birth as suffering
from a congenitally dislocated hip.   The orthopædic treatment had
been successfully completed by the time the infant went home from the
premature baby unit at the age of 10 weeks, when the weight was 6 lb.

Talipes Equino-varus (Club Feet)

The cause of this is unknown; associated congenital deformities
are not uncommon, whilst some cases are familial.   Treatment
should be commenced as soon after birth as possible, with manipula-
tions and splinting.

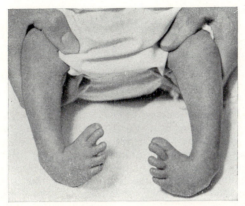

Fig. 70.—Talipes.

Flat-foot and Valgus Ankle

In overweight infants there is a tendency for the ankles to bend inward, and, if the muscles be soft, the feet are everted (valgus ankles). Such children should be given shoes with slight wedges on the inner side, say one-sixth of an inch, or valgus insoles with stiffening of the inner side of the shoe. Exercises designed to strengthen the muscles of the feet are helpful.

Knock-knee (Genu Valgum)

This is extremely common in childhood, and is probably a mechanical condition, due to an overweight child walking with weak (valgus) ankles. Rickets may, however, be a contributing factor. When such a child bears his weight on everted ankles, the weight causes knock-knee to develop as a secondary condition. Shoes with valgus wedges to soles and heels will aid the cure of both the valgus ankles and the knock-knee.

In severe cases, suitable night splints are a great help. In older children, renal rickets (*see* p. 375) should be borne in mind.

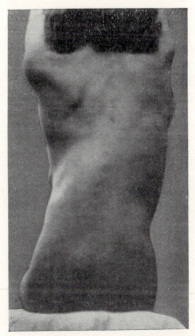

Fig. 71.—Spinal curvature in a girl with 14 ribs on the right side and 12 on the left,

Bow-leg (Genu Varum)

This is rare, and may be secondary to rickets or, when slight, it may be an inherited defect from one of the parents. Treatment is usually expectant; orthopædic measures may be necessary for the more severe cases.

Scoliosis (Lateral Deviation of the Spine)

This may be congenital or due to wedged vertebræ, or extra ribs (*see* Fig. 71). Poliomyelitis, torticollis, empyema and congenital short-leg are all causes of the acquired form. Many cases, however, have no apparent cause other than faulty posture from weakness of the spinal muscles. In such cases, before structural damage has occurred, the curve undoes itself when the child is suspended or bends the trunk.

Treatment. The results of orthopædic treatment for scoliosis have in the past been disappointing. Recent treatment with corrective plasters, which can be progressively modified to produce a steady correction of the scoliosis, combined with the use of a Milwaukee brace, and, at a later stage, spinal fusion operations seem to offer the best results.

Kyphosis and Lordosis (Antero-posterior Deviations of the Spine)

This is a less common condition. Spinal caries should be excluded by x-rays and tuberculin skin-tests. Marked round-shoulder may be seen in rapidly growing children, but is most marked in children with bilateral pulmonary emphysema, as in chronic asthmatics.

Intensive physiotherapy offers the best results in treatment.

CHAPTER 22

Diseases of the Skin

CONGENITAL DEFECTS OF THE SKIN

NÆVI (BIRTH MARKS)

THE term is applied not only to vascular nævi but also to congenital localized overgrowth of any of the elements of the skin.

In the past, insufficient attention has been given to the natural tendency of many forms of vascular nævi to disappear spontaneously, with the result that much unnecessary treatment has been undertaken and many children have been left with permanent scars as a result of that treatment. When a vascular nævus disappears spontaneously no mark remains on the skin. This applies particularly to cavernous hæmangioma (strawberry nævi), but not to capillary nævi (port-wine stain).

Capillary Nævi (Port-wine Mark)

These appear as a flat purple stain on the skin, usually the face. The birth mark grows in proportion to the size of the child. In the past, treatment has been unsatisfactory, the mark often being made more unsightly than before, but skin grafting in well-selected cases gives good cosmetic results.

Nævus Flammeus

At birth there may be a pink discoloration of the skin of the nape of the neck or of the forehead or upper eyelids. Such marks usually disappear spontaneously during the first year of life.

Cavernous Hæmangioma (Strawberry Mark)

At birth a small red or bluish patch may be present in the skin. This increases in size for a time and then gradually disappears in most cases. A spontaneous resolution of this kind is clearly preferable to any form of active treatment, which, however skilfully applied, is likely to leave a scar. The parents should be reassured and the reason for withholding treatment given. Whilst such a nævus is still enlarging, the child should be seen from time to time.

Some cavernous hæmangioma extend beneath the skin, or mucous membranes may be involved. Thrombosis is an occasional com-

plication and ulceration may occur. There is a high rate of spontaneous cure and no treatment is usually necessary. When treatment
is required sclerosing injections can be used.

Stellate Nævi (Spider Nævi)

A solitary spider nævus occurring on the face may, for cosmetic
reasons, be treated with electro-cautery. Multiple spider nævi are
seen in patients with hepatic cirrhosis.

Lymphangiomata

These are present from birth, or shortly after birth, and are often
found in the neck, or along the trunk, upper limbs, or occasionally on
the tongue. They appear as greyish translucent vesicles, capillary
lymphangiomata, or as soft, translucent swellings, cavernous lymphangiomata. Treatment, where necessary, is surgical.

Moles or Pigmented Nævi and Hairy Nævi

These may occur on almost any part of the body, and may be
single or multiple. Excision is the treatment, if any is desired.

Hereditary Telangiectasia (Osler-Weber-Rendu Syndrome)

This is inherited as a dominant genetic characteristic and is expressed
by the presence of aggregations of innumerable small blood vessels
visible through the skin and mucous membranes. They appear
during childhood and later increase in number. Small repeated
hæmorrhages occur from the skin, mucous membrane lesions or renal
tract. Hepatic cirrhosis may occur in this syndrome.

Ichthyosis

This is a congenital and often hereditary dryness and roughness of
the skin accompanied by undue scaliness. It is often but by no means
always found in allergic subjects. Pathologically there is a deficiency
of sweat and of sebaceous glands, and a thickening of the horny layer.

The clinical picture may be merely a dry skin (xeroderma), except
in the flexor areas, where the skin is smooth. The palms show an
exaggeration of the natural creases and lines. Chapping and roughness is common. The condition may be so severe that the body is
covered with scales, and the term " crocodile hide " has been used.
The condition persists throughout life. The skin may be kept soft
with a preparation such as unguentum aquosum.[1]

Collodion Skin of the Newborn

In this condition, the infant is born with a smooth yellowish covering
which is likened to parchment, oiled skin, varnish or collodion. This
covering interferes with facial movement and may cause difficulty in

[1] A water-in-oil emulsion of 50 per cent. w/w of water and wool alcohols ointment (wool alcohols
6 per cent., with hard paraffin, soft paraffin and liquid paraffin).

sucking or in either opening or closing the eyes. After a few days, cracks appear and the covering desquamates leaving a beefy red skin which may bleed a little.

Collodion skin may be due to a persistence of the epitrichium which normally desquamates by the 6th month of fœtal life. If so, the underlying skin will be quite normal by the age of a year. Alternatively, it may be due to ichthyosis (ichthyosiform erythrodermia, *see* below). Then the skin will never be normal and there is the risk of death in early infancy. Unfortunately, it is impossible to distinguish these two types at birth.

Treatment consists of protecting the eyes from infection and applying warm sterile oil to the skin.

Ichthyosiform Erythrodermia (Brock's Disease)

Infants with this disease are born with no superficial layers to their skin. Their bodies appear red and raw with thin bullous cysts in some areas. The disease may be mistaken for an acute infective illness such as pemphigus neonatorum (Ritter's Disease). If the infant survives more than a few days a more adequate skin covering develops, although constant desquamation occurs and some raw areas remain. Skin biopsy shows a vacuolation of the prickle layer of the skin from which the more superficial skin layers strip away extremely rapidly. The disease can be distinguished from epidermolysis bullosa by the normality of the nails. Few cases survive infancy.

Albinism

Total albinism is a complete failure of melanin formation due to absence of tyrosinase in melanocytes, caused by an autosomal recessive. There is a virtual absence of skin, hair and uveal pigment; it is often associated with mental impairment. Nystagmus and photophobia occur.

Partial albinism exists in several varieties (for example, white forelocks, piebald, etc.), transmitted as mendelian dominants; not associated with mental impairment.

Ehlers-Danlos Syndrome

Individuals with this disease have an inherent abnormality of collagen which permits excessive mobility of joints and causes a remarkable elasticity and fragility of the skin. Curious scars appear on the body where the skin has been stretched. The blood vessels are unusually fragile, again as the result of the abnormal collagen in the vessel wall, and hæmorrhages are likely to occur.

Congenital Ectodermal Dysplasia

In this inherited disorder (autosomal dominant), there may be a partial or complete failure of development of the nails, hair and teeth. In addition the facial bones are poorly formed with underdevelopment of the jaws and a flattened nasal bridge.

Epidermolysis Bullosa

There are two forms of this disease.   The *severe type* is inherited as a dominant characteristic.   Widespread bullæ appear on the skin in infancy, either spontaneously or in response to the slightest pressure, and may become hæmorrhagic.   The mucous membranes are also involved.   In the few individuals who survive infancy, permanent scarring, contractures and crippling deformities develop.

The *mild type* is recessively inherited, the bullæ healing without scarring.   The nails are frequently involved and are usually lost in the first years of life.   The mucous membranes, particularly of the con-junctivæ and the anal margin, are liable to recurrent ulceration.

Incontinentia Pigmenti (Block-Sulzberger Disease)

Vesicles appear on the skin soon after birth and later shrink to form grey or brown warty macules or papules.   It is seen more commonly in girls than boys and may be associated with congenital malforma-tions of the eyes, teeth and hair.

Mast-cell Disease[1]

Mast cells are found in many normal tissues, particularly in loose connective tissue, synovial membrane, gastro-intestinal submucosa, bladder wall, lymph nodes and dermal layer of the skin.   They are irregularly shaped, pleomorphic cells not easily identified in sections without special staining methods; they have a pale cytoplasm packed with large granules arranged about a round or oval nucleus.   Although the physiological function of mast cells is not understood, it is agreed that the granules contain histamine and heparin, perhaps loosely bonded, and on stimulation mast cells release histamine and heparin locally with effects on surrounding tissues.   In *mast-cell disease*, focal or diffuse mast-cell infiltrations occur in certain tissues, the skin being the most commonly affected.

For tissue biopsy to reveal the nature of the disease, it is necessary to overcome the considerable technical difficulties of identifying mast cells in sections.   The response of the skin to stroking or trauma provides a useful clinical aid because it results in whealing of the skin with sparing of the intervening areas.

URTICARIA PIGMENTOSA: CUTANEOUS MAST-CELL DISEASE

This, the commonest type of mast-cell disease, was described in 1869[2] as a disorder of the skin characterized by urticaria following slight skin trauma and leading to pigmentation.   Although it may begin at any age, it usually appears in infancy with successive crops of urticarial or bullous lesions which end as pigmented macules or

---

[1] Stutzman, L., Urbach, F. (1961).   Mast-cell disease.   *Pediat. Clin. N. Amer.*, **8**, No. 3, 857.
[2] Nettleship, E. (1869).   Rare forms of urticaria.   *Brit. med. J.*, 2, 323.

papules. The diagnosis is difficult at the onset because the disease is rare and the initial attacks are easily mistaken for the more usual types of urticaria. Recurring crops of urticarial spots and persisting pigmented macules or papules should suggest urticaria pigmentosa.

TREATMENT

There is no useful treatment except the avoidance of scratching and other minor skin trauma. The value of cortisone analogues has not been worked out. Oral administration of antihistamine drugs does not prevent urtication and may not even relieve itching. Heparin antagonists are ineffective. But the prognosis in children is favourable with an expectation of spontaneous involution of the lesions by puberty, unless there is also systemic involvement.

POLYSYSTEMIC MAST-CELL DISEASE

This type is less common than cutaneous urticaria pigmentosa. It causes involvement of bone[1] and other systems as well as the skin. The manifestations are variable, the salient features being hepato-splenomegaly, lymphadenopathy, rarefaction and sclerosis of ribs or other bones (lacework appearance) and the skin changes of urticaria pigmentosa. Pruritis occurs, especially in areas of skin exposed to trauma (collar, belt, etc.). There may be changes in the peripheral blood[2] and leukæmia occasionally develops.

SOLITARY MASTOCYTOMA

A single cutaneous nodule may occur without other lesions. The nodule may be some centimetres in diameter and topped with vesicles containing mast cells. It generally resolves slowly.

REACTIONS DUE TO PHYSICAL CAUSES

Napkin Eruptions

EXCORIATION of the buttocks may be due to:

(a) *Simple Intertrigo.* This condition may arise when a child is left for long periods in a wet napkin; it may be aggravated by rubber pants, which poultice the buttocks with warm urine and fæces. The folds of the skin are chiefly affected and are pink and moist and may become secondarily infected. The essential treatment of this condition is to *leave the buttocks exposed* thus keeping the skin dry; the affected area is kept well powdered and, if a secondary infection is present, a simple lotion, such as benzalkonium chloride (Roccal) is used.

(b) *Acid Stools.* An excess of fat or sugar in the diet will tend to produce acid stools. These are acrid or bubbly, and however frequently the baby is changed there is a tendency for the buttocks to be

[1] Lees, M. H., Stroud, C. E. (1959). Bone lesions of urticaria pigmentosa in childhood. *Arch. Dis. Childh.*, **34**, 205.
[2] Stutzman, L., Urbach, F. (1961). Mast-cell disease. *Pediat. Clin. N. Amer.*, **8**, No. 3, 857.

burned. Regulation of the diet is necessary together with local applications of zinc and castor oil ointment or benzalkonium chloride. If the skin remains moist, it can be toughened and made less sore by the application of 2 per cent. tannic acid in soft paraffin.

(*c*) *Ammonia Dermatitis.* Some infants smell strongly of ammonia, especially when changed in the morning. The thighs and the buttocks are reddened, and may actually receive a slight burn if the condition persists. This effect is commonly due to bacteria derived from the large bowel, such as *B. ammoniagenes*, which in an alkaline medium liberate ammonia from the urea contained in the urine retained in the wet napkins, setting up a local ammonia dermatitis. *Preventive* treatment consists in changing the napkins frequently, together with the addition of bicarbonate of soda one drachm to each pint of water in which they are rinsed after washing. This prevents bacterial decomposition and formation of ammonia. Meatal ulcers can be smeared with soft paraffin; they heal with the dermatitis.

Chilblains (Erythema pernio)

Chilblains manifest themselves by localized swellings, redness and tenderness of some or all of the extremities. These swellings are irritating, and itch, and they may form vesicles and ulcerate or break open. They should be regarded as a minor form of frostbite. The individuals affected have a poor natural circulation, and cold weather intensifies the condition. Usually, the hands and feet are warmed too suddenly by being plunged into very warm water, or toasted before a hot fire.

TREATMENT

The extremities should be protected from chill by warm socks and gloves. In cold weather two pairs of gloves and thick socks together with fleece-lined boots should be worn. Sudden changes from cold to warm should be avoided and very hot baths and hot-water bottles should be forbidden. Measures should be taken to improve the circulation; nicotinic acid may be helpful, as Pernivit (B.D.H.) 25 mg. daily. Where the skin is broken, a nicotinic acid ester in a water-miscible base may be used. Trafuril cream (Ciba) is a satisfactory application.

INFANTILE ECZEMA

BOTH allergy and trauma play a part in the ætiology of this condition. It is well known that a large proportion of children with eczema afterwards develop asthma, hay-fever or migraine. There is often a familial history of allergic disorders. Specific sensitivities, particularly to lactalbumin, casein, egg-white, egg-yolk, cereals, fruit juices or other foods have all been blamed as the causative factor in infantile eczema. Very occasionally, removal of one of these dietary constituents brings about clinical improvement. More often no change is found.   Rare cases show a marked sensitivity to cows' milk, which has then, in all its forms, to be rigorously excluded from the diet.

Abrasions and friction of the skin causing a local inflammation frequently precede eczema, or the skin may become sensitive to wool or soap.   In some cases, the condition is maintained by a low-grade secondary infection, coupled with constant rubbing and scratching.

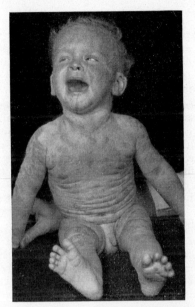

Fig. 72.—Infantile eczema in a child of 11 months.

CLINICAL PICTURE

The age of onset is commonly between six months and two years (the dentitional period), but eczema may commence when the infant is only a month or two old.   There are two common clinical varieties, of which the more frequent is that in which the lesions appear on the cheeks, forehead and scalp and subsequently affects other parts. This merges into the second variety or flexural type (Besnier's prurigo), frequently associated with asthma; here the lesions mostly affect the flexures, especially the bends of the elbows and behind the knees.

In both cases the essential lesions are a characteristic group of vesico-papules.   The child rubs or scratches these, causing them to burst and weep.   This is followed by the formation of a crust.   In Besnier's prurigo intense irritation may occur before the skin lesions, which are often produced by scratching, become visible.

When eczema is extensive, the infant is much upset and may be reduced to a pitiful state. In severe cases there is constant rolling of the head, and a wriggling movement of the body, feet and hands in an effort to get relief from the irritation. If the hands are free, the child tears at the face and body. Diarrhœa may occur, associated with transient improvement in the eczema. Infections of all sorts are easily acquired, and badly borne, by these infants.

TREATMENT

It should be explained to the mother at the start that this condition is not infectious, and is not due to neglect on her part. The greatest care should be taken that the eczema is not treated so strenuously that the regular gain is impeded or the general health neglected. The child must come first and the eczema second.

Prevention of Scratching. This is the most important principle in treatment, and once it is achieved considerable improvement in the condition may confidently be expected. Adequate sedation (*see* below) remains the prime method of relieving pruritus and thus reducing the otherwise uncontrollable desire to scratch. Secondly, some form of splintage for the arms and often the legs, together with securely fastened cotton gloves or mittens, is needed in severe cases.

The clothing should be light and the infant kept as cool as possible in hot weather. Wool should not be allowed next to the skin and dressings should be made of thin linen or cotton.

Local Applications. If the face is affected and if it is the dry type of eczema, the lesions will respond best to a simple cream or ointment. If, on the other hand, it tends to weep or is already moist, a soothing lotion is usually better as it will help to dry up the exudate and prevent secondary infection, for example:

> Liq. picis carb. 1 ml. (15 minims)
> Calamine lotion to 30 ml. (1 oz.).

Occasionally tar is not tolerated, and then 2 per cent. of ichthammol may be used instead.

During an acute exudative stage, the application of one or, in resistant cases, two per cent. hydrocortisone ointment may improve the condition in a dramatic way.

Cleansing the Skin. Soap and water should not be used on an eczematous skin, which is best cleansed with emulsifying ointment (B.P.).

Diet. It is most exceptional to find any true milk allergy, although it is claimed that the use of Velactim (*see* p. 514) has occasionally improved matters. Alternatively, cows' milk may be treated in the following way: boil cows' milk for one minute, then remove the skin from the top. Now add 1½ drops of dilute hydrochloric acid (B.P.) for each ounce of cows' milk. Add the hydrochloric acid just before using the milk, to prevent curdling. Children may very occasionally be sensitive to egg, either the yolk or the white, or indeed to any other article of diet. The offending allergen, when discovered, should be excluded entirely. There should be no delay in getting the child on to a good mixed weaning diet (p. 40).

Sedatives. These are essential. Sodium amytal or phenobarbitone, syrup of chloral, promethazine or hydroxyzine hydrochloride (Atarax) may all be used (for dosages, *see* p. 665). Infants and small children quickly become tolerant of the original dosage which usually has to be increased after an interval. A good method is to try to anticipate such tolerance by changing the form of sedation every three to four weeks.

General directions for the mother are:

1. Eczema should be looked upon as an inherited, sensitive skin and not a disease. It is not a sign of neglect or mismanagement on the part of the mother or nurse, and the mother can be reassured that it will become less troublesome by the age of three years, although a number of the children may continue to show less severe eczema until about the age of puberty. It is not infectious.

2. Warmth will invariably bring out and aggravate the eczema. Keep as cool as possible and tend to underclothe the infant.

3. The infant should have silk or cotton material next to the skin; wool is not allowed to touch the skin.

4. Where the eczema is dry let it remain dry. Where it is broken or weeping use a cream or lotion, and keep bandaged as far as possible to prevent scratching. Keep the child's finger nails clipped short.

5. The infant should not be allowed to scratch. To prevent this, light cardboard splints can be applied to the arms, so as to prevent the infant from reaching the face. Securely fastened cotton gloves are essential.

6. Avoid soap and water on the skin; emulsifying ointment should be used for cleaning the skin.

7. See that the child has a sleeping draught at night. Keep the doctor informed of its effectiveness so that he may change the prescription if the skin irritation is not allayed.

8. Do not have the baby vaccinated when eczema is present on account of the danger of generalized vaccinia (*see* p. 516).

PROGNOSIS

The mother of a child with eczema may be assured that scars will not be left from patches of eczema; in fact the skin remains singularly clear and soft afterwards. Many cases of eczema improve by the age of three or four years. Even if the eczema remains somewhat longer it is much easier to deal with in an older child.

Seborrhœa and Seborrhœic Dermatitis

In infants, scurf tends to form down the centre of the scalp, especially over the anterior fontanelle. In simple cases, the scalp should be anointed with oil and subsequently shampooed with water containing bicarbonate of soda. In resistant cases, half per cent. salicylic acid in petroleum jelly should be applied before the shampoo. The daily use of a fine tooth comb will facilitate removal of crusts.

In older children, " dandruff " and scaliness of the skin of the scalp may be seen. Exudative lesions with crust formation may occur, together with a tendency to a generalized dermatitis over the whole body.

Soap and water cleansing is permissible and then a lotion (2 per cent. precipitated sulphur in calamine lotion) or a cream (such as 10 per cent. ichthammol) can be applied.

PARASITIC ERUPTIONS

Scabies

THE infection is caused by the female acarus which burrows into the skin and causes a bleb-like eruption. The eruption is seen on the hands and feet, most commonly between the fingers and toes, and on the ulnar surface of the palms of the hands and soles of the feet; also on the palms and soles themselves. The burrows are also found in the folds behind the knees, in the groins, beneath the arms, and on the buttocks. There is frequent itching, and, as a result, the bleb is torn open, leaving a tiny abrasion. The irritation is greatest during the night or when the child is warm. Infections from the skin are apt to be superimposed on these burrows, masking the true state of affairs; for instance, impetigo commonly accompanies scabies. Scabies is seldom seen on the face. The disease resembling it most closely is lichen urticatus or urticaria papulosa. This latter condition is seldom seen between the fingers and toes, however, and is often found scattered over the trunk, especially in the loin.

TREATMENT

Scabies is effectively treated by benzyl benzoate in the form of:

Application of Benzyl Benzoate B.P.C.
Contains benzyl benzoate 25 per cent. w/v with emulsifying wax, and water.

This should be applied after thorough washing with soap and water all over the body. The application is repeated next day. The treatment should be carried out as soon as the diagnosis of scabies is suspected, and irrespective of whether any secondary infection, such as impetigo, is present or not. When one member of a family is found to be infected, the rest of the family should be regarded with suspicion and treated if possible.

Pediculosis Capitis

This condition was at one time very common but is now much less so, owing to the fashion of keeping girls' hair short. " Nits " are easily distinguished from scurf or dandruff, which is not fastened to the hair. Infestation leads to scratching, and erythematous rashes may be present over the neck and forehead, or there may actually be ulceration of the scalp. Pediculosis capitis may be accompanied by impetigo of the scalp with large crusted areas. The glands of the scalp and neck draining the infected area are often enlarged.

Lethane hair oil or oil of sassafras is the treatment of choice, but the application of any simple oil, followed by shampooing with carbolic soap and combing, should control the infection. DDT powder is an effective louse removing agent for potentially infected clothing.

Ringworm

TINEA CORPORIS (RINGWORM OF THE BODY: TINEA CIRCINATA)

This is often communicated from one child to another, or by a cat or dog. It does not spread to the scalp or nails. Small areas with a raised edge, aptly described by the name *tinea circinata*, form on the forehead, chest, back, arms and legs and spread rapidly. The diagnosis is best made by the microscopic examination of scales of epidermis for the mycelium.

The application of an antiseptic ointment, such as Merthiolate cream or Whitfield's ointment (salicylic acid 3 per cent., benzoic acid 6 per cent., emulsifying ointment 91 per cent.), is standard treatment. Rubbing the area with silver nitrate, 2 per cent., followed by tincture of iodine, thus forming silver iodide, is successful. The introduction of griseofulvin (*see* p. 508) as a systemic treatment makes the cure much more certain and rapid.

TINEA CRURIS (SCHOOLBOYS' ITCH: DHOBIE ITCH)

This may be recognized by a circinate eruption with a slight, definitely scaly edge, affecting the groin, thigh or axillæ. The eruption is also common on the feet (tinea pedis). The application of 1 per cent. gentian violet, dilute tincture of iodine, or Merthiolate cream, avoiding the scrotum, is effective treatment.

For tinea pedis, soaking the feet in a solution of potassium permanganate (1 in 8,000) is extremely useful or Castellani's paint may be applied.

TINEA CAPITIS (RINGWORM OF THE SCALP: TINEA TONSURANS)

This is sometimes seen in children in poor home conditions; it is transferred from child to child by hair-brushes, combs or caps. In small or large areas most of the hairs are broken short. Gradually, the whole scalp becomes involved, and the denuded areas may be scaly or crusted.

Wood's glass filter and an ultra-violet light will reveal a microsporon infection of the scalp with great ease, the affected hairs showing butterfly-wing fluorescence.

Hair which is affected is shaved and a three week course of griseo-fulvin is given (for dosage, *see* below).

TINEA UNGUUM (RINGWORM OF THE NAILS)

In this manifestation of ringworm the nails are wrinkled, pitted and discoloured. Removal of the nails used to be the surest way of curing the condition, for otherwise the infection persisted for months or years.

Griseofulvin has recently been introduced as a most effective fungi-static for this type of infection. The daily dosage is 0·25–0·5 G. until all the abnormal nail has been shed.

MICROBIC INFECTIONS

Impetigo Contagiosa

THIS is due to a streptococcal or staphylococcal infection of the skin; the lesions are various, and may appear as simple scabby sores placed on an inflamed base, circinate and imitating ringworm, or dry and scaly, like seborrhœic dermatitis or early ulcerative dermatitis. Bullous impetigo is seen in younger children and may require differen-tiation from the Stevens-Johnson syndrome (p. 513). In general, impetigo tends to appear on the face or in the skin folds or behind the ears. Once established, the infection may spread to other parts of the body, particularly in households where hygiene is poor.

Local applications of antibiotics, such as neomycin, tetracycline, or chloramphenicol, have largely replaced the older remedies which relied upon antiseptics, such as 1 per cent. aqueous gentian violet or 1/1,000 acriflavine solution. Chlorhexidene, either as a 1 in 2,000 solution or in the form of a dusting powder, is of value for skin infections in infancy. Where persistent nasal infection is found, a combination of 0·1 per cent. chlorhexidine and 0·5 per cent. neomycin (Naseptin Cream) is often effective.

A course of systemic penicillin (for dosage, *see* Appendix 1) or other appropriate antibiotic is a great help when the infection is widespread and the sensitivity of the infecting organism is known. Penicillin cream should never be applied locally, but one per cent. aureomycin or neomycin ointment is of great value. For the rapid clearance of small infected skin lesions Dequadin cream with one per cent. hydro-cortisone is often very effective.

Pemphigus

In the newborn infant, a widespread bullous eruption which may rapidly progress to a fatal conclusion has in the past been labelled as pemphigus neonatorum. It seems probable that the majority of these cases are examples of acute *Staph. pyogenes* infection giving rise to bullous impetigo and staphylococcal septicæmia. Intensive treatment with an antibiotic to which the organism is sensitive is given, and systemic steroid therapy (for dosage, *see* Appendix 2) must be added immediately if toxæmia has led to peripheral circulatory failure. Ritter's disease is probably the same condition under another name (Fig. 7, p. 106).

Furunculosis (Boils)

This disease is usually due to the *Staph. pyogenes*, the infection being in or round a hair follicle. The lesions may take the form of very fine pustules or even of indurated boils. Common sites are the buttocks, the perineum, under the arms, the back of the neck, or the chin. Boils are especially common in children who wet the bed and in school-children who get an insufficient number of baths. The urine should always be investigated for possible glycosuria in cases of recurrent boils.

For the prevention of recurrent boils on the napkin area, treatment for enuresis should be instituted in older children, and the treatment for napkin dermatitis (described on p. 501) for infants. At the very earliest sign of a boil, it should be covered with an adhesive plaster dressing. Hexachlorophane soap can be used for prevention.

For any severe staphylococcal skin infection, particularly in the newborn, the organism should be cultured in the laboratory and its sensitivity to the antibiotics noted. Then, if the infection is producing any general reaction or suspicion of septicæmia, the appropriate antibiotic, usually either penicillin or tetracycline (for dosage, *see* p. 656), should be given. Where the clinical condition warrants it, a broad-spectrum antibiotic should be started without waiting for the sensitivity report from the laboratory. Penicillin should never be applied locally to the skin, as in this way a tendency to the production of drug-resistant organisms is encouraged.

Erysipelas

Erysipelas may start from some trivial abrasion or, on the other hand, it may occasionally follow circumcision, or be found in the skin surrounding the navel, or after opening some superficial abscess of the scalp or face. The organism is, as a rule, the hæmolytic streptococcus. The skin round the site of infection becomes firm, indurated and dark red, and there is a very definite edge to the indurated area. It spreads rapidly and may involve the whole of a limb, or the head and neck. The temperature is high, the tongue dry and furred, and vomiting and diarrhœa are common.

A course of sulphonamide or systemic penicillin effectively controls such an infection.

Warts (Verrucæ)

Warts are contagious, and have been shown to be due to a filter-passing virus.

Electric cauterization is most effective treatment. Glacial acetic acid with 1 per cent perchloride of mercury, applied with a match stick, or 10 per cent. salicylic acid in collodion may be used.

PLANTAR WARTS

Plantar warts, most commonly affecting children of school age, are thought to be acquired through using swimming baths, common changing rooms or the same bath mat as an infected child. They form on the soles of the feet or on the heels. They are vascular and tender on pressure; this helps to distinguish them from corns which are hard and avascular.

Under general or local anæsthetic, warts may be dissected out completely, or curetted, with subsequent cauterization of the base with pure phenol. Superficial x-ray therapy has also been used as has carbon dioxide snow.

Molluscum Contagiosum

This is also a virus infection and may be acquired at public baths. The papules are small pearly-white tumours, usually umbilicated, and may appear anywhere on the body.

Curettage and cauterization of the cavity is the best treatment, but when the lesions are small, erythema doses of ultra-violet light may be effective.

Lupus Vulgaris (Tuberculosis of the Skin)

Lupus is comparatively rare in children. It usually appears on the cheeks and nose and may be due to direct infection from phthisical parents kissing their children, but also arises from a glandular infection, particularly when tuberculous abscesses, or glands in the softened stage, have been incised. It may appear in any part of the body. At first there is a small tuberculous nodule; this gives rise to an indurated patch which under slight pressure from a glass slide takes on the appearance of apple jelly. The lesion is often a chronic one and full investigation for other tuberculous lesions should be undertaken.

General treatment for tuberculosis is often necessary. The local lesion is best treated by INH powder.

Herpes Zoster (Shingles)

This is due to an infection of the posterior root ganglia by an ultramicroscopic virus. It is interesting to note the connection between chickenpox and herpes. Very often after an adult case of herpes a case of chickenpox follows in the household, or vice versa.

It is now practically certain that the viruses of herpes zoster and varicella are related.

The eruption consists of a group of vesicles on an inflamed base and is distributed along the sensory fibres of a posterior nerve root. The chest, abdomen, thighs, neck or forehead may be involved. An erythematous rash appears first, and becomes vesicular, the vesicles containing clear fluid. Later, crusts dry up and fall off, this stage being accompanied by a slight fever and some malaise, and occasionally by neuralgic pains. Scarring does not occur if the scabs are left alone. Herpes of the fifth nerve may be accompanied by corneal ulcer and iritis, in which event great damage to the eye occasionally results.

Lumbar puncture shows lymphocytosis of the cerebrospinal fluid, and the posterior root ganglia on section show inflammation and hæmorrhage.

Friction and scratching should be prevented, and the lesion should be kept dry with 2 per cent. phenol in calamine lotion. Painting with collodion is also useful. Aspirin may be given at bedtime if the child is restless.

Herpes Simplex

The commonest manifestation of infection with this virus is shown as a crop of small vesicles, usually appearing about the mouth or nose, as an accompaniment of the common cold. Other sites are the cheeks, ears, neck or fingers. It may accompany pneumonia, meningococcal meningitis, tonsillitis or intestinal upsets. The crusts dry up in a few days and fall off. It tends to recur at the same site. The virus can be isolated on culture.

There is no preventive treatment, but when the herpetic spots occur they can be covered with cetrimide cream or dusted with one per cent. chlorhexidene in talc powder.

Other manifestations of herpes simplex infection include ulcerative stomatitis (p. 188), and the very rare generalized infections of the newborn where hepatitis or encephalitis may sometimes have fatal results. In infants already subject to infantile eczema, herpes simplex infection of the skin may give rise to a generalized vesicular reaction (Kaposi's varicelliform eruption, see p. 516).

Cutaneous Signs of Congenital Syphilis

Very rarely a syphilitic infant is born with a bullous rash on the palms of the hands and soles of the feet; more usually between the fourth and eighth weeks a rash appears on the buttocks. The skin appears glazed, and has a peculiar copper-coloured hue. The rash tends to spread down the legs and up on to the abdomen, and may become widespread and extend to the face and trunk. The palms of the hands and soles of the feet may have a shiny, glazed appearance. Condylomata appear about the anus and vulva at the same time.

The cutaneous manifestations of congenital syphilis are likely to be associated with other lesions of congenital syphilis (*see* p. 564).

TOXIC ERUPTIONS—ERYTHEMATA

THESE are rashes due to some toxin circulating in the blood, either a product of defective metabolism, or a food or drug poison, or the result of microbic infection:

1. The rashes of acute infectious fevers, such as scarlet fever, measles, German measles. These are dealt with in Chapter 24.
2. Morbilliform and scarlatiniform rashes due to food allergy or associated with infections other than the specific fevers.
3. Erythema nodosum.
4. Erythema multiforme.
5. Vaccination rashes.
6. Certain drug rashes.

Erythema Nodosum

Erythema nodosum is a symptom complex, and not a disease in itself. It occurs at all ages, but is seldom seen before the age of one year.

Large red blotches or nodes appear on the front of the shins, especially on the inner surface over the tibiæ, and also, but less frequently, on

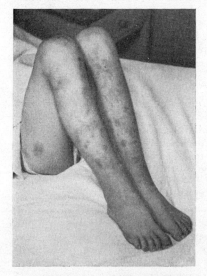

the thighs, extensor surfaces of the forearms and the malar regions. They are tender on pressure but otherwise do not give rise to pain. At the same time the temperature is raised and the child shows lassitude and a poor appetite. The fever may last for two or three weeks, but the rash ceases in about 10 days or less, on the average.

A proportion of cases are due to a tuberculous sensitization as shown by a strongly positive tuberculin reaction (*see* p. 573); in others, the streptococcus is the sensitizing agent, and more rarely the meningococcus. The administration of sulphathiazole has also given rise to the condition. In America, coccidioidomycosis (San Joaquin fever) has produced a similar eruption, and other possible causes include histoplasmosis and sarcoidosis.

Fig. 73.—Erythema nodosum resulting from a streptococcal tonsillitis in a boy aged 9 years. The lesions are seen on the shins and there is one on the right thigh.

In every case a very dilute Mantoux tuberculin test, say one in ten thousand, should be done, and, if positive, a search should be made by x-rays for the infecting focus. In other cases the appropriate treatment for the underlying cause is begun. In cases due to tuberculosis sulphathiazole may cause a recrudescence of erythema nodosum.

Erythema Multiforme

This erythematous eruption is characterized by symmetrical distribution on the limbs and face, and by the exudative nature of the erythema. The cause is unknown.

The lesion appears on the backs of the hands and forearms, sides of the face and neck, and on the legs. There are disc-like dark-red erythematous patches, usually somewhat raised. There may be vesicles or bullæ at their summits. The central portion may fade, producing a ring-like appearance resembling a pupil and iris. This variety—erythema iris—is very liable to frequent relapse.

The condition lasts from a few days to a week, and then fades, but it may recur over and over again. A rise of temperature is observed at each eruption, and the eruption may appear in the mouth.

STEVENS-JOHNSON SYNDROME

In this condition there is an acute reaction both of the skin and mucous membranes. In a matter of hours, large vesicles appear on the skin sometimes involving the greater part of the body. The remaining skin on the trunk may become friable and easily separated from the deeper layers of the dermis by gentle pressure with the finger (Nicolski's sign). At the same time the mucous membranes of the conjunctivæ, buccal mucosa, tongue, penile meatus, vulva and anal margin may become hyperæmic and may ulcerate. A distressing stomatitis may develop.

The cause of this syndrome is unknown. It may be a viral infection or possibly an auto-immune reaction to a foreign substance. Once established, secondary infection with resulting severe toxæmia may cause death within a few days.

Such patients must be carefully isolated and nursed by a meticulous aseptic technique. Steroids (Appendix 2) should be given in full dosage together with a broad-spectrum antibiotic as a prophylactic against infection. The child is best nursed naked in a warmed cubicle. The skin should be sprayed with Polybactrin, after which a sterile dusting powder should be applied. Treated in this way, the patient should be restored to normal health in two to three weeks, and the mortality should be negligible.

Papular Urticaria (Lichen Urticatus, Heat-spots, Nettle-rash, Hives)

There is little doubt that, in the past, children exposed to repeated insect bites or bed-bugs have been incorrectly diagnosed as suffering from papular urticaria.   Many such children come from homes where hygienic standards are poor and in these particularly the diagnosis of true papular urticaria should be treated with considerable suspicion. The lesions usually diagnosed as papular urticaria consist of pink papules, sometimes showing vesicle formation, occurring mainly on the limbs and lower part of the trunk.   There is intense pruritus.

It is thought that the bites of parasites, e.g. cat-fleas, bird-fleas and dog-fleas, in specifically sensitive children is the usual cause.

It seems very doubtful whether food allergy ever plays a part in their origin since the most drastic restriction of possible dietary causes is seldom effective.   In general terms a soothing lotion, such as one per cent. Benadryl in calamine lotion, should be applied to the skin. Household pets should be cleansed with DDT powder and the possibility of bed-bugs remembered.

True *urticaria* is sometimes seen in the child, as in the adult, in response to well defined food allergies such as shell fish or fruits such as strawberries or plums.   The lesion produced may be a generalized swelling of the face or hands with a blotchy erythema extending on to the trunk.   Occasionally no obvious cause is found for such urticarial eruptions.

Where a true food allergy exists it is best to exclude this substance from the diet.   In the attack ephedrine, a quarter of a grain twice a day, or one of the antihistamine drugs, such as Anthisan, 25 mg. twice daily, may be tried for a child of three years.   Calamine lotion containing 1 per cent. Benadryl is a useful local application to the affected part, relieving the irritation.   A sedative such as phenobarbitone may be necessary.

Milk Allergy

There is a rare but well-defined group of infants who show a true allergy to cows' milk.   In such an infant within a few minutes of the taking of the first feed of cows' milk one of two things may happen. Either the infant develops an urticarial swelling of the face and limbs, with an associated erythema, or in the more severe form may become ashen pale and shocked so that death appears imminent.   Recovery occurs in about fifteen to thirty minutes.   The symptoms recur each time cows' milk is given.   In the more severe type the infant's life is clearly endangered and experimentation with further feeds must not be permitted.

Treatment must provide for an adequate diet free of cows' milk and later a carefully controlled desensitization regime.   Substitutes for cows' milk include stored human milk, goats' milk or Velactim (Wander).

In the subsequent desensitization against cows' milk, minute quantities of the order of one ml. of a 1 in 1,000 solution of cows' milk should first be given, the amount each day being increased by 1 ml. Subsequently the strength of the milk solution can be carefully increased until ultimately the infant can tolerate small amounts of whole milk which are again gradually increased. The whole process may take 3 to 6 months to complete.

Drug Rashes

Many drugs may in idiosyncratic subjects produce an eruption. The rashes are like those described as toxic erythemata but the abrupt onset and absence of any constitutional disturbances may give a clue to the diagnosis. A few of the common drug eruptions are given as examples of these rashes.

BROMIDE RASH

Bromide has been supplied in the form of " gripe water " or soothing powders, or the mother may be taking the drug for some purpose and excreting it in her milk. The rash appears as vesicles or pustules on the face, body and limbs, and later these become hard, raised crusts, varying from the size of a pea to that of an almond. In some cases the eruption is suspected to be smallpox. When the crusts fall off they leave no scar, and usually the lesions disappear rapidly with the cessation of the drug, but occasionally a rather slow resolution takes place.

SULPHONAMIDE RASH

After the administration of any of the sulphonamide group a toxic rash may occasionally appear. This may be purpuric, scarlatiniform, morbilliform or maculopapular, and the distribution may be general or patchy. Pruritus is uncommon. The rashes are toxic in type and disappear rapidly when the drug is withdrawn. Eruptions are quite often provoked by local sulphonamide applications, and an intractable eczema or dermatitis may result. Such a result is commonly seen in tropical climates where the local application of sulphonamides should never be made in any circumstances.

BARBITURATE RASH

The barbiturates may produce a blotchy erythema, particularly over the joints, in susceptible individuals. Quite often the eruption simulates German measles.

OTHER DRUG RASHES

Sodium hydantoin may produce a morbilliform rash and temperature, but the glands are not swollen. This subsides with its withdrawal.

Other drugs which may give rise to rashes include chloral, quinine, opium, iodides, antipyrine, salicylates and digitalis. A rash may occasionally follow the systemic administration of penicillin. Sedormid may give rise to purpura.

DERMATITIS VENENATA

Many individuals react to external poisons in plants, e.g. poison ivy (*Rhus toxicodendron*) and the primrose (*Primula obconica*), and to aromatic oils or other applications. The hands, face or legs may come in contact with the plant, and a severe dermatitis result. There may be a simple redness and swelling, but often large bullæ or vesicles are formed, and irritation is marked. The illness lasts from one to three weeks.

If there is much constitutional upset, the child is best put to bed, and sedatives and antihistamines should be given. A local application of bicarbonate of soda, or washing with strongly alkaline soap, may lessen the spread.

Serum Rash (Serum Sickness)

A rash may follow injections of tetanus or diphtheria antitoxin, horse serum or other antisera. As a rule, it appears about ten days after the injection, but it may come earlier or later. The first symptom may be an urticarial rash, which may be blotchy and erythematous, resembling measles. There is tenderness in the joints, a temperature, malaise and occasionally actual vomiting. The danger of an immediate and potentially fatal *anaphylactoid reaction* will almost always be avoided, if serum is given only after a preliminary subcutaneous test-dose has produced no local response. When major anaphylaxis has occurred there is shock and peripheral circulatory failure, which may require full resuscitation with intravenous noradrenaline and hydrocortisone, oxygen and artificial respiration. The milder delayed serum reactions are helped by promethazine, ephedrine, and sedatives such as phenobarbitone (for dosages, *see* p. 663).

Vaccination Eruptions

Seven to fourteen days after the primary vaccination a generalized vaccinia may occur; it is a sparse eruption of umbilicated papular pustules resembling smallpox. Auto-infection from the primary vaccination lesion may result in an acute secondary vaccinal eruption which is very severe, and the skin may be markedly œdematous. Infants with infantile eczema are particularly liable to develop a generalized vesicular rash following vaccination (Kaposi's varicelliform eruption), and for this reason vaccination is contra-indicated in such children. A similar reaction is sometimes seen in eczematous children exposed to herpes simplex infection. This widespread vesicular eruption follows a benign self-limited course unless secondary infection occurs, which may require intensive antibiotic treatment.

There may be superadded infection at the site of vaccination, and erysipelas may result. In children with agammaglobulinæmia (p. 134) a gangrenous reaction may ensue, progressing to a fatal outcome.

OTHER SKIN CONDITIONS

Psoriasis

THIS is a recurring eruption, with a hereditary or familial history in a large number of cases. It has a characteristic appearance and is rare before the age of five or six years. The causation is unknown.

The clinical picture is of a child in good health who develops either an extensive eruption, usually on the body, or the eruption may be limited to the extensor aspects of the limbs, especially the elbows and knees. The scalp and nails may also be affected. The lesions consist of small pale, scaly, pink papules. They start as tiny points or patches, and extend to patches an inch or more in diameter. The following points are characteristic:

1. The circumscribed patches grow by extension at the margin, not by coalescence of smaller patches.
2. They remain always dry.
3. On scraping, the scales first become more obvious; at length a level is reached where there are no more scales, but a dry, red smooth surface, which bleeds on further scraping.
4. The red patch which remains after the scales have been removed shows no infiltration, and fades on firm pressure; that is, the lesion is a scaly macule, not a papule.
5. On the scalp the patches are usually thicker, and more scaly.

Dieting and general treatment do not seem of value. A very useful ointment for local treatment is:

> Liq. picis carb. 2 ml. (30 minims).
> Zinc paste to 30 G. (1 oz.).

The older applications such as chrysarobin and Cignolin have been generally discarded; instead, where the lesions fail to respond to simple treatment, 30 per cent. hydrocortisone may be applied and kept in place by a polyethylene covering. An improvement may be expected in about a fortnight, but it must be realized that the disease is a recurrent one with spontaneous remissions and relapses, probably for the rest of the patient's life.

Pityriasis Capitis

Scurf is probably due to a mild infection of the scalp with the organism called *Pityrosporom ovale*. In susceptible subjects the infection may produce either a seborrhœic dermatitis or an eczematous process which spreads from the scalp to the face and flexures. It is important therefore to treat the scurfy scalp; 2 per cent. of sulphur and salicylic acid in coconut oil is a suitable application, and frequent shampoos should be given until the scalp is clear.

Pityriasis Rosea

Pityriasis rosea is uncommon in children. The characteristic features are:

1. It commences as a solitary patch called the " herald patch." This may appear on the chest, neck, abdomen, arm, or thigh.
2. A week or ten days later similar patches in great number appear over the body, particularly the trunk.
3. The patches are the size of a finger-nail, and show three zones: a central yellowish zone of finely wrinkled epidermis, outside this a narrow scaly band, and a fine smooth pink margin. The patches are irritating.
4. The eruption lasts about six weeks, and constitutional disturbances are slight or absent.

No treatment is required.

Alopecia (Baldness)

BALDNESS may occur over a wide area, due to depression of the general health of the child by some febrile illness. Thus, after measles, scarlet fever, typhus or typhoid, the hair may come out, but with improvement in the general health a fresh growth occurs. Alopecia may also follow chronic metabolic diseases such as subacute nephritis, renal rickets, or other chronic diseases such as ulcerative colitis. Baldness may also occur about an inflamed area of the scalp, such as a boil or ringworm patch.

ALOPECIA AREATA

The characteristic of this form of baldness is that it occurs in patches, and may be mistaken for ringworm. Constitutional factors—toxic, nervous or endocrine—probably form the ætiological basis.

Diagnosis. The bald patch is usually smooth, shiny and devoid of scales, unlike that of ringworm. The eyebrows may also be affected.

Recovery in children usually occurs in six to eighteen months (Adamson). When alopecia is widespread the prognosis is less good.

Seborrhœa Oleosa

This is a condition of hypersecretion of *sebum*, the subjects of which have large sebaceous glands, especially about the sides of the nose and central parts of the face. Seborrhœic subjects are also very liable to acne, boils, eczema and infections of the mucous membranes. This appears to be a permanent condition, and an inborn characteristic rather than a disease; treatment is only palliative, e.g. frequent use of soap and hot water, and sulphur lotions.

Acne Vulgaris

Acne vulgaris occurs in those who suffer from seborrhœa oleosa, and is due to an infection of the pilo-sebaceous apparatus.

Between puberty and the age of about eighteen hypertrophy of the sebaceous glands is usual. Acne is common therefore at this age but it may also appear in young children or even in infants if greasy preparations are constantly applied to the skin. Both males and females are affected. The sebaceous glands become blocked because of inflammation, and blackheads are formed. These in turn may become infected and develop into small pustules. It is worse at the menstrual periods.

The spots appear on the forehead, cheeks, sides of the nose, temples, chin, chest, back of the neck, and between the shoulder-blades.

Since acne may leave permanent scarring and disfigurement and produces an inferiority complex in some individuals, the treatment is important. The sheet anchor is soap and hot water to remove the excessive grease from the skin and scalp. A lotion, such as 2 per cent. sulphur in calamine lotion is indicated. This should be applied with the hand two or three times daily, after washing, and should be allowed to dry on the skin.

Once daily, the following cream is used:

> Ung. acid. salicyl. (2%), 31 G. (1 oz.).
> Glycer. amyli, 31 G. (1 oz.).
> Aqua ros. geran., q.s.

Broad spectrum antibiotics may be helpful in severe pustular cases.

Ultra-violet light, and especially x-rays, will be found of real value. Quarter pastille (100γ) doses of x-rays, from three to five doses in all, at weekly intervals, are recommended by Roxburgh.

Localized Sclerema Neonatorum (Fat Necrosis)

This condition is sometimes seen in newly-born infants. Extensive, brawny, lard-like lumps may be felt on the thighs, shoulders and back. The skin is firmly adherent to the patches, which are occasionally purplish-red.

The condition is due to localized subcutaneous fat necrosis. It is an entirely benign condition with an excellent prognosis, although several weeks may elapse before the subcutaneous masses disappear completely.

The condition is not to be confused with the generalized form of œdema or sclerœdema (*see* p. 108) sometimes seen in premature infants or other newly-born full term infants suffering from *hypothermia* or *severe infections*.

Scleroderma

This condition is identical with that in adults and is very rare in children. The affected areas are indurated, have a yellowish waxen surface, and calcification may appear in the skin. Signs of Raynaud phenomena often develop in the hands. There may be dilatation and hypertrophy of the capillaries at the base of the nail beds.

It is probable that *dermatomyositis* (p. 323) is a different disorder, being less uncommon in young people. It affects striped muscle, leading ultimately to calcification, and has a high incidence of complicating carcinoma when adult life is reached.

Vitiligo (Leucoderma)

A child with this condition shows patches of skin from which the pigment has disappeared. They are most noticeable in the summer months, when the surrounding skin is pigmented. As a rule, they are symmetrically distributed, such as on both knees, or a patch on both shoulder-blades. The health of the child is unaffected. The cause is unknown.

No specific treatment is known or necessary, but if a cosmetic improvement is required the pale areas may be toned to match the surrounding skin; dihydroxyacetone (DHA)[1] can be applied as a lotion. Recently, a group of Asian and African children and adolescents with vitiligo was treated orally with 8-methoxypsoralen and sunlight with encouraging results.[2]

[1] Annotation (1960). *Brit. med. J.*, 1, 285.
[2] Lanceley, J. L., Lanceley, E. S., Jeliffe, D. B. (1962). *J. Pediat.*, **60**, 572.

CHAPTER 23

Diseases of the Eye

Blindness and Partial Sightedness

THE statutory definition of blindness is " so blind as to be unable to perform any work for which eyesight is essential." In actual practice this means that the visual acuity is 3/60 or less. Most registered blind persons have some degree of vision and only about 5 per cent. of newly registered persons are totally blind.

There are about 100,000 registered blind persons in England and Wales, of which about 2,500 (2·5 per cent.) are under sixteen years of age. About 85 per cent. are over the age of fifty.

There is no sharp division between " blindness " and " partial sightedness." The latter term usually refers to persons whose visual acuity is less than 6/24 in both eyes. In childhood it means that such individuals are likely to require special methods of education because of their visual disability. The number of registered partially sighted persons in England and Wales is about 20,000 of whom about 2,200 (11 per cent.) are under sixteen years old.

ÆTIOLOGY

There has been a complete change in the relative importance of the various causes of blindness in childhood in the United Kingdom in the last fifty years. Previously, ophthalmia neonatorum and syphilis were the usual factors; they have both now virtually disappeared. Retrolental fibroplasia (p. 83) was frequently responsible for blindness between 1942–1954, but since its cause was recognized it has steadily declined in incidence. Congenital malformations of the eyes are now the commonest cause of blindness and it is likely that with better obstetric and pædiatric care more such children are now surviving than in the past. The causes of congenital malformations of the eyes have a similar range of ætiology to that already described for congenital malformations in general (p. 97), maternal rubella in the first trimester of pregnancy being a clearly identifiable if infrequent example. Among the other causes, fœtal anoxia is probably the commonest explanation. Visual defects are frequently associated with other congenital malformations, such as cerebral palsy and mongolism, in addition to the characteristic multiple malformations seen in the

521

rubella syndrome.   Genetically determined causes of blindness include retinitis pigmentosa and albinism.

Although the blindness seldom occurs in childhood, the incidence of severe visual defect in young adults who developed diabetes mellitus in childhood is a serious cause for concern (*see* p. 172).

Injuries to the eyes are usually unilateral but may occasionally affect both eyes.   In the world population trachoma (p. 529) remains the commonest single cause of blindness.

DIAGNOSIS

Parents are generally quick to detect blindness in an otherwise normal infant.   Partial sightedness, however, may often be un-suspected in the first eighteen months of life.   On the other hand parents of brain-damaged or mentally defective children may suspect blindness in infancy which does not in fact exist.   A backward child may be able to see but often does not bother to look.

Poor vision should always be looked for in children with other known malformations.   It is found, for example, that nearly half the children with cerebral palsy have visual defects of a greater or lesser degree.

The specific diagnostic criteria are described under the appropriate lesion giving rise to the blindness.

GENERAL MANAGEMENT

In all cases of blindness and partial sight, it is imperative that the child should be given the maximum help to lead a life as nearly as possible approaching normality.   Relatives of blind children through mistaken kindness or anxiety tend to over-protect them, restricting their activities and tending to isolate them from society so that they remain emotionally dependent and more severely incapacitated than necessary.

The Local Authorities in the United Kingdom wish to be notified of all such children so that their social welfare services and the various voluntary organizations may provide the maximum help.   Special schools are provided for such children from the age of two years onwards.   Later on, special help is required in arranging suitable employment.

CONGENITAL MALFORMATIONS OF THE EYES

MALFORMATIONS may involve the whole or any part of the eye.

Anophthalmos and Microphthalmia

In some infants, the eyeball may apparently be completely deficient, being replaced by a cystic swelling of the lower lid (orbito-palpebral cyst).   In fact microscopical remnants of ocular tissue are always present in such cases, which are due to a failure of fusion of the surface ectoderm and the optic vesicle.

In other instances the eyeballs are present but are much reduced in size, with a similar failure of development of the eyelids. In such cases vision is very defective, if not totally absent. There may be an associated persistence of the hyaloid artery, which with its vascular sheath obscures the retina from the lens.

Congenital Malformation of the Lens

Coloboma of lens. In this malformation there is a deficiency of the inferior margin of the lens due to a failure of development of the suspensory ligament.

Congenital Dislocation of the Lens

In the congenital form this is a bilateral condition and is associated with gross interference with vision. The lens, which is unduly small, is shifted upwards and medially; the edge, however, is not usually visible unless the pupil is dilated, when it immediately becomes visible and the extent of the displacement can be assessed.

The disorder, which may be inherited as an incompletely expressed dominant genetic characteristic, is a component of Marfan's syndrome (*see* p. 479).

Congenital Cataract

By definition any opacity in the lens or its capsule is called a cataract; it is not surprising that there are many causes of lens opacity, some of which are of congenital, some genetic and some of acquired origin.

Cataracts may be due to factors operative in fœtal life, as shown by the inclusion of congenital cataract as one of the abnormalities seen in the rubella syndrome (*see* p. 540). In mongolism also, cataracts of congenital origin are more common than in the general population. It may well be that other abnormalities of fœtal environment, such as fœtal anoxia, may cause a nutritional failure in lens development and subsequent cataract. Whilst cataract may occur as an isolated abnormality, it may be seen in association with other congenital abnormalities such as cerebral palsy or congenital heart disease.

The development of cataract in infancy is commonly associated with biochemical anomalies. Thus cataracts may develop during the first months of life in untreated galactosæmia (p. 131), idiopathic hypoparathyroidism (p. 158) or may be a feature of Lowe's syndrome. In this latter syndrome the symptoms of mental deficiency and congenital cataract are associated with a generalized amino-aciduria and a raised blood-urea level. The cause of this metabolic and renal tubular disorder is not known.

Finally, cataracts in childhood may be of hereditary origin, the characteristic being inherited as a dominant genetic trait.

Cataracts become increasingly obvious as the lens becomes more opaque. In the early stages, however, the condition may be unsuspected. The authors recall one infant referred to them as a possible case of chronic meningitis on account of persistent head retraction. On examination bilateral congenital cataracts were present with only a small area of translucent lens remaining in the lower margin. By retracting his head the child was still able to use such vision as remained in this area.

The treatment is operative, but it must be co-ordinated with general treatment in the cases of biochemical origin.

Infiltrations of the lens, not amounting to frank cataract, are found in gargoylism (p. 480) and in cystinosis (p. 130).

Congenital Malformation of the Iris

The usual defect of development (*coloboma*) of the iris is a triangular defect of the iris continuous with the pupil, the apex of the triangle pointing away from the centre.

Congenital Malformations of the Retina

COLOBOMA

A coloboma of the retina is seen as a localized white or pigmented patch on the retina which may or may not involve the optic disc. A few blood vessels arising from the posterior ciliary arteries may be seen on the surface. The vision from this area of the retina is deficient, giving rise to a localized visual field defect (scotoma). If bilateral and extensive, the condition may need to be distinguished from congenital toxoplasmosis (p. 413).

OPAQUE NERVE FIBRES

Occasionally some fibres of the optic nerve retain their medullary sheaths after passing beyond the lamina cribrosa. They appear on the surface of the retina as white patches with striated (frayed out) edges. They are usually close to the optic disc and may involve it. They may be bilateral. No blood vessels are visible on their retinal surface. As with the coloboma, they give rise to scotomata corresponding with the position of the medullated fibres.

Colour Blindness

Complete colour blindness in which all colours appear as greys of varying shades is extremely rare. More common is partial colour blindness which affects about four per cent. of males but is more rare (less than a half per cent.) in females. It is an inherited condition of a sex-linked character (p. 14). Partial colour blindness may often remain undiscovered unless special tests are made, the individual learning to compensate for his defect by paying attention to shades and textures. In most cases reds and greens are confused. Colour blindness involving blue colour sensation is extremely rare.

The condition becomes a problem in certain occupations in adult life, but is seldom encountered as a clinical problem of childhood.

Infantile Glaucoma (Buphthalmos)

In infancy raised intra-ocular pressure usually occurs because of an obstruction of flow of the aqueous content of the eye at the angle of the anterior chamber. This is usually due to a failure of separation of the iris and cornea, which remain joined by embryonic tissue. Some circulation of fluid is maintained by the anterior ciliary veins but there is a consistently raised intra-ocular tension. The condition is bilateral.

The first result of the rise of pressure is a generalized enlargement of the globe which may at first mask the rise in pressure. Subsequently œdema of the cornea occurs and corneal opacities may develop. There is raised ocular tension and intense photophobia, and vascular congestion becomes obvious around the cornea.

TREATMENT

The pupil must be kept contracted with eserine, 0·25 per cent. drops, to facilitate drainage, but operative treatment is usually essential to relieve the obstruction.

Refractive Errors

For a description of the refractive errors of childhood the reader is referred to the text-books of ophthalmology. In childhood, myopia and astigmatism are most liable to require treatment since hypermetropic errors are unlikely to cause symptoms until later life, apart from their tendency to bring out a convergent strabismus (*see* below).

Squint in Childhood

Squint may be organic or functional. The former, due to some lesion of the brain or of the nerves supplying the muscles to the eyeball, may follow congenital defects, or hæmorrhage and injury during birth, or infection such as meningitis or encephalitis, or brain tumours. The latter, which may be convergent or divergent, is the common type of squint found in infancy or early childhood. A debilitating illness, such as measles, whooping-cough, or influenza, may bring out or greatly accentuate such a squint.

Some infants at birth are hypermetropic; the eyeball being small, rays of light entering the cornea focus behind the retina rather than on it, thus making an indistinct image. Subsequently, binocular vision is acquired, and the infant is able to fix objects.

If the eye remains hypermetropic there is a tendency to *convergent* squint; the infant, in an effort to fix near objects, attempts to exert accommodation by contraction of the ciliary muscles to allow the lens to become more convex and thus bring the rays to focus on the retina.

Divergent squint is much less common, and is usually associated with myopia. It generally develops at school age in a short-sighted child.

TREATMENT

A squinting child should be referred for treatment by the age of six months or one year, or as soon as the squint is noticed after this. Disease of the eyes, including developmental defects, birth injury and optic atrophy, should first be excluded. The majority of the remaining cases are found to be hypermetropic, and should be treated appropriately. Unless treatment is instituted at an early age, a squinting eye may become blind. Full treatment includes (*a*) the prescription of the proper glasses; (*b*) orthoptic examination, or investigation for binocular vision; (*c*) orthoptic or squint training, for the purpose of obtaining binocular vision; (*d*) occlusion of the non-squinting eye; and (*e*) perhaps, operation.

Blocked Lacrimal or Tear-duct (Dacrocystitis)

Frequently, advice is sought because an infant has a " running eye." The tears continually run over the cheek, and in the morning a slight discharge is seen on the affected side. In such cases the tear-duct will be found to be blocked somewhere in its course, but usually at its exit into the nose. It will be found that the infant has a slight nasal catarrh.

The mother should be told to squeeze the side of the bridge of the nose several times a day in order to empty the lacrimal sac. The duct opening will then become less inflamed, and patency will be re-established. Usually, nothing further is required, but meanwhile the eye may be bathed twice daily, and an ophthalmic cream may be applied at bedtime. In cases which fail to respond to this treatment, probing of the naso-lacrimal duct may be necessary.

INFECTIONS OF THE EYE

CONJUNCTIVITIS

IN its mildest form, namely congestion or hyperæmia, this may be due to (*a*) foreign bodies, (*b*) glare of strong light, (*c*) irritants, such as smoke or gaseous products, in the surrounding atmosphere, (*d*) pollens, as in hay-fever, (*e*) blocking of the lacrimal duct.

General treatment consists in removing the cause. Local treatment consists in bathing the eyes with zinc sulphate solution, one grain to the ounce. An antihistamine preparation (for dosage, *see* p. 664) gives relief in allergic cases.

Acute Conjunctivitis (" Cold in the Eye," " Pink Eye ")

In acute conjunctivitis the discharge is muco-purulent. The eye is fiery red and congested, and the vessels engorged. The lids are stuck together in the morning, and the lashes are matted. Usually, such infections reach their height in three or four days, and are better in a week to ten days.

The organism most commonly found is the " Koch-Weeks bacillus," which is a slender Gram-negative rod. It is infectious to others, but is killed on drying. *Staph. pyogenes* or pneumococci may cause epidemics of conjunctivitis and it is a common complication of measles and scarlet fever.

TREATMENT

Frequent bathing with a simple solution of warm normal saline should be undertaken at once. In infants and young children the lids should be held apart, and the lotion dropped in freely. Sulphacetamide drops are an effective local application. In more severe cases, the appropriate antibiotic should be given locally in ointment form or together with systemic treatment.

Ophthalmia Neonatorum

This is a preventable disease which in the past was responsible for 50 per cent. of all blind children. Infection occurs during birth from the mother's passages or discharges. The eye infection is noted about the third day, both eyes being involved as a rule. The lids are swollen, and there is much congestion. There is a risk of corneal ulceration, and even perforation. Gonococcal infection is now only an occasional cause in the United Kingdom, the organism more often responsible being *Staphylococcus pyogenes*.

TREATMENT

Local treatment to the eyes for non-gonorrhœal cases is usually effective: bathing with warm normal saline every two hours, and the application of sodium sulphacetamide drops.

Chemotherapy or antibiotics may be required for the more severe cases; a culture should be taken immediately the infection is first noted so that the appropriate antibiotic to which the organism is sensitive may be administered; this is of particular importance in maternity units where penicillin- and tetracycline-resistant staphylococci are common. Chloramphenicol ophthalmic ointment is applied after the saline irrigations. This treatment is preferred to local penicillin in view of the likelihood of breeding out the penicillin-resistant cases, particularly following its local application. Penicillin should be reserved therefore for cases where the organism has been proved to be sensitive to the drug.

For gonococcal cases, however, penicillin is the treatment of choice, and should be used in full doses (*see* Appendix 1), systemically and locally. As a preventive measure, a 5 per cent. solution of argyrol is sometimes instilled into the infant's eyes at birth.

Diphtheritic Conjunctivitis

In this disease membranes are formed on the surface of the conjunctiva. The diagnosis is settled by culture and examination of a direct smear. The full treatment for diphtheria should be given (*see* p. 552), and atropine instilled locally.

Phlyctenular Conjunctivitis

Small, round, grey or yellow nodules appear on the conjunctiva, surrounded by leashes of congested vessels. The condition may, however, be complicated by a general conjunctivitis. It is most frequent between the ages of 6 and 12 years.

Phlyctenular conjunctivitis is an occasional manifestation of tuberculous infection due to the development of an allergic reaction.

TREATMENT

Locally, this consists in bathing the eye with boric lotion and applying yellow oxide of mercury ointment. Full anti-tuberculous therapy with local streptomycin and systemic PAS and INH (for dosage, *see* p. 665) should be given for a minimum of six months. Full investigation and appropriate treatment for tuberculosis in other sites should be undertaken.

Angular Conjunctivitis

The area affected is limited to the intermarginal strip of conjunctiva at the inner and outer canthus. The organism is the bacillus of Morax-Axenfeld, a rod-shaped Gram-negative diplobacillus. Zinc sulphate, 2 grains to the ounce, is the specific treatment.

INFLAMMATION OF THE CORNEA (KERATITIS)

THIS is usually the result of an injury to the cornea by a foreign body and follows acute ulceration. Since perforation or permanent clouding of the cornea, with partial blindness, may be the outcome, detailed examination and treatment by an ophthalmologist is essential.

Phlyctenular Keratitis (Strumous Keratitis)

This condition occurs as an extension of phlyctenular conjunctivitis to the cornea, where it may give rise to ulceration and permanent opacities or nebulæ, with varying degrees of blindness. Treatment is as for phlyctenular conjunctivitis.

Interstitial Keratitis (Syphilitic Keratitis)

See p. 566.

Trachoma

Although very rare in the United Kingdom, trachoma is the commonest cause of blindness in the world population. Being spread by dirty fingers and flies, it is found wherever there is widespread lack of hygiene.

PATHOGENESIS

The infecting organism is a virus, *Chlamydozoon trachomatis*, which can be recovered from the conjunctival secretion of infected persons. The commonly associated purulent conjunctivitis from other organisms increases the conjunctival secretion and therefore the risk of contagion.

SYMPTOMS

The clinical picture of trachoma is almost invariably complicated by a long-standing purulent conjunctivitis from such organisms as the Koch-Weeks bacillus, gonococcus or other pyogenic organisms. The initial infection involves the conjunctiva and the cornea. Trachoma follicles appear on the upper tarsus, later extending to the palpebral conjunctiva. They are much larger in size than the small follicles seen in simple conjunctivitis. They heal by extensive scarring and cicatrization.

Clouding of the cornea occurs as a result of numerous epithelial erosions, and indolent corneal ulcers are common. Trachomatous pannus refers to the lymphoid infiltration and vascular engorgement of the margin of the cornea which later extends to involve the whole of the cornea itself.

TREATMENT

Wherever adequate standards of hygiene are maintained the disease can be prevented.

In the early stages of the disease, together with efforts to inculcate hygienic standards into the patient's personal habits, systemic treatment with tetracyclines and local treatment with sodium sulphacetamide drops are essential and may need to be continued for at least six months. In more established cases additional local applications of copper sulphate or silver nitrate may be required, as well as destruction of the follicles by scarification or diathermy. Operative treatment may also be required in advanced cases to remove the tarsal plate or excise the fornix.

The mass treatment campaigns against trachoma sponsored by WHO have been highly successful.

UVEITIS

THE uveal tract consists of the iris, the ciliary body and the choroid. Inflammation tends to involve the whole rather than one part of the tract. The term irido-cyclitis thus relates to anterior uveitis, and choroiditis to posterior uveitis.

ÆTIOLOGY

The condition may arise from exogenous causes, usually secondary to infection of other ocular tissues, or may follow a penetrating eye injury. It may also result from endogenous infections which give rise to blood-borne spread. Syphilis, brucellosis, mumps and toxoplasmosis are typical examples. Uveitis may also occur as a complication of rheumatoid arthritis, erythema multiforme and Stevens-Johnson syndrome.

Irido-cyclitis

DIAGNOSIS

Duke-Elder[1] gives a most helpful differentiation of the three main types of ocular inflammation, namely conjunctivitis, iritis and glaucoma.

	Conjunctivitis	Iritis	Glaucoma
Vascular Injection	Superficial	Deep ciliary	Deep ciliary
Secretion	Muco-purulent	Watery	Watery
Pupil	Normal	Small and irregular	Large and oval
Media	Clear	Sometimes opaque	Corneal œdema
Tension	Normal	Normal	Raised
Pain	Mild discomfort	Moderate (first division of trigeminal nerve)	Severe (entire trigeminal distribution)
Tenderness	Absent	Marked	Marked
Vision	Good	Fair	Poor
Onset	Gradual	Gradual	Sudden

The differentiation of irido-cyclitis and glaucoma is vitally important in relation to treatment. Dilatation of the pupil is essential in iritis but is strongly contra-indicated in glaucoma (p. 525).

TREATMENT

Dilatation of the pupil with atropine, fomentations, steroids and antibiotics form the basis of treatment. For a detailed description, the reader must refer to ophthalmological text-books.

Choroidoretinitis

Since the nutrition of the outer parts of the retina is derived from the choroid, a choroiditis of any severity will always involve the retina. By contrast, primary diseases of the retina may occur without involvement of the choroid.

[1] Duke-Elder, Sir Stewart (1959). " Diseases of the Eye." London: Churchill.

Congenital syphilis may give rise to a disseminated choroiditis in which scattered areas of inflammation are seen in the retina; these progress to a white atrophic stage. In *miliary tuberculosis* a few pinkish raised spots may be seen on the retina in juxtaposition to the retinal arteries. As they heal, these miliary tubercles become yellowish white in colour.

In *congenital toxoplasmosis* (p. 413), the severe choroidoretinitis leaves multiple punched-out heavily pigmented scars in both retinæ. *Cytomegalic inclusion-body disease* is another cause (p. 99).

Panophthalmitis

Following a deep corneal ulcer or penetrating wound of the eye, a purulent uveitis may lead to inflammation of the whole eye, including the vitreous in addition to the entire uveal tract and retina. An endogenous form of panophthalmitis may sometimes occur from an infective embolus of the retinal artery in overwhelming septicæmia. This acute form is likely to lead to loss of the eye, unless intensive treatment is started early with antibiotics, steroids and local treatment by a skilled ophthalmologist.

The term *pseudoglioma* refers to a subacute form of panophthalmitis. There may be no history of eye trouble until it is noticed that there is a white reflection from the pupil. Examination reveals extensive disease of all the ocular tissues. The condition has to be distinguished from retinoblastoma (p. 534). The treatment is excision of the eye.

A proportion of these cases has been shown to be due to visceral larva migrans (p. 630) with actual deposition of the *Toxocara canis* larva within the eye.

INHERITED DISEASES OF THE RETINA

Retinitis Pigmentosa

This disorder appears in childhood and commences with night blindness. Subsequently the visual fields become progressively contracted until ultimately in middle age the field is restricted to a small area around the fixation point. By this time the individual is severely handicapped visually, and by the age of sixty even central vision may be lost.

The retinæ show punctate black areas with a sheath of black pigment along the retinal veins. Gradually the remainder of the retina becomes decolourized and the retinal arteries and veins become threadlike in appearance. The disc takes on a waxy yellow appearance. Finally cataract formation may occur in the lens.

The disease is usually inherited as a recessive genetic characteristic. A few families are known in which the disorder is seen in the heterozygotes. In some families the disorder is associated with obesity, mental retardation, hypogonadism and polydactyly (Laurence-Moon-Biedl Syndrome, *see* p. 149).

Familial Lipoid Degenerations

Amaurotic Familial Idiocy (Tay-Sachs Disease, p. 444). This recessively inherited disorder of Jewish children commences in the first year of life. Apart from the ocular changes, the child is weak and wasted and seldom survives beyond the age of two to three years.

The retinal appearance is characteristic, with a white area at the macula in the centre of which is a cherry red circular spot. There is associated optic atrophy.

Maculo-cerebral Familial Degeneration (Batten-Mayou Disease). This represents a delayed or juvenile form of Tay-Sachs disease. It is also recessively inherited but is not restricted to the Jewish race. The disease commences at about six to ten years of age. The symptoms of cerebral degeneration include spasticity, convulsions and mental deterioration. The retinæ show yellowish grey spots in the region of the macula with some generalized retinal pigmentation. The discs are pale. The cherry-red spot at the macula is not a constant feature.

Optic Atrophy

In some infants blindness occurs as a result of a primary optic atrophy. The infant is blind from birth and on examination the optic disc is seen to be contracted and white in colour. The vessels are thin and atrophic. The cause is unknown.

Secondary optic atrophy occurs as a result of raised intracranial pressure from any cause, e.g. hydrocephalus, cerebral tumour, etc.

DISORDERS OF THE EYE-LIDS

Blepharitis

THIS may be acute, accompanying an acute or chronic conjunctivitis. The chronic form is often found in eczematous children. It is common in mongols and is also found in children who live in surroundings where there is much smoke or other irritating substance in the atmosphere. In some children the blepharitis is kept up by allergy to some outside irritant; feathers, dust and pollens, as well as dusting-powder, face-powder and flour have all produced a state of chronic blepharitis.

Constant rubbing of the eyes should be prevented, and the underlying cause of the inflammation should, as far as possible, be removed. The eyes should be kept well bathed with normal saline, and the crusts removed with hydrogen peroxide. Yellow oxide of mercury is then applied locally. In the chronic cases, the affected areas are painted daily with half per cent. brilliant green or two per cent. silver nitrate, after careful removal of all the crusts with hydrogen peroxide.

Styes

These are due to an infection, usually by the staphylococcus, of the Zeis's glands, resulting in the formation of minute abscesses. Hot bathing and pulling out the appropriate eye-lashes will give relief. Occasionally the abscesses may require incising.

In recurrent cases, a full systemic course of the appropriate antibiotic is required.

Chalazion

This is a chronic granulomatous inflammation of one of the Meibomian glands. Small ones may be left alone, the larger varieties should be incised and thoroughly scraped out.

Entropion

In small infants it is not uncommon to see the cilia directed inwards and rubbing against the scleral conjunctiva. This appears to cause no irritation. The condition of trichiasis, in which the lids are markedly inverted and the cilia irritate the cornea, is more commonly seen in adults. It may occur in trachoma, where surgical correction may be indicated.

Ectropion

Eversion of the lids may be seen following long-standing blepharitis, in lid distortion from trachoma or associated with proptosis. Plastic surgery may be necessary.

PROPTOSIS OR EXOPHTHALMOS

EXOPHTHALMOS may be found in the following conditions in children:

Exophthalmic goitre is uncommon before the age of 12 to 14 years.

Occasionally, the condition is unilateral. Along with this there are other signs of Graves's disease, such as flushing, tachycardia, and tremors of the extremities.

In *scurvy* there may be hæmorrhages round about and behind the eyeball, causing protrusion. This is not seen before the sixth month and is uncommon after one year. A diet defective in vitamin c will have been given to the infant, who will also show other signs of the disease (p. 117).

In *new growths*, such as neuroblastoma (*see* p. 377), metastases appear in the retro-orbital space and may cause proptosis. Other portions of the skull and some long bones are also involved.

Ethmoidal sinusitis may give rise to orbital cellulitis, with abscess formation. The eye is pushed forward, and the surrounding tissues are red and œdematous. Such cases may require incision, with drainage of the abscess. This is often done at the inner angle of the eye, and, in those cases seen by the authors, it has been most successful. Systemic penicillin is advisable in such cases.

NEW GROWTHS OF THE EYE

Retinoblastoma

THIS tumour is probably always embryonic in origin being due to proliferation of undifferentiated neural cells in the retina. It is invariably multiple. The second eye is affected in about a quarter of the cases. Several siblings may be similarly affected.

The symptoms usually become obvious at about six or seven years of age. The leading symptom is frequently the observation of a yellow reflex from the pupil. Subsequently the globe enlarges, often with proptosis. There may be pain in the eye until the tumour actually bursts through the sclera. This is followed by fungation of the whole globe. Metastases occur along the optic nerves and in cranial and other bones. Retinoblastoma has to be distinguished from pseudoglioma (p. 531).

TREATMENT

Excision of the eye should be carried out immediately. Where only one eye is affected, a watch must be kept on the second eye for many years after enucleation of the first eye. Recurrence in the orbit is possible. The siblings of the patient must also be watched.

CHAPTER 24

Infectious Diseases

INFECTIOUS disease plays an important part among the diseases of childhood. In former times the children of even the well-to-do had some, if not most, of the infectious diseases before school age. Now, as a result of immunization, care of contacts, observance of quarantine and, among other factors, better ventilation and hygiene, children may reach secondary or public school having had only one or two infections. In England, putting off certain infectious diseases, such as measles, until a child is over five is an advantage, because the mortality of most infectious fevers is much higher among children of the pre-school age than among those above it. This is borne out in the following mortality statistics:

TABLE XX
INCIDENCE AND MORTALITY OF INFECTIOUS DISEASES

Disease	Incidence and Mortality 1945 0–4 years	Incidence and Mortality 1960 0–4 years	Incidence and Mortality 1945 5–14 years	Incidence and Mortality 1960 5–14 years
Measles	Notifications 233,334	Notifications 84,533	Notifications 196,807	Notifications 74,045
	Deaths 632	Deaths 25	Deaths 69	Deaths 4
Scarlet Fever	Notifications 16,517	Notifications 9,454	Notifications 46,826	Notifications 21,556
	Deaths 30	Deaths 0	Deaths 31	Deaths 0
Whooping-Cough	Notifications 41,449	Notifications 24,738	Notifications 19,868	Notifications 25,184
	Deaths 666	Deaths 34	Deaths 22	Deaths 2
Typhoid Fever	Notifications 20	Notifications 10	Notifications 49	Notifications 13
	Deaths 1	Deaths 0	Deaths 1	Deaths 0

Incidence and Mortality, 1945–60, in England and Wales of Measles, Scarlet Fever, Whooping-Cough and Typhoid Fever. Registrar-General's returns.

However, these circumstances do not apply in all countries; for example, in Lagos, Nigeria, where the state of nutrition was *worse among the older children*, then mortality from measles was greater.[1]

SCARLET FEVER

IN the past fifty years, scarlet fever has declined considerably in importance as a cause of mortality in childhood. It is still responsible, however, by virtue of its more important complications, namely nephritis, rheumatic fever and carditis, for a definite though decreasing amount of chronic ill-health in the young.

Scarlet fever is most prevalent in the late summer and early autumn, but may occur in epidemic form at any time of the year. It is uncommon in infants under one year, and is most common between five and nine years.

INCUBATION PERIOD

This is from 1 to 7 days, but usually 2 to 4 days. Once the hæmolytic streptococcal infection of the upper respiratory tract has been effectively treated by penicillin (negative nasal and throat swabs), isolation of the patient is no longer necessary. Without such treatment, 21 days isolation was the rule.

MODE OF INFECTION

This is either by droplet spread from some infected individual or carrier to a healthy person, or by direct contact with infectious discharges, or through milk. It can also be transmitted on infected articles of clothing and dusts.

ÆTIOLOGY

Scarlet fever is caused by the hæmolytic streptococcus; the general effects, including the rash, being largely the result of systemic invasion by the erythrogenic toxin of the hæmolytic streptococcus. The throat is the usual site of attack, but infection of wounds by the same organism produces surgical scarlet fever.

SYMPTOMS AND CLINICAL PICTURE

In very mild cases nothing may be seen beyond a very slight soreness of the throat and a rise of temperature, with a transient rash, the whole illness subsiding in 3 or 4 days and ending in complete recovery. In the more severe cases there is an abrupt onset, usually with vomiting, and both headache and intense sore throat. The child is ill and toxic. The pulse and respiration-rate are increased, the skin is hot, the temperature considerably raised and the cheeks are flushed. The rash appears in 24 to 48 hours, but occasionally not until the third or fourth day. In some cases, however, it occurs first of all. There is usually only one vomit. A very rapid pulse, out of

[1] Gans, B. (1961). " Pædiatric problems in Lagos." *W. Afr. med. J.*, **10**, 33.

proportion to the temperature, is characteristic (Trousseau's sign) and may suggest the diagnosis.

The rash is erythematous and comes out on the trunk and limbs (except the palms of the hands and soles of the feet), and on the neck towards the lower borders of the jaw, where it merges with the flush on the face. Pastia's sign is described as linear petechial markings around the elbows. Round about the mouth there is a pale area, the so-called " circumoral pallor." The rash may last for a few hours or as long as a week.

At the end of a week or ten days the skin begins to peel, starting round the neck and upper part of the chest, then generally. The skin of the hands and feet peels last; the tags of skin can be seen for some time afterwards at the roots of the nails. The peeling is generally in proportion to the intensity of the rash and lasts from 4 to 8 weeks. It is not a sign of infectivity.

The so-called " strawberry tongue " can be seen on the first or second day—a white tongue with red papillæ showing through. As the disease progresses, the tongue becomes red all over (" raspberry tongue "), the throat being painful and the tonsils enlarged and fiery red, with enlarged glands at the angle of the jaw. The younger the child, the greater the glandular enlargement.

DIAGNOSIS

The diagnosis may sometimes be extremely difficult, as it depends on the rash, which can be simulated by a toxic, food-poisoning or sulphonamide rash. The sore throat in no way differs from that in a streptococcal infection unaccompanied by scarlet fever. The Dick test (see p. 538) is always positive in the first few days, but changes to negative in the second or third week. Peeling, a late sign, is pathognomonic of scarlet fever.

The *Schultz-Charlton test*, which is performed by injecting intradermally 0·2 ml. of a 1-in-10 dilution of streptococcal antitoxin, is a useful diagnostic measure. The antitoxin is injected into the skin of patients exhibiting a rash, and where the rash is due to scarlet fever there is a blanching about the point of injection 4 to 10 hours later, which persists for from 12 to 72 hours.

PROGNOSIS

In the now rare fatal cases, where the infection has been especially virulent, death is due to a general septicæmia, with an accompanying myocarditis, or to some complication such as pneumonia or nephritis. Generally speaking, the prognosis for life is excellent. Hæmorrhagic rashes are a bad prognostic sign.

TREATMENT

The patient is nursed in bed from the beginning and isolated from other children. The diet should be the fever diet described on p. 563. If the temperature is unduly high, tepid sponging should be given.

The fluid intake must be maintained at a high level. A careful examination of the urine for albumin should be made daily and a watch must be kept on the ears for any signs of otitis media. The child should be kept in bed until the temperature and pulse-rate are normal. If there is any suggestion of involvement of the heart, the patient should be kept at rest in bed for a long period.

Chemotherapy. Penicillin and the sulphonamides are the drugs of choice for this condition, and one of them should be given in full dosage. When persistent vomiting makes the retention of oral sulphonamide doubtful, or when nephritis is suspected, penicillin becomes the drug of choice.

Antitoxin. Before the introduction of antibiotics and sulphonamides, antitoxin provided the only specific treatment. Nowadays its use is rarely indicated, being restricted to the very occasional fulminating case presenting with complications, such as myocarditis, already present.

COMPLICATIONS

The most common complications are otitis media and cervical adenitis. Glomerulo-nephritis is a sequel to a small but definite proportion. Rheumatic carditis or arthritis following scarlet fever differs in no way from other cases of rheumatic fever. It rarely occurs under six years of age, and probably in not more than 0·5 per cent. of cases.

Relapse, due to re-infection of children with another and probably more potent type of streptococcus, may occur and can be prevented by nursing children separately or in wards where only one type is present, and by adequate chemotherapy.

PROPHYLAXIS

In a community such as a school individuals susceptible to scarlet fever may be detected by means of the Dick test (*see* below). This procedure was valuable when active and passive immunization against scarlet fever was widely practised. The use of penicillin, both as an effective prophylactic and as a therapeutic agent for the disease, has replaced these procedures. Oral penicillin V, 125 mg. twice daily, provides an effective prophylaxis for contacts.

The Dick Test. This is performed by injecting intradermally 0·2 ml. of diluted filtrate obtained from a broth-culture of the streptococcus of scarlet fever; it has been found to cause erythema 1 cm. in diameter when injected into susceptible subjects. This is called the skin-test dose. Heated filtrate is used as a control to be certain that the patient is not reacting to the horse serum. If the patient is susceptible to scarlet fever a reddened area appears in from 6 to 24 hours round about the site of the injection.

RUBELLA (GERMAN MEASLES)

THIS condition is one of the mildest of the infectious fevers and its importance at the present time arises mainly from the " rubella syndrome," whereby children born of mothers who have had rubella during the first three months of the pregnancy are likely to reveal multiple congenital deformities. RA virus was identified in 1962 by several groups of workers by means of monkey-cell cultures using interference techniques.

INCUBATION PERIOD

This is from 10 to 21 days, but is usually 17 or 18 days, the child being infectious from 1 to 4 days before the appearance of the rash or other symptoms. *Isolation* of cases is to be deprecated, as it is advisable that all females should have acquired an immunity to the disease before they reach the child-bearing age, but contact with cases of rubella should be avoided by any woman during the first three months of pregnancy.

CLINICAL PICTURE AND SYMPTOMS

The disease commences with very slight constitutional symptoms, the temperature rising shortly before the rash comes out. There may be coryza and sore throat, and there is usually enlargement of the glands behind the sternomastoid, and round the occipital and mastoid regions. The axillary and inguinal glands often share in the glandular enlargement. As a rule, however, the rash is the first indication. Occasionally conjunctivitis (pink-eye) accompanies the disease. The complications which are all uncommon, include encephalitis and polyarthritis.

The distribution of the rash is on the face and scalp, trunk and extremities. It may be morbilliform or erythematous, but is not usually as generalized as that of scarlet fever. Occasionally, it is urticarial. It rarely lasts longer than three days and may have completely disappeared in 24 hours. The disease may be mistaken for measles or, on the other hand, it may resemble urticaria or nettle-rash, due to some food or drug. In measles, unlike rubella, there is some indisposition and coryza two or three days before the appearance of the rash. Glandular fever is sometimes mistaken for rubella and vice versa.

TREATMENT

The child should be kept in bed until the temperature has become normal. Usually no specific treatment is necessary.

The mortality is negligible. Second attacks occur, but one attack confers immunity probably in 90 per cent. of cases.

RUBELLA SYNDROME

In 1941 Gregg[1] first drew attention to the association of congenital cataract and maternal rubella during the early months of pregnancy. Since then numerous surveys have been carried out, and it has been shown that there is a small but significant chance that multiple congenital defects may occur in children when maternal rubella has developed during the first trimester of the pregnancy, the precise nature of the defects varying according to the actual week of pregnancy in which rubella developed. Thus, congenital cataract is most common if rubella developed between the fifth and eighth weeks of pregnancy, congenital heart lesions between the fourth and ninth weeks, and congenital nerve deafness between the seventh and twelfth weeks. The ear and eye defects may be unilateral or bilateral. Other defects include microphthalmos, dotted pigmentary stippling of the retina, microcephaly, mental retardation, cleft palate, congenital obliteration of the bile ducts, and diaphragmatic hernia. The most common congenital cardiac anomalies are acyanotic disorders, such as patent ductus, or atrial or ventricular septal defects.

The likelihood of the infant being born with such disabilities appears to vary from epidemic to epidemic of rubella. In the original epidemics reported from Australia the incidence of affected children appeared to be 20–25 per cent. of those at risk, but in epidemics reported subsequently the incidence has been very much less. Therefore it seems hard to justify the case for termination of pregnancy where the mother develops rubella even in the first trimester of pregnancy.

If a susceptible woman is in contact with a case of rubella during the early weeks of pregnancy, it is advisable to administer specially prepared gammaglobulin at the earliest possible moment.

MEASLES (MORBILLI)

INCUBATION PERIOD

THIS is from 7 to 21 days, usually 10 days, the child being infectious at least 4 days before the appearance of the rash or other symptoms. Passive immunization prolongs the incubation period. A child may return to school when 16 clear days have elapsed from the last date of exposure to infection, but if he has himself been infected, he cannot return until 14 days after the appearance of the rash. The causal agent is a virus. One attack almost always confers permanent immunity.

CLINICAL PICTURE

Four to five days before the rash appears there is fever and malaise (prodromal period). The fever may then subside only to return with the appearance of the rash and an exaggeration of the symptoms. During the prodromal stage the eyes and nose run, and the face is

[1] Gregg, N. McA. (1941). *Trans. ophthal. Soc. Aust.*, **3**, 35

puffy. The child looks heavy and appears to have a bad cold. The inside of the mouth and cheeks shows Koplik's spots (*see* below), and a troublesome cough develops. The rash appears behind the ears and round the mouth, and then spreads rapidly over the rest of the body. The throat is sore, and there is an associated catarrhal

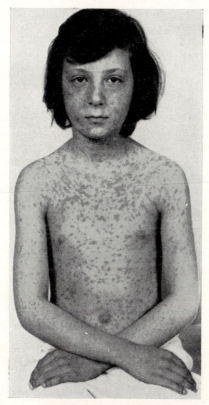

Fig. 74—The rash in measles

bronchitis. There is a conjunctivitis, so that the eyes are sore and tend to discharge. Photophobia may occur without conjunctivitis. The glands of the neck, particularly those behind the sternomastoid, become enlarged and tender. The child improves as the rash fades, when the temperature falls quickly.

Koplik's Spots. These appear on the first, second or third day of the prodromal period, and are best seen inside the cheeks, especially towards the posterior part of the mouth. They are small, about the size of a pinhead, raised, and bluish-white, surrounded by a red areola. Their absence, unfortunately, does not in any way exclude a diagnosis of measles.

The *rash* of measles is characteristic. It starts behind the ears as small pink macules which rapidly form larger, irregular-shaped patches or blotches. The rash spreads quickly to involve the face and front of the chest; within twenty-four hours it has spread to the rest of the body. Large areas may become involved, giving an erythematous appearance. This rash may last from 3 to 5 days, and often leaves a faint brown, stained appearance behind it. The temperature falls with the fading of the rash. Prodromal rashes occur during the period of incubation. They are usually blotchy and erythematous.

TREATMENT

The child should be put to bed, and the room darkened if photophobia is troublesome. A fever diet (*see* p. 563) with plenty of fluids is given.

Chemotherapy. The introduction of the sulphonamides and penicillin has greatly reduced both the mortality and the frequency of the complications of measles. In all children under two years, and in weakly children over this age, and in all those with signs of respiratory complications, sulphonamides or penicillin should be given from the beginning and continued for at least five days.

COMPLICATIONS

The most common are pneumonia, otitis media, mastoiditis, conjunctivitis and gastro-enteritis. An extreme rarity is measles encephalomyelitis with a mortality of about 10 per cent. Transverse myelitis sometimes occurs. Convulsions may accompany the prodromal symptoms of measles. If the rash becomes hæmorrhagic (black measles), the prognosis is greatly worsened; such cases are seen in tropical countries where the basic nutrition of the children is poor and where the immunity to the exanthematous infections is particularly low (*see* p. 536).

PROPHYLAXIS

Passive immunity can be conveyed by intramuscular injection of human gammaglobulin. A smaller dosage is given for attenuation and a larger one for prevention; for children between one and three years, 4·0 ml. is given for prevention within three days of exposure and 2·0 ml. for attenuation; the earlier gammaglobulin is given the more certain is prevention.

Active immunity is conferred by an attenuated attack. Following the isolation of measles virus by Enders and his colleagues, several types of measles virus vaccine are on trial.[1] Katz[2] has reported that

[1] Vaccination against measles (1961). *Brit. med. J.*, 2, 1246 and 1250.
[2] Bethesda International Conference on Measles Immunization (1961). *Lancet* 2, 246,

Enders measles-vaccine B induced attenuated measles in a form sometimes too severe to warrant general use unless gammaglobulin was given simultaneously at a separate injection site.

MUMPS (EPIDEMIC PAROTITIS)

MUMPS is a virus infection. The virus can be recovered from saliva and cerebrospinal fluid. It may occur at any age, but is most common between the ages of 5 and 15, and is conveyed by droplet spread from one child to another; second attacks are rare. The commonest clinical manifestation is parotitis.

INCUBATION PERIOD

This is from 14 to 28 days, but is on the average 18 days, and the child may be infectious 1 day before the appearance of the symptoms. Cases are regarded as infectious until 7 days after all swelling has disappeared, and not less than 14 days from the start of the illness. In schools, complete isolation of contacts for the optimal 28 days is usually impracticable and not altogether desirable, as it is preferable for a boy to contract the disease before, rather than after puberty, owing to the small risk of orchitis.

CLINICAL PICTURE AND SYMPTOMS

The disease commences with pain in the region of one parotid gland, which begins to swell, the pain being more marked on opening or shutting the mouth. At the same time there is some fever. The submaxillary and sublingual glands are often involved in addition. After 4 or 5 days, the other parotid gland may become involved, the first rapidly subsiding. In a mild case both swellings have subsided in from 10 days to a fortnight. In more severe cases the child is very ill, with a high temperature and a dirty tongue, and unable to open the mouth sufficiently to take food other than liquids. The blood shows a lymphocytosis.

TREATMENT

The child should be confined to bed on a fever diet (*see* p. 563). If opening the mouth is painful, it is helpful for the patient to take fluids through a straw. A simple mouth-wash, such as compound glycerin of thymol (B.P.C.), keeps the mouth clean.

COMPLICATIONS

Orchitis is the commonest complication, and the most severe, the testicles becoming greatly swollen, usually about the time the parotid swelling is at its height, but this varies. Orchitis rarely occurs before puberty, and there is approximately a 20 per cent. incidence among those past puberty. There is a danger afterwards, when the swellings have subsided, of atrophy. In the female, the breasts and also the ovaries may be involved. No case of sterility after mumps in the female has been recorded.

Occasionally *acute pancreatitis* occurs, usually as the parotitis subsides; it is ushered in by acute upper abdominal pain and vomiting. Mumps arthritis[1] is an uncommon variation.

A rare complication is *mumps meningitis* or encephalitis. Drowsiness, vomiting and sometimes convulsions are accompanied by neck rigidity and occasionally focal signs of paralysis, together with an increase of lymphocytes in the cerebrospinal fluid. The prognosis is usually good. On the whole, the complications, apart from sterility following orchitis, are not serious, and usually mumps is to be considered a mild disease.

Treatment of Complications. Orchitis is best treated by confining the patient to bed and supporting the scrotum with a T-bandage. In adolescent patients diethylstilbœstrol, 2–5 mg. 4 times a day, can be given to lessen the symptoms and duration of orchitis, and a smaller dose (1–2 mg.) helps to prevent this complication. Mumps meningitis requires no specific treatment although lumbar puncture often provides relief from the intense headache, and the outlook is usually excellent. Pancreatitis is treated symptomatically.

WHOOPING-COUGH (PERTUSSIS)

This, together with measles, is one of the more serious diseases of childhood, although the statistics in Table XX show the considerable decline in mortality in the last fifteen years, even in early childhood. In older children it is comparatively mild. In the United Kingdom, the greatest number of cases occurs during the first quarter of the year.

The disease occurs most commonly between the ages of two and five years, but affects infants under the age of one year more frequently than any other of the acute infectious fevers, there being little transmission of passive immunity from mother to infant as is the case with most other acute specific fevers.

INCUBATION PERIOD

This is usually about 7 to 10 days, but may vary from 5 to 14 days. Whooping-cough is infectious as soon as the first cough appears. Contacts may return to school when 14 clear days have elapsed from the last date of exposure to infection, but an infected child may not return for 5 weeks from the commencement of the illness.

BACTERIOLOGY AND PATHOLOGY

Whooping-cough is due to the Gram-negative Bordet-Gengou bacillus (*Hæmophilus pertussis*). The infection is essentially a laryngitis and tracheitis, much semi-purulent material mixed with mucus being produced. A help in the diagnosis may be found in the blood-count, where a distinct lymphocytosis occurs. The white-cell count may

[1] Lass, R., Shephard, E. (1961). *Brit. med. J.* 1, 1613.

rise to 20,000 or 30,000 per c.mm., with a proportion of 60 or 70 per cent. of lymphocytes. If the child coughs spontaneously on to specially prepared media, such as the Bordet-Gengou preparation, which is composed of blood-agar containing glycerin and potato, or if per-nasal or laryngeal swabs are cultured in this way, the organism can be isolated in a large proportion of cases, provided the specimens are taken in the early stages of the disease.

ONSET AND CLINICAL PICTURE

Generally speaking, whooping-cough may be divided into three phases: the catarrhal or onset stage; the paroxysmal stage; and the phase of recovery. In a classical case these three stages last approximately a fortnight each, but there is very great variation.

1. *The Catarrhal Phase.* The disease starts with congestion of the upper respiratory mucous membranes. There is a slight fever, and a persistent hacking cough gradually becomes worse, especially at night. The nose runs and sneezing may be a marked feature, particularly in cases under two years of age, the face is puffy, and a little albumin may appear in the urine. A blood-count shows an increase of the leucocytes to 15,000 or 30,000, a high proportion being lymphocytes. Gradually, the cough becomes more and more spasmodic, i.e. it occurs in sudden severe spasms, followed by a comparatively long period quite free of cough. The child is wakened by the cough more and more frequently during the night. A small ulcer may appear on the frenum of the tongue, where the frenum impinges on the lower incisors. The duration of this phase varies considerably, in some cases being as short as 4 or 5 days.

2. *The Paroxysmal Phase.* At about this time, or just before, whooping-cough is strongly suspected and is usually diagnosed when the child begins to whoop and vomit. Young children, who seem able to anticipate an attack of coughing, run to their mother or nurse for support. Along with the bout of coughing the last food taken may be mechanically vomited. Each paroxysm of coughing ends in such a spasm that, on inspiration, a long drawn-out whoop may be heard, the face becoming cyanosed and the eyes bloodshot. A typical paroxysm may be said to consist of a series of short expiratory coughs, with a long inspiratory whoop, which is repeated until the spasm ceases. Mucus and saliva stream from the nose and mouth during the attack. This phase generally lasts about a fortnight but in some cases may be almost, or entirely, absent or last for many weeks.

3. *The Phase of Recovery.* During the last fortnight, the whole process rapidly retrogresses. The whoops become less frequent at night, so that the child's sleep is less disturbed. During the day there is less vomiting, and consequently the child begins to gain weight. By the end of this fortnight, in the average case, the cough has practically ceased.

In young infants the diagnosis may not be easy, as the characteristic whoop may never develop. Paroxysms of sneezing may usher in the attack, and sometimes repeated vomiting with occasional coughing may be the only symptoms.

Attacks Attenuated by Previous Immunization. In older children previously immunized against whooping-cough the attack may be so modified as to be almost unrecognizable. The whoop may never develop and vomiting may be slight, indeed a spasmodic cough may be the only sign of the disease. Nevertheless, such cases are infectious and should be suspected particularly when associated cases of the disease are known.

Recurrences. In some cases there is a continuance of the whoop, and bouts of coughing occur for many months. There seems no explanation, except that the child has acquired a habit or trick of whooping. Other children, who seem to recover completely, have a return of what appears to be a typical whoop whenever a respiratory infection is contracted during the next few months.

COMPLICATIONS

Undoubtedly one of the most distressing complications is convulsions. At the end of a bout of coughing the child, now extremely cyanosed, passes rapidly into a convulsion, which continues for some minutes. Such cases on the whole do extremely badly, and there appears to be a tendency to minute cerebral hæmorrhages at this time. Certainly, cases of hemiplegia are not unknown after whooping-cough convulsions.

Epistaxis is another quite common complication. It should be treated by keeping the child sitting up, and by applying cold compresses. Conjunctival hæmorrhages may also occur. Rarely hæmorrhages into vital organs such as the brain develop.

Wasting, due to vomiting, may be a serious complication in infants suffering from severe attacks. It is advisable during the stage when vomiting is most frequent either to feed the child again immediately after the vomit or to give frequent small feeds of thin fluids containing glucose, which can rapidly pass out of the stomach.

Primary tuberculosis is sometimes a co-incidental infection. In such circumstances what might have been a silent and benign Ghon focus may become a widespread and serious infection (*see* p. 580). Thus a tuberculin test is desirable and, if positive, a chest x-ray to exclude the possibility of an active infection.

Broncho-pneumonia is probably the most serious complication of whooping-cough. It occurs particularly in infants, and still has a definite mortality in this age-group.

Atelectasis is a frequent complication of whooping-cough, the right middle lobe and the lingular segment of the left upper lobe being most frequently affected. Such atelectasis may be responsible for persistence of the cough beyond the usual period. If re-expansion of the affected pulmonary segments does not occur *bronchiectasis* may develop.

Prolapse of the rectum, and umbilical and inguinal hernia may occur as a result of the abnormal strain imposed by the repeated coughing.

TREATMENT

In the catarrhal phase, the child is often best kept in bed, or at least off his legs. This is even more essential in the paroxysmal phase of the severe type of case as, with much whooping and vomiting, the child suffers from loss of weight and exhaustion. In a mild case, if the child is afebrile, he should be up and about, and in the garden if the weather is suitable. Cough sedatives may be used.

The diet should be light and essentially non-irritating to the pharynx; by this is meant the avoidance of dry or crumbly foods, such as toast or biscuits. Milky foods, such as junkets, milk puddings, custards, cereals well soaked in milk, gravy and potato, and nutritious soups, are best. It may be necessary to discontinue the regular times of meals for a short time, and feed young children immediately after a bout of whooping and vomiting. A sedative such as phenobarbitone or chlorpromazine may be given in an attempt to reduce the number of coughing spasms, particularly at night. Atropine and its derivatives are to be avoided in the early stages.

Chemotherapy. The introduction of chloramphenicol and the tetracyclines provided the first specific remedies for whooping-cough. They should be given during the first week of the disease to obtain the optimum effect.

For older children, the use of antibiotics is usually reserved for the most severe cases, particularly those in which broncho-pneumonia is present, and for children who are suffering from additional illnesses.

PROPHYLAXIS

Active Immunization. The best results are obtained from the use of dissolved vaccines prepared from strains of *H. pertussis* of the " type 1 phase " which have been proved to be capable of producing antibodies. Three injections are required at three- to four-week intervals. Such immunization should be undertaken at about 3–6 months of age, with a boosting dose at the age of five years. It is convenient to incorporate pertussis immunization in the triple inoculation which includes diphtheria and tetanus toxoid.

Immunization procedures should not be carried out during epidemics of poliomyelitis, owing to the risk of local paralysis occurring at the site of injection. Pertussis immunization is also contra-indicated in children who have had convulsions, as there may be further convulsions following injections, and occasionally permanent neurological sequelæ have occurred. It must be said, however, that such cases are extremely rare and in no way form a contra-indication to immunization among the rest of the child population.

CHICKENPOX (VARICELLA)

INCUBATION PERIOD

THIS is from 12 to 20 days, the child being infectious for two days before the vesicles appear. Cases are usually regarded as infectious for 14 days from the start of the rash, but in fact the risk of infection is very slight after the end of the first week. During the first week, however, it is one of the most highly infectious of all the acute specific fevers. Isolation in cubicles within a ward is rarely proof against infection. Chickenpox is caused by a filter-passing virus.

SYMPTOMS AND CLINICAL PICTURE

Chickenpox is one of the mildest diseases of childhood, but may occasionally take a very severe form. As a rule, the first signs of infection are the vesicles, but the child may have been out of sorts for a day or two previously. The rash appears as a series of red papules, which rapidly become vesicles or blisters. The temperature is usually 100°–102°F.

Distribution of Rash. The rash appears first on the trunk, face and scalp, then on the limbs, sometimes in the mouth. It is moderately itchy.

Fever develops with the appearance of the rash, but the temperature falls to normal within a day or two. Successive crops of the eruption may appear for several days, and pocks may be seen alongside one another in different stages of development.

TREATMENT

The child should be kept in bed during the period of fever. The main treatment should be directed towards the prevention of scratching, in order that scarring (particularly of the face) does not occur and the lesions do not become infected. This is best done by wearing loose, soft, smooth clothing, by the application of dusting powder or calamine lotion, and by keeping the child very cool.

COMPLICATIONS

The very rare encephalitis is the only serious complication.

DIPHTHERIA

DIPHTHERIA remains one of the most serious potential causes of mortality in childhood, and only widespread immunization is responsible for the great reduction in morbidity and mortality that has taken place over the last twenty years. In England and Wales, during 1959, 87 children under fifteen years of age were notified as suffering from diphtheria. There were no deaths. Nevertheless, there is apprehension that whilst the percentage of infants immunized against the disease remains as low as its present level of 56 per cent. of the total child population there is a real danger of a return of the large epidemics of the past. A further immunization should be given on school entry at five years of age.

INCUBATION PERIOD

This is between one to seven days, but is usually two to five days.

ÆTIOLOGY

Diphtheria is caused by infection with the *Corynebacterium diphtheriæ*. This can be differentiated into at least three culturally and serologically different types. They are termed *mitis, intermedius* and *gravis*. These different species are associated with clinical variations in the disease. The mitis type tends to produce a considerable volume of exudate and membrane at the site of infection, and thus when it affects the larynx, particularly of infants, is likely to cause death from respiratory obstruction. On the other hand, the intermedius and gravis strains produce less membrane but penetrate deeply into surrounding tissues, producing considerable œdema and the release of large quantities of toxin into the blood-stream, giving rise to generalized toxæmia, myocardial effects and subsequent neurological complications.

INCIDENCE

Diphtheria may occur at any age; it is rarely seen before one year, because passive immunity is transmitted from the mother.

PATHOLOGY

The organism tends to remain localized at the site of infection and does not invade the tissues deeply.[1] The toxins, however, are absorbed into the blood-stream and lymphatics. The intermedius and gravis strains show more tendency to local invasiveness and toxin production than the mitis form. The faucial membrane consists of fibrin, masses of necrotic cells and bacteria. The heart shows acute parenchymatous degeneration; the kidneys and liver cloudy swelling and fatty degeneration.

SYMPTOMS

The three chief forms of diphtheria are faucial, laryngeal and nasal; they may occur separately or in combination. Very occasionally, the ear, anus, vulva or skin abrasions may be infected.

CLINICAL PICTURE

Faucial Diphtheria. The onset is insidious, and although older children may complain of a sore throat such a lesion may not be suspected in the young child who complains only of general malaise, anorexia and pains in the limbs. Vomiting may occur.

In the early stages one or more patches of membrane resembling old ivory or washleather appear on the tonsils, rapidly spreading to the uvula; the fauces are red and œdematous. The membrane is firmly attached to the subjacent mucosa, and attempts to remove it cause bleeding. The cervical glands are enlarged and may be much enlarged with surrounding œdema, resulting in the so-called " bull-neck." The odour from the throat is fœtid and characteristic, and there is often a blood-stained nasal discharge.

The temperature is usually only slightly raised or may be normal throughout. The pulse-rate is rapid, being raised out of proportion to the temperature.

Although the face may be flushed in mild cases, in those of any severity, with much toxæmia, the complexion is pallid and grey. The patient may have a bloated appearance.

Laryngeal Diphtheria. The first sign of the onset of this is a change in the character of the voice. Later, the breathing becomes more difficult, with indrawing of the suprasternal space and recession of the ribs, and over-action of the muscles of respiration. Laryngeal inspiratory stridor develops and becomes increasingly severe. The lumen of the larynx is progressively reduced in size by œdema of its wall, and by the presence of necrotic exudate within. Cyanosis becomes obvious and steadily deepens. In severe cases, if untreated, death occurs from asphyxia or heart failure.

Nasal Diphtheria. This is usually an extension of the faucial form but may occur by itself, in which case it is comparatively benign. In the isolated nasal form, the lesion is in the anterior portion of the nares and may be accompanied by general symptoms, such as head-ache, shivering and vomiting, or with no symptoms apart from a profuse, watery or purulent blood-stained discharge, which may be unilateral. The cervical glands may be enlarged.

Cutaneous Diphtheria. Although rarely seen in the United Kingdom, diphtheritic infection of chronic skin lesions is not uncommon in tropical climates. Such lesions produce indolent ulceration and are subsequently attended by a high incidence of neurological complications.

About 2 per cent. of diphtheria cases used to suffer second attacks. It should be clear, therefore, that an attack of diphtheria does not necessarily render a person immune.

DIAGNOSIS

The clinical diagnosis is of much more importance—since on it treatment must be instituted—than the bacteriological diagnosis, which will not be available for 24 hours. A small dose of antitoxin given on the first day of the disease is of more value to a child than a large dose given 24 hours later. The clinical diagnosis is made on the appearance of the membrane covering the tonsils, uvula and soft palate, together with enlarged glands, nasal discharge, fœtor, and the fact that the membrane cannot be separated from its bed without causing bleeding. When the diagnosis is suspected clinically, the giving of antitoxin should never be delayed until the bacteriological confirmation of a suspected case is available.

Differential Diagnosis. The chief conditions likely to be mistaken for faucial diphtheria are acute follicular tonsillitis, Vincent's angina, acute leukæmia, glandular fever, streptococcal cervical adenitis and mumps.

Laryngeal diphtheria should be differentiated from simple laryngitis or croup and laryngo-tracheo-bronchitis; and nasal diphtheria from acute rhinitis and foreign body in the nostril.

The Schick Test. This test makes it possible to determine whether an individual is susceptible or immune to diphtheria. It is performed by injecting 0·2 ml. of a diluted diphtheria toxin into the skin of the forearm, intracutaneously. A control of heated toxin is used on the opposite arm. If the patient is not immune to diphtheria, a reaction appears round the injection, indicating that he is susceptible and should therefore be actively immunized. If the result is negative, nothing further need be done.

COMPLICATIONS

Various *neurological sequelæ* may develop as a consequence of diphtheria; they are described on pp. 423 and 553.

Cardiovascular system. During the initial stage of toxæmia a condition resembling shock may develop with evidence of peripheral circulatory failure. The patient is grey, cold, sweating, and collapsed, with a feeble pulse and a fall in blood-pressure. Subsequently signs of myocarditis may become apparent, with cardiac dilatation, weakness of the first sound at the apex, tic-tac rhythm and extrasystoles. Some degree of heart block is likely to occur, through damage to the conducting fibres, which may take the form of a complete or partial heart block or of bundle-branch block. Simple prolongation of the P–R interval, with or without dropped beats, may occur. An electrocardiogram taken early on will form a basis for comparison with subsequent examinations.

Vomiting occurring in association with other evidence of myocarditis is of severe prognostic importance. There is often a critical period at the end of the second week, but once this is survived the prognosis improves.

Other complications include *broncho-pneumonia, otitis media* and *albuminuria.*

PROGNOSIS

This depends on (1) the age of the child; in general, the younger the child the higher the mortality; (2) the day of the disease on which antitoxin is given; it is found that the mortality rises steeply for each day the antitoxin is delayed; (3) the type of infection and severity of reaction to the infecting organism, e.g. where the infecting organism is of the " gravis " type there is a correspondingly serious prognosis. Some children react badly to diphtheria; from the start they show palatal œdema, profuse nasal discharge, much glandular enlargement, oral fœtor and hæmorrhages into the skin, and despite big doses of antitoxin these fail to clear up.

Other signs of bad prognostic significance are: cardiac failure; thready pulse; persistent vomiting with signs of peripheral circulatory collapse; and early palatal paralysis, particularly if associated with paralysis of the diaphragm or pharyngeal muscles.

In an immunized patient diphtheria is a very mild condition, the exudate often being so slight as to make the diagnosis seem unlikely.

TREATMENT

Antitoxin. The prompt administration of diphtheria *antitoxin* is of prime importance and the aim should be to give all that is required in a single dose. A total dosage of 50,000–200,000 units is required, which may be given partly by intramuscular and partly by intravenous injection depending upon the severity of the case. The smaller dose is given for a simple nasal infection, the higher dose being used for a severe faucial and laryngeal infection. A preliminary intramuscular injection of 0·2 ml. is given and followed half an hour later by the full dose, provided that no reaction has occurred. In case of a reaction, adrenaline, antihistamines, and chlorpromazine should be immediately available. If a reaction occurs to the test dose, a series of graduated amounts of antitoxin are given under antihistamine coverage.

Antibiotics. Penicillin, although in no way replacing antitoxin, is a most useful ancillary treatment, especially in preventing secondary infection. It should be started at once, and continued until the membrane has cleared.

GENERAL MANAGEMENT

The patient should be isolated for as long as infection persists, and full barrier-nursing precautions employed. Absolute rest in bed, together with the early and adequate administration of antitoxin, are the keystones of successful treatment. The length of time for which absolute rest is necessary varies from case to case, but three weeks is probably the minimum for a mild case, whilst in severe cases ten or twelve weeks of complete rest may be required. For children, absolute rest is best obtained by allowing the child a pillow so that he can watch the activities around him without the temptation of continually wishing to raise his head from the pillow.

In cases in which palatal and pharyngeal paralysis develop, tube-feeding becomes necessary, and it is an essential part of treatment to watch for signs of such paralysis, so that inhalation of diet or vomitus can be avoided and tracheostomy, together with assisted respiration, undertaken in time.

Circulatory failure. During the early stages of the disease, circulatory failure may develop and may be associated with hæmorrhage into the suprarenals. Absolute rest, warmth and oxygen are necessary. Digoxin (for dosage, *see* Appendix 3) should be started if congestive cardiac failure develops. In the most severe cases, where the danger of acute suprarenal hæmorrhage seems likely, Eucortone (5 ml.) or desoxycorticosterone acetate (5 mg.) may be given daily as a prophylactic. If persistent vomiting and general collapse occur, indicating acute suprarenal failure, then intravenous cortisone acetate 50–100 mg. should be given immediately and repeated at least every four hours. Intravenous saline should be given also to combat the associated loss of salt and water.

Laryngeal Diphtheria. A moist atmosphere is helpful, and may be obtained by means of a steam kettle or by an atomizer. If respiratory obstruction becomes severe, with extreme restlessness, cyanosis and marked recession of the chest-wall, active measures are required. If skilled assistance is available, laryngeal intubation under direct vision and sucking out of the membrane is the treatment of choice. Such treatment may have to be repeated on several occasions. If no such treatment is available, or if laryngoscopy reveals that the obstruction is due to œdema rather than to exudate, tracheostomy is indicated and should be carried out without delay.

Neurological Complications. The necessity for tube-feeding in cases of palatal and pharyngeal paralysis has already been mentioned. In the rare cases of diaphragmatic paralysis the use of a respirator may be required, together with oxygen if the cyanosis is not controlled. If limb palsies develop, splintage and good nursing are required to prevent deformities.

Physiotherapy. For cases with limb palsies, active physiotherapy will be necessary.

FREEDOM FROM INFECTION

Before release from quarantine, cultures of the throat, nose and of any discharges should be taken; two successive negative results are a fair indication of freedom from infection.

PROPHYLAXIS AND IMMUNIZATION AGAINST DIPHTHERIA

Most infants carry over from their mother some immunity to the disease for the first few months, but rapidly lose this towards the end of the first year. It is customary to immunize infants between the ages of three and six months, except during epidemics of poliomyelitis, when the immunization should be delayed until the epidemic has ceased. For routine prophylaxis, the triple immunization which includes diphtheria pertussis and tetanus toxoid is advised. This is given as three injections of 1·0 ml. of the triple antigens at monthly intervals. For infants who have undergone convulsions it is inadvisable to use pertussis antigen, and in such circumstances a preparation containing only the diphtheria and tetanus toxoids should be used. A " boosting " dose of 1·0 ml. of triple antigen in normal circumstances should be given during the fourth year, before the child starts school.

For older children not previously immunized, who require only immunization against diphtheria, the combined toxin-antitoxin floccule (TAF) should be used, three doses of 1·0 ml. at four-weekly intervals being given. Three months after the initial immunization the child should have a Schick test done to make certain that immunity has been gained.

TYPHOID FEVER (ENTERIC FEVER)

THIS disease is caused by the *Salmonella typhi*.

Incubation is commonly 10 to 15 days, but may be from 5 to 23 days. As a rule, the patient is infected by means of water, milk, or milk products, such as ice-cream or cream, by shellfish, meat or fish, or by direct contact with a typhoid patient or " carrier." Outbreaks in institutions have occasionally been traced to a " carrier " in the kitchen. Ice and salads have both been found infected, the latter from contaminated soil.

CLINICAL PICTURE

Generally, the onset of the attack is gradual, with a slight headache, epistaxis and staircase-like rise of temperature. In a moderately severe case there is a gradual onset of delirium and drowsiness, followed by extreme prostration and toxæmia. The disease may be ushered in by acute diarrhœa and vomiting. The period of fever may continue for 3 weeks and sometimes longer. There is almost invariably some intestinal disturbance, either diarrhœa and vomiting at the beginning, or, later on, some degree of looseness of the bowels with pea-soup stools. Occasionally, however, there is obstinate constipation. Gradually, in the third or fourth week, the temperature settles, the tongue becomes clean, the appetite improves, the delirium ceases, and the patient begins to recover.

During the first few days of the illness, in the majority of cases the spleen is found to be enlarged, a sign which should always be sought.

The white count shows a normal number of white cells or a leucopenia.

The agglutination (Widal) test is seldom positive before the tenth day and reaches its maximum about the sixteenth day. It should not be considered positive unless it agglutinates the typhoid organism in a dilution of 1 in 25. As a rule, the test gives a positive agglutination in a dilution of from 1 in 250 to 1 in 1,000. Two specimens should be examined; the first taken as soon as the diagnosis is suspected, the second, two weeks later in order to demonstrate a rise in the titre at which agglutination takes place.

Cultures of the blood and urine may be positive during the first 4 or 5 days of the illness. The stool culture may be positive during the first weeks of the disease.

In a classical case of typhoid the pulse is slow and bounding, but this cannot be relied upon. The so-called " rose-spots " are diagnostic and appear at the beginning of the second week, usually over the abdomen, chest and back. They are round and are about the size of split peas or smaller, and disappear on pressure. They are few in number, usually not more than 4 or 6 being present at a time. Headache is, as a rule, very severe and, coupled with epistaxis, is most suggestive. One of the most alarming features of typhoid fever is the tendency to wasting. A limited quantity of food only can be administered and digested; in spite of a high continuous temperature, restlessness and delirium, the caloric requirements of the patient are extraordinarily high and in consequence wasting invariably occurs.

DIFFERENTIAL DIAGNOSIS

This is from pneumonia, meningitis, paratyphoid fever, brucellosis, subacute bacterial endocarditis, malaria, mononucleosis and miliary tuberculosis.

PATHOLOGY

There is a septicæmic stage during the first week and *S. typhi* is recoverable from the blood and urine as well as from the stools. Then the infection localizes in the intestine, especially in the lymphoid tissues, causing hyperplasia and ulceration of the Peyer's patches and swelling of the mesenteric glands and spleen. Evidence of toxicity is shown by cloudy swelling throughout all the organs and there may be a severe peripheral neuritis or encephalitis. The Peyer's patches slough and separate, leaving shallow ulcers, which tend to perforate. The sloughs may show a tendency to hæmorrhage.

TREATMENT

As soon as the diagnosis has been established, chloramphenicol should be started in full dosage (*see* p. 655) for one week and continued on a reduced dosage for a further ten days.

The patient should be isolated with full barrier-nursing precautions and kept in bed for at least three weeks. He should be given an abundance of sugar-water or fruit juice and water, and fed regularly on diluted milk thickened with some cereal preparation, such as Benger's Food, groats, cornflour, arrowroot, or broth thickened with potato. When the temperature subsides, soft solids should be added and soon a liberal nutritious diet is given.

The general management includes careful attention to the mouth, control of fever, prevention of bed-sores and treatment of constipation, for which petroleum emulsion is safest, aperients being avoided until there is no longer fear of perforation. As soon as the acute stage is over the child will require occupation in bed so as to avoid boredom. Convalescence is slow.

COMPLICATIONS

The chief complications are bronchitis, broncho-pneumonia, myocarditis, intestinal hæmorrhage and intestinal perforation; meningitis, thrombosis, osteomyelitis or neuritis are occasional.

PROPHYLAXIS

Combined typhoid and paratyphoid A and B vaccine is employed in routine immunization procedure. For a child of 5 to 10 years two doses of 0·2 ml. and 0·4 ml., with a two-weekly interval, should be given. The immunity conferred is of short duration, and if the patient is living in a country where contact with typhoid is probable, yearly " booster " doses of 0·4 ml. are required. A sharp febrile reaction may occur; to counteract this aspirin may be given two hours after the injection and repeated again after four hours.

PROGNOSIS

In children the mortality is extremely low, the complications of perforation and hæmorrhage of the bowel being less commonly seen than in adult patients. An exception to this good prognosis must be made in the case of infants.

PARATYPHOID FEVER

THIS is commoner in the United Kingdom than typhoid fever, and most of the epidemics of recent years have been of this variety. Paratyphoid has a clinical picture like that of a very mild form of typhoid. The duration of the fever is shorter, being from two to three weeks at most (Fig. 75). The feeling of malaise and general upset may be severe, but is more often mild or even slight. The organisms responsible are the *Salmonella paratyphi A*, *B* and *C*, and these can be demonstrated on culture of blood, urine and stools; later a positive agglutination (Widal) test is obtained.

UNDULANT FEVER (BRUCELLOSIS)

THIS is a preventable infection caused by *Brucella melitensis* and *Brucella abortus* and acquired from unpasteurized milk, milk products or meat, or less commonly from cattle or goats. It should not be overlooked when dealing with a rural community where the risk of the milk being unpasteurized is greater than in urban areas.

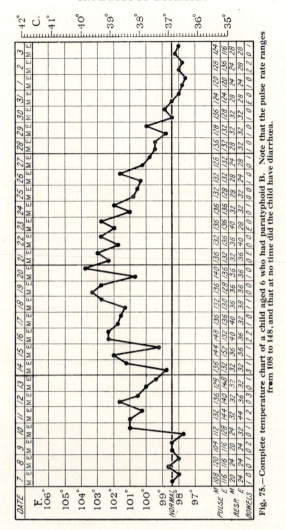

Fig. 75.—Complete temperature chart of a child aged 6 who had paratyphoid B. Note that the pulse rate ranges from 108 to 148, and that at no time did the child have diarrhoea.

CLINICAL COURSE

After an incubation of 5–30 days, this infection causes fever, malaise, sweating, mental depression and lassitude. The temperature fluctuates, sometimes being up continuously, but at other times undulating. It may rise slowly to a peak, and then come down over a period of days, then stay normal for a few days, and once more undulate; it may continue for many months. The spleen is usually palpable and pain in the limbs and acute arthritis coinciding with the episodes of fever may be a feature.

DIAGNOSIS

A positive blood culture is diagnostic. Failing this, an agglutination test should be carried out. When the patient is seen early in the course of the illness, it may be possible, by making two estimations with a two week interval, to demonstrate a rising agglutination titre. For cases seen later in the disease an agglutination titre of 1 in 4 or 1 in 16 should not be regarded as significant of active disease particularly in a rural community. A positive reaction to the intradermal injection of brucellin antigen is not of itself indicative of active disease. Indeed this procedure is of dubious value, as it may cause a subsequent slight rise in the agglutination titre and cause further difficulties in diagnosis.

TREATMENT

Combined therapy with tetracyclines, streptomycin and sulpha-diazine is recommended. It should be continued for at least 3 weeks. Relapses are common.

PROPHYLAXIS

Efficient pasteurization of milk affords protection.

INFLUENZA

INFLUENZA may be either of the epidemic type, in which event a large proportion of the population is affected, or sporadic. The incubation period is 1–3 days. It is highly infectious.

ÆTIOLOGY AND PATHOLOGY

Influenza is due to a *filter-passing virus*, which can be obtained in nasal washings from the patient. Two main groups of influenza virus have so far been isolated and are named influenza A and B; within each group numerous minor sub-groups exist, each with slightly different antigenic properties but with a common property of inducing either the influenza A or B antibody in the infected person. Influenza C virus has more recently been differentiated, giving rise to a mild febrile illness, and there is no doubt that numerous allied viruses are as yet unidentified. Both influenza A and B can give rise to widespread epidemics or remain endemic in a community. In general, however, influenza A shows more epidemic propensities than influenza B.

CLINICAL PICTURE

This may show great variations, both with the particular epidemic and from year to year. Usually, the onset is acute, the temperature rising suddenly to 102° or 103°F, with aching all over, a disinclination for food and a tendency to vomit. There may be a slight coryza or sore throat, and the tongue is dry and coated. Mild cases subside in two or three days, but the more severe cases may last for a week or longer. In addition to a general toxæmia, there is also, it is believed, a viræmia. The respiratory system is often affected, usually only the upper respiratory tract, but sometimes extending down to the smaller tubes, giving rise to bronchitis, bronchiolitis or broncho-pneumonia.

Epidemic nausea and vomiting, also called *epidemic viral gastro-enteritis*, is caused by a separate virus which has its main effect on the stomach. It has been described as an epidemic disease in hospitals, schools and other institutions. The symptoms come on very suddenly and are of short duration. The infection has been produced experimentally in human volunteers by feeding fæcal filtrates and throat washings.

DIAGNOSIS

The chief difficulty in diagnosis arises in sporadic infections, and the name " influenza " is often given without justification because the symptoms are so indefinite. Later, the true nature of the complaint is disclosed, and the mistake becomes apparent. The diagnosis of influenza should not be made without a thorough examination to exclude more serious diseases. There is no greater trap for the unwary physician than a small child presenting with appendicitis in the midst of an influenza epidemic in which vomiting is one of the predominating symptoms. In difficult cases the white-cell count may be helpful, since influenza shares with typhoid fever the peculiarity that there is no leucocytosis, but rather a tendency to leucopenia.

Confirmation of the diagnosis in the laboratory is still complex and not yet in routine use. Direct culture of the virus from nasal washings and stools is possible on special media. A rise in the titre of influenza A or B antibody between the start of the disease and the convalescent stage can also be demonstrated.

PROGNOSIS

On the whole the prognosis in children is excellent, the mortality being restricted to certain virulent epidemics in which a fulminating bronchiolitis is a feature. Occasionally encephalitis (p. 411) is seen in particular epidemics and this also gives rise to fatalities.

TREATMENT

The child should, where possible, be kept apart from other members of the family.

Where the respiratory tract involvement is extensive, penicillin or a broad spectrum antibiotic may be given from the start; although this treatment has no effect on the virus, secondary infections with hæmolytic streptococci, *Staph. pyogenes* and pneumococci may be suppressed.

In the acute stage the child must be made to drink.   With defervescence, light diet is introduced.

Where the symptoms are largely gastro-intestinal, infants will require the therapy described on p. 195 to make good their dehydration.

COMPLICATIONS AND SEQUELÆ

Bronchitis, pneumonia, otitis media and nasal sinusitis are the chief complications.

OTHER VIRUS INFECTIONS

IN recent years progress has been made in the laboratory identification of a number of the viruses responsible for some of the mild febrile illnesses so commonly seen in general practice.   At present the laboratory techniques used are difficult and costly and are thus not generally available for routine use.   In the United Kingdom, the Public Health Laboratory Service obtain sufficient material in the form of nasal washings and paired samples of sera to determine the degree of prevalence of the identifiable virus infections in the community at any particular time.   In addition, material from epidemics at the time unidentifiable is stored at low temperatures so that, as new viruses are identified, improved techniques can be applied to provide retrospective diagnosis of past epidemics.   Undoubtedly much work remains to be done, both in the identification of viruses at present unknown and in the simplification of present virus laboratory techniques.

ADENOVIRUS GROUP

A GROUP of antigenically similar viruses is now described under this name.   They include a number of allied viruses of which one was initially known as the APC virus.   Clinically, the type of infection varies from a pharyngitis or upper respiratory catarrhal infection to a type in which cervical glandular enlargement predominates.   At least 18 types of adenovirus have been isolated; type 8 gives rise to an epidemic kerato-conjunctivitis.   A remarkable feature of the adenoviruses is their ability to persist in lymphoid tissue for a long time and thus provide a continuing source of infection.   The incubation period is thought to be 5–7 days.

ENTEROVIRUS GROUP

THESE include Coxsackie, ECHO, and the poliomyelitis viruses.

Within the Coxsackie virus group at least 25 substrains have been identified, of which 19 are classified as Coxsackie A virus and 6 under Coxsackie B virus type.   Although complete clinical correlation with the laboratory strains is still not possible, certain clinical groupings can be described.

Coxsackie A Virus Infection

There are three main forms of clinical infection caused by the antigenic types of Coxsackie A virus:

1. *Herpangina.* The child becomes feverish with a vesicular eruption limited to the posterior pharynx and soft palate. The back of the tongue may also be involved. As the vesicles rupture, shallow ulcers develop comparable to those seen on the anterior part of the tongue and buccal mucosa in acute ulcerative stomatitis due to herpes simplex infection (p. 188). The infection runs a benign course but there may be associated cases of Coxsackie A meningitis (*see* below) so that the condition has epidemiological significance.

2. *Acute lymphadenitis.* Coxsackie A virus may also give rise to fever and enlargement of the lymphatic glands in the neck, groins and axillæ resembling glandular fever. A particular feature of the illness may be muscle spasm adjacent to the enlarged glands. The illness may run a relapsing course for six or eight weeks during which time a low-grade fever may persist.

3. *Benign lymphocytic meningitis.* This clinical reaction is less common than in Coxsackie B virus infection but cases due to the A strains have been described, particularly in South Africa. The clinical picture is described on p. 410.

Coxsackie B Virus Infection

There are six antigenic types. Among the clinical conditions associated with Coxsackie B virus infection are included:

1. *Bornholm Disease* or *Epidemic Pleurodynia.* After an incubation of two to four days, there is a sudden onset of acute pain usually localized either in the chest or anterior abdominal wall. In the former case a mistaken diagnosis of pleurisy may be made and, in the latter, surgeons have been known to open the abdomen, suspecting a perforated peptic ulcer or other abdominal emergency. A dromedary type of temperature chart is commonly seen, in which the first "hump" of temperature lasts for forty-eight hours followed, after a twenty-four hour period of normality, by a second hump of similar duration to the first. There is usually localized muscle tenderness at the site of the pain, and the condition is considered to be the result of a focal myositis. The condition is entirely benign and runs a self-limited course.

2. *Benign Lymphocytic Meningitis.* Coxsackie B virus probably accounts for a fairly large proportion of the cases of benign viral meningitis as described on p. 409. There is no doubt that in a small number of cases due to this infection paralysis of muscles may occur, thus giving a close resemblance to poliomyelitis.

3. *Infantile Myocarditis.* Small infants exposed to Coxsackie B virus infection may develop an overwhelming viræmia with encephalitis, hepatitis and severe myocarditis. In a number of such cases the diagnosis has been confirmed at autopsy by direct identification of the virus.

Echo Virus Group

About twenty viruses of this group (enteric cytopathogenic virus of human origin) have been recovered from patients suffering from febrile exanthemata, diarrhœa or benign lymphocytic meningitis (p. 409). Biologically the virus is similar to though antigenically different from the poliomyelitis and Coxsackie viruses. ECHO virus from pharyngeal secretions, fæces and cerebrospinal fluid can be grown in tissue culture.

Poliomyelitis Virus Group *(see p. 417)*

SG Virus (Cytomegalic Inclusion-duty Disease)

This virus is separate from the other groups. For clinical features *see* p. 99.

Cat Scratch Fever

This is a viral infection which usually follows a cat scratch or bite. After an incubation period of 3–10 days fever develops, the lymph nodes draining the affected area of skin enlarge, and usually pus forms. A diagnostic skin test, using Forshay's antigen prepared from affected glands of other patients, can be applied intradermally. No treatment other than incision of an abscess, if formed, is required. The pus is sterile. Spontaneous resolution of the infection takes 2–6 weeks.

Smallpox (Variola). *See* p. 620.

Vaccination

Vaccination remains the chief method of prophylaxis against smallpox, and children who have been recently vaccinated are almost entirely immune to the disease. Complications *(see* p. 516) are least common when it is undertaken between one and two years of age. It is contraindicated in infants suffering from infantile eczema in view of the possible complication of a generalized eruption *(see* p. 505). There is even a potential danger to such children if other members of the household are vaccinated; thus it is necessary to warn the family of the dangers of contagious infection by means of towels or direct contact between the vaccinated person and the child with infantile eczema.

METHOD

The arm should be cleansed with Cetavlon and the calf lymph applied at one spot. Then, with a sterile needle or scalpel, held flush with the skin, a tiny scratch should be made just through the epidermis, insufficient to draw blood; alternatively the skin may be penetrated by means of a special vaccination applicator. Immediately after this, a sterile dressing should be applied and firmly strapped in place with adhesive plaster. In girls, the leg, preferably the outer surface of the thigh, may be used; if the buttock is chosen, the site of vaccination is more likely to be infected. The following directions should be given to the mother:

1. The arm must be kept absolutely dry. If it should get wet in bathing, the dressing must be changed at once. Do not use boracic lint or powder.

2. Once the vaccination " takes," it reaches its height in 9 or 10 days and then commences to heal rapidly.

Post-vaccinal Encephalitis

Encephalitis is a rare complication, symptoms commencing about 7–14 days after vaccination. It may start with drowsiness, vomiting and convulsions. The complication occurs most commonly in older children, not in the infant and young child, or in those who have been previously vaccinated. After a short illness the child usually recovers completely, though the condition may be fatal. For management, see p. 412.

Other complications of vaccination include *eczema vaccination* or *Kaposi's varicelliform* eruption (p. 516) and *vaccinia gangrenosa* (p. 516). The vaccination of the pregnant mother may very occasionally cause a generalized vaccinial reaction in the fœtus.

FEVER DIET

IN acute febrile disturbances that are likely to run a short and fierce course, one of the most important considerations, from the standpoint of patient, nurse and doctor, is the diet. As a rule, the child refuses food and wants drinks only. The tongue is dirty and coated, the breath offensive, and constipation is present, due partly to confinement in bed but chiefly to dehydration and lack of solid diet.

The constituents of the diet which throw least work on digestion, and yet supply it with the calories it demands in the most readily assimilable form, are sugar and cereal.

At least two pints of plain water, sugar-water, barley-water or well-sweetened fruit juice and water should be taken every 24 hours (2 to 4 years of age). It is as well to keep a jug of such drinks within the child's sight as an invitation to him to take more. If the child is able to take sufficient quantities at a time, the regular times of feeding (breakfast, dinner and tea) should be adhered to, but more frequent drinks should also be offered. At first, cornflour or other cereal preparations, made with water, should be administered, since they have a very high caloric value and can be made palatable. These foods can be made up with skimmed milk if desired, but certainly not more than half to three-quarters of a pint of milk should be given in the day. Bovril or beef tea is useful. Broth, made from veal, chicken or beef bones, is recommended, preferably thickened with breadcrumbs or potato or other starchy substance. Plain water-ices are permitted.

In chronic conditions, such as rheumatoid arthritis and tuberculosis, the patient will, on the other hand, require " feeding up " almost from the first. The maximum caloric intake which the patient is capable of digesting may be given, and protein is essential. (For further details *see under* each individual disease.)

CONGENITAL SYPHILIS

THE incidence of congenital syphilis has declined markedly with improvements in the treatment of acquired syphilis and the serological testing of pregnant women as a routine in the ante-natal clinic.

In 1913 the death rate in England and Wales from syphilis in infants under one year was 146 per 100,000 live births; by 1938 it had declined to 20, and by 1959 to 0·3 per 100,000 live births. The number of new cases seen in the treatment centres under one year of age in 1959 was 20, and between the ages of 1 year and 14 years 48. Congenital syphilis is therefore no longer a major problem in pædiatrics in the United Kingdom and has in fact become a clinical rarity.

ÆTIOLOGY

Syphilis is the result of an infection by the *Treponema pallidum*. In most cases the father has contracted syphilis and has passed on the infection to the mother who has given birth to a syphilitic infant. It is an interesting fact that very often the mother shows no clinical signs of the disease, although she may have a positive Wassermann reaction. Wassermann and Kahn tests should be applied to both mother and child; as a rule, if positive in one they will be positive in the other also. Although the Wassermann reaction in the father may be negative, this does not prove that he was not the primary infecting agent, as he may have had treatment after infecting his wife.

There is no doubt that congenital syphilis is potentially infectious but recorded instances of cross-infection to other children are extremely rare.

PATHOLOGY

The *Treponema pallidum* causes an inflammation near the blood-vessel, the reaction to which shows the presence of round cells; later, fibrosis occurs. *T. pallidum* is best demonstrated in the liver, but a confirmation of the diagnosis depends largely on the Wassermann reaction. The cerebrospinal fluid will often reveal a positive reaction.

CLINICAL PICTURE

A syphilitic infant may be born dead, either at full term or prematurely. It may be a macerated fœtus, the placenta being infected, friable and containing infarcts. A history marked by such events as the following is quite common: first, an abortion at 2 or 3 months; then possibly another at 5 months; then a premature birth or stillbirth at 7 months; and finally a full-term child apparently quite healthy. At birth, as a rule, the infant shows no signs of syphilis. In a very few cases, the rash is present at birth or develops within the first week; in the great majority of cases, it develops between the fourth and eighth weeks. The rash may be a *macular* one, which appears on the buttocks, the palms of the hands, the soles of the feet and the legs; it is pale-red or *copper-coloured*, and has a shiny, dry, silky appearance. It may be present over the whole body, but this is uncommon. (Fig. 76.)

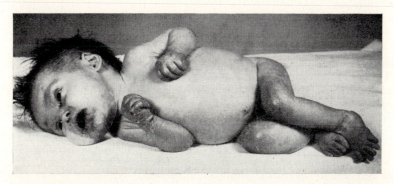

Fig. 76.—An infant with congenital syphilis. Observe the distribution of the rash; it is present round the mouth, where there is also some fissuring, and on the hands and feet, with peeling of the fingers and toes. Sometimes this rash has a rather coppery colour, and there may be moderate œdema. In this case the rash has extended to the thighs.

Syphilitic pemphigus, which occurs on the soles of the feet, palms of the hands, the knees and sometimes the face, does not usually appear for two or three weeks, but occasionally the infant is born with it. There may be a syphilitic wig, that is, the hair may be thick, black and straight, but this is of no great importance, as many normal infants have a profuse growth of hair. *Snuffles* is one of the earliest symptoms; it may be present at birth or appear within a few days, or develop after some weeks. Snuffles is due to a syphilis of the septum and turbinate bones, in which other organisms take part, causing a muco-purulent discharge and destruction of the nasal bones. The

19

bridge of the nose then falls in, and the flat, saddle-shaped nose results. *Rhagades*, or scarring about the mouth, in its most typical form is best seen in older children. In the younger child it assumes the picture of sores about the mouth or merely roughness. In older children a syphilitic perforation of the soft palate may very occasionally be seen. In young infants with syphilis the cry is often hoarse, due to *syphilitic laryngitis*. In about half the cases there is an enlargement of the spleen within a few weeks of birth. A newborn infant with an enlarged spleen, whether it has any of the other manifestations of syphilis or not, is suspect; combined with other manifestations of syphilis, this renders the diagnosis almost certain.

Syphilis of the Bones. One of the earliest manifestations of syphilis is that of Parrot's pseudo-paralysis. The child develops acute syphilitic *epiphysitis*, usually at the upper end of the humerus, but it may be elsewhere. The arm is not used, and the question is raised whether a fracture may have occurred at birth unnoticed. As a rule, however, there are other manifestations of syphilis which help in the diagnosis. The commonest lesion in congenital syphilis is *osteitis*, best seen in the tibiæ, which show bowing and forward curving, and in the thickened skull-bones, especially in the bossing over the frontal and occipital regions. A syphilitic dactylitis shows a typical periostitis in the x-ray (*see also* p. 491).

Syphilitic Meningitis. Cases of syphilitic meningitis, as a rule, manifest themselves by hydrocephalus of the communicating type. The head becomes larger and larger, the spleen may be palpable, and the child may show other signs of syphilis. The Wassermann and Kahn reactions will be positive in the blood or cerebrospinal fluid. It is always advisable to test the mother at the same time.

Mental Deficiency. In syphilitic meningitis there is likely to be accompanying damage to the cerebrum (meningo-encephalitis). Mental deficiency is also possible even in the absence of these evidences of cerebral involvement, although, in general, syphilis is a very rare cause of such deficiency.

Lesions of the Eyes. The commonest lesion is *choroiditis*, when black or dark patches may be seen scattered over the choroid. This is possible at any age. *Interstitial keratitis* comes on, as a rule, during second dentition, between the ages of six and twelve. With photo-phobia, opacities of the cornea, and peg-shaped teeth or some other manifestation of syphilis, the diagnosis is comparatively easy.

Syphilitic Hepatitis. In this there are often two processes at work: (*a*) miliary gummata with fine, intercellular cirrhosis; (*b*) localized patches of gummatous material, sometimes beneath the capsule.

Among other manifestations of congenital syphilis, though rare, are dactylitis, diffuse infiltration of the testis, and involvement of the heart or kidneys.

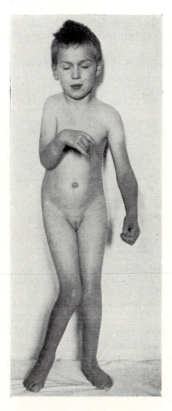

Fig. 77.—Right-sided hemiplegia in an 8-year-old girl who was the sub-ject of congenital syphilis.

White pneumonia in the newborn infant is also extremely rare; there is an interstitial fibrosis of syphilitic origin, involving the whole of one lung.

The Teeth. Peg-shaped or Hutchinsonian teeth (Fig. 78) are extremely characteristic of congenital syphilis. These appear in the second dentition only. The broadest portion of the peg is next to the gum, the free edge being narrow in all dimensions, with a characteristic crescentic notch.

TREATMENT

Just as in adult syphilis, the longer the lesion has existed the harder it is to eradicate the infection from the body, and the more likelihood there is of permanent damage. In congenital syphilis the infection has been acquired *in utero* and has existed for some months before the child's birth. The infection is therefore very widely spead throughout the tissues and some of the vital organs are already grossly damaged.

Penicillin, as the primary therapeutic agent, has replaced the older treatments in both acquired and congenital syphilis. Many workers consider that penicillin alone provides adequate cure of congenital lesions whilst others, more cautious and perhaps recalling the false

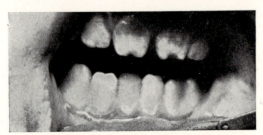

Fig. 78.—Hutchinsonian teeth of congenital syphilis.

prophets of short cures with other drugs, still advise subsequent treatment with bismuth or arsenic or both.

Penicillin is given intramuscularly in doses of 1 mega unit twice each day for fourteen days to a patient in whom the diagnosis has been made within the first few weeks of life. For older children increased dosage is required for a rather longer period, i.e. up to twenty-eight days.

PROGNOSIS

Infants in whom there are gross manifestations of syphilis at or shortly after birth show a high mortality and, if they survive, exhibit, as a rule, some permanent disability. If the manifestations are delayed for some weeks or months and treatment is begun immediately they commence, there is good hope of the child being quite cured; that is, the clinical manifestations clear up, there is a permanently negative result to the Wassermann reaction, and no further recurrences take place. Of all the manifestations, eye symptoms are the most difficult to eradicate. In the mentally defective child improvement but not recovery takes place. It is obvious that the ultimate prognosis depends entirely on the organs affected and the duration of infection before treatment is instituted.

CHAPTER 25

Tuberculosis

TUBERCULOSIS affecting children should not be considered as an isolated problem but one in relation to the health of the community, for the incidence and severity of the disease in childhood is determined by its prevalence in the child's environment, the natural resistance of the individual and of the general population, and by the success of preventive work, including case-finding and case-treatment, vaccination with BGG, and the elimination of bovine tuberculosis.

The most common tuberculous lesion in childhood is, of course, *primary tuberculosis* occurring as a result of the child's first infection with the tubercle bacillus. In most cases, no further evidence of the disease is seen, but, in a minority, signs of hæmatogenous dissemination occur, giving rise to foci of infection in organs remote from the site of the original primary lesion or even to *miliary tuberculosis.* Alternatively, or in addition, local complications may develop around the primary lesion. Finally, *post-primary lesions* may develop in the lungs, which may be either *early* or *late*, according to their time relation to the initial infection. Among the latter, *adult phthisis* is to be included, for although the possibility that an individual in the post-primary stage may develop adult phthisis through further contact with infected persons cannot be entirely dismissed (exogenous re-infection), it seems probable that most cases arise either from a hæmatogenous or local spread from the original lesion (endogenous re-activation).

Bacteriology

The tubercle bacillus, *M. tuberculosis,* was first isolated by Robert Koch in 1882. It is a slender rod-shaped bacillus, staining with basic dyes and retaining these stains despite treatment with acid and alcohol. Various types of *M. tuberculosis* have now been recognized: human, bovine, avian, and vole, of which only the first two are pathogenic to man.

In pulmonary lesions, the bacilli may be recovered from sputum or, in children who swallow their secretions, from gastric washings and sometimes from the stool. It may be recovered from lesions in other parts of the body; from caseous glands, tuberculous abscesses; in urological lesions from the urine; and in tuberculous meningitis from the cerebrospinal fluid. The organism can be recognized by direct staining by the Ziehl-Neelsen method, or by culture on special media such as the Lowenstein slope, or by animal inoculation of infected material, the guinea-pig being the test animal usually selected.

Pathology

PRIMARY TUBERCULOSIS

The initial tuberculous infection in a child or young adult gives rise to a *primary complex*, consisting of a primary focus of entry of bacilli and involvement of regional lymph nodes. The primary complex may be derived from a primary focus in the lungs, intestine, pharynx or skin. The most common site is the lung, where the primary focus is usually found in a peripheral (sub-pleural) position, the apices rarely being affected. Multiple primary foci may sometimes occur. The focus consists of a small area of tuberculous pneumonia, which later forms a small central area of caseation surrounded by granulation tissue containing tuberculous giant-cells, small round-cells, plasma-cells and, later, fibrous tissue. This is often termed a *Ghon focus*. Later, the lesion resolves into a small area of calcification surrounded by fibrous tissue. In some cases a necrotic centre persists, in which viable tubercle bacilli may remain as a potential source of endogenous re-activation should the lesion break down. Shortly after the primary focus has arisen, the lymphatic gland draining the area becomes infected, and enlargement, often associated with tuberculous caseation and the production of giant cells, occurs. In the case of primary intra-thoracic lesions the broncho-pulmonary glands will be so affected. These glands may either heal by calcification or develop necrotic centres, sometimes with ulceration into the lumen of the bronchus.

The term "primary complex" refers to both the primary tuberculous focus and also to the infected draining lymphatic gland. Primary tuberculous complexes in parts of the body other than the lung retain the same basic pathological pattern. The primary focus, when it occurs on the skin or mucous membrane, takes the form of an ulcer, consisting of tuberculous granulation tissue, which slowly heals and is always associated, as in the lungs, with infection and enlargement of the appropriate draining lymphatic gland.

Extensions from the Primary Complex. Extensions from the primary complex may occur in various ways; there may be a local extension from the pulmonary lesion by infiltration or bronchogenic spread; alternatively, generalized hæmatogenous or lymphatic dissemination may occur. Similar dissemination may arise from an infected lymphatic gland. In addition, mechanical complications may develop in the lung in the form of *atelectasis*, due to occlusion of a bronchus by tuberculous lymphadenitis, either by external pressure or, more usually, by an endobronchial lesion; there may even be ulceration by the gland through the wall of the bronchus and the formation of tuberculous granulation tissue within the lumen of the bronchus.

Owing to the usual sub-pleural position of the Ghon focus, involvement of the pleura may occur, with the subsequent development of *pleurisy* and *effusion*.

DISSEMINATED TUBERCULOSIS

This may occur as a result of hæmatogenous or lymphatic spread. If such spread is initially lymphatic in origin, hæmatogenous spread occasionally follows as a result of spill-over of tubercle bacilli via the thoracic duct into the blood-stream. Such spread may only be manifest in the lungs, either as multiple small apical foci which heal by scarring or calcification (*Simon foci*), or as single large foci which form necrotic centres (*Assmann foci*), again usually in the apical region.

More intense hæmatogenous dissemination may also occur. This may take the form of miliary tuberculosis, or seeding may take place in certain sites. It appears that some organs are favourable places for such metastatic infections; these include the meninges and central nervous system, the kidneys, adrenal glands, the epididymis and Fallopian tubes (usually in young adults rather than children), spleen, bones and joints. The pathology of these lesions is described under the appropriate section.

ADULT TYPE PHTHISIS

Usually this is due to the formation of a fibrocaseous lesion, situated characteristically in one or both lung apices. Some cases of adult-type phthisis derive from the extension or re-activation of some part of a primary complex, while others develop from an incompletely healed hæmatogenous lung focus (*Simon focus*) which becomes transformed into an *Assmann focus* (*see* above).

Resistance and Immunity

The natural resistance of the individual and his ability to develop specific immunity to the disease play a large part in determining the course which the primary infection will take and the frequency with which complications will occur. This resistance is partly determined by the inherited resistance of the stock from which the child springs, and partly by his own state of nutrition and the presence of inter-current infections.

Active immunity develops during the stage of recovery from the primary infection, but tends to fall off over a period of years. Artificial active immunity may be induced by the use of BCG (*see* p. 586) in patients who have not undergone a primary infection. Immunity is to be regarded as distinct from tuberculin sensitivity (*see* p. 572).

TUBERCULIN SENSITIVITY (ALLERGY)

Following a primary tuberculous infection or successful BCG vaccination, a greater or lesser degree of sensitivity towards tuberculin is acquired, and subsequent percutaneous or intradermal inoculation with tuberculin produces an inflammatory reaction at the site of the inoculation (for details of tuberculin testing, *see* p. 573). This tuberculin sensitivity or allergy develops soon after the beginning of a natural primary infection and also after a successful BCG vaccination. High degrees of allergy are shown by exaggerated responses to tuberculin. Similarly, allergic responses indicating hypersensitivity to tuberculosis may occur during the course of a primary infection in the form of erythema nodosum (*see* p. 577). It is probable also that similar inflammatory exudates can occur locally in the lung tissue as a result of hypersensitivity. A high degree of allergy, however, is not quantitatively related to immunity, since such patients may develop complicated and progressive lesions. After a number of years the degree of allergy to tuberculosis often begins to wane. A person who, with the passage of time, has lost his tuberculin sensitivity and most of his specific immunity could, in theory, acquire primary tuberculosis a second time; this has, in fact, occasionally been observed.

Epidemiology and Incidence

Infection by the human type of bacillus accounts for the great majority of cases, and in a large proportion of infected children a direct contact can be traced among the relatives or neighbours of the patient. Droplet infection is by far the most common mode of transmission. Discharges from infected sinuses or other infected material are far less frequent causes. Overcrowding, poor ventilation and poor nutrition make such spread more likely. Until recent years there was a considerable incidence of bovine tuberculosis; unsterilized cows' milk frequently contained living tubercle bacilli and therefore infection with bovine-type bacilli was common. In most Western countries bovine tuberculosis has now been eliminated; in others, compulsory sterilization or pasteurization has made bovine-type infection rare.

Since effective chemotherapy has become available, the decline in the incidence of tuberculosis has become steeper. There are now plenty of sanatorium beds for " open " cases and therefore the hazard of the sanatorium " waiting list " has been removed. With these reduced risks of acquiring primary infections, primary tuberculosis in children has become a comparatively uncommon condition in many parts of the United Kingdom and in the Scandinavian countries. Vaccination with BCG is a further prophylactic weapon (*see* p. 586).

DIAGNOSIS

THE following methods of diagnosis are available:

(*a*) Tuberculin skin tests.

(*b*) Search for tubercle bacilli in sputum, stomach washings, stools, urine or purulent discharges.

(*c*) X-rays.

(*d*) Sedimentation rate.

Skin Tests

INTRACUTANEOUS TUBERCULIN TEST (MANTOUX TEST)

This is performed by injecting 0·1 ml. of a solution of 1 in 10,000, 1 in 1,000, or 1 in 100 dilution of old tuberculin *into* the skin, just as in the Schick test. 0·1 ml. of 1 in 100 O.T. contains 100 tuberculin units. The test should be read after 48 hours and the reaction is usually present up to a fortnight thereafter. Where tuberculous infection is strongly suspected, the more dilute solutions are first used but, when negative, the stronger solutions should then be tried. The solution of old tuberculin should be freshly prepared for use; a solution that has been kept for longer than a week, even in a refrigerator, begins to lose its potency and becomes unreliable.

MULTIPLE-PUNCTURE TUBERCULIN TEST (HEAF-GUN TEST)

The Heaf gun is a simple device with a trigger which makes multiple pricks in the skin to a suitable depth through a drop of tuberculin solution. It is comparable in accuracy to a Mantoux test.

TUBERCULIN-JELLY TEST

A convenient method of tuberculin testing is by the use of a jelly containing old tuberculin. The skin between the shoulder blades is cleaned with acetone and the jelly applied in some characteristic shape, such as a " V " or " T." A piece of adhesive (*e.g.* 2 in. by 1 in.) is then applied immediately, directly over the jelly, and left on for 48 hours; after its removal the site of the application is noted daily for several days (Fig. 79). A control jelly is used in exactly similar fashion to avoid misinterpretation of results. The positive reaction approximates to that of the Mantoux (1 in 1,000 dilution) intradermal test, with about 95 per cent. of its accuracy. It is less reliable in adolescents and adults than an intradermal test.

VALUE OF THE SKIN TESTS

The greatest value can be attached to either a positive or negative reaction in infancy or early childhood—say, below the age of six or eight years. In older children the possibility of the child having had his primary infection some time before is greater. Tuberculin sensitivity, once established, usually persists for a period of years and sometimes for life. Thus, a positive reaction may either indicate recent and active infection or an old and inactive one. An inquiry must be made concerning previous BCG inoculation. Where doubt exists a history of contact, x-ray examination, and the ESR will help in evaluating the position.

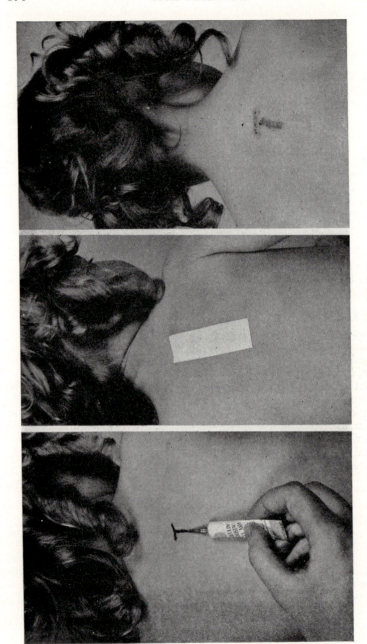

Fig. 79.—Tuberculin-jelly test.

Left: Application after cleansing the skin with acetone. *Centre:* Adhesive plaster has been applied over the tuberculin jelly. *Right:* The adhesive plaster was removed after 48 hours and, on the third day, the test is seen to be positive.

Search for Tubercle Bacilli in Stomach Washings and Stools

Where tuberculosis is suspected because of contact and the tuberculin tests are positive, or a lesion in the chest or abdomen is thought to be actively tuberculous, the assistance of the pathologist should be sought. Since it is impossible to obtain a fair sample of sputum from infants and young children in the ordinary way, gastric lavage is performed to obtain the swallowed secretions. In a high percentage of cases the organism may be found. It may, however, be necessary to inoculate a guinea-pig with the sediment. The stools can also be examined in this way after antiformin has been added. Occasionally tubercle bacilli may be recovered from the urine of patients with primary intrathoracic tuberculosis during the stage of hæmatogenous dissemination.

X-rays

The value of x-rays in the diagnosis is very great indeed. With a positive skin test, even without physical signs in the chest, every child should be x-rayed. It cannot be overstressed that it is characteristic for the physical signs to be few or entirely absent in the early stages, although quite a gross and obvious lesion may be seen by x-rays. In primary tuberculosis in other sites the x-ray is of less assistance. Only in the healing stage of abdominal tuberculosis will the x-ray reveal retrospective evidence of infection as calcification becomes obvious in mesenteric glands.

Sedimentation Rate

If the lesion be an old healed one, the erythrocyte sedimentation rate will be normal. If, however, it is recent and active, the sedimentation rate will usually be raised from the normal (3 to 10 mm.) to 20 or 30 mm. or more in the hour. As long as the sedimentation rate is raised, the lesion should be considered active. The sedimentation rate is often a more certain guide to the activity of the lesion than the temperature or the clinical and general condition.

PRIMARY INFECTION OF THE LUNGS
(Primary Tuberculosis)

MODE OF INFECTION

THE tubercle bacilli are air-borne from infected sputum and are inhaled by the infant or child. The bacilli lodge in the wall of a bronchiole, beneath the pleural surface, and cause the initial lesion known as the *primary focus*.

Sometimes the source of the infection may be obvious, such as one or other of the parents. Often, the infant is infected by a visiting grandparent who is apparently in good health but has a long-standing cough, or by a kindly well-meaning neighbour. Careful inquiry will almost always reveal a contact in the case of a young child.

MODE OF SPREAD

Once the lung focus is established, the organisms multiply and invade the neighbouring alveoli, producing a localized pneumonic process which may affect a few alveoli only or, sometimes, in the case of an infant, a large part of a lobe.

Next, the tubercle bacilli spread from the primary focus along the lymphatics (causing a lymphangitis) to the glands draining the

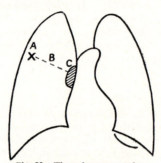

Fig. 80.—The primary complex.
A. Subpleural tuberculous lesion
       of the lung (primary focus).
B. Tuberculous lymphangitis.
C. Hilar gland.

adjacent area. These are most commonly the broncho-pulmonary, tracheo-bronchial and paratracheal glands. The primary focus, the tuberculous lymphangitis and the glandular lesion are known as the *primary complex*.

INCUBATION PERIOD

This is the period between the first introduction of the organisms into the body and their passage into the glands with an inflammatory reaction sufficient to cause tuberculin allergy, including the development of hypersensitivity of the skin. This period lasts *from three to twelve weeks* (*see* Fig. 81).

During these three to twelve weeks the child remains perfectly well; there is no cough or wasting or other sign or symptom on which to base a diagnosis. The tuberculin tests are negative and the x-ray picture has not sufficiently developed to demonstrate the primary focus. Actually, however, even during this early period, tubercle bacilli may be obtained from stomach washings.

Coincident with the development of immunity, there is an increased sensitivity to tuberculo-protein. This shows itself by the tuberculin skin reactions and such manifestations as erythema nodosum and, occasionally, phlyctenular conjunctivitis.

At the end of the incubation period a sudden inflammatory reaction develops about the primary focus. Hyperæmia, œdema and lympho-

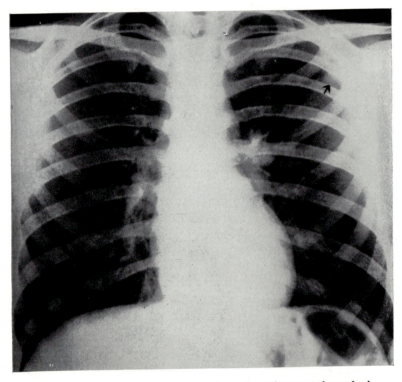

PLATE XIX. X-ray appearances in early primary tuberculosis.
The primary focus (Ghon focus) is in the second left interspace
(indicated by an arrow). There is also left hilar adenitis. The
patient, a youth of 14 years, had no symptoms.

cytes surround it. The reaction also occurs about the lymphatics and the hilar glands (*see* Plate XIX). An x-ray will show a definite lesion; the original focus may be lost in the centre of quite a large lobular shadow, and other shadows are seen about the inflamed hilar glands. Simultaneously, the skin tests to tuberculin become strongly positive.

CLINICAL PICTURE

The majority of children, particularly the older ones, remain afebrile and show no clinical upset. The lesion may be so slight that they do not even develop a cough, and it heals completely and gives rise to no symptoms throughout life.

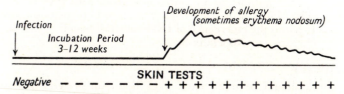

Fig 81.—Relation between incubation, allergy and fever, shown diagramatically

A smaller proportion have a benign fever lasting from one to four weeks. The symptoms are vague and non-specific, although in a few patients the temperature may rise at the beginning to 104° F. The majority of cases subside in a few weeks. In addition to fever, other symptoms which develop are lassitude, headache, loss of appetite and weight, and sometimes a slight cough. Occasionally the cough is accompanied by stridor, caused by bronchial or tracheal obstruction, and wheezing may accompany the stridor in cases of obstructive emphysema (*see* Plate XXI), especially in infants. On examination physical signs are absent or meagre; this must be stressed. An ailing child with unilateral bronchitis should always be suspected of tuberculosis. The lesion may be situated deeply in the hilar region, with healthy lung tissue over it, and neither by percussion nor by auscultation can gross abnormality be detected. The positive tuberculin test, however, should lead to radiography and the diagnosis will become clear.

In a small proportion of cases, as the fever and skin sensitivity (allergy) develop, so *erythema nodosum* (*see* p. 512) appears. This syndrome is a great help in the diagnosis of the primary infection. The majority of cases of erythema nodosum due to tuberculous infection arise soon after the end of the incubation period when tuberculin allergy suddenly develops. A small proportion are post-primary in time, usually following coincident infections. It is considered that if a coincident illness arises shortly after or during a primary tuberculous illness, tuberculous allergy can be temporarily depressed; as recovery occurs tuberculin sensitivity is re-established and erythema nodosum may develop.

COURSE AND TREATMENT OF THE PRIMARY TUBERCULOUS INFECTION

In the slight cases in older children the whole process passes unnoticed. Such individuals seem to have gained immunity from this slight infection. In the more severe cases and in the very young, the fever subsides in 2 to 4 weeks, but such a child should be kept in bed until the ESR is normal. Chemotherapy should be instituted at once, and maintained for 6–12 months. If this is done, treatment in hospital can be shortened or avoided altogether. Except in the few instances in which the source-case is known to be infected with an INH-resistant strain, the treatment of choice is to give INH, either alone or, as the authors advise, in combination with PAS or streptomycin. The object of giving a combination of two chemotherapeutic agents is to avoid the emergence of INH-resistant bacilli. (For dosage of chemotherapy, *see* Appendix 3.)

FOLLOW-UP

A check should be made each week upon the weight, and about each month, at first, upon the chest x-ray and the sedimentation rate. A return to bed-rest should be ordered if progress is not satisfactory. The danger period in relation to hæmatogenous dissemination is in the first three months of the illness, and during this time careful supervision is necessary although it has been shown that adequate chemotherapy almost entirely eliminates this special risk.

The following table, which gives the interval in untreated cases between the primary infection and the occurrence of tuberculous meningitis, illustrates the importance of treatment:—

	Months								Total
Interval ..	0–1	1–2	2–3	3–4	4–5	5–6	6–7	7–13	
Cases .. (Wallgren)[1]	15	25	12	4	2	3	2	1	64

From this it is seen that most cases of tuberculous meningitis occurred one to two months after the first manifestations of primary tuberculosis. It seldom occurred later than three months after the primary infection had shown itself. These three months are clearly a period of danger.

WHAT HAPPENS TO THE PRIMARY FOCUS?

(1) In the majority of cases the lesions in the lung parenchyma, lymphatics and tracheo-bronchial glands calcify (Plate XX), or become surrounded with fibrous tissue and almost disappear.

(2) In a small proportion of children, however, an infection such

[1] Wallgren, A. (1941). *Amer. J. Dis. Child.*, **61**, 577.

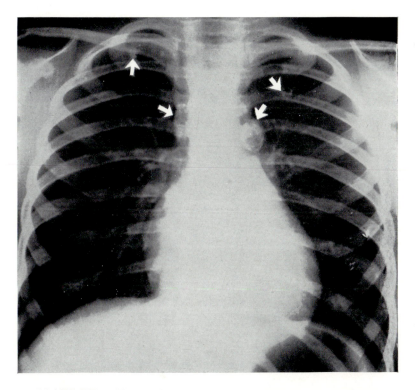

PLATE XX.   X-ray changes after healing in a case of primary
intrathoracic tuberculosis.   Bilateral calcification of paratracheal
and tracheobronchial lymph nodes is present, and foci of
calcification in right upper lobe (probable " Simon focus ").   From
a girl, aged 5 years, who had had an illness of three weeks' duration (fever, sweating and anorexia) two years previously.

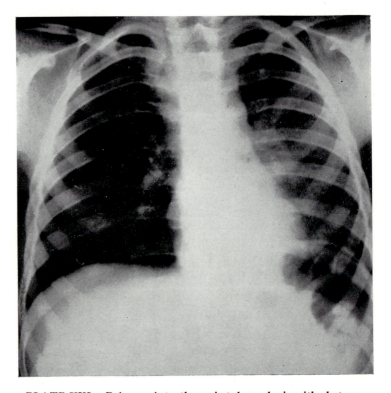

PLATE XXI. Primary intrathoracic tuberculosis with obstructive emphysema of the right lung. This x-ray shows right
paratracheal and left hilar lymphadenitis.   There is also displacement of the trachea and mediastinum to the left, and downward displacement of the right diaphragm.   Note the increased
translucency of the emphysematous right lung. From a
boy, aged 5 years, with stridor and a wheezy cough.

cytes surround it.   The reaction also occurs about the lymphatics and the hilar glands (*see* Plate XIX).   An x-ray will show a definite lesion; the original focus may be lost in the centre of quite a large lobular shadow, and other shadows are seen about the inflamed hilar glands. Simultaneously, the skin tests to tuberculin become strongly positive.

CLINICAL PICTURE

The majority of children, particularly the older ones, remain afebrile and show no clinical upset.   The lesion may be so slight that they do not even develop a cough, and it heals completely and gives rise to no symptoms throughout life.

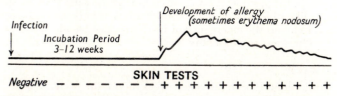

Fig 81.—Relation between incubation, allergy and fever, shown diagramatically

A smaller proportion have a benign fever lasting from one to four weeks.   The symptoms are vague and non-specific, although in a few patients the temperature may rise at the beginning to 104° F. The majority of cases subside in a few weeks.   In addition to fever, other symptoms which develop are lassitude, headache, loss of appetite and weight, and sometimes a slight cough.   Occasionally the cough is accompanied by stridor, caused by bronchial or tracheal obstruction, and wheezing may accompany the stridor in cases of obstructive emphysema (*see* Plate XXI), especially in infants.   On examination physical signs are absent or meagre; this must be stressed.   An ailing child with unilateral bronchitis should always be suspected of tuberculosis.   The lesion may be situated deeply in the hilar region, with healthy lung tissue over it, and neither by percussion nor by auscultation can gross abnormality be detected.   The positive tuberculin test, however, should lead to radiography and the diagnosis will become clear.

In a small proportion of cases, as the fever and skin sensitivity (allergy) develop, so *erythema nodosum* (*see* p. 512) appears.   This syndrome is a great help in the diagnosis of the primary infection. The majority of cases of erythema nodosum due to tuberculous infection arise soon after the end of the incubation period when tuberculin allergy suddenly develops.   A small proportion are post-primary in time, usually following coincident infections.   It is considered that if a coincident illness arises shortly after or during a primary tuberculous illness, tuberculous allergy can be temporarily depressed; as recovery occurs tuberculin sensitivity is re-established and erythema nodosum may develop.

COURSE AND TREATMENT OF THE PRIMARY TUBERCULOUS
INFECTION

In the slight cases in older children the whole process passes unnoticed. Such individuals seem to have gained immunity from this
slight infection. In the more severe cases and in the very young, the
fever subsides in 2 to 4 weeks, but such a child should be kept in
bed until the ESR is normal. Chemotherapy should be instituted
at once, and maintained for 6–12 months. If this is done, treatment
in hospital can be shortened or avoided altogether. Except in the
few instances in which the source-case is known to be infected with an
INH-resistant strain, the treatment of choice is to give INH, either
alone or, as the authors advise, in combination with PAS or streptomycin. The object of giving a combination of two chemotherapeutic
agents is to avoid the emergence of INH-resistant bacilli. (For dosage
of chemotherapy, see Appendix 3.)

FOLLOW-UP

A check should be made each week upon the weight, and about
each month, at first, upon the chest x-ray and the sedimentation rate.
A return to bed-rest should be ordered if progress is not satisfactory.
The danger period in relation to hæmatogenous dissemination is in
the first three months of the illness, and during this time careful
supervision is necessary although it has been shown that adequate
chemotherapy almost entirely eliminates this special risk.

The following table, which gives the interval in untreated cases
between the primary infection and the occurrence of tuberculous
meningitis, illustrates the importance of treatment:—

	Months								Total
Interval ..	0–1	1–2	2–3	3–4	4–5	5–6	6–7	7–13	
Cases .. (Wallgren)[1]	15	25	12	4	2	3	2	1	64

From this it is seen that most cases of tuberculous meningitis occurred
one to two months after the first manifestations of primary tuberculosis.
It seldom occurred later than three months after the primary infection
had shown itself. These three months are clearly a period of danger.

WHAT HAPPENS TO THE PRIMARY FOCUS?

(1) In the majority of cases the lesions in the lung parenchyma,
lymphatics and tracheo-bronchial glands calcify (Plate XX), or become surrounded with fibrous tissue and almost disappear.

(2) In a small proportion of children, however, an infection such

[1] Wallgren, A. (1941). *Amer. J. Dis. Child.*, **61**, 577.

as broncho-pneumonia or whooping-cough may re-activate the primary complex and a sudden extension of the disease results. This most often occurs under the age of two or at puberty, which are danger periods when there is particular susceptibility to such extension.

(3) Bronchial obstruction from the pressure of enlarged glands or from endobronchial œdema and granulations may cause segmental or lobar collapse of lung. In the majority of such cases, as the adenitis resolves during the healing stage, the bronchus becomes patent again and pulmonary re-expansion occurs. Occasionally partial occlusion causes obstructive emphysema (Plate XXI). If the paratracheal or the carinal (bifurcation) glands are involved, gross dyspnœa may occur, sometimes with alarming suddenness. In such cases it is often found that the bronchial wall has been eroded by the gland and that the lumen of the bronchus is filled with tuberculous granulation tissue and caseous material. In these cases immediate bronchoscopy is essential. It is also advisable in less severe ones in which the collapse persists for more than a few weeks, because a lobar type of bronchiectasis may result from prolonged bronchial obstruction. There is a place for surgical removal of enlarged hilar glands in carefully selected cases, when bronchial obstruction and erosion would otherwise do irreparable damage to the affected lung.

Tuberculous Pleurisy

ÆTIOLOGY AND PATHOLOGY

A subpleural primary focus or a caseous hilar gland often involves the pleura, causing localized thickening. Occasionally there is a serous pleural effusion and clear straw-coloured fluid collects. Both the visceral and parietal pleuræ are thickened, red, and shaggy, with a tendency to form adhesions between the adjacent surfaces.

The usual time interval between the initial infection and a pleural effusion is about 6–7 months and the commonest age for it is 6–15 years.

SYMPTOMS AND CLINICAL PICTURE

The patient sometimes complains of a sharp pain in the affected side, and there is fever and a persistent cough. Friction may be heard at the onset. More characteristically, absent breath-sounds and dullness to percussion, with displacement of the heart and trachea, suggest the presence of fluid. The blood-count is usually normal, but may also show an initial polymorphonuclear leucocytosis, but not such as is found in purulent empyema. The skin tests give a positive reaction to tuberculin, and an x-ray confirms the diagnosis (Plate XXII).

PROGNOSIS AND TREATMENT

The prognosis is usually excellent. INH and PAS or streptomycin should be given. The child should be kept in bed and nursed in the fresh air if possible. If the effusion is gross and there is much displacement of the heart so as to occasion distress, it may be necessary to withdraw fluid with a needle and syringe. Usually this is not necessary, however, and the fluid is gradually absorbed.

As the fluid disappears, the primary complex may be visible in the x-ray. Further x-rays should be taken, together with sedimentation rates, to check subsequent progress.

Progressive Pulmonary Infiltration

Occasionally, after the primary infection, the primary lung lesion and adjacent infected glands fail to resolve. The lesions of the primary complex may spread and involve the whole lobe of a lung, or caseous glands may ulcerate and discharge bacilli into the adjacent bronchus with the possibility of a bronchogenic spread.

CLINICAL PICTURE

This " adult " type of the disease is comparatively rare in early childhood, being more often found at or after puberty. The fever is high and swinging, and there is persistent cough, with sputum, especially when cavitation has occurred. The physical signs are those of consolidation as seen in the adult.

PROGNOSIS AND TREATMENT

Without chemotherapy the outlook in these cases was bad. Death from hæmoptysis, exhaustion or generalized infection was not very uncommon. Early and effective treatment with INH and PAS or streptomycin will do much to prevent all this. Intercurrent pulmonary infection due to other organisms may require the use of penicillin and other antibiotics.

In well-selected cases, surgery has a valuable part in treatment. Lobectomy, or in rare instances pneumonectomy, may be undertaken to remove irremediably damaged lung segments. Full chemotherapeutic coverage is essential.

Pulmonary Collapse (" Epituberculosis ")

There has been much speculation on the pathology of this clinical picture. Since these children almost invariably recover, autopsies have been very few indeed. " Epituberculosis " signifies the radiological finding of a wedge-like shadow projecting out from the hilum of the lung towards the periphery. Such a shadow may conform to a segmental or lobar pulmonary distribution. It seems probable that the appearance is due to collapse, for on bronchoscopy the bronchus supplying the affected area is nearly always occluded, either from without by pressure from a mediastinal gland, or from within by tuberculous granulation tissue due to a gland eroding into the lumen of the bronchus. Careful examination of the x-ray will usually reveal an area of compensatory emphysema in another part of the lung (Plate XXIII).

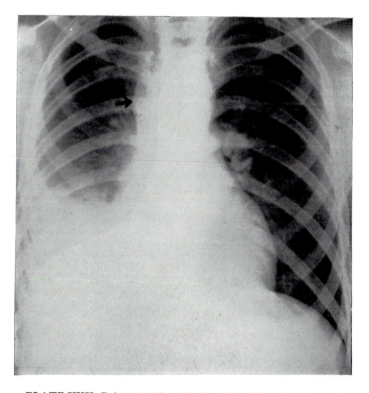

PLATE XXII. Primary tuberculosis with right-sided pleural
effusion in a boy of 7 years with a short history of cough,
pain in the right side and fever. The x-ray shows an
effusion not large enough to cause mediastinal displacement.
An arrow indicates the position of an enlarged right paratracheal gland.

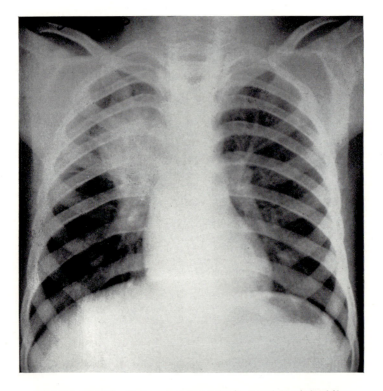

PLATE XXIII. Primary tuberculosis causing right hilar adenitis. There is also collapse and consolidation of the right upper lobe. Note the thickened interlobar pleura in the lesser fissure and compensatory emphysema below on the same side. From a boy aged 4 years. Tubercle bacilli were found in the gastric washings.

CLINICAL PICTURE

It is typical of the condition that it is unsuspected and discovered only by routine x-ray examination. Usually the child is afebrile and appears to be in reasonably good health. The physical signs are either minimal or absent; if present they resemble those of lobar consolidation. Such signs and radiographic picture may last for many weeks or months and then appear to clear up completely, or leave minor evidence of fibrosis or calcification only. In such cases the tuberculin skin-tests are strongly positive. The treatment is similar to other tuberculous infections; chemotherapy, rest in bed, a good diet and fresh air. In rare instances in which there is much residual damage to the affected lobe or segment, surgical removal may be indicated; but in general the prognosis is good.

HÆMATOGENOUS SPREAD OF TUBERCULOUS INFECTION

It is claimed that there is some spread to the blood-stream via the thoracic duct in all cases of primary infection. Gross hæmatogenous infection, however, occurs when a caseous gland has eroded the wall of a vein and emptied its contents into the vein, either all at once or at intervals. Then there is a general or partial hæmatogenous spread, but certain situations are more commonly affected than others. These are:

Lungs, where miliary tuberculosis occurs.
Brain, where tuberculomata may be found.
Bones and joints, giving rise to tuberculous osteitis and arthritis.
Visceral organs, such as kidney, spleen, epididymis and Fallopian tubes.

Miliary Tuberculosis

PATHOGENESIS

Miliary tuberculosis results when tubercle bacilli invade the blood-stream in sufficient number. Gross disseminated tuberculosis is ordinarily an acute process, always fatal without treatment, but very occasionally it follows a chronic course and then spontaneous recovery is a possibility.

The bacilli responsible for miliary tuberculosis can come directly from a primary complex but more often the process is the result of a terminal meningitis with the following sequence of events: (1) " seeding " of bacilli takes place from a primary complex to the brain, where minute tuberculomata (called " Rich foci ") may be found; (2) in the neighbourhood of one of these foci involvement of the meninges may occur; (3) the bacilli then pass into the cerebrospinal fluid reaching the longitudinal sinus and the systemic circulation (*see also* p. 405).

The disease is most commonly found between the ages of one and three years (*see* Fig. 82).

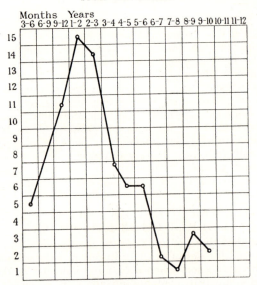

Fig. 82.—Age inc'dence of miliary tuberculosis and tuberculous meningitis in 70 post-mortem examinations.

CLINICAL PICTURE

The symptoms may be either insidious or those of an acute illness. There may be little else than listlessness, anorexia, and loss of weight. In other cases there may be a high swinging temperature, extreme irritability, prostration, and possibly cough, with rapid respiration and even cyanosis.

On examination, a feature of the picture is the paucity of physical signs in a child who is obviously ill. There may be a few moist sounds scattered over the chest. In the abdomen, the spleen can often be felt, a very significant finding. The temperature may be continually up, but in the early stages there are short bouts of pyrexia only. There is progressive loss of weight.

DIAGNOSIS

This is often difficult, especially early in the disease, because of the lack of physical signs. An x-ray of the chest shows typical fine, mottled or stippled appearances. On washing out the stomach or examining the stools, tubercle bacilli may be discovered. Whether or not symptoms and signs of tuberculous meningitis are present (*see* p. 405) a lumbar puncture should be carried out and will often reveal the presence of an early meningeal infection. A most helpful point in diagnosis is the presence of choroidal tubercles. These take the form of oval, yellowish-white or yellowish-pink raised areas along the line of the retinal vessels. They are usually about a third of the size of the optic disc. As they heal they become white in colour and usually shrink in size. If they are seen, the diagnosis of miliary tuberculosis is established.

Very often typhoid or paratyphoid fever is suspected but can be ruled out by a negative Widal test. Examination of the urine excludes pyelitis. Other infections, e.g. brucellosis and Still's disease, may have to be considered. In the early stages the Mantoux and tuberculin jelly tests are positive. In the late stages, however, skin sensitivity may wane.

PROGNOSIS AND TREATMENT

Chemotherapy has revolutionized the prognosis in this disease which was almost always fatal in its outcome. Such cases as did recover were of a chronic type, healing by multiple calcification in all tissues involved.

As soon as the diagnosis is made, INH with streptomycin should be given; this is followed later by treatment with PAS which should be continued for 6 to 12 months. It is wise to examine the cerebrospinal fluid at the beginning of treatment and to repeat the examination if there is suspicion of meningeal involvement. The patient should be nursed in the best possible conditions and carefully observed. Long-term follow-up is essential.

Tuberculous Meningitis (*see* p. 405).

Tuberculosis of Bones and Joints (*see* p. 487).

Abdominal Tuberculosis

This includes tuberculous ulceration of the bowel, tuberculosis of abdominal lymph nodes (*tabes mesenterica*), and both the ascitic and plastic forms of tuberculous peritonitis. It is usual to find two or more of them at the same time; in fact they develop one from the other and all will have been present to some extent in most cases.

Abdominal tuberculosis is usually due to a primary focus in the bowel, spreading to the mesenteric glands or peritoneum; but sometimes, especially in the much older child, there is a previous pulmonary lesion which has secondarily infected the bowel. The disease is most common during the second, third and fourth years.

ÆTIOLOGY

Abdominal tuberculosis has become rare in Britain. It has a geographical incidence which can be attributed to a difference in milk supply, for in most cases it is due to the bovine rather than the human tubercle bacillus. Certainly abdominal tuberculosis has occasionally developed in children who have had all their milk boiled, and in such cases the disease is due to the human bacillus, but in the majority of cases the organism is found to be of bovine origin.

Eradication of tuberculosis from cattle, successfully achieved in some
countries, is the logical method of prevention; failing this all milk
should be heat-treated before being drunk. The geographical distribution of abdominal tuberculosis shows that the disease is found in
areas where raw milk, which has been taken from herds where tuberculin testing is not carried out, is drunk, or where elimination of infected cows from the herd is not insisted upon. In large cities where
the milk is properly pasteurized before delivery, abdominal tuberculosis
is rarely seen.

PATHOLOGY

The infection gains entry through a primary focus in the intestinal
mucosa, spreads by way of the lymphatics to the mesenteric glands or
to the peritoneum of the bowel, and thence perhaps to the rest of the
peritoneal cavity.

SYMPTOMS AND PHYSICAL FINDINGS

Abdominal pain and perhaps fever are the commonest symptoms.
The pain is probably caused by inflammation in the glands in the
mesentery and their overlying peritoneum. Apart from this a primary
complex, as it forms in the abdomen, produces little in the way of
defined symptoms, although exceptionally there may be considerable
fever. In a few cases there is a history of colicky pain and diarrhœa;
sometimes mucus and a little blood is noted. Sometimes the clinical
picture resembles that of cœliac disease on account of the passage of
pale, loose and offensive stools, possibly due to interference with the
absorption of fat.

In *tabes mesenterica* colicky pains in the abdomen, lassitude and
failure to gain weight are the usual symptoms. On palpation little
can be made out unless the child is asleep, or under an anæsthetic, or
will allow the abdominal wall to relax completely; then the enlarged
mesenteric glands may be found; in healing cases x-ray reveals calcification.

In the *ascitic form* there is abdominal enlargement and discomfort
which directs attention to the abdomen. There is fullness in the
flanks, the umbilicus may unfold and shifting dullness is elicited. A
mass of enlarged glands and rolled-up omentum may be felt on deep
palpation. The child himself is pale, wasted and languid.

In the *plastic form of peritonitis* the abdomen feels doughy and loops
of bowel are adherent. With relaxation of the abdominal wall,
large caseous glands and the rolled-up omentum are made out.
Very often there is an irregular temperature, especially when the
patient is not progressing well.

TREATMENT

Rest in bed is necessary and it will usually give relief from abdominal
pain.

With tuberculous ulceration of the bowel there is interference with absorption from the intestine, further complicated by intestinal hurry and imperfect digestion. This should be treated by offering the child those foodstuffs which are easily digested and assimilated. A diet high in protein, low in fat, and moderately high in carbohydrates is therefore suitable. As the child improves and the stools become normal, butter, milk, cream and eggs may be added.

The general measures of treatment described on p. 578 should be adopted together with anti-tuberculous chemotherapy.

OTHER PRIMARY INFECTIONS

Tuberculous Cervical Adenitis

IN tuberculous cervical adenitis the primary lesion is, as a rule, situated in the lymphoid tissue of the tonsils and adenoids.

CLINICAL PICTURE

Occasionally there is a history of sore throats but usually nothing has been noted until a unilateral swelling appears. This may develop slowly, or perhaps more acutely as the result of an intercurrent attack of ordinary throat infection. Unless there is secondary infection of the gland, there is no great tenderness and there is no fluctuation in the early stages. Later, as the pus nears the surface, the skin becomes red and shiny and distinct fluctuation is noticed. If no treatment is instituted the skin breaks down and a sinus is formed. Differentiation between streptococcal (or other pyogenic adenitis) and tuberculous glands may be difficult clinically, and a tuberculin test is required.

TREATMENT

Chemotherapy against tuberculosis, and the other measures described on p. 578 should be followed. If there is any evidence that the tonsils are infected, tonsillectomy should be advised. If an abscess is present it must be incised and its contents expressed; repeated aspirations are not advised. A mass of adherent tuberculous glands can be locally excised in order to hasten recovery.

Rare Sites for the Primary Complex

Although the lungs, intestine and neck form the sites for the great majority of primary tuberculous complexes, on rare occasions the primary complex is found elsewhere. The palpebral conjunctivæ, tooth sockets, lips, and even normal skin surfaces, may on occasion be the site of the primary tuberculous focus. In such sites the lesion takes the form of a chronic granulomatous ulcer and, as with any primary tuberculous focus, is associated with infection and enlargement of the draining lymphatic gland. Complications may follow such a primary complex in the same way as with the lesions already described,

Renal Tuberculosis

Early in the evolution of primary tuberculosis a transient tubercle bacillæmia often occurs, perhaps leading to a focal lesion in one or other kidney.   Such a focus usually heals without giving rise to any symptoms, or it may settle and become latent; but if the process is extensive there are likely to be clinical manifestations, particularly painless hæmaturia, or a subacute or chronic urinary infection, and there may be loss of weight, lassitude and fever.   Renal tuberculosis has become extremely uncommon in childhood in the United Kingdom.

DIAGNOSIS

A persistent and sterile pyuria is suggestive of renal tuberculosis. Tuberculin testing and examination of several 24-hour collections of urine are necessary, together with a complete urological investigation; a search should be made for signs of tuberculosis in other situations.

TREATMENT

Tuberculosis chemotherapy and the general measures outlined on p. 578 should be instituted.   Surgery, either of a conservative or radical nature, may be necessary in advanced cases.

Congenital Tuberculosis

On rare occasions infected mothers may give birth to infants already showing evidence of tuberculosis.   In such cases the mode of entry is the umbilical vein, and the brunt of the disease falls upon the liver, with gland enlargement in the *porta hepatis*.   Such congenital lesions have not usually been compatible with life for more than a few days at the most.

PROPHYLAXIS AGAINST TUBERCULOSIS WITH BCG VACCINE

INOCULATION against tuberculosis by means of BCG is in general use in many parts of the world.   The vaccine is prepared from a strain of avirulent tubercle bacilli originally used by Calmette and Guérin.

Successful BCG vaccination in a tuberculin-negative person results in Mantoux conversion in six to twelve weeks, with persistence of positivity for about four years.   The great value of BCG inoculation appears to be the subsequent decrease in the incidence of all forms of tuberculosis in persons successfully inoculated, and in particular the virtual abolition of tuberculous meningitis in children in this group.

There are two main methods of applying BCG inoculation to a community.   Either all tuberculin-negative reactors are immunized, infants being inoculated at the age of three months (such a practice is almost universal in Scandinavia), or else BCG is reserved for certain groups of people who are likely to undergo special risk: (*a*) nurses and medical students who, on starting their training, are found to be tuberculin-negative; (*b*) persons who are contacts of known cases of tuberculosis and are found to be tuberculin-negative; and (*c*) pupils about to leave school who are found to be negative reactors. In contacts, it is important to know that the child is not already in the process of developing a primary lesion at the time of the inoculation. Ideally, he should be isolated from the contact for six weeks before BCG inoculation is carried out and afterwards until Mantoux conversion occurs.

BCG inoculation does not protect entirely from subsequent tuberculosis, but it does appear to reduce the mortality and the incidence

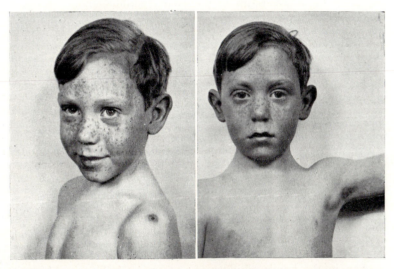

Fig. 83.—A normal BCG reaction over the left deltoid region with enlarged lymph nodes in the axilla. Vaccination in this area is preferred to the thigh, because suppuration in the glands is less likely.

of the severer forms of the the disease, as well as practically eliminating tuberculous meningitis.

Technique. Intradermal vaccination is better than oral vaccine. It may be given by intracutaneous injection or by multiple puncture using the Heaf gun. The intradermal injection consists in giving 0·1 ml. of vaccine into the skin over the deltoid region (Fig. 83). Afterwards the axillary lymph nodes enlarge and occasionally a sinus forms, but this is only a nuisance and never a danger.

CHAPTER 26

Diseases of Children in the Tropics

CHILD health is the result of the total environment, a complex of biological and living conditions. In general, climatic factors are of less importance to health than those factors which can be brought gradually under human control; these include economic conditions in the community, the standard of living and education of the parents, housing, water supply, sanitation, food availability and food habits, clothing, animal parasites, insect pests, the family traditions, religious or cultural persuasions, and the availability and standard of medical care. It follows that both curative and preventive medicine have special opportunities in the many countries where mortality and morbidity among children are high.

The most important causes of ill-health are not malaria, tuberculosis, cholera, plague and other communicable diseases, but poverty, malnutrition, lack of education, and of personal and community hygiene. Curative and preventive work must go hand-in-hand in the task of improving child health. Child-care services must be well-balanced and properly integrated with all curative work, and health expenditure should be budgeted for with this end in view.

In many tropical countries vital statistics are not available or else they are grossly inaccurate, and the registration of births and deaths is often in the hands of illiterate or inexpert persons. Moreover, curative pædiatrics has received little attention and in some areas only small numbers of the many diseased children are brought to the hospitals and dispensaries. Interest in research is of recent growth, and there are many common clinical conditions demanding investigation, as well as a great variety of less common ones. Post-mortem examinations are often forbidden by religion and tradition; vital statistics, medical education and research are affected by this.

There is much to be learned from the experience of pædiatricians working in tropical countries. An underfed child in the tropics requires smaller doses of drugs than does his better nourished counterpart in Western countries. He is also a worse surgical risk and operations should only take place on competent advice.

CLINICAL ASPECTS

THERE are certain points to be noted in regard to the differing pattern of disease in different areas. In most tropical countries the native children show a high incidence of malnutrition and parasitic disease, whereas diabetes mellitus and obesity—diseases associated with dietetic plenty—are rarely seen. It is rare for allergic conditions to appear in a comparatively undernourished population, but some cases of asthma or asthmatic bronchitis may improve with the eradication of ascariasis. Appendicitis is uncommon in undernourished populations.

When a young child needs to be in hospital, there is, in all countries, much to be said for admitting his mother as well. There is even more reason for this in backward countries, because it creates opportunities for teaching her how her children should be fed, clothed and cared for; and it often affords an opportunity of dealing with defects in her own health at the same time. In this way hospitals can play a vital part in preventive care.

Children of unsophisticated races are usually treated with ready affection, in spite of their being sometimes submitted to seemingly cruel customs. However, little allowance is made for the special requirements of children, either in general or in dietary matters, and this has the effect of developing their limited maturity at an early age.

Psychological disorders are seemingly rare amongst primitive tribes. Individuals who are mentally retarded or abnormal will nearly always find some form of occupation, and are generally taken for granted by the community. The arrival of Western culture and the growth of modern towns have produced conditions in which mental and emotional instability may be encouraged, particularly among adolescents.

Mongolism occurs in every race, and there is no difficulty in recognizing it, even in a Chinese baby. Paralysis from muscular dystrophies and poliomyelitis is common in Egypt and Middle East countries; suitable arrangements for rehabilitation are rarely found. Rheumatic fever is not by any means uncommon, though it is unusual to find rheumatic nodules. Conjunctivitis from dust, smoke and infection is common. Blindness, acquired through keratomalacia, parasitic diseases, trachoma, gonorrhœa and pyogenic infection, is a vast problem.

The diseases of children in Ceylon may be taken as fairly representative of those of a tropical country. Prematurity continues to be the commonest cause of infant death under one week of age. In infants over one week and under one year, the most frequently certified causes of death (diarrhœa and enteritis, pneumonia, debility and convulsions) do not reflect the significant part still played by malnutrition, infestation, malaria and tuberculosis. In a recent preliminary survey of the child population in the Kurunegala District, 50 per cent. of the children showed positive evidence of hookworm infestation and 45 per cent. of roundworm infestation; salmonellosis was present in 4 per cent. of the children, shigellosis in 5 per cent., and amœbic infection in 14 per cent.

In the chief towns of Ceylon there are good, though very over-crowded, hospitals and one medical practitioner to about 5,600 population. The birth rate per 1,000 population was 38·2 in 1959, and it is interesting to compare this figure with the present rate of 17·4 for England and Wales. Although decreasing steadily, the Cingalese maternal mortality rate is still relatively high at 3·4 per 1,000 live births. Infant mortality (deaths under one year of age per 1,000 live births) has fallen as follows:

[1] 1921–25	..	..	.. 190
1941–45	..	..	.. 131
1955	..	..	.. 71
1959	..	..	.. 58

In Western countries we are often warned against the danger of making a double diagnosis. In many tropical countries it is common to find several concomitant pathological conditions, and each must be explained in simple language if the parents are to be taught how to care for the health of their children. This point is well illustrated by experience in Malaya where the " Singapore syndrome " is made up of infestation with ascaris and scabies, together with malnutrition causing anæmia, beri-beri and rickets, a combination that often leads to pneumonia or enteritis.

CHILD HEALTH IN DEVELOPING COUNTRIES

In the more advanced Western countries, the hospital pædiatric services are now reasonably adequate and the child welfare and other services have raised the general standard of child health in remarkable degree. It is not surprising, therefore, that general morbidity and mortality rates have shown immense improvements during the present century. In 1900, the infant mortality rate for England and Wales was no less than 154 per 1,000 live births; by 1962 the rate had fallen to 20·7 per 1,000.

In the " developing " countries the background is entirely different. In many places there is scant medical treatment, and little attention is paid to sick children. The infant mortality rate may be as high as 400 per 1,000 live births, while the mortality rate of children between 1 and 4 years bears even worse comparison with that of Western countries. In these regions the babies are often born small and weakly because of maternal conditions resulting from early marriage, repeated pregnancies, malnutrition, anæmia and over-work.

Child-health work should aim at supervision of the pregnant and lactating mother, and of the child from birth up to and including

[1] Administrative Report of the Director of Health Services (1960). Colombo: Government Publications Bureau.

school age. The other obvious need is for medical treatment; any system in which hospitals are under one authority and " welfare " is under another is irrational and should be avoided. The welfare or health services should be an extension of the hospital services. The patients and the parents more readily accept advice about the prevention of disease if they have confidence in those who they know have the ability to treat it.

PERSONNEL AND THEIR TRAINING

Lack of trained personnel is a problem in all tropical countries, and education must be one of the doctor's chief duties. Adequate attention must be given to the training of nurses and medical assistants in the care of children; thus, midwives should be instructed not only in the details of obstetrics but also in antenatal and postnatal care. In countries where malnutrition is common, all trained staff should have a thorough knowledge of how to improve dietary standards. Moreover, present methods of training nurses and midwives often pay insufficient attention to the background from which the pupils originate, and thus they have great difficulty in learning procedures which are foreign to them. Training should therefore be accompanied by detailed and repeated explanations; it is better to cultivate habits of observation and imagination than to impart ill-understood techniques. In certain instances a proper sense of responsibility is lacking, and it may be necessary to insist on the ethics of medical care to a degree not required in regions where they are taken for granted.

When nurses and others work in welfare centres and homes as well as in hospital, they learn to correlate the diseases with the environmental conditions which give rise to those diseases and to take a more intelligent and responsible interest in their patients. To follow the same families through periods of health and disease is more valuable than to learn only the diagnosis and treatment of each " case " as it presents itself.

CHILD CARE AND NUTRITION

It is rash to generalize about infant care, because customs vary from place to place. It is wise to interfere with established customs as little as possible, and then only when they are harmful.

Unsophisticated people are generally successful in establishing and maintaining breast-feeding, in securing a good mother-child relationship, and in fostering child development during the first 8 to 12 months. The baby is near the mother, constantly handled, and fed at frequent and irregular intervals. The mother rarely experiences any trouble with engorged breasts or abscesses. The child grows, perhaps not very rapidly, but he gains initiative and neuromuscular control. It is true that among many primitive peoples there are customs which imperil him. Very unsuitable and infected substances may be applied to the umbilicus; chewed-up rice or banana may be given even during the first week of life; twins, or a motherless baby, may be looked upon as undesirable or as non-viable and may die from neglect; forced feeding with water or with curious infusions may be practised. The young child may be given a highly-spiced or indigestible diet, or allowed to eat heavily contaminated food. A sick child may not be brought for treatment until traditional medications have failed, and even then our instructions may not be understood and followed. It is only by observing habits and customs that such things are learned, and we can give advice that is practical and likely to be followed.

In hospital, as in home deliveries, it is better to keep the newborn baby with the mother. Breast-feeding is then easily established because mother and baby quickly learn to indicate to each other when another feed is desirable.

There are many countries where it is necessary to teach the value of cleanliness, sunlight and fresh air, because the babies are over-clothed, kept too much indoors, and not properly washed. Education in mothercraft should start in pregnancy and be continued throughout childhood.

WEANING

At 3–5 months a baby can be given bone and vegetable broth (*see* p. 54), the juice of orange, grapefruit, tangerine, mangoe, tomato, or guava, and mashed paw paw or mashed ripe banana.

From the fifth month other foods may be used to supplement breast feeding until lactation ceases, for example, soups made without pepper or spices; purées made from peas, beans, sweet potatoes or green leaves, such as the leaves of sweet potatoes, cassava, pumpkin, groundnuts or spinach; porridge made from well-ground and well-cooked wheat, maize, rice or other cereal or green bananas. These foods may be enriched with egg, milk or milk powders.

By the age of 9 months other vegetables and fruits can be offered, and a biscuit or crust to chew, each new food being given in small amounts at first. It is essential to choose the foodstuffs locally available in so far as they are suitable at this age. Thus, it is useless to advocate leeks, carrots and cabbages when there are local forms of spinach, sweet potatoes and their leaves, peas, groundnuts, red palm oil, egg-plant, guavas and bananas readily available but often being wrongly used.

The welfare of children and families should be supervised wherever possible. In many communities, when a new baby is born the mother takes too little interest in her deposed baby, and the mortality is unduly high in children aged 1 to 5 years. Government administrations of some countries, faced with the problems associated with rapidly increasing population, would perhaps like to inculcate birth control and " family planning," but they know that it is not possible to force reluctant and uneducated people to undertake family planning except by totalitarian means. Many families not only lack the knowledge and self-control necessary for the techniques of birth control but, owing to the non-survival of so many infants, they do not want to limit family size.   Only when parents can rely on the survival of their children, will they wish to restrict their families and learn to take more interest in their children's upbringing.

DISEASES OF THE NEWBORN

Prematurity and Debility
ONE of the major tasks of child care in the tropics is the reduction of neonatal mortality and morbidity, for they are unduly high.   In many tropical countries the average birth weight is found to be $\frac{1}{2}$ lb. to $1\frac{1}{2}$ lb. less than in England.   This initial difference may be partly racial, but many of the babies are immature or weakly because of adverse maternal factors, such as malnutrition, excessive physical labour, untreated anæmia, malaria, helminthiasis, and repeated child-bearing.

The prevention of prematurity depends in the first place on know-ledge of the causes, and so medical and nursing personnel must study the œcological problems involved.   In the adverse circumstances obtaining in the tropics, a premature or weakly baby has little chance of survival; the infant may have to contend with ritual incisions after birth; if breast-milk is not available, the main food may be bananas and boiled rice; artificial feeding of any kind carries a high risk of infection.

Diseases of the Umbilicus
Methods of tying, cutting and treating the cord are curious and often very dirty.   Dressings vary from nothing at all to sandalwood dust, cowdung, ashes, mud, and saliva.   All things considered, infec-tion is less common than might be expected, but many instances of omphalitis occur, as well as *tetanus neonatorum*.   It is rare to find any sort of bandage applied, and the cord usually dries up and drops off earlier than it does with orthodox techniques.   Umbilical infection should be treated by the usual methods (*see* p. 106).   When infection persists, the abdominal wall may be weakened, and it is as well to apply an adhesive plaster bandage, encircling the back, but divided in front, where tapes attached to the ends keep the dressing in place and give the necessary support.

Umbilical hernia rarely causes symptoms and usually undergoes spontaneous cure.   In African babies it appears to be almost a genetic characteristic; it is as common among those given orthodox treatment in hospital as it is in the rest of the population.   Treatment is seldom required.   Umbilical hernia tends to persist if the child is wrongly fed and suffers from abdominal distension.

Tetanus Neonatorum
In some countries this is an appallingly common disease; usually it is fatal.   Considering the curious applications sometimes used for the

cord, it is remarkable that even more babies do not die from it. The treatment of tetanus is described in Chapter 19 (p. 428).

There is no greater challenge to preventive medicine than the education of native populations in simple matters of elementary hygiene.

MALNUTRITION

DEFECTS in nutrition may be either quantitative or qualitative, and infestation and infection often combine to produce a cumulative complex of symptoms. The economic life of families largely determines their degree of undernutrition, although local customs, only to be corrected by patient teaching, may often be even more important. In countries blessed with a good standard of hygiene, artificial feeding may be used without much danger, but in those where the elementary rules of hygiene are unknown and the supply of artificial milk poor, it may easily become a deadly menace. Unhappily, propaganda issued by less principled agents of milk firms has begun to fall on the too-ready ears of mothers compelled for traditional or economic reasons to go out to work.

In areas where breast-feeding is customary, the infant at the breast usually looks healthy, even when the mother's diet is far from satisfactory. Sometimes a mother may go through her pregnancy with a subclinical vitamin deficiency, and subsequently her milk may be unequal to the task of preventing the newborn baby from developing obvious avitaminosis. In one such instance a baby had been put on sweetened condensed milk, because the mother had died in childbirth, and when ten days old it was already blind with keratomalacia.

Despite deficiencies in the maternal diet, the babies who are being naturally fed often do well on a system of " demand feeding " which sometimes amounts almost to non-stop nutrition. Later, in the period of weaning, the additional defects begin to appear. The weaning diet is usually from from ideal and frequently contains no extra milk. The adult diet, which is that usually given to the children, may be indigestible and totally unsuitable, yet it is seldom modified for them. It consists mainly of coarse, bulky carbohydrates, dried fish, highly seasoned soup and roasted vegetables, which, even if their chemical constituents are reasonable, are often highly undesirable in their physical characteristics. The undernourished bodies and distended abdomens of the children can present a pitiful picture, and their constant abdominal discomfort and complaints are frequently assuaged with yet another roasted yam, another tough chappati made of coarse flour or gram, or another green banana. The sheer bulk of this diet may distend the digestive tract, interfere with assimilation, and result in wasting. There may be attacks of colic, of diarrhœa, or of dysentery. The intestine becomes atonic and later atrophic. A large proportion of the cases of malnutrition arises from food that predisposes to indigestion or diarrhœa; in general, it is comparatively rare to find cases due to feeding that is inadequate in quantity or in essential chemical components.

It is always important to distinguish between cases of primary malnutrition (due to defects in the food) and secondary malnutrition (due to infections, such as dysentery, or infestations, such as ancylostoma caused by poor sanitation and soil-pollution). As soon as the baby learns to crawl, he is allowed to sit about on the ground and to stuff his mouth with indescribably unpleasant substances.

If the child survives, he gradually becomes accustomed to the traditional diet, and by the age of eight or ten the abdomen begins to assume a more normal outline. However, one may still detect the signs of malnutrition (glossitis, phrynoderma, gingivitis, hypochromatotrichia, Bitot's spots, and mosaic dermatoses), while symptoms of riboflavine deficiency (cheilosis, perlèche, fissuring of the tongue, and vascularization of the cornea) remain common.

An excess of carbohydrate in the diet will cause intestinal fermentation and diarrhœa. When enough of such food is absorbed, it often results in a fat, cheerful, rachitic and bronchitic baby, subject to pneumonia and infections of the skin. Sometimes exclusive breast-feeding is continued long past infancy, and iron-deficiency anæmia results.

Non-specific Signs of Malnutrition. The non-specific signs of malnutrition vary with the degree of dietary defect and with the accompanying diseases. Most cases of malnutrition show growth-failure and some show emaciation, with or without œdema. In nearly all chronic cases hair changes will be found. The severity, variety and extent of dyspigmentation of hair and skin will depend on such factors as (*a*) original genetic pigmentation; (*b*) exposure to sun and water, especially salt water; (*c*) habitual protection by oily inunctions; (*d*) the fat content of the diet. In most cases of defective nutrition the skin becomes dry and inelastic and loses its natural gloss. Certain areas, particularly the anterior aspect of the tibiæ, become dry, cracking, or mosaic. These changes of the integument occur in children over 2 years but are rare in infants. In all cases of malnutrition the skin becomes more liable to infection, and wounds are slow in healing.

Even short periods of undernutrition may give rise to mental changes —irritability, misery and apathy.

Children suffering from severe malnutrition show increased susceptibility to certain infections, and the response to them is more bizarre and damaging than in a well-fed child. For instance, a malnourished child may develop *cancrum oris* (or noma) from a slight stomatitis. This condition was often fatal before the days of antibiotics. Now, if the child is brought to hospital in time, modern treatment can overcome the infection, and can be followed at a later stage by skin-grafting; but in neglected cases the damage is such that even the most skilled plastic surgery cannot correct the deformities that result.

Convulsions

In the tropics " convulsions " are often certified as a cause of death. Rickets is an important predisposing cause; exciting causes are numerous. In young babies repeated convulsions may signify *tetanus*. In children they may be associated with intestinal infestations, chronic beri-beri, tetany, meningitis, as well as the non-specific febrile illnesses. In some regions they may signify cerebral malaria; in others, such as Jamaica, hypoglycæmia is an important cause of convulsions. When the liver is damaged by protein malnutrition, there is defective storage of glycogen so that a severe hypoglycæmia may result from even a mild attack of gastro-enteritis.

Stomatitis

Thrush and other forms of stomatitis are very common in some areas and are potentially dangerous illnesses leading to cancrum oris or to widespread moniliasis of the alimentary or respiratory tract. The majority of cases respond well to adequate and early treatment (*see* p. 188).

Chronic Parotitis

This seldom occurs in children under the age of 3 years. It may then be a sign of chronic malnutrition. It is not generally accompanied by fever or pain, nor associated with oral infection. Treatment is dietary, and the swelling is slow to disappear.

Treatment of Malnutrition

The customary diet in backward areas is often ill-balanced and unsuitable for children, and it is hard to improve it because of local tradition and age-long fatalism. The objective should be to encourage and assist the families to grow vegetables, raise chickens, keep milch goats, as well as to teach them how to prepare meals and how to give the available food supplements. The less radically we attempt to alter the traditional diet, the more success we shall have. For instance, instead of giving the dyspeptic toddler a tough, leathery chappati, the parents may be persuaded to give peas or coarse flour boiled as a porridge, perhaps with an egg beaten in. Instead of giving the sweet-potato leaves in a curry, they can make them into an unseasoned purée by rubbing the leaves through a tin with holes punched in the bottom. Instead of giving the green banana roasted hard, they can learn to make banana flour or to give well-mashed ripe banana. And instead of giving all the available water-buffalo milk (8 to 12 per cent. fat content) to the grandfather, they may give some, mixed with their rice kanji (soft-boiled rice), to the small children.

Modifications of this sort will suggest themselves to anyone with a practical knowledge of the local diet.   In nearly all regions, green-leaf vegetables are obtainable; although often not sufficiently used, they are a valuable addition to a diet and useful at almost every age.

Contributing factors also need attention; for example, intestinal infections and parasites, malaria, tuberculosis, syphilis, yaws and leprosy.   The attempt should always be made to determine how far the malnourished state is due to primary defects in the diet, and how far it is secondary to underlying diseases.

SPECIFIC NUTRITIONAL DISEASES

Rickets (*see also* p. 119).

FŒTAL rickets has been described in the children of mothers suffering from osteomalacia.   Ordinary infantile rickets, sometimes occurring in equatorial regions (Fig. 84), is much commoner and is frequently present in premature babies.   It is also seen among full-term babies

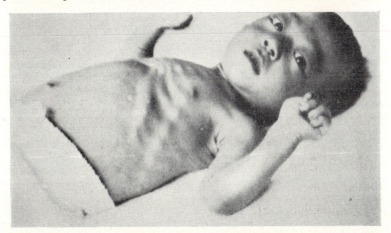

Fig. 84.—Rickets in a Chinese child, aged 15 months, in Singapore.   Note the characteristic beading of the costochondral junctions.

that get insufficient sunlight, and is common among those fed on sweetened condensed milk.   Some people keep their babies indoors because they admire a fair complexion; others believe there is danger out of doors from evil spirits.   Sometimes the mother has to go out to work, yet rarely takes the baby outside her room.   Rickets is seen early in infancy (six to twelve weeks) because the mother's diet has been defective; in the tropics it is less usual to see active signs of it in older children.   If the baby survives death from the usual inter-current diseases, the rachitic lesions usually disappear as soon as he is old enough to take himself out of doors.   But even the minor sequels of rickets will render an infant more liable to disorders of the respiratory

20

and digestive systems. There may be histological evidence of rickets in infants examined after death from intercurrent diseases, even though there is no radiological evidence. Both *treatment* and *prevention* are the same all over the world, although in regions where little milk is available the provision of calcium, fat, and fat-soluble vitamins becomes very important.

Beri-beri (Thiamine Deficiency)

This deficiency disease is most commonly encountered among people eating large quantities of polished rice, especially in China and Malaya. It exists in acute and chronic forms, and the more carbohydrate consumed the greater is the need for vitamin B_1 (*thiamine*).

(*a*) INFANTILE BERI-BERI is generally seen in its acute cardiac form. The prodromal symptoms are mild or absent. A fine healthy-looking baby may stop gaining weight for a week or two, or there may be slight restlessness, cough or diarrhœa. Cardiac failure suddenly appears, with cyanosis, tachycardia and dyspnœa, and may cause sudden death. The heart is dilated and a little hypertrophied, chiefly on the right, and the venous circulation is engorged. The lungs are usually congested and may be œdematous. Usually there is oliguria or anuria; œdema may be extreme in the more chronic cases; often pericardial effusion and ascites may be found; vomiting is common. The symptoms may appear at any time after birth, or the disease may be the cause of a stillbirth.

The nervous system is less affected, only atonia being conspicuous; the knee-jerks may be absent, increased, or unchanged. Convulsions sometimes occur. There is often an increased cerebrospinal fluid pressure (sometimes with increase of cells). At post-mortem examination the brain is found to be œdematous and engorged. Frequently there is considerable œdema of the internal organs, even when none is present externally. Œdema of the gall bladder, or of the neck of the gall bladder, is characteristic of beri-beri, as well as the dilatation and hypertrophy of the right side of the heart.

The *treatment* of infantile beri-beri is a medical emergency. A routine that has proved successful is to give 5 to 10 mg. of thiamine, first intracardiac, then intravenously and intramuscularly, as promptly as possible. Sometimes preliminary venesection seems to be of assistance. If available, oxygen should be given. Nothing should be offered by mouth, except occasional sips of water, until the kidneys are working and the œdema is disappearing. A hot-air cradle helps to eliminate fluid. Such emergency treatment may have to be repeated; in any case, 5 to 10 mg. of thiamine should be given daily for 3 to 5 days, and a smaller dose by mouth continued over several weeks.

If breast-feeding is abandoned, the danger to the child is greatly increased; instead, the mother, even in the absence of clinical signs, should be given massive doses of vitamin B_1 and her diet improved. She should be persuaded to eat undermilled rice, vegetables and eggs.

(*b*) CHRONIC BERI-BERI is more often a condition seen in late infancy and childhood. The child may be undersized and malnourished, or may be suffering from severe œdema. Often the most prominent symptom is aphonia, due to œdema of the vocal cords. Sometimes gaseous intestinal distension is marked and intractable; this needs repeated deflation by catheter *per os* and *per rectum*. Some cases have shown marked head retraction (comparable to the experimentally deprived pigeon). The lower motor-neurone paralysis, typical of chronic beri-beri in adults, is seldom seen in children though atonia may be extreme and the knee-jerks variable or absent. Chronic cases seldom require intracardiac or intravenous treatment with vitamin B_1, but intramuscular injections of B_1 concentrates should be given for some days and the diet improved. When œdema is due to beri-beri, diuresis will start within an hour or two of giving the intramuscular injections.

PROGNOSIS

In promptly treated acute cases, the prognosis is good; but in many of the chronic, and in some of the subacute ones, the child recovers only after many months, or not at all. Between these two types there are numerous subacute cases.

Vitamin B_{12}-Deficiency Syndrome in Infants[1]

In India, megaloblastic anæmia with hyperpigmentation and cerebral signs, *responsive to B_{12}*, has been seen in breast-fed infants of mothers with this anæmia. B_{12}-deficiency is occasionally found in infants elsewhere. In infants, megaloblastic anæmia is usually ascribed to *folic-acid deficiency* (or to mixed deficiencies); however, treatment with folic acid alone is dangerous in B_{12}-deficiency because of possible neurological effects.

Keratomalacia from Vitamin-A Deficiency

Many tropical diets are poor in fat, particularly in animal fats; some kinds of tinned milk are prepared from stall-fed cows and are poor in vitamins A and D. Vitamin-A deficiency is a cause of blindness; thus it is not rare to find severe cases of keratomalacia in artificially-fed babies. All 26 babies seen in Singapore Hospital who were blind from keratomalacia had been fed on sweetened condensed milk. In older children, it was common to find some swelling and wrinkling of the conjunctiva and injection of the blood-vessels; in the dry and dusty territories, even minor degrees of this deficiency may lead to conjunctivitis, corneal ulceration and trachoma.

Phrynoderma

Phrynoderma, or *hyperkeratosis pilaris*, is also thought to be due to lack of vitamin A, although some cases will clear up with local treatment. Possibly the lack of vitamin A renders the skin more liable to

[1] Malati, J., Webb, J. K. G., Sarla, V., Baker, S. J. (1962). *Lancet*, 2, 903.

infections. This condition is never found in young babies but is met with in varying severity from the age of five years onwards.

Pellagra

Pellagra is unknown in infants on a milk diet and it is extremely rare in children under the age of 3 years. It occurs mainly in areas where maize is eaten in large quantities and without additional foods containing niacin and tryptophane. It used to be common in Italy, Rumania, Yugoslavia and the Southern States of the U.S.A. and now occurs mainly in certain areas in Africa, Asia and the West Indies. The rash may be difficult to recognize in cases of multiple deficiency. In people whose diet is deficient in milk, fresh vegetables, and therefore in nicotinic acid, the skin becomes photosensitive; those areas which are exposed to sunlight become red, inflamed, tender and irritating, and have a well-defined edge. Severe lesions may proceed to blistering and desquamation. In chronic cases, there is no blistering but there is dry, branny desquamation of the exposed skin, which is darkly pigmented, and mental deterioration and diarrhœa are present. In pellagrous children the skin signs appear early and may be obvious long before there is any constitutional disturbance. Kwashiorkor may be associated with pellagra.

TREATMENT

Except in the most chronic cases, pellagra is readily cured with nicotinamide. Careful revision of the diet is necessary.

Protein Malnutrition: Kwashiorkor

AETIOLOGY

This condition exists in many areas and has been recognized in most tropical and some non-tropical countries. It is a complex one of protein deficiency, often in association with other conditions, both dietetic and infective. Kwashiorkor is a name applied by the *Ga* people of Ghana, and it has been defined as " the sickness the elder child gets when the next baby is born ", because in this area, where cows' milk is not available though food is abundant, the diet offered to the toddler is (without the protection of breast-milk) injurious through lack of protein. Dietary deficiency in the mother is another predisposing factor. The disease usually occurs between 10 months and 4 years of age, since it is in this age bracket that the diet is apt to be lacking in protein. Other diseases which can interfere with digestion and absorption, including intestinal infections and infestations, may also be present, and the clinical picture may be further complicated by multiple vitamin deficiencies.

Furthermore, an inadequate protein diet disturbs enzymic digestion and the activity of intestinal flora. It may be difficult to judge how far the malnutrition is due to diarrhœa and how far diarrhœa is due to malnutrition.

CLINICAL PICTURE

The condition may be seen in acute and chronic forms. In acute cases early enlargement of the liver may occur. Then follow slight swelling of the dorsum of the feet, shininess of the skin, flabbiness of tissues and an alteration of temperament, with anorexia, peevishness and apathy. The extremities are often noticeably cold, even in hot weather. Sometimes, when the mother is suffering from protein deficiency, these signs may arise while the baby is still on the breast. Acute symptoms are apt to be precipitated by an infection, such as gastro-enteritis, malaria or measles. In such a case, œdema appears and the skin changes characteristic of acute kwashiorkor may develop in a spectacular way (Fig. 85). The distribution of the lesions has no relation to light exposure: they are seen especially on the extensor surfaces, pressure areas and the perineum; the face is not usually affected (Fig. 86), though it may be pale. The lesions take the form of dark-brown thickened patches which tend to peel off easily leaving a pale, almost raw, surface.

The chronic forms of the disease are generally found in older children. In an African child, for example, the dark skin lightens to become more coffee-coloured, or there may be a patchy dyspigmentation. The black hair loses its curl and lustre, and a reddish dyspigmentation gradually appears. Wasting is often obscured by œdema. There may be anæmia, diarrhœa or respiratory infection. Ascariasis is an important complicating or precipitating factor in some areas, hookworm infestation in others. Abdominal distention may be prominent. Some infants show severe marasmus; others, more acutely affected, may die before emaciation has set in and even before there is much œdema.

PATHOLOGY

Fatty degeneration of the liver is conspicuous at some stage, and is always present if there is much hepatomegaly. In the later stages the liver may be much reduced in size; some cases go on to fibrosis. Liver changes are accompanied, and sometimes preceded, by degeneration in pancreatic cells, while the enzymes lipase, amylase and trypsin are reduced. In the plasma, total proteins and albumin are low, while the globulins, especially the gammaglobulin, are high. The blood urea and cholesterol are low, as are amylase, alkaline phosphatase and cholinesterase.

TREATMENT

Treatment varies according to the acuteness and the severity of the condition, and according to the age of the child and other diseases present. Good nursing is essential. It is best to admit the mother to hospital as well as the baby, so that by improving her diet, it is

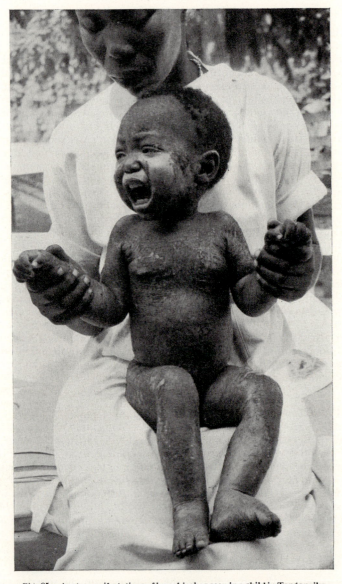

Fig. 85.—Acute manifestations of kwashiorkor seen in a child in Tanganyika. Note his look of misery. Much of the wasting is masked by the presence of œdema, which is seen especially in the legs. In this case the skin manifestations developed suddenly after an attack of measles. *By permission Public Relations Department, Dar-es-Salaam, Tanganyika.*

possible also to improve the quantity and quality of the supply of breast-milk.

The child must be kept warm, perhaps with a radiant-heat cradle. Hypoglycæmia may be present and must receive adequate treatment. Dietary protein must be increased; in mild cases, dried skimmed milk is useful, and may be added to the soups, stews, rice, maize, and banana or cassava porridge which form the child's accustomed diet. In more serious cases pure milk protein should be used, and in cases

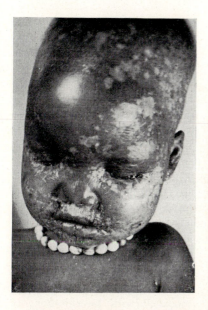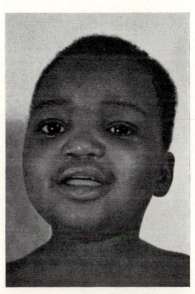

Fig. 86.—Kwashiorkor. *Left :* **Although the face is not usually affected, in this case there is œdema with areas of dyspigmentation and some exfoliation ; mucocutaneous lesions are seen in the region of the mouth, nose and eyes.** *Right :* **The same child a few months later.**

with much vomiting tube feeding by slow drip may be needed. Brock has recently reported improved results by withholding food for the first day and by giving potassium. If there is accompanying beri-beri, œdema will quickly respond to injections of thiamine. Dean reports good results by using soya bean protein, and mashed ripe banana is well assimilated. Bean-porridge, groundnut or green leaf soups, minced or pounded meat and fish, eggs, and cheese or curds should be added to the diet.

As the condition improves, the child's diet should be varied and well balanced, and the parents fully instructed about this. All observers agree that these children may die or relapse with the most unexpected suddenness, and therefore supervision is important. The older and more chronic cases can be treated as out-patients. Careful follow-up and attention to infections, infestations and other deficiencies is essential.

The dietetic factors underlying this condition, which is common in many parts of the world, should be investigated and the diet corrected. It is important for all health workers to be able to diagnose it in its early stages while it is still curable.

Infantile Hepatic Cirrhosis

This is common in many parts of India, and particularly so among the more wealthy of the strictly vegetarian families. It generally starts between the ages of 1 to 4 years, and is often fatal. It has been regarded as a nutritional disorder, although some of the patients have received a fair amount of milk (possibly defective in quality). An alternative explanation is an infection (perhaps allied to hepatitis virus, because a considerable proportion of asymptomatic siblings also show enlarged livers), but K. C. Chaudhuri suspects genetic factors.

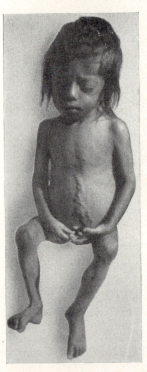

Fig. 87.—An Indian child, aged 4 years, with advanced hepatic cirrhosis. Her family were high-caste and strictly vegetarian. The father was a farmer and the child had plenty of milk, but the cows were thin and their milk may have been poor in quality.

CLINICAL PICTURE

The patient is usually well nourished. The liver is enlarged and hard; the spleen is also palpable. Ascites develops, then jaundice, and bile appears in the urine. There is often some fever. The skin conditions associated with kwashiorkor are absent. Children who appear to recover may later show signs of portal obstruction (Fig. 87). The disease seems to be more common in the first-born, and more common in boys than in girls. In advanced cases the superficial abdominal veins are prominent.

Veno-occlusive Disease of the Liver

Bras and his co-workers in Jamaica have described a disease of the liver in children on a low-protein diet. It is probable that some of the popular " bush teas " may contain a toxin which results in this disease. The chief lesion is a gradually increasing fibrosis of the hepatic veins, with diffuse collagenosis and fibrosis. Enlargement of the liver and spleen, and ascites occur.

Epidemic Dropsy (*Argemone Mexicana* Poisoning)

This is confined to the areas in India where mustard-seed oil is used for cooking.   The symptoms appear slowly, and weakness and œdema develop.   There may be fever, signs in the lungs, and disturbances of vision.   The swelling of legs and feet is generally well marked and with a nodular rash that is very like erythema nodosum.   The condition is rare in children.   It is due to the seeds of a weed, *Argemone mexicana*, being mixed with those of the mustard plant, which they resemble. Treatment consists in stopping the adulterated mustard oil and giving a high-protein diet with calcium lactate.

Urinary Calculus

In some areas, kidney stones are extraordinarily common, even in babies of a few months old.   They have been ascribed to dehydration and to lack of vitamin A, but these are certainly not the only factors concerned and the matter needs investigation.

INTESTINAL DISEASES

Enteritis (*see also* p. 192).

INTESTINAL disorders are common in all tropical and sub-tropical countries on account of temperature, living conditions, the prevalence of flies and intestinal worms, and poor toilet hygiene.   Unsuitable food is another factor, since enteritis is not only caused by infections but also by the irritant nature of a coarse diet.

In non-dysenteric and non-enteric diarrhœas, the treatment usually begins with a low-calorie, residue-free diet with plenty of fluid, and the child is kept in bed.   It is important to exclude the entero-dysenteric group of infections whenever possible by bacteriological examination, and the stools should be examined for parasites.

The Dysenteries

Bacillary dysenteries are common in hot countries.   They respond well to the usual sulphonamide treatment when used early in the disease (*see* Appendix 1).   Rest in bed and low-residue diet are also necessary (*see also* pp. 194–198).

Amœbic Dysentery (Amœbiasis)

This is caused by *Entamœba histolytica* transmitted by fæcally contaminated food and water, human carriers being the source.   Affected persons may be symptomless or may have recurrent dysentery with blood in the stool.   The diagnosis is made microscopically by identification of cysts or motile forms of *E. histolytica* in fresh stools; often many specimens have to be examined.

In *hepatic amœbiasis*, amœbæ reach the liver, via the portal vein, setting up small liver abscesses, which are usually multiple. There is irregular fever and discomfort over the liver, with some tenderness and enlargement on examination. Such a case may progress to a fully established *liver abscess* with increasing liver enlargement, pain, high swinging temperature and loss of weight.

TREATMENT

The *dysenteric form* is treated as follows:

(1) Emetine hydrochloride is given by intramuscular injection (1·0 mg. ($\frac{1}{60}$ grain) per Kg. body-weight once daily) for six days.

(2) Iodochlorhydroxyquinoline 0·125–0·25 G. (1$\frac{1}{2}$–4 grains) three times daily for ten to fourteen days.

(3) Oxytetracycline (for dosage, *see* Appendix 1) for seven to ten days.

Hepatic amœbiasis is treated as follows:

(1) Emetine hydrochloride (as above).

(2) This is followed by chloroquine for two to three weeks. Dosage is as follows:

1–5 years	0·125–0·25 G. (2–4 grains) twice daily.
5–10 years	twice the above dose.

Chloroquine may be repeated at three-monthly intervals for four courses.

Amœbic abscess formation in its early stages responds to the above treatment; only when the abscess has reached large proportions will surgical drainage be required. Specific anti-amœbic treatment must never be omitted despite adequate surgical drainage.

Enteric Fevers. (*See also* p. 554.)

Typhoid is common in many tropical and sub-tropical regions. Protective inoculation is effective, and should be routinely employed and repeated every two years. Enteric infections are somewhat less serious and less fatal in children than in adults, and they follow a rather different course. Thus, the period of bradycardia may be short and the temperature is more irregular in type than that usually described. Treatment with chloramphenicol is indicated.

Paratyphoid and other salmonella infections are also encountered, either as more or less mild enteritis, or, with greater severity, as fulminating septicæmia. Chloramphenicol has given good results.

Intestinal Myiasis

Sometimes the stools of a child are found to be crawling with maggots. This is an indication of the gross contamination to which food is exposed, the maggots usually being those of the common house-fly. No special treatment is necessary except to give an aperient to the child and a serious talk to the mother.

"Vomiting Sickness" of Jamaica and Hypoglycæmia

" Vomiting sickness " is a local name used to describe a number of diseases that are associated with acute vomiting and end frequently in death.

The cause is unknown but has been attributed to the ackee (an excellent culture medium for *Staphylococcus aureus*) and to toxins from immature yams. However, experimental work has shown that it takes a very large quantity of ackee fruit to produce lethal quantities of toxin. Perhaps chronic undernutrition followed by a period of starvation (or near starvation) is more important than toxin contained in ackees; it is possible that certain other local Jamaican herbs may contain toxins causing hypoglycæmia.

The onset is characterized by acute vomiting and hypoglycæmia and, in severe cases, convulsions and coma. Most of the fatalities are amongst children suffering from intestinal parasites and malnutrition. There is a high incidence of marasmus and liver disease. Hypoglycæmia should be suspected in cases of rapidly developing coma or convulsions. Treatment consists first in raising the blood-sugar content by intravenous dextrose, then dealing with the underlying malnutrition.

HELMINTHIASIS

HELMINTHIASIS is a serious public-health problem in all parts where sanitation is poor. The more important intestinal parasites are described in Chapter 27.

Schistosoma (Bilharzia)

These flukes or trematode worms are responsible for a great deal of ill-health in some regions. The intermediate host is a snail, and infection is caused by contact with snail-infested water. The larval flukes enter through the skin, and grow to adults in the portal, mesenteric and pelvic veins. The eggs they deposit ulcerate through nearby organs.

There are three main varieties of schistosome:

(1) *Schistosoma hæmatobium* is common in Egypt, Equatorial Africa and the Near East; it produces mainly genito-urinary symptoms, such as hæmaturia. The ova usually appear in urine.

(2) *S. mansoni* (Egypt, Equatorial Africa, South America and West Indies) produces dysenteric symptoms. The ova usually appear in stools.

(3) *S. japonicum* (China, Japan, and the Philippines) often causes general symptoms with fever, cough and diarrhœa. The diagnosis is made by complement-fixation test or by finding ova in stools.

These infestations occasionally manifest with initial itchy rash, then with malaise, fever and *eosinophilia*, and later with enlargement of liver and spleen.   Often the condition heals spontaneously, but some of the victims become gradually and seriously ill.

TREATMENT

Preventive. Bathing and paddling should not be allowed in any freshwater ponds and lakes in which the snail vector exists.   Sometimes infection occurs through the capsizing of a boat on fresh water. There is no risk of bilharzial infection in seawater.

Curative. Antimony lithium thiomalate (Anthiomaline) or lucanthone hydrochloride (Miracil D) are usually employed.   The treatment, which may be unpleasant, has to be maintained for a considerable time.

A great deal of money is being spent in trying to control the breeding of the snails, which are the intermediate hosts, and in educating people to keep their water supplies free from human excreta.

Filaria

This name covers a group of small nematodes that live in the lymphatics and connective tissue in man.   They produce large numbers of embryos, or " microfilariæ."   These inhabit chiefly the skin or the blood-stream, from which they may be transferred to other individuals by the appropriate insect vector—a Culicini mosquito, Simulium fly, Chrysops, or Culicoides.   The infection may be present for years before causing symptoms, but in many cases they block the lymphatics, and give rise to elephantiasis, chyluria or blindness.

The following are the most important varieties:

(1) *Wuchereria bancrofti.* In some areas the microfilariæ are found in the blood only at night and in others only in the daytime (nocturnal or diurnal periodicity).   The vector is usually a mosquito.   Infection may give rise to transient swellings, but it is unusual for serious symptoms to arise for some years or until the adult nematodes produce elephantiasis, chyluria or lymphangitis.

(2) *Wuchereria malayi.* Similar to above, occurring mainly in the Western Pacific region.

(3) *Loa loa* occurs especially in Central and West Africa and the microfilariæ are diurnal.   The adult parasite wanders about the body and may cause swellings.   It may be seen crossing the eye under the conjunctiva, from which position it can be excised.

(4) *Onchocerca volvulus.* (Central and West Africa, West Indies, and Mexico).   The diagnosis is generally made by examination of skin clips.   The disease may be contracted in early life and has in the past been regarded as a cause of " river blindness ".   The vector is a small fly—*Simulium damnosum*— the eradication of which is a vast public health problem.

TREATMENT

Diethylcarbamazine citrate (Banocide) is the most potent antifilarial drug available (2–3 mg./Kg. thrice daily for 21 days). *Prevention* lies in avoiding the bites of the insect vector.

MALARIA

MALARIA affects about one per cent. of the world's population, and within the last 10 years, with international support, control and eradication operations have been organized. These are mainly effected by residual spraying of houses with DDT to destroy the mosquito vector.

In areas where mosquitoes have shown DDT-resistance, other methods of control, including elimination of breeding grounds, larvicides and rigorous treatment of malaria patients, have been brought into use. The disease is especially dangerous and prevalent in children between the ages of three months and three years. The possibility of transplacental infection has been established, but "congenital malaria" is very rare.

Infection is almost invariably conveyed by the bite of certain mosquitoes of the *Anopheles* varieties, in which the parasite undergoes a sexual phase of development. The chief forms are: benign tertian malaria—*Plasmodium vivax*; subtertian (malignant) malaria—*Plasmodium falciparum;* quartan malaria—*Plasmodium ovale. Plasmodium ovale* is rare except in W. Africa. Unless there is reinfection, parasites will die out in the human host within two years but quartan malaria may recur even after several years.

Mechanism of Immunity. Work in the Gambia has shown that the development of specific antimalarial immunity is associated with an elevation of serum gammaglobulin level; also that gammaglobulin prepared from the blood of immune subjects rapidly cures malaria when injected into severely infected children. In endemic areas many adults, and perhaps some children, become tolerant, getting attacks of fever only when ill from other causes, such as injury, infection, or malnutrition. Immunity, which is specific for the plasmodial strain, is reduced by living outside endemic areas.

SYMPTOMATOLOGY

Acute and chronic forms are seen. In the acute form there is pyrexia and, occasionally, hyperpyrexia; convulsions are common in young children; rigors are comparatively rare. The attack is generally accompanied by anorexia, gastritis or gastro-enteritis. In cerebral types there is hyperpyrexia, meningism, convulsions and coma. Bronchitis is a common complication. The liver enlarges and there may be jaundice. Splenomegaly develops more rapidly than in the adult; there may be pain, tenderness and rigidity over the spleen. In a young baby, the spleen will sometimes enlarge within a week almost to the level of the umbilicus and, when the attack is treated, will decrease again in size. The fibrotic splenomegaly of chronic malaria is more persistent. Anæmia is caused by the destruction of erythrocytes and damage to the bone-marrow. In children it may be much more sudden and severe than in adults, and transfusions are frequently indicated. There is an acute, fulminating form of anæmia which may be rapidly fatal.

In the more chronic forms of malaria, fever occurs at intervals. There is persistent splenomegaly and a variable degree of anæmia. Traces of albumin may be found in the urine. Cachexia sometimes develops. Many of the children in malarious areas are malnourished, and the algid form of malaria sometimes occurs.

DIAGNOSIS

To detect malarial parasites, the blood should be examined on thick and thin films taken, if possible, during fever. The incidence of the disease in a community may be roughly assessed by surveying the " spleen rate ", that is, the percentage of children between 2 and 10 years with an enlarged spleen.

TREATMENT

The synthetic antimalarials now in general use have largely replaced quinine both in the prevention and cure of malaria, although a few authorities still consider quinine to be the best treatment for acute attacks in children for all types of malaria.

Of the synthetic antimalarials, chloroquine and amodiaquine, which are both schizonticides, provide the first choices of treatment for acute attacks. Proguanil (Paludrine) and mepacrine, also schizonticides, are useful alternatives. In addition, proguanil and pamaquin are true causal prophylactics of falciparum malaria, acting in the pre-erythrocyte phase and thus preventing invasion of the red blood cells. Pamaquin also has an inhibiting effect upon the pre-erythrocyte phase of benign tertia malaria. Pyrimethamine acts on the pre-erythrocyte forms of falciparum malaria and also on the asexual erythrocytic forms of the disease, but some falciparum strains have already proved relatively insensitive to this drug.

For prophylaxis, chloroquine, amodiaquine, and proguanil are all widely used, as is pyrimethamine in some areas. These preparations are generally considered to be less toxic than quinine and mepacrine and have tended to replace them. The protagonists of quinine claim that it is generally well tolerated by children in spite of its bitter taste, quinine sulphate being less likely to cause vomiting than the more rapidly dissociated hydrochloride.

DOSAGE OF ANTIMALARIAL DRUGS

Chloroquine Di-phosphate: Acute Attack. 25 mg. ($\frac{2}{5}$ grain) per Kg. body-weight orally initially, followed by half this dose daily for a further four days. In unconscious patients 6–12 mg. ($\frac{1}{10}$–$\frac{1}{5}$ grain) per Kg. body-weight of the dihydrochloride may be given intramuscularly or slowly by intravenous drip as initial treatment.

Suppressant. 250 mg. (4 grains) at weekly intervals over the age of six years; below this age half that dose (no casual prophylactic action).

Amodiaquine (Camoquine): Acute Attack. 10 mg. ($\frac{1}{6}$ grain) of base per Kg. body-weight orally initially, followed by half this dose daily for a further four days.

Prophylaxis. 6 mg. ($\frac{1}{10}$ grain) of base per Kg. body-weight as a weekly suppressant dose.

Proguanil (Paludrine): Acute Attack. This drug has some schizonticidal activity. It is effective against *P. falciparum* but its chief value is in prophylaxis.

Prophylaxis. 2 mg. ($\frac{1}{30}$ grain) per Kg. body-weight daily.

Pyrimethamine: Prophylaxis. 6·25 mg. ($\frac{1}{10}$ grain) weekly under 6 years of age, 12·5 mg. ($\frac{1}{5}$ grain) over 6 years of age at weekly intervals.

Mepacrine: Acute Attack. For children over 6 years of age: 1st day 0·3–0·5 G. (5–8 grains) thrice daily; 2nd day 0·15–0·3 G. (2$\frac{1}{2}$–5 grains) thrice daily; succeeding days 0·15 G. (2$\frac{1}{2}$ grains) thrice daily.

Children under 6 years take half this dosage.

Prophylaxis. Mepacrine is not recommended for children.

Quinine: Acute Attack. For oral treatment the following mixture is used.

Quinine sulphate	120 mg. (2 grains)
Ferrous sulphate	60 mg. (1 grain)
Glucose	600 mg. (10 grains)
Dilute sulphuric acid	as required
Chloroform water	to 4 ml. (1 drachm)

This mixture can be given three times daily to an infant. An increased dose is indicated for older children.

When a child is unconscious chloroquine dihydrochloride can be given parenterally (*see* above).

Where hyperpyrexia is a feature, the child is treated by tepid sponging. Cold sponging is to be avoided, especially in young children.

PREVENTION

In endemic areas young children should sleep under a mosquito net. Control of anopheline mosquitoes by "residual spraying" with the newer insecticides can be achieved successfully and economically provided local conditions are properly studied.

It is unwise to give suppressive antimalarial therapy to children in endemic areas, unless it is certain that this can be continued regularly and indefinitely. On the other hand, every effort should be made to provide for rapid and effective treatment when attacks of fever occur.

Blackwater Fever

This occurs chiefly in Europeans, who have little or no immunity, and only rarely in indigenous people living in malarious areas. It is associated with use of quinine for chronic falciparum infections—a double infection with *P. vivax* and unrecognized *P. falciparum* may easily be overlooked. The malarial infection should be treated with chloroquine or amodiaquine (never quinine). Primaquine and pamaquin should be avoided. Rest in bed is essential. A carefully matched blood transfusion may be carried out. Prednisone (Deltacortone) may terminate the hæmolytic process. Afterwards Paludrine should be used for prophylaxis.

LEISHMANIASIS

THE three clinical varieties are kala-azar, oriental sore and espundia.

Kala-azar (Visceral Leishmaniasis)

This disease is caused by the protozoa *Leishmania donovani*, which is transmitted by a sandfly. The incubation period is normally 2–6 months but may be up to 6 years.

It occurs in the Mediterranean area, Turkey, Iran, Egypt, India, and China. It is more common in hot, dry regions, and may start at any age, but is rare before six months. The symptoms are fever, splenomegaly, lymphadenitis, progressive anæmia and cachexia. Diagnosis is generally made by spleen, liver, bone-marrow or gland puncture.

TREATMENT

Treatment with antimony compounds is generally successful. Trivalent compounds have proved to be much less effective than pentavalent compounds, such as ethylstibamine, given either intramuscularly or intravenously. (For a child of one year, the dose is given on alternate days increasing through 0·05 G., 0·075 G., 0·1 G., to a total of 2·5 G. within six weeks.) The course may be repeated in two months. A single course of ethylstibamine lasts about one month. It may be given intramuscularly to infants (0·01 to 0·08 G. in distilled water to a total of 0·65 G.). Pentamidine isethionate is an alternative form of treatment, but it may cause peripheral neuritis. The maximum single dose is 3 mg. per Kg. body-weight by intramuscular injection, but preceded by one or two smaller doses.

Prevention consists in protection from exposure to sandfly bites, control of sandfly breeding places, and destruction of dogs or other animals infected with the disease.

Oriental Sore (Dermal Leishmaniasis)

The indolent lesions of dermal leishmaniasis result in scarring. The geographical distribution is the same as kala-azar. Pentavalent antimony compounds and treatment for secondary pyogenic infection are given.

Espundia (Naso-pharyngeal Leishmaniasis)

The disease is found in South and Central America, sometimes appearing in epidemics. The sores may be extremely serious and proceed to gangrene. Treatment is by pentavalent antimony compounds.

AFRICAN TRYPANOSOMIASIS (SLEEPING SICKNESS)

AFRICAN trypanosomiasis is transmitted by various types of tsetse flies (or *Glossina*). *T. rhodesiense*, the more serious type of infection, is conveyed by *G. morsitans* and *G. swynnertoni*, both of which breed at considerable distances from water and are widely distributed in East and Central Africa. *T. rhodesiense* is derived from reservoirs of infection in certain wild game. *T. gambiense* is conveyed by *G. palpalis* and *G. tachinoides*, which reproduce only near water, and infection occurs chiefly in West Africa where the principle reservoir of infection is probably man.

Children are commonly infected and in proportion to their exposure to tsetse flies.

The usual manifestations are irregular fever; a rash, which may be patchy, erythematous and transient; neuralgia; adenitis, particularly of the cervical glands; anæmia; headache; insomnia and cardiac changes. There may be periods of quiescence, or the patient may develop increasing coma. Trypanosoma may be found by examination of blood, gland puncture or cerebrospinal fluid. Rise of protein or cells in the CSF is significant. In *Trypanosoma rhodesiense* infections, adenitis is not as common or as pronounced; this disease, both in its sporadic and epidemic forms, is more severe and is very often fatal. It is very rare for recovery to take place after the somnolence has developed. Mania and convulsions are not infrequent.

TREATMENT

Pentamidine and suramin are used for blood and lymphatic forms; tryparsamide for nervous system involvement. Suramin (Antrypol) is of chief value in the early stages and of little use in later ones. Tryparsamide penetrates into the central nervous system and is therefore of value in the later stages, especially in *T. gambiense* infections, whilst *T. rhodesiense* are more resistant to arsenicals. Treatment must be prolonged and surviving patients followed up for three or four years.

SOUTH AMERICAN TRYPANOSOMIASIS
(CHAGAS' DISEASE)

CHAGAS' disease, caused by *T. cruzi*, is found in Mexico, Central America, and South America. It occurs predominantly among children and is transmitted to them by reduviid bugs. These are often 3 cm. in length and become infected by feeding on an animal or a person having *T. cruzi* in the blood; afterwards their excreta is capable of infecting man through abrasions of the skin and mucosæ. The bugs infest cracks in mud-walled houses and they feed at night by biting exposed areas of sleeping persons; thus poor people are chiefly affected because the bugs are found in primitive houses. Various small animals (rats, pigs, armadillos and opossums) are the reservoirs of infection.

The manifestations are fever, palpebral œdema, conjunctivitis, lymphocytosis, lymphadenopathy and splenomegaly. Involvement of the heart causes tachycardia and cardiac irregularity. There may be encephalitis. The outcome may be fatal in the acute stage, or recovery from this stage may leave sequelæ in the heart, brain or viscera.

In Chagas' disease the arsenic and antimony compounds are useless, and an effective drug treatment is awaited. Tetracycline in combination with primaquine has given some encouraging results, and there is a recently reported case of an adult having been successfully treated with nitrofurazone.[1] Control depends on improved housing, the destruction of bug-infested huts, the use of insecticides, such as Gammexane, and the prevention of bug bites at night.

SPIROCHÆTAL DISEASES
Relapsing Fever (Spirillum Fever, Tick Fever)

THE *epidemic* form of the disease is due to *Spirochæta recurrentis* conveyed by the body louse. The patient scratches and the spirochæte enters the skin from the fæces or from the crushed body of the louse. This type is mainly found in overcrowded conditions in Asia.

The *endemic* form of the disease, due to the *S. duttoni*, is transmitted by a tick—*Ornithodorus moubata*. As this tick can live for many months without food, it forms a long-term reservoir for the infection in certain parts of Africa.

Symptoms are a fulminating pyrexia or irregular fever. Headache, somnolence, sweating, an enlarged spleen, diarrhœa or constipation, abdominal pain, an occasional erythematous rash, jaundice and prostration are the symptoms that have been described. Hæmorrhages into the skin and the internal organs, and albuminuria may occur.

Treatment with penicillin, alone or combined with acetarsol or arsphenamine, was frequently successful, but has now been replaced by the tetracyclines. Mortality in young children is high.

Prophylaxis is by control of insect vectors.

[1] Melzer, H., Kollert, W. (1963). *Dtsch. med. Wschr.*, **88**, 188, *et seq.*

Leptospirosis Icterohaemorrhagica (Weil's Disease)

This infection is generally caused by contact with water that contains the excreta of animals. It is a common infection of rats and may be picked up by those working in damp places, in sewers and in some areas in forest pools; thus to some extent it is an occupational disease. *Leptospira canicola* is occasionally transmitted by dogs to children through close contact. It is a less common and less severe infection than Weil's disease.

Weil's disease has been found in almost every country; many cases occur in Malaya and Indonesia. As a rule, the symptoms start with fever, vomiting, muscular pains, rigors and injected conjunctivæ. Jaundice often starts a day or two after the onset, and the liver enlarges. Albumin and bile pigments appear in the urine. Diagnosis is made by examination of the blood and urine for leptospira, by culture and by agglutination tests. The urine gives a green colour when added to a small quantity of acetic acid.

Treatment consists of rest and combating the possibility of renal failure (p. 374). Penicillin has been used with success. Prophylaxis is by sterilization of urine and fæces from all patients and by control of rodents. Pools that may be infected should be prohibited for swimming.

Spirillary Rat-bite Fever

Rat-bite fever occurs in children of any age and the mortality may be as high as 10 per cent. There is always a history of a rat bite or bite of some other animal (dog, cat, mouse, or ferret). After incubation of one to four weeks, there is a renewal of inflammation in the bite accompanied by rash and regional adenitis. The rash returns with recurrences of fever. Diagnosis should be confirmed by guinea-pig inoculation, as it may be difficult to find the spirillum in the blood. A relapsing or intermittent type of fever may be severe, and there is considerable prostration. Without treatment the infection may last for some weeks. It responds to penicillin or tetra-cyclines, especially the latter.

Yaws (Frambœsia)

This is due to the *Treponema pertenuis* which is morphologically indistinguishable from *T. pallidum*. Yaws may be epidemic or endemic but has not been proved to exist in a congenital form.

Yaws occurs in tropical Africa, the West Indies, Central and South America, the East Indies and Malaya, and in certain localities in India and China; it has also been described among the aborigines of Australia. In areas where treatment is neglected, yaws increases and becomes a grave health problem. It is more common in damp areas. It occurs in children of 2 to 10 years and may even appear in infants of 2 to 3 months. Symptoms may persist or reappear even 20 or 30 years after the primary attack.

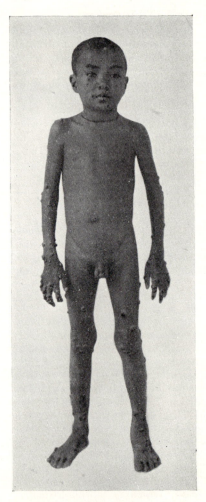

Fig. 88.—Yaws. Note typical secondary rash and its distribution.

SYMPTOMS

A soft gelatinous blister develops (Fig. 88), which soon breaks and becomes a raised, fungating, purulent sore. The sores multiply and may become extensive; secondary infection is common and various stages of the disease may be found in one individual. General symptoms, which may be slight or severe, include fever, pain, and general misery.

In later stages, the primary lesions may dry up, leaving patchy discoloration and scarring, or they may become chronic ulcers or lichenous, hyperkeratotic lesions. Pustules, not unlike those of other poxes, may develop. Later osseous changes are granulomatous deformity, dactylitis, periosteal nodule formation and sabre tibia. The latter, and a similar condition of the ulna, are common in children. *Goundou* (enlargement of the nasal bones), *gangosa* (destructive granuloma of the nose and palate), and juxta-articular nodules may appear at a late stage. Chronic granulomatous ulcers on the feet and thickening of the plantar and palmar epidermis with desquamation and fissuring (crab yaws) are common.

TREATMENT

Yaws responds to penicillin, the tetracyclines and chloramphenicol. Penicillin is probably the treatment of choice at present. In recent years yaws eradication campaigns have proved remarkably successful in a number of countries.

BACTERIAL DISEASES

Plague (Pestis)

THIS is an acute infectious fever, primarily of rats, but transferred to man through fleas infected by the rodents with *Pasteurella pestis*. The incidence and severity of the disease is often less in children than in adults. The bubonic type is a toxæmia or bacteriæmia, and is acquired by the bite of the infected flea. The more fatal pneumonic type is acquired by droplet infection and becomes a septicæmia. The disease is apt to appear in epidemics where a disorganized population is living in overcrowded and insanitary conditions. In parts of Asia the disease is endemic.

Cases of fever and adenitis, either during an epidemic or in endemic areas, must be regarded with suspicion. The typical cocco-bacillus, with bipolar staining, may be demonstrated in the blood, glands, sputum, etc. and may be cultivated by Haffkine's method, or animal inoculation may be used.

Treatment with sulphonamides or, better, intramuscular streptomycin is dramatically effective; tetracyclines have also been successful.

Prophylaxis is by means of: (*a*) quarantine of ships from plague areas, especially with respect to the rats they may carry; (*b*) destruction of rats; (*c*) treatment of patients, contacts and houses in a plague area with DDT in order to kill the fleas; (*d*) prophylactic inoculation, a valuable measure indicated for children of any age; (*e*) prophylactic sulphonamides given to those working on health measures; (*f*) protective clothing for workers.

Cholera

This acute infectious enteritis is caused by Koch's comma bacillus, or vibrio. The disease is endemic in certain parts of Asia; outbreaks occur very often in the wake of pilgrimages and are more likely after periods of high absolute humidity. The bacillus is transmitted through contaminated food and water. Children who acquire the disease generally die so quickly that relatively few are seen in hospitals.

The incubation is 1 to 5 days. The onset is abrupt and the symptoms are diarrhœa, becoming profuse and watery, vomiting, muscle cramps and intense dehydration. The typical stools are of the " rice water " appearance and consistency, but may be blood-stained.

Treatment consists in combating the infection with sulphonamides and antibiotics (sulphaguanidine, succinylsulphathiazole, chloramphenicol or tetracycline), and the dehydration by intravenous saline. Normal saline is the basic solution to which is added lactate, to correct associated acidosis, and potassium once the initial dehydration is overcome (*see* p. 194). In small children intragastric and subcutaneous drips may, in the absence of skilled ward supervisors, be preferable to intravenous therapy. Cramps and pains may be relieved by hot-water bottles, gentle friction, or with codeine, etc. Thirst may be relieved by giving ice to suck, or hot drinks if collapse is threatened. Noradrenaline and corticosteroids have been used. Rest and warmth are essential.

Cholera should be prevented by the normal quarantine precautions. In endemic areas it has proved impossible to end the disease merely by providing a good water supply. Where personal hygiene is of a low standard, the disease is not likely to be eliminated without patient and thorough education.

Patients should be carefully isolated and all discharges disinfected. Water supplies must be chlorinated or treated with permanganate of potash 1: 500,000. All drinking water should be boiled. Food must be carefully prepared and protected from flies and dust. Prophylactic inoculation is recommended for travel to or through endemic areas and booster injections every five months in areas where danger exists.

TABLE XXI
PROPHYLATIC INOCULATION AGAINST CHOLERA

Age	1st Dose	2nd Dose	3rd Dose
6 months to 4 years	0·1 ml. (1½ minims)	0·3 ml. (5 minims)	0·3 ml. (5 minims)
5–9 years	0·3 ml. (5 minims)	0·5 ml. (8 minims)	0·5 ml. (8 minims)
10 years and over	0·5 ml. (8 minims)	0·5 ml. (8 minims)	

Leprosy

Leprosy is nowadays generally confined to those countries that have a low standard of personal and domestic hygiene. The first manifestations often appear in children or adolescents, who are more susceptible than adults. The incubation period may be as long as seven years. The diagnosis is made by nasal swabs and skin clippings and by the appearance of the lesions.

Treatment is *dapsone* (diaminodiphenyl-sulphone) given by mouth over a minimum period of two years but always used with care because of possible toxic effects. PAS and streptomycin are less effective. Chaulmoogra oil was used formerly and was effective in early lesions; advanced lesions, however, showed little response.

The children born of lepers should be separated from the mother at or very soon after birth.

The presence of leprosy in any area makes it supremely important to exercise the greatest care in sterilizing syringes and needles.

RICKETTSIAL DISEASES

THE typhus fevers, with the exception of the Rocky Mountain type, are uncommon in children and less severe than in adults. The following are the chief varieties that have been described:

Epidemic Typhus

The infection is carried from man to man by the louse and occurs most frequently when crowds of people are living in congested, insanitary conditions. It is characterized by a rash and severe prostration. Chloramphenicol is effective; other antibiotics are on trial.

Scrub Typhus (Japanese River, or Tsutsugamushi Fever)

Mite borne, it is found in rural areas mainly in Malaya and the Far East. Field mice and rats are the usual hosts. Untreated, the infection has a high mortality. Chloramphenicol and the tetracyclines have proved to be of value.

Endemic (Murine) Typhus

Typhus, which is flea-borne, has a wide distribution. The rat is the usual host. The same antibiotics are used.

Rocky Mountain Spotted Fever

This occurs in parts of the U.S.A. The rash is well marked. Children often are sufferers. It is carried by the dog tick, and various rodents are the hosts. Tetracyclines are more effective than chloramphenicol.

South African Tick Typhus

The fever may be mild or severe. Dogs are probably a reservoir of infection.

Q Fever

Occurring mainly in Australia and the U.S.A., this is tick-borne and wild rodents form the reservoir of infection. Although rare in children, infection may come through dust (dried tick fæces).

Diagnosis is by complement-fixation test and treatment with tetracyclines. Prophylaxis is by the use of DDT and the newer insecticides to control the insect vectors; control of the animal reservoirs is often difficult. Protective vaccine has been prepared but is not generally available.

VIRUS DISEASES

Yellow Fever

A FILTERABLE virus is responsible, and in the past severe epidemics have taken place in West Africa, the West Indies and in the Southern States of the U.S.A. The disease also exists in Central and East Africa and in South America. It may be exceedingly difficult to recognize in young children, the symptoms being either atypical or completely absent. Apparently, children from endemic areas nearly all have a life-long immunity to the disease. The virus is conveyed by certain mosquitoes, usually *Aëdes ægtypi*.

The typical symptoms develop, after an incubation period of about five days, in the form of a severe illness with prostration, fever, headache, slow pulse, " black vomit," injected conjunctivæ, albuminuria and jaundice.   The treatment consists of fluids, glucose and calcium. A purgative may be necessary in the early stages and barbiturates or codeine to relieve the restlessness and intense pain.

In the past, the disease has been controlled by rigid anti-mosquito measures, and now that a very successful form of protective inoculation exists newcomers to these areas rarely get the disease.   Inoculation should be repeated every six years.

Dengue

This fever is rare in children.   It is accompanied by severe pains in the back, head, and joints, but has no mortality.   Newcomers to a country are often the only victims, but sometimes it appears in epidemic form.   The incubation period is 5 to 9 days.   The fever is of the " saddle back " variety, the typical morbilliform rash occurring with the recrudescence of the fever.   There is no specific treatment. It is a virus infection carried by mosquitoes of the genus *Aëdes*; prevention is by mosquito eradication and the use of insect repellents.

Sandfly Fever (Phlebotomus Fever)

The virus is transmitted by sandfly bites.   This infection is not seen in children indigenous to the country.   The symptoms are very like those of dengue, except that the fever in this case is more irregular and the conjunctivæ are often more injected.   There is no secondary rise of temperature and no exanthem.

Smallpox (Variola)

In some areas in the tropics and in some parts of India and China this disease has been common.   Even where vaccination is freely available the indifference, fatalism or conservatism of the population prevents them from appreciating its value.   It is not uncommon to find babies and young children with florid smallpox being carried around in the usual way.

The incubation period is 10 to 14 days.   Small children often get the disease.   The severity varies from that of a mild " alastrim " to a rapidly fatal condition.   The earliest symptoms are generally those of headache, restlessness and vomiting, allied with a prodromal rise of temperature which then subsides.   Between two and five days later the temperature rises again and the rash appears.   This differs from that of chickenpox in that it is profuse on the face and on the extremities, and often on the back, being less so on the chest and abdomen.   The pox may appear on the palms, soles, inside the mouth, and on the cornea (which may lead to blindness).   The pock is deep-seated and has a " shotty " feel.   The patient is in acute distress with pain, discomfort and thirst.   All the spots come out at one time, so they are more or less all in the same stage of development. After a few days the small pustules that have developed become umbilicated and in favourable cases they may gradually dry up and the scabs fall off, very often leaving pitted scars.

The confluent and hæmorrhagic forms of the disease are usually fatal. In sporadic cases, the condition may be difficult to distinguish from chickenpox, particularly if it is in a modified form due to vaccination.

TREATMENT

Treatment consists of rest and warmth, penicillin for the secondary infection which is present, plenty of fluid, and some bland, moist dressing, such as weak solution of potassium permanganate, to protect the skin. Preliminary reports of the therapeutic use of N-methylisatin beta-thiosemicarbazone suggest that it may be of value in smallpox. The child must be prevented from scratching, or scarring will be severe. Cases should be isolated. Vaccination should be advised for the whole population and repeated every three years. If vaccination is performed in early childhood, the reaction is less severe than if the primary vaccination is deferred until later years (*see* p. 562).

Cases of symmetrical osteomyelitis, generally of the elbows, have been reported by MacGregor[1] as a sequel to smallpox, and may possibly be associated with malnutrition or with yaws. The treatment for this complication is surgical, together with appropriate antibiotics.

NEOPLASMS

CERTAIN neoplasms appear to be more prevalent in some tropical countries than elsewhere in the world. Thus, malignant lymphoma,[2] commonly involving the jaw, is seen in a belt of African territory stretching across the continent south of the Sahara, from west to east coast, while similar tumours have been encountered in children in Bombay and Hong Kong. Kaposi's sarcoma,[3] presenting as one or more bluish-red skin nodules on the legs or arms, has a similar geographical distribution in Africa to malignant lymphoma. In young children, the course may be fulminating with widespread lymphadenopathy and involvement of the eyelids and salivary glands. Treatment is palliative. Cytotoxic preparations may induce partial remissions.

DISEASES AND CARE OF THE SKIN

MANY of the infections and other disorders of the integument are attributable to lack of washing facilities and soap, overcrowding and ignorance of personal hygiene. Sometimes neglect is responsible and this tends especially to affect infants. Under such conditions careful

[1] MacGregor, M. (1958). *Arch. Dis. Childh.*, **33**, 383.
[2] Annotation (1961). *Lancet*, 1, 1156.
[3] Jeliffe, D. B., Cook, J., Davies, J. N. P. (1962). *J. Pediat.*, **61**, 452.

teaching must be given in the cleaning of eyes, nose, ears, and perineum, Too often the secretions are not wiped away, the face of the child remains plastered with remnants of food and is soon crawling with flies. It is not surprising that sore eyes and all manner of skin infections are rife, especially those due to staphylococci and tinea. The baby's skin may even be attacked by ants, cockroaches and rats.

Many of the nutritional diseases affect the skin, especially kwashiorkor, pellagra, phrynoderma, purpura and a mosaic dermatosis which is most frequently seen over the tibia. A low-fat diet, or gross undernutrition may render the skin dry, harsh and inelastic and will delay healing. Mixed conditions often arise, and a dark skin does not make diagnosis easier.

Follicular Hyperkeratosis (Phrynoderma)

This is ascribed by nutritionists to lack of vitamin A (p. 115) and by dermatologists to an infection. It is comparatively rare in children on a balanced diet and it generally clears up on a salicylic acid ointment, so that it is probable that both factors are concerned. The characteristic distribution is a patchy one on the extensor surfaces, but it may be more generalized. It does not appear before the age of four or five.

Prickly Heat (Miliaria, Strophulus)

This is liable to be troublesome in babies and young children, whether indigenous or European. It should be treated by keeping the baby and any clothing as cool, clean, and free from perspiration as possible. Applications of a lotion containing salicylic acid and alcohol are useful, or a powder containing zinc oxide and menthol. Air-conditioning is a wonderful therapeutic agent when available.

Scabies

Scabies is apt to be more active in hot weather than in cold. It is a serious condition in babies and children, in whom exhaustion produced by constant and intense irritation can cause death. The lesions are liable to secondary infections. The belief that *Sarcoptes scabiei* is only carried by personal contact and not by fomites is not in accord with experience in the tropics. Spraying with DDT, scrubbing floors and furniture with soap and water and antiseptic, and boiling or exposing clothing and bedding to strong sunlight will eventually get rid of the infestation.

A mild sulphur ointment is applied daily for 3 to 4 days and again at the end of a week, or benzyl benzoate emulsion can be used (*see* p. 506). If there is secondary infection, a suitable mild antiseptic ointment should also be applied. The mother must be taught in the simplest terms and shown how the child should be thoroughly washed and scrubbed all over before the treatment is applied and how he must be put into clean clothes and bedclothes afterwards. Every health centre should have facilities for demonstrating the process. Contacts should be examined and treated.

Larva Migrans (Creeping Eruption)

The larval form of a hookworm (*Ancylostoma braziliense*) that normally infests cats and dogs is found in Africa and other tropical countries. In man it forms burrows under the skin, leaving a wayward, complicated, irritating and often ulcerating track that looks like a thread of cotton just below the skin. It is not uncommon in children, especially if they have been playing about on infected ground. The most effective method of attack is to inject, with a fine needle, a few minims of absolute alcohol into the advancing head of the larva. This may cause a pin head area of necrosis, but it heals readily under a small adhesive dressing.

Dermal Myiasis

In South America the " ver macaque " (*Dermatobia cyaniventris*) and in tropical Africa the tumbu fly (*Cordylobia anthropophaga*) deposit their eggs on human beings. The larval worm develops under the skin and produces a painful swelling. Children are more liable to suffer from this condition than adults who have generally developed an immunity. A few drops of alcohol should be dropped on to the opening of the swelling and the larva squeezed out. The aperture heals readily.

Leech Infection

In areas where the water is infested with leeches, only boiled water should be used for drinking. Cases have occurred in which a leech, imbibed with water, has attached itself to the nasopharynx of a baby and caused a fatal hæmorrhage.

Tropical Ulcers

In some areas " tropical " ulcers are common. They are associated with a poor or unbalanced diet, and very frequently with yaws and a primitive environment. Sometimes a diphtheritic infection (p. 550) is found. The ulcers are usually started by insect bites or some slight trauma, the most common site being perhaps the shins. Neglected cases become chronic and resistant.

In treatment, penicillin is used and a generous diet provided. When the base of the ulcer has been cleaned and begins to granulate, it can be covered with an adhesive dressing, which may remain on for 10 to 14 days and be repeated until healing is complete. Rest and the treatment of worms and anæmia are important.   Skin grafting may be necessary.

Tinea Imbricata

This condition is very common in some regions.   It can be treated with a lotion of salicylic acid 10 per cent., strong tincture of iodine 5 per cent. and alcohol 90 per cent.

DISEASES DUE TO HEAT

It used to be considered dangerous for Caucasians to go about in the tropics unless protected with helmets, veils and spine pads.   These are no longer considered desirable.   Children coming from more northern climates should gradually get accustomed to the sun, and, except in extremes of temperature, it will be found that most children stand up well to a tropical climate.

Over-exposure to heat, with perspiration and salt depletion, may produce fever, severe headache, nausea and cramps.   The child should be kept in a darkened room and sponged with water, the temperature of which is gradually reduced by adding ice.   Cold or iced rectal washouts, and cold compresses to the head may be indicated in hyperpyrexia.   Salt and fluid depletion should be treated, and, if there is coma, subcutaneous and intravenous fluids may be necessary, care being taken to avoid water intoxication (*see* p. 196).   A wet sheet covering the patient, with a fan playing on it, is a simple method of reducing the temperature.

Heat exhaustion may be more gradual in its manifestations.   It is marked by increasing malaise, anorexia and oliguria.   The child should be kept sheltered as far as possible from excessive heat, and increased fluids and *salt* administered.   Some children are much affected by glare and should be encouraged to use dark glasses.

In hot climates, European children may appear pale and listless, but as long as they have good appetites and display the expected energy and boisterousness at some part of the day, they are probably coming to no harm.   Many of these children become rosy and vigorous within a day or two of reaching a cool climate.

There is no foundation for the legend that children reach physical maturity earlier in the tropics than in colder climates.   Life on a farm in East Africa or in the suburbs of Panama is likely to be more varied and colourful, both for the local and for the European population, than that in a northern town or boarding school, and the children are apt to seem sophisticated compared with those brought up in the more conventional atmosphere of the countries of Western Europe or North America.

The effects of heat, particularly when associated with a low humidity, are apt to be dangerous for small and premature babies; dehydration fever and collapse readily occur.   Dust is also a serious embarrassment to a small child.

DENTAL DISEASES

INTERESTING differences are often to be found in dental health, even between members of the same family eating the same food, drinking the same water and exposed to the same environment.

Most rural peoples, eating the food they produce and having little access to refined sugars or grains, have few or no caries, even when economic conditions appear poor. Where the diet lacks calcium, and the mother during her pregnancy has taken little or no milk, the first dentition of the offspring may be markedly hypoplastic. But breast-feeding, often prolonged, is the general rule, and the second teeth are remarkably good, even when the child suffers from a number of diseases such as malnutrition, worms and yaws. Even children with severe rickets may have perfect teeth. However, although the second dentition may be well formed, these rural populations are often seriously affected with spongy gums that bleed on pressure, with a great deal of tartar formation, gingivosis, gingivitis and severe pyor-rhœa, and they may become edentulous at an early age.

Usually, urban populations are far more subject to caries, but in general breast-fed babies later develop better permanent teeth than those who are artificially fed.

In many countries the chewing of betel leaf, areca nut, kola nut and the rest is very prevalent. In some cases lime and various spices are included in the mixture. The betel leaf and the lime contain useful additions to the diet, but the profuse expectoration that generally accompanies this habit prevents the possibility of their absorption. These substances are astringent, but they do not seem to prevent the development of pyorrhœa and they lead to a high incidence of buccal carcinoma.

CICELY D. WILLIAMS

" Diseases of Children in the Subtropics and Tropics " by H. C. Trowell and D. B. Jeliffe (1958, London: Edward Arnold) may be read for fuller details of tropical disorders.

CHAPTER 27

Intestinal Parasites

HELMINTHIASIS is a serious public health problem in those parts of the world where sanitation is poor. It is best tackled by raising the standard of environmental hygiene and, through education, of personal hygiene as well. There is also the possibility of mass treatment for certain infestations, but this is never the complete answer and may be unsuitable for young children owing to the attendant risk.

Well-nourished individuals often harbour helminths without much apparent inconvenience. The effects are much more serious in poorly nourished children.

Of the helminths to be described, only threadworm, tapeworm, roundworm and *Giardia lamblia* are commonly seen in the United Kingdom.

Tænia Saginata (Mediocanellata) (Beef Tapeworm)

This worm inhabits the intestine of human beings, but the larvæ inhabit, as an intermediate host, the muscles and solid organs of cattle. Infection is found in individuals of any age who eat uncooked meat, and where cattle have access to fodder contaminated with human fæces. The adult worm in man may reach a total length of 15–20 feet. In adult form it consists of a minute head or scolex with four hooks. From this develop the segments or proglottides which may number up to 2,000 in a chain. The oldest segments (measuring some 2 cm. in length and 0·5–1 cm. in breadth) break off and appear in the stools. The segments contain the ova.

SYMPTOMS AND DIAGNOSIS

Symptoms may be absent, or there may be anæmia and wasting. The appetite may be voracious. Sometimes the patient's skin has an earthy hue. The diagnosis is made by recognition of the whitish segments in the stools.

TREATMENT

Male fern extract remains the most reliable remedy. It is important that the following treatment, which is suitable for a child aged 5 to 7 years, be rigidly followed in every detail.

For forty-eight hours a diet as far as possible in liquid form should be given. If treatment is to be effective, high residue foods *must* be excluded.

On the third day, the specific treatment is carried out. At, say, 7 a.m. the child may have a little weak tea with a lump of sugar in it, but nothing more. At 9 a.m. a capsule containing 1·0 ml. of extract of filix mas should be given, and this dose repeated at half-hourly intervals until four doses have been given. (Should the first treatment have failed, six doses may safely be given during a subsequent treatment, provided the after-treatment is rigidly adhered to.) This means that the fourth capsule has been given at 10.30 a.m. At 11 a.m. 15 G. of magnesium sulphate is administered and the worm may be expected within an hour. Castor oil should not be given as this would facilitate the absorption of filix mas with subsequent toxic effects. Black crêpe is placed over the chamber pot and the motion passed directly onto it. This is then washed through, and the white segments of worm, standing out plainly on the black crêpe, are easily distinguishable. As a rule, the larger portion of the worm will be found to have been passed unbroken, and search should then be made among the short slim portions for the head.

Should the treatment fail it must not be repeated for six to eight weeks.

Alternatively, *mepacrine hydrochloride* 250 mg. in 50 ml. of water is given on an empty stomach and repeated in half an hour; a further half hour later the same dose of magnesium sulphate is given as with male fern extract. Such treatment is usually tried only if male fern extract has not been effective. Yomesan ($\frac{1}{2}$ tablet at 1 year; 1 tablet at 5 years; 2 tablets at 10 years), taken before breakfast and repeated after half an hour, is an effective and non-toxic remedy.

Tænia Solium (Pork Tapeworm)

Man acquires the adult tapeworm by eating measly pork which is undercooked. As with *Tænia saginata*, the adult worm inhabits the small intestine; it is smaller in size, but the head has a number of hooklets in addition to the four suckers. The ova may penetrate the wall of the intestine and give rise to cysticercosis (*see below*).

The symptoms and treatment of this intestinal infestation are similar to that described for *Tænia saginata*.

Cysticercosis

Cysticercosis is caused by eating uncooked pork or pork sausage which contains the larval form or cysticercus of *Tænia solium*. The embryos migrate to any part of the body, very often to the brain where they may later give rise to epileptic attacks. Cysticercosis is found only among pork-eating communities. In recent years a number of cases have been met with in England.

The cysts form small hard nodules, from 2–5 cm. in size, which may be palpated in the tissues. Radiology may help in diagnosis, but as it may take some years before the cysts calcify they are seldom demonstrated in young children.

There is no specific treatment, but prevention is simple if " measly pork " is avoided and if all pork is thoroughly cooked.

Diphyllobothrium Latum

Man and animals acquire this large tapeworm by eating fish containing the worm in its larval stage. Apart from the general symptoms of tæniasis (see p. 626), the patient may develop a macrocytic anæmia. It has been shown that the worm absorbs vitamin B_{12}; if attached high up in the intestine, it may divert to itself this vitamin before the human host has been able to absorb it. The treatment is the same as for other tapeworms.

Tænia Echinococcus and Hydatid Disease

The adult worm, 3–6 mm. in length, infests the gut of dogs, jackals, wolves, foxes and cats. These animals infect pastures, and the eggs are taken in by sheep, pigs, horses and cattle. In the intestine of the animal host, the eggs develop into larval worms which pierce the intestinal mucosa and then enter the blood stream, lodging eventually in almost any organ and giving rise to hydatid cysts. Human infection is most common in countries where children are in close contact with dogs that have access to the viscera of slaughtered animals. In some countries jackals are often responsible for soiling pastures with the eggs of *T. echinococcus*; elsewhere dogs are chiefly responsible. The disease occurs in Africa, South America and the Middle Eastern countries; it is seen only very occasionally in England, but more commonly in Wales.

In man, cysts are found in liver, lungs, brain and bone. They may enlarge to attain a size of 15 cm. or more in diameter and are then found to contain an enormous number of daughter and granddaughter cysts. The cysts contain antigens which provoke the formation of antibodies and an eosinophilia. The diagnosis is confirmed by a complement fixation test and the intradermal Casoni test. In the lungs, hydatid cysts present characteristic radiological appearances. Treatment of hydatid cyst is surgical.

Since the fæces of infected animals provide the source of human infection, children should avoid contact with contaminated material and hand washing before meals should be taught. Vegetables, if eaten uncooked, and salads should first be washed in dilute potassium permanganate solution.

Ascaris Lumbricoides (Roundworm)

In the United Kingdom roundworms are not very common, but in tropical countries ascariasis is one of the most serious causes of morbidity and mortality in children; in some areas the incidence of ascariasis is over 90 per cent. of the population. Its seriousness is not nearly as well recognized as that of ancylostoma. An infant can be infected at any moment after birth by the entry of the ascaris ova into the mouth on the dirty hand of the mother or other attendant, or by means of dust, flies and dirty utensils. During and after the first dentition the incidence is very high.

PATHOGENESIS

The egg is ingested into the stomach. The larva hatches out and enters a tributary of the vena mesenterica; then by the pulmonary circulation it finds its way into the lungs whence it passes up a bronchus and so into the trachea and mouth. It is then swallowed in the sputum, and in the intestines it grows into an adult worm. The female lays thousands of eggs which pass out with the fæces. The eggs survive heating and drying, and they are not killed in septic tanks or by freezing, nor by ordinary methods of composting, and so may, under favourable circumstances, remain viable for many years.

CLINICAL PICTURE

In tropical countries the effects of the worms are manifold. The larvæ during their passage through the respiratory system may cause bronchitis or fatal pneumonia. The presence of the worms in the

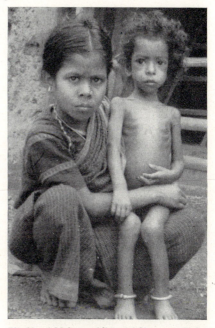

Fig. 89.—A Malayan child aged 2½ years suffering from ascariasis. Note expression, emaciation, dyspigmentation of skin and hair, œdema of extremities and cheeks (not of eyelids), distended abdomen, and dry and staring hair. The other child was exposed to the same conditions, and may even have gone through these same stages, and acquired some immunity.

stomach and intestines gives rise to diarrhœa, colic, malabsorption and anæmia, or indigestion and constipation. Attacks of enteritis are frequent and tend to be serious. The abdominal wall is often flaccid and the intestine distended. There is œdema of the extremities and of the face—mainly of the cheeks, and not of the eyelids. The skin becomes dusky and loses the healthy gloss that is normal in pigmented races. The hair becomes dry, sparse and staring, and loses its normal curl and pigmentation (*see* Fig. 89) as in protein malnutrition.

There may be symptoms referable to the nervous system, such as meningism, convulsions and even coma. In long-standing cases the mental outlook of the child becomes completely altered. He is stolid

21

and indifferent, with peevish intervals, and finally develops such stupidity as to suggest mental deterioration.

Sometimes symptoms arise through the entry of one or more worms into the common bile duct; in this way a prolonged attack of obstructive jaundice may be caused, and then hepatitis or even multiple liver abscesses may follow. Masses of worms may cause intestinal obstruction; peritonitis is an occasional development. Worms may be produced startlingly from the mouth or they may enter the nose or the larynx.

In 1948, De Silva found that 25 per cent. of the children under six years old in hospital in Singapore had ascariasis. Adults and some children in good condition develop a certain degree of immunity towards the worm (Fig. 89).

DIAGNOSIS

This is not always easy, unless the worms are seen or the eggs are found in the stool. Repeated examination should be made by concentration methods if there is any cause to suspect worms. In a chronic case the child's appearance may be characteristic, and sometimes worms can be palpated through the abdominal wall.

TREATMENT

(a) *General Measures.* If the child is seriously ill, it may be preferable to postpone de-worming until the general condition has been improved by rest in bed, vitamins, concentrated foods, iron tonic and so forth. Sometimes the abdominal musculature has become so lax that aperients produce little effect. In these cases a firm binder, applied after rectal irrigation, gives support, promotes digestion and relieves discomfort.

(b) *Drugs.* Piperazine salts is the most effective treatment. The action is to narcotize the worm without causing stimulation which thus minimises the risk of obstruction in heavily infected cases (for dosage, *see* p. 632).

Visceral Larva Migrans

The roundworms of dogs and cats, *Toxocara canis* and *Toxocara cati* may occasionally affect the human. The eggs of *T. canis* are excreted in large numbers by puppies undergoing their initial infection. If the eggs are swallowed by man, the larvæ may leave the intestinal tract and migrate via the blood-stream to somatic tissues.

The clinical features are of fever, pulmonary infiltration, massive eosinophilia and hypergammaglobulinæmia. Larvæ show a particular predilection for the eye, giving rise to an endophthalmitis with total retinal detachment and blindness.

Prevention lies in adequate de-worming of puppies with piperazine and in preventing their too close association with children until this has been done.

Trichiniasis

This infestation is caused by a minute roundworm, *Trichinella spiralis*. The adult worm inhabits the intestine of the pig. The embryo forms produced burrow through the wall of the intestine and ultimately migrate to muscle where they form cysts, which contain the larval worm. No further development occurs unless the flesh is eaten. If such flesh is eaten by man in an undercooked condition, the larvæ hatch out in the intestine to form adult worms. These adult worms in the human intestine produce embryo forms which pass through the intestinal wall to invade muscle tissue in particular.

SYMPTOMS

After an initial gastro-intestinal disturbance following the eating of the undercooked pork, there is a latent interval of a week. This is followed by a generalized illness with fever, urticaria œdema of the eyelids and considerable muscle tenderness. The blood shows a marked eosinophilia.

Recovery occurs over a period of weeks but there may be residual muscle pains for many years. Minute areas of calcification may develop.

TREATMENT

The cysts are destroyed by heat; therefore any pork-containing food can be rendered harmless by adequate cooking.

There is no specific treatment for the disease itself.

Oxyuris Vermicularis (Threadworm)

This infestation is not uncommon in the United Kingdom and is greater in girls than boys.

The threadworm is white, 0·5–1 cm. long and about the thickness of a fine cotton thread. A single worm produces, on average, 11,000 eggs. The eggs are found in the dust of rooms and clinging to the walls. As a rule, more than one other individual in each family is infested. The diagnosis is made by finding the threadworms or the eggs in the stools, or in a scraping from the perineum which has been swabbed with a Cellophane-tipped swab. The Cellophane is detached from the rod, mounted in water or $\frac{1}{10}$ normal sodium hydroxide solution, and examined under the microscope for the eggs. The swab is best taken immediately after the patient gets up in the morning and before bath or motion. It is generally considered that seven negative peri-anal swabs are necessary before the child is considered cured.

SYMPTOMS

The chief symptom is irritation about the anus and vulva, and threadworms may be considered a common cause of vulvo-vaginitis.

Other symptoms are restlessness and sleeplessness from the irritation, vague abdominal pain and a tendency to unexplained diarrhœa. Thumb-sucking and nail-biting tend to cause reinfection. On examination of the anus, threadworms can often be observed extruding themselves, and are frequently seen moving about in the motions. Sometimes at operation, an appendix full of worms is found.

Errors in diagnosis are made by mothers who mistake particles of food debris for threadworms.

TREATMENT

Since more than one individual in the household is usually infested, it is necessary to examine the stools or peri-anal swabs from each member. All infested members of the family should then be treated. Piperazine is the treatment of choice.

TABLE XXII

DOSAGE OF PIPERAZINE ACCORDING TO AGE

Threadworms: Daily Dose for One Week (given in 2 or 3 divided doses)	Piperazine	
	Adipate	Citrate (elixir)
1–2 years	600 mg. (10 grains)	4 ml. (60 minims)
2–6 years	1·0 G. (15 grains)	8 ml. (120 minims)
6–12 years	1·5 G. (22 grains)	12 ml. (180 minims)
Roundworms: Single Dose		
Under 5 years	3·0 G. (45 grains)	20 ml. (300 minims)
Over 5 years	5·0 G. (75 grains)	30 ml. (450 minims)

Giardia Intestinalis (Lamblia Intestinalis)

This infestation is no longer common in England, but in many parts of the world the carrier rate is high.

Giardia inhabits especially the duodenum and jejunum, and adheres, by means of large, oblique, sucker-like depressions, to the mucous membrane. The tail terminates in two flagella; there are three other pairs of flagella; it is motile in recently passed stools and varies in length from 12 to 18 μ. The encysted forms are passed in the fæces in enormous numbers, the free form being found usually only during attacks of diarrhœa. The cysts are ovoid in shape.

SYMPTOMS

The child has chronic diarrhœa or bouts of diarrhœa at intervals. Blood may sometimes be passed in the stools. The stools contain mucus and are large, bulky, offensive, high in fat content (the fat is, however, well split), and somewhat resemble those of cœliac disease. After treatment, the fat-content of the stool returns to normal.

The abdomen is large and, in time, the child's growth may be retarded. As a rule, the appetite is good and the child is thin and lively.

TREATMENT

Mepacrine hydrochloride B.P., given orally, is the treatment of choice. The dosage, according to age, is given below:

Age in Years	Daily Dose in 0·1 G tablets	Course in Days	Total Dose
½–2	¼ × 2	3–5	0·15–0·25 G. (2½–4 grains)
2–6	½ × 2	3–5	0·30–0·50 G. (5–8 grains)
6–9	½ × 3	4–5	0·60–0·75 G. (10–12 grains)
9–10	1 × 2	5	1·0 G. (15 grains)
Adult	1 × 3	5	1·5 G. (25 grains)

The cysts disappear from the stools in five days as a rule, and the diarrhœa clears up. The drug is non-toxic, but the child may very occasionally become yellow, and, if he should vomit, the stain on the bed clothes is permanent. A further course is sometimes necessary.

Ancylostoma (Hookworm)

Hookworm disease, due to the several varieties of ancylostoma, is exceedingly common in East and West Africa, India, Ceylon, Malaya, South America and in the southern United States. It is occasionally found in Europe, usually in mine-workers. It tends to show its greatest effects in undernourished subjects. The infection is contracted by the larva entering through the intact skin, and is therefore not usual in children before they are old enough to wander about in swampy or muddy ground where the larvæ are likely to be found. Thus it is very rare in young babies and is more common in country than in urban populations. Its effects are serious, particularly when associated with nutritional deficiency diseases, such as kwashiorkor (p. 600).

The ova hatch in warm water or moist mud; the larvæ thus formed have the ability to pass through the intact skin of the feet or ankles if unprotected by boots or shoes. The larvæ then pass via the blood-stream to the lungs, whence they escape into the bronchi; thence to the trachea, œsophagus, and stomach, to lodge finally in the duodenum, where the adult worm develops. Numerous eggs are hatched which are passed in the stools to complete the life cycle.

SYMPTOMS

Penetration of the skin by the larvæ often occurs unnoticed, or there may be local irritation with transient dermatitis adjacent to the toes and around the ankles.

The chief manifestation is anæmia. This appears especially in children living on a protein-deficient diet. This anæmia is produced by many hookworms feeding on the blood of the intestinal mucosa; its severity depends on the number of worms and the degree of dietary deficiency; it is usually microcytic and hypochromic. The children affected have a muddy-coloured complexion, complain of epigastric discomfort and are listless. Eosinophilia occurs, especially during the stages of invasion.

The loss of plasma protein which occurs in a mass infestation can be replaced only out of the child's protein intake; this often contributes to protein-deficiency, and kwashiorkor may be seen in association with hookworm anæmia.

Diagnosis is by demonstration of eggs in the stool. Repeated examination by concentration methods may be necessary.

TREATMENT

Of the several drugs available hexylresorcinol and bephenium hydroxinaphthoate (Alcopar) are recommended. In order to make sure that treatment is adequate, the child should be admitted to hospital. Unfortunately, many of the children in the tropics who have been treated become re-infected when they return home and visit that part of the " bush " reserved as the latrine area, where the soil is heavily contaminated with hookworm larvæ.

The essence of *prevention* is to see that hygienic habits are followed and that shoes are worn. Attention to nutrition can prevent the occurrence of anæmia.

Strongyloides

This parasite is a human pathogen and the whole life-cycle may take place within a single host. The larvæ of *Strongyloides stercoralis* are very similar to the hookworm larvæ but enter the host either through the skin or with contaminated food. The adult female parasite is small (2 to 3 mm.) and lives buried in the wall of the small intestine. The parasite produces respiratory symptoms and a chronic, watery, sometimes blood-stained diarrhœa. The disease may be serious, especially in young children, though a light infection may produce no symptoms at all. Gentian violet appears to be the most effective treatment. It is prescribed in enteric-coated capsules (10 mg. (one-sixth of a grain) per year of the child's age, each day, for five consecutive days).

CHAPTER 28

Accidents in Childhood

WHILST the morbidity and mortality rates of most childhood disorders have been falling rapidly, accident rates have kept up. In Western countries accidents are the great cause of mortality between the ages of one and fourteen years[1].

TABLE XXIII

TOTAL NUMBER OF DEATHS IN ENGLAND AND WALES (REGISTRAR-GENERAL'S RETURNS) IN 1960, IN EACH OF THE FIVE COMMONEST CAUSATIVE-GROUPS, IN CHILDREN AGED ONE TO FOURTEEN YEARS

	All Deaths	Accidents of all Kinds	Diseases of the Respiratory System	Congenital Malformations	Neoplasms (including Leukæmia	Diseases of the Digestive System
Boys aged 1–4 ..	1,362	335	326	185	158	98
Girls aged 1–4 ..	1,069	192	233	168	143	78
Boys aged 5–9 ..	881	349	86	70	177	44
Girls aged 5–9 ..	545	150	57	79	111	30
Boys aged 10–14 ..	722	301	56	59	115	32
Girls aged 10–14 ..	467	117	29	49	112	27

In England and Wales the percentage of the total childhood mortality due to accidents at different ages is as follows:

AGE	PERCENTAGE OF TOTAL CHILDHOOD MORTALITY
0–1 Years	2·7
1–4 Years	22·0
5–9 Years	35·0
10–14 Years	35·0

[1] Lightwood, R. (1960). Accidents and accident prevention in childhood. " Pædiatrics for the Practitioner " (Supplement). Ed. Gaisford and Lightwood. London: Butterworth.

It has been estimated that, for every fatal accident to a child, there are one hundred non-fatal accidents requiring admission to hospital and a further one hundred and fifty accidents severe enough to cause some restriction of activity.

ÆTIOLOGY

THE relative mortality due to the commoner types of childhood accident is shown in Table XXIV.

TABLE XXIV

NUMBER OF DEATHS DUE TO VARIOUS TYPES OF ACCIDENTS IN CHILDREN AGED ONE TO FOURTEEN YEARS IN ENGLAND AND WALES IN 1960 (REGISTRAR-GENERAL'S RETURNS)

	Accidents of all Kinds	Road Accidents	Drown-ing	Burns and Ex-plosions	Accidental Falls	Accidental Poison-ings
Boys aged 1–4 ..	335	112	83	35	18	14
Girls aged 1–4 ..	192	71	20	41	12	13
Boys aged 5–9 ..	349	181	89	9	9	2
Girls aged 5–9 ..	150	79	12	31	8	3
Boys aged 10–14 ..	301	124	61	3	32	3
Girls aged 10–14 ..	117	66	18	6	4	9

SEX INCIDENCE

As shown in Table XXIII, there is a marked male preponderance even in the pre-school age group. Yet, when types of accidents are separately considered, the male preponderance is seen to be most marked first in drowning accidents and secondly in road accidents; fatal falls and accidental poisoning show little sex differentiation, whilst fatal burns are commoner in girls.

ACCIDENT PRONENESS

An innate proneness to accidents is particularly difficult to determine in the case of children, because of parental and environmental influences. Preliminary studies of children[1] who have already had accidents suggest that they are generally more careless than other children, and, at the same time, reveal that a high proportion of these children

(1957). *Wld Hlth Org. techn. Rep. Ser.*, No. 118.

TABLE XXV

Fatal and Serious Road Accidents to Children in 1960 according to Age and Class of Road User in Great Britain

Age (Years)	Pedestrians		Pedal Cyclists		Passengers		Total	
	Killed	Seriously Injured	Killed	Seriously Injured	Killed	Seriously Injured	Killed	Seriously Injured
Under 1	2	5	—	—	10	41	12	46
1	28	63	—	—	8	91	36	154
2	60	355	1	5	10	111	71	471
3	60	668	2	4	3	105	65	777
4	49	768	1	12	8	115	58	895
5	73	901	—	22	3	99	76	1,022
6	60	812	1	36	5	121	66	969
7	47	810	5	76	4	115	56	1,001
8	45	671	6	143	8	120	59	934
9	25	574	9	183	9	115	43	872
10	23	468	8	244	4	134	35	846
11	18	384	20	346	8	120	46	850
12	11	346	25	464	6	134	42	944
13	14	253	27	589	8	176	49	1,018
14	7	188	19	654	6	190	32	1,032
Total	522	7,266	124	2,778	100	1,787	746	11,831

In addition, one child driver was killed and five child riders of motor-cycles and scooters and 21 child drivers were seriously injured.

come from broken homes. Thus, their apparent carelessness and disregard of consequences may be the result of emotional disturbance expressed in physical behaviour. Research into this subject is needed, but it seems probable, with the exception of mentally sub-normal children, that the intrinsic intelligence may be of less importance than childhood training and home environment.

ENVIRONMENT

Burns are more common in conditions of overcrowding or bad housing,[1] whilst ill-health in the family, particularly in the mother, renders a child more vulnerable to accidents of all kinds.[2]

PHYSICAL HANDICAPS

Impairment of vision or hearing, cerebral palsy, and subnormal intelligence all predispose to accidents; epileptic children are also at special risk.

Road Accidents

As with other common accidents, there is a depressing similarity in the causes of most fatal road accidents to children. The circumstances commonly are:

(1) Crossing the road in the path of an approaching vehicle.
(2) Leaving the footpath unexpectedly as a vehicle approaches.
(3) Crossing the road from behind a stationary vehicle.
(4) Boarding or leaving a public transport vehicle.
(5) Playing around a vehicle as it is about to move off.

With regard to cyclists, the common causes of accidents are inattention, turning right recklessly (in countries where driving on the left side of the road is the rule), crossing road junctions carelessly, and inadequate maintenance of the bicycle.

Prevention lies in better planning of towns whereby small children have play areas away from public highways, and in intensive training in road sense from a very early age. Much has been achieved by local campaigns to encourage road safety in young cyclists.

Despite the great increase in the number of vehicles on the roads, the number of fatal road accidents to children in Great Britain has fallen during the last thirty-five years, although but little in the last decade. By contrast, the fatality rate in adults has risen markedly.

On the other hand, the number of non-fatal road accidents has increased in respect of both children and adults.

[1] Tempest, M. H. (1956). *Brit. med. J.*, 1, 1387.
[2] Backett, E. M., Johnston, A. M. (1959). *Brit. med. J.*, 1, 409.

TABLE XXVI

Child Road Accident Deaths in Great Britain 1926–1960 (0-15 years)

Year	Killed	Year	Killed	Year	Killed
1926	1,232	1938	1,130	1950	868
1927	1,334	1939	1,100	1951	914
1928	1,503	1940	1,255	1952	786
1929	1,621	1941	1,510	1953	797
1930	1,685	1942	1,370	1954	662
1931	1,525	1943	1,200	1955	764
1932	1,439	1944	1,395	1956	717
1933	1,474	1945	1,282	1957	629
1934	1,438	1946	1,060	1958	717
1935	1,243	1947	958	1959	680
1936	1,206	1948	1,035	1960	747
1937	1,115	1949	965	1961	767

TABLE XXVII

Fatal and Non-fatal Road Casualties in Children (0-15 years) and Adults in Great Britain during the decade 1951–1960

All Children	Fatal	Serious	Slight	Total
Year 1951	914	8,988	32,774	42,676
1952	786	8,630	31,511	40,927
1953	797	9,689	33,760	44,246
1954	662	9,370	34,101	44,133
1955	764	9,951	37,995	48,710
1956	717	9,592	36,700	47,009
1957	629	9,300	35,401	45,330
1958	717	10,331	38,815	49,863
1959	680	10,907	40,101	51,688
1960	747	11,857	41,063	53,667
All Adults	**Fatal**	**Serious**	**Slight**	**Total**
Year 1951	4,336	43,381	126,100	173,817
1952	3,920	41,721	121,444	167,085
1953	4,293	46,833	131,398	182,524
1954	4,348	47,831	141,969	194,148
1955	4,762	52,155	162,295	219,212
1956	4,650	51,863	164,438	220,951
1957	4,921	54,406	169,201	228,528
1958	5,253	58,835	185,816	249,904
1959	5,840	69,765	206,160	281,765
1960	6,223	72,586	215,075	293,884

Drowning

Deaths from drowning are exceeded in number only by deaths from road accidents. They are very much more common in boys of all ages, between one and fourteen years, than in girls.

Prevention lies in teaching children to swim from a very early age. More awareness is also needed by parents of the danger to children who are non-swimmers of being allowed to use canoes and other light craft; insufficient attention is paid to notices regarding bathing precautions on dangerous beaches, but " life guards " on beaches do much to promote the safety of bathers of all ages.

Drowning accidents are even more common in Scandinavia and the Netherlands[1], where efforts are being made as a part of the public health programme to increase the proportion of school children who are able to swim.

Small children require constant supervision whenever playing near water. Children under the age of three are sometimes found drowned in no more than twelve to eighteen inches of water.

Burns

The causes of the more severe and often fatal burns in childhood are different from the causes of the commoner and usually milder scalds.[2] The former are mainly due to open fires and to inadequately protected heaters. The British Standards Institution (1956) has specified desirable requirements for fireguards, and legislation makes it illegal to leave a child of under twelve years of age alone in a room with an unguarded fire; yet, basically, it is upon the wisdom and carefulness of parents that the prevention of serious burns depends. Publicity, including television as a means of disseminating information about such subjects as non-inflammable night clothing, is of great value in parent education.

Scalds, though generally less severe, are much more frequent than burns and tend to be particularly common in younger children. All the activities associated with the preparation of cups of tea, once the water has been heated, are potentially dangerous to young children, as is the use of coppers for washing clothing. Saucepans within reach of small children provide another danger.

Hot-water bottles continue to be a source of scalds, particularly in children already ill or in a state of unconsciousness.

TREATMENT

The immediate treatment of a burn has two objectives: the prevention of shock and the prevention of infection. A badly burned child should be wrapped in a clean sheet, kept warm with blankets and be taken straight to hospital. A state of clinical shock is likely to develop if there is full- or partial-thickness skin involvement of more than 10–15 per cent. of the body surface.

Early transfusion can prevent or minimize shock and the attendant danger of renal failure. Plasma or dextran is used, but whole blood

[1] Van der berg, B. J. (1959). *Nederlands Institut voor Preventieve Geneeskunde*, p. 162.
[2] McLauchlan, G. P., Irvine, E. D., Keen, J. H., Brimblecombe, F. S. W. (1961). *Med. Offr*, **105**, 115.

is also needed in severe cases or where extensive shock is present. The transfusion is maintained throughout the period in which exudation of fluid from the burned areas continues—amounting in most cases to 36–48 hours. The quantity of fluid transfused will depend upon the extent of the burn, the degree of clinical shock, the urine output and the hæmatocrit. Each patient needs individual assessment, but as a rough guide a child with a burn involving fifteen per cent. of the skin surface is likely to require a total amount of plasma and dextran equal to his own plasma volume (plasma volume 60–65 per cent. of the total blood volume), of which half the amount will be needed in the first eight hours. A child with a thirty per cent. skin surface burn would be likely to need about twice this amount.

In the local treatment of burns, there is a place for both the *exposure* and the *closed* methods. The exposure method is suitable only in hospital, but is particularly valuable in cases where the site of the burn makes the application and renewal of dressings difficult; the avoidance of repeated dressings also relieves the child of much apprehension and discomfort. Spraying the burned area with Polybactrin (Calmic) containing neomycin sulphate, polymixin B sulphate, and zinc bacitracin helps to prevent infection, whilst exposure to the air allows the burn to dry rapidly and to remain cool. A closed method of treating burns is advisable in domiciliary practice, but is difficult where burns involve the buttocks or genitalia of small children and in hot climates. In general, dressings should be changed as infrequently as possible.

Consideration should be given, in all severe burns where skin grafting is needed, as to whether this should be undertaken immediately in order to reduce the risk of infection, i.e. as soon as the state of shock has been corrected, or after an interval of two or three weeks. Early skin grafting is particularly successful in full-thickness burns involving less than fifteen per cent. of the body surface.

Accidental Poisoning [1,2]

For every fatal accidental poisoning in a child, there are about 100 non-fatal accidental poisonings requiring a child's admission to hospital. Among the causes, the most usual is *the ingestion of tablets* of one kind or another, aspirin, barbiturates, laxatives and iron, in that order, being the most frequently implicated. Children between the ages of one and three are by far the most commonly affected. *Household substances*, in particular kerosene, turpentine, washing soda, and disinfectants, form the second major cause of poisoning. Other causes of accidental poisoning include the whole range of *medical products found in private houses other than tablets*, whether intended for internal or external use, camphorated oil and surgical spirit being among the most

[1] Heasman, M. A. (1961). *Arch. Dis. Childh.*, **36**, 390.
[2] Emergency Treatment in Hospital of Cases of Acute Poisoning (1962). London: H.M.S.O.

frequent offenders; vegetable substances, in particular *berries and seeds*, and *carbon monoxide poisoning* also require special mention.

PREVENTION

Inquiries into the circumstances[1] of individual cases show that the great majority of accidental poisonings of young children might be prevented by:

(1) Keeping substances known to be poisonous in locked cupboards. All new houses should be designed to contain at least two safety cupboards.

(2) Remembering to put away poisonous substances after use.

(3) Never putting poisonous substances into fresh containers without placing on them an appropriate label including the word POISON.

(4) The use of special labels, with such phrases as KEEP OUT OF THE REACH OF CHILDREN, for household substances which are potentially poisonous.

(5) A reversal of the present trend of drug firms to make up potentially poisonous tablets in shapes and sizes that resemble children's sweets.

(6) The use by pharmacists of containers incorporating safety devices when dispensing drugs that are potentially dangerous.

(7) The nature of all pharmaceutical preparations being fully described on the label on the container.

TREATMENT

The number of Regional Information Centres for doctors wishing to identify the properties and ingredients of a substance known to have been accidentally ingested needs to be increased. From such a centre it is possible to obtain details of the composition of the innumerable proprietary preparations, medicinal and otherwise, and also of the appropriate treatment. In this Chapter, the treatment of the commoner causes of accidental poisoning in childhood only are considered.

Gastric Lavage. In the case of all swallowed poisons, the stomach is washed out as soon as possible with several pints of plain water. If the patient is unconscious or if kerosene has been swallowed, a cuffed endotracheal tube is first passed to prevent inhalation into the lungs. In the case of corrosives, such as lysol or soda, gastric lavage is likely to be helpful only if the poison has been swallowed for less than fifteen minutes.

In all cases of poisoning the gastric contents should be preserved for subsequent laboratory identification.

[1] McKendrick ,T. (1959). *Arch. Dis. Childh.*, **35**, 127.

Aspirin Poisoning

The great majority of cases of aspirin poisoning in childhood reach hospital and receive gastric lavage sufficiently quickly to prevent the onset of the more serious symptoms. Where large quantities of aspirin have been absorbed, the clinical picture is one of hyperventilation, sweating, nausea, vomiting, sometimes with hæmatemesis, tinnitus, deafness, hypotension and dehydration. The ferric chloride test in the urine is positive.

The electrolyte disturbance is a complex one, involving a respiratory alkalosis secondary to the hyperventilation and a metabolic acidosis from the direct absorption of salicylate. Intravenous therapy, using 5 per cent. dextrose, is required to overcome dehydration; sodium bicarbonate is added if severe metabolic acidosis is present. In such circumstances sodium bicarbonate in 1·25 per cent. solution is used, of which 30 ml. per Kg. body-weight is calculated to raise the CO_2-combining power about 15 vols. per cent. Dialysis has proved a successful treatment in severe aspirin poisoning.

Barbiturate Poisoning

In severe and established cases, the child is unconscious with flaccid limbs and extensor plantar responses. Short-acting barbiturates, e.g. pentobarbitone, amylobarbitone and butobarbitone, cause a rapid onset of deep coma of relatively short duration; the longer-acting barbiturates, e.g. methyl-phenobarbitone, phenobarbitone and barbitone, cause a relatively less deep coma of later onset and longer duration. The minimum potentially fatal dose of a barbiturate is approximately five times its maximum therapeutic dose.

The priorities of treatment, where coma is already present, are:

(1) Establishment and maintenance of an airway.
(2) Gastric lavage.
(3) The use of stimulants (bemegride).
(4) Prevention of pneumonia.

Where the child is seen before the onset of symptoms, gastric lavage alone, using plain water (bicarbonate should be avoided owing to the solubility of barbiturates in alkali), will usually prevent the absorption of toxic amounts.

Where unconsciousness is already present, it is essential to maintain the airway and to nurse in the prone position. Care must be taken to prevent inhalation of fluid during and after gastric lavage. In the most severe cases, bemegride is the stimulant of choice; 10 mg. by intravenous injection every 10 minutes is suggested as a scheme of treatment which may be continued until improvement has begun to occur. A total of up to 200 mg. of bemegride may be required for an individual patient before the depth of unconsciousness is reduced to the comparatively safe state of light anæsthesia.

Other treatment includes fluids by stomach tube or intravenously, and the avoidance of acute retention of urine.   Antibiotics are given routinely to prevent pneumonia.

Ferrous-Sulphate Poisoning

Ferrous-sulphate poisoning occurs when the pleasantly coloured tablets supplied to mothers during pregnancy are mistaken for sweets by a two- or three-year-old child.   Death has occurred in a child aged nineteen months after taking 2 G. (30 grains) of ferrous sulphate.

Vomiting is the first symptom, progressing frequently to hæmate-mesis and shock as a result of gastric erosions.   This is succeeded by a period of apparent improvement until the second to fourth day when, in cases where considerable systemic absorption of iron has taken place, there may be a sudden relapse into unconsciousness, followed by death.

TREATMENT

The stomach is washed out with large quantities of water at the earliest opportunity.   Palliative treatment, including blood transfusion, is given as indicated.   Vitamins, especially alpha tocopherol, have been recommended.

Lead Poisoning (see p. 414).

Kerosene and Petrol Poisoning

The severity of the symptoms depends upon the degree to which ingestion has been complicated by inhalation.   In the most severe cases, there are signs of pulmonary œdema with dyspnœa and cyanosis. Central nervous involvement is shown by drowsiness or coma with a feeble pulse and failing respiration.   If the first 24 hours are survived the patient is likely to recover.

Milder cases show simply a repetitive cough initially, but subse-quently evidence of oil aspiration pneumonia appears.   Clinical signs may be minimal, but the radiological changes are extensive (p. 254).

TREATMENT

The stomach is washed out as soon as possible.   Care must be taken to avoid further inhalation during this procedure.   In the severe cases, oxygen, atropine, and hypertonic glucose intravenously are given.   For the milder cases an antibiotic, such as penicillin or tetra-cycline, is used to minimize secondary bacterial infection of the lipoid pneumonia.

Other Accidents to Children

Suffocation figures largely in infant mortality statistics.   The true state of affairs is not easy to determine, but careful histology of post-mortem material indicates that many infants, found dead in their cots, have not died of accidental suffocation but of overwhelming respiratory infections. Others have inhaled vomited milk or gastric secretions into their respiratory tree and died of acute shock, anaphylaxis or asphyxia. Infants should be laid well over on their side in their cot; pillows, if used at all, should be placed under the bottom sheet.

Other hazards to toddlers include falls inside the house or from windows, and suffocation from plastic bags. In the United Kingdom the health visitor has the opportunity, during her visits to the home of each newborn infant in her district, to advise the parents about elementary safety precautions, such as the protection of upper-floor windows by safety bars and the top of steep stairways by gates. Precautions against burns and scalds and against accidental poisoning can also be explained. Suffocation from plastic bags is now a well-recognized danger, but one which has to be restated to all young parents.

When accidents, such as a fall out of a cot or a burn from a hot-water bottle, occur in hospital, those in authority should immediately be informed. In addition to any treatment, the doctor must record in detail the nature of any injury and the nurse who saw the accident must write a report of the circumstances. The parents should be informed at once of what has happened.

In the education of the schoolchild, the opportunity exists to provide an awareness of the risks of the common road and home accidents without necessarily imposing tedious restraints. Similarly, the dangers of cigarette-smoking should be brought home to all children of secondary school age.

APPENDIX 1

Sulphonamides and Antibiotic Preparations

IN the treatment of infections great care must be exercised in the choice and dosage of antibiotic drugs. This is important because the increased use of these drugs has led to the emergence of resistant strains of certain pathogenic organisms which have become a special danger. The *Staph. pyogenes* organism is a case in point. When penicillin and the tetracyclines were first used, almost all strains of *Staph. pyogenes* were sensitive to these antibiotics, but soon there began to emerge mutant insensitive strains which became more prevalent, while the sensitive strains became relatively less common. This situation is found particularly in hospitals where antibiotics are inevitably most widely used. Wherever possible, therefore, the specific infecting organism should be isolated in the laboratory and its sensitivity to the different antibiotics ascertained. There should be restraint in the use of antibiotics for mild infections in which the child's own powers of resistance will lead to a rapid spontaneous recovery.

Theoretically, the emergence of resistant strains should be rendered less likely when two antibiotics are used together, but caution should be exercised in using antibiotics in certain combinations since, although there can be synergistic action, some combinations may be mutually antagonistic in the treatment of some bacterial infections. Generally speaking, it may be said that penicillin and streptomycin act in combination with each other whereas, if penicillin is used simultaneously with chloramphenicol or with chlortetracycline, antagonism may result, particularly in pneumococcal meningitis.

A plan for the administration of each drug is given in Tables XXVIII and XXIX. Whilst excessive use of these drugs may produce complications, insufficient treatment should be avoided, not only on account of probable failure to overcome the infection but also because of the danger of encouraging resistant bacteria. Once a treatment has been started, it should be continued for a minimum of five days, unless drug complications occur.

Prevention of cross-infection by meticulous application of hygienic principles together with the use of local antiseptics remains as important today, in all aspects of medical practice, as in the pre-antibiotic era.

CHEMOTHERAPY

Sulphonamides

WHILST for many infections antibiotic drugs have tended to replace sulphonamides, this group retains its place in the treatment of others. Cheapness and ease of administration will always be important factors.

646

INDICATIONS FOR USE OF SULPHONAMIDES

The place of sulphonamides can be summarized as follows:

As the Drug of Choice

1. *Urinary Infections.* Sulphonamides are effective for the treatment of most strains of *E. coli* infection of the urinary tract. The urine should be rendered alkaline with a potassium citrate or sodium citrate mixture, and the fluid intake should be liberal in order to avoid the crystallization of the sulphonamide in the urine (*see* below). Infections of the urinary tract by other organisms, or by *E. coli* resistant to sulphonamides, usually require the use of antibiotics or nitrofurantoin, after *in vitro* testing of the bacteria has determined their specific sensitivity. Urinary-tract infections require a minimum of two to three weeks' treatment, subsequent recurrence is an indication that full investigation should be undertaken to exclude a malformation of the urological tract.

2. *Acute Meningitis.* Sulphonamides, due to the ease with which they pass across the blood-brain barrier, play an important part in the treatment of many varieties of acute meningitis. Thus a sulphonamide, usually sulphadiazine, remains the principal therapeutic agent in meningococcal meningitis, although penicillin is usually given as additional supportive treatment. For other forms of meningitis (streptococcal, staphylococcal, pneumococcal and *H. influenzæ*) sulphonamides form a part of the treatment, being used in combination with appropriate antibiotics.

3. *Bacillary Dysentery.* Sulphonamides are satisfactory for Flexner and Sonne dysentery, although certain subtypes of the Sonne group may prove resistant to them. Sulphadiazine is probably as effective as the less soluble sulphonamides, such as sulphaguanidine, succinylsulphathiazole or phthalylsulphathiazole.

As an Alternative Drug or for Supportive Treatment

4. *Streptococcal Infections.* For hæmolytic streptococcal infections of the throat and for erysipelas, sulphonamides provide an alternative to penicillin. It is to be remembered that penicillin is bactericidal and sulphonamides bacteriostatic.

5. *Pneumonia.* Sulphonamides are effective for pneumococcal or streptococcal pneumonia. They may be used in combination with systemic penicillin.

PROPHYLACTIC TREATMENT

1. After an attack of rheumatic fever or rheumatic carditis, a long-term scheme of prophylaxis is essential. Penicillin is the treatment of choice, but sulphonamides provide an alternative, when, for example, a particular patient proves to be allergic to penicillin.

2. In severe cases of measles in infants or young children already ill with other diseases, a short course of sulphonamides can be employed to reduce the risk of complications.

ADMINISTRATION AND DOSE

Sulphonamides are usually given orally, either in the form of tablets (0·5 G.) or as a flavoured suspension. Either a single sulphonamide, such as sulphadiazine, is given or a triple preparation, sulphathiazole, sulphadiazine and sulphamerazine, is used. In the latter triad, the fact that each type of sulphonamide is present in reduced amounts theoretically lessens the risk of crystalluria, whilst maintaining the equivalent chemotherapeutic effect. Nevertheless, the inclusion of sulphamerazine in most of the proprietary triple sulphonamide preparations makes their usage undesirable, since sulphamerazine is particularly likely to cause hæmaturia. It is important that plenty of fluid should also be given and dehydration must be actively corrected.

TABLE XXVIII

DOSAGE FOR SULPHONAMIDES
(other than for particular sulphonamides specified below)

Age	Initial Dose	Four-hourly Dose
0–1 year	0·5 G.	0·25 G.
1–2 years	0·5 G.	0·5 G.
2–5 years	1·0 G.	0·5 G.
5–10 years	1·5 G.	0·75 G.

The above dosage is suitable for sulphathiazole, sulphadiazine, sulphadimidine, sulphafurazole (Gantrisin) and sulphasomidine (Elkosin). A course of sulphonamide treatment is usually given for five to seven days, except in cases of urinary-tract infections or meningitis when more prolonged treatment is necessary.

Alternatively, the total dose may be calculated as 1 to 3 grains per pound body-weight per 24 hours, or 0·1 to 0·3 G. per Kg. body-weight per 24 hours, divided into four- or six-hourly doses; the larger dose is used in severe infections such as meningitis. In severe infections, and especially in meningococcal meningitis and septicæmia, intravenous or intramuscular administration may be necessary at first, particularly if vomiting is present; the same dose as that used by mouth is given and soluble sulphathiazole or sulphadiazine is available for this purpose. If, as is commonly necessary, fluids have to be given intravenously, it is convenient to inject a soluble sulphonamide into the intravenous drip.

Sulphamethizole (Urolucosil). This preparation, which is used particularly for infections of the urinary tract, requires only one-eighth of the standard sulphonamide dosage mentioned above.

Succinylsulphathiazole, Sulphaguanidine and Phthalylsulphathiazole. These drugs are poorly absorbed from the alimentary tract and are thus used particularly for gastro-intestinal infections. The dose is twice that of the standard sulphonamide dosage mentioned above, except for phthalylsulphathiazole which is the same as the standard dosage.

Sulphasalazine (Salazopyrine). This contains a combination of sulphapyridine and salicylic acid. It has been found to be effective for inflammatory lesions of the bowel wall and particularly for ulcerative colitis (p. 204). Under the age of 7 years 0·25–0·5 G., and over the age of 7 years 0·5–1·0 G., four times a day, is recommended.

Sulphamethoxypyridazine (Lederkyn, Midicel). Due to its slow rate of excretion, a single daily dose of this preparation is claimed to be sufficient to maintain a blood level of sulphonamide comparable with other sulphonamides given in standard dosage. The initial dose is half the initial dose recommended for the standard sulphonamides followed by half the maintenance dose given *once* daily.

TOXIC EFFECTS OF SULPHONAMIDES

Malaise, vomiting and slight cyanosis may occur with some sulphonamides. Vomiting may cause dehydration and a change to antibiotic therapy may be required.

Hæmatological Complications. Purpura, hæmolytic anæmia and agranulocytosis occasionally occur. If repeated courses of sulphonamides are given, a careful watch should be kept on the leucocyte count to give warning of granulocytopenia.

Kernicterus. The use of sulphafurazole (Gantrisin) in the first week is contra-indicated in view of the danger of producing jaundice and kernicterus.

Renal Complications. Diuresis should always be encouraged during sulphonamide therapy because precipitation of acetylated sulphonamide crystals may give rise to hæmaturia. Sulphamerazine and sulphadiazine are chiefly responsible for this, and it is an indication for stopping treatment immediately, otherwise anuria may develop. Plenty of fluid should be given promptly, parenterally if required. In order to offset the difficulty of low solubility, smaller amounts of several different sulphonamide preparations may be given, since each retains its own solubility irrespective of the presence of other preparations. Sulphonamides of high solubility, such as sulphafurazole, do not cause renal damage unless there is oliguria.

Sensitization. Sensitization to a sulphonamide is a possibility. Fever may occur early or may be delayed until about the tenth day of treatment. Drug fever usually disappears on stopping sulphonamide, but may persist for several days. Occasionally a rash due to sulphonamides is seen. The risk of sulphonamide dermatitis contra-indicates all local application to the skin.

ANTIBIOTIC PREPARATIONS
Penicillin

DESPITE recent discoveries, penicillin remains the outstanding antibiotic. It is effective against a wide range of organisms and is relatively free from toxic effects. The antibiotic range of penicillin is extremely wide, but it must be borne in mind that not all organisms are equally sensitive to it and that some, in particular the staphylococcus, produce resistant strains (due to the presence of a penicillinase in their structure), which go on multiplying when the sensitive strains have been destroyed. More recently methicillin, which is resistant to the penicillinase produced by these organisms, has come into clinical usage. Even so, certain strains of *Staph. pyogenes* still show a resistance even to methicillin. Widespread and indiscriminate use of methicillin will undoubtedly tend to favour the multiplication of such organisms and thus reduce the value of this antibiotic.

INDICATIONS FOR PENICILLIN

1. Hæmolytic streptococcal and pneumococcal infections, including especially meningitis, septicæmia, bacterial endocarditis and pneumonia.
2. Gonorrhœa.
3. Diphtheria, tetanus and gas gangrene (in combination with antitoxin).
4. Syphilis (*see* p. 568).
5. *H. influenzæ* meningitis (in combination with streptomycin and sulphonamides).

6. For local treatment of empyema, abscesses and pneumococcal meningitis.
7. For inhalation (aerosol) in chronic pulmonary infections, bronchitis and bronchiectasis.
8. For prophylaxis before and after tonsillectomy and other operations, and in severe forms of measles.

Long-term Prophylaxis

The place of long-term oral treatment with phenoxymethylpenicillin in prevention of further attacks of Group A streptococcal infections in patients who have already had rheumatic carditis or acute nephritis is now well established.   In the case of rheumatic carditis patients, it is recommended that daily treatment should be continued for five or six years, whilst in the case of acute nephritis a shorter period of preventive treatment (between six to twelve months) is more commonly employed.

VARIETIES OF PENICILLIN

Benzylpenicillin (Penicillin G)

This type of penicillin is the one commonly given by injection.   It is prepared in crystalline form either as its sodium or potassium salt.   Procaine benzylpenicillin is also prepared and provides a longer effective blood level (up to twenty-four hours between injections) than the other benzylpenicillins which need six- to twelve-hourly injections.

Benzathine Penicillin

This is a more insoluble preparation of penicillin and will give effective blood levels of up to three to four days between injections.   The injections, however, tend to be somewhat painful.

Phenoxymethylpenicillin (Penicillin V)

This preparation is stable in acid solutions such as gastric juice and is thus suitable for oral use.   With optimum dosage, adequate blood levels are maintained for four hours after each oral administration.

Phenethicillin (Broxil)
Propicillin (Brocillin, Ultrapen)
Ampicillin (Penbritin)

Synthetic penicillins which are resistant to the action of acid are available for oral use.   It is claimed that higher blood levels are obtained than with phenoxymethylpenicillin.   The antibacterial range is similar except in the case of ampicillin, which is claimed to have a bacteriocidal action against the typhoid group as well as against Gram-positive organisms.

Methicillin (Celbenin)

The recent introduction of methicillin, which is itself resistant to the penicillinase produced by certain strains of *Staph. pyogenes*, has provided a valuable antibiotic against those *Staph. pyogenes* which are so prevalent in many hospitals. Widespread use of methicillin could rapidly reduce its value since rare strains of *Staph. pyogenes*, already resistant to it, would multiply rapidly if the more general strains of *Staph. pyogenes* were eliminated.   Methicillin is effective only by intramuscular injection.

Cloxacillin (Orbenin) is said to be comparable with methicillin and can be given orally.

DOSAGE (*see* Table **XXIX**)

TOXIC EFFECTS OF PENICILLIN

Occasionally drug rashes and fever occur, though these are seldom so serious as to warrant changing the treatment except in the case of urticaria. A troublesome stomatitis may develop in allergic subjects following treatment with an oral penicillin.

Streptomycin

INDICATIONS FOR STREPTOMYCIN

As the Drug of Choice

1. Miliary tuberculosis, tuberculous meningitis, peritonitis, bone and joint lesions, and certain severe cases of primary tuberculosis. Streptomycin is usually given in combination with sodium aminosalicylate and isoniazid (for dosage, *see* Appendix 3), to lessen the risk of bacterial resistance.
2. *H. influenzæ* meningitis, in combination with penicillin and sulphonamides and with specific antisera.

As an Alternative Drug

3. Urinary infections (sulphonamides remain the initial drug of choice). Bacillary dysentery (as an alternative to sulphonamides).

It should be noted that certain bacteria easily become resistant to streptomycin; *H. influenzæ* may become insensitive to it in a few days, tubercle bacilli within a few weeks. Streptomycin should not be used indiscriminately; it is of chief value when bacteria show a high degree of sensitivity and the infection can be quickly overcome.

DOSAGE (*see* Table **XXIX**, p. 656)

TOXIC EFFECTS

The most important toxic effects are vestibular damage and deafness. In children, the former effect, though probably as frequent as in adults, is not as serious, as the patients quickly learn to compensate for their lack of vestibular function; deafness, however, is a serious problem, especially after prolonged courses of intrathecal streptomycin for the treatment of tuberculous meningitis. It seems probable that most cases of serious deafness or vestibular damage have followed the use of too high a dosage of streptomycin or the use of dihydrostreptomycin, a preparation which is no longer recommended. Sensitivity reactions also occur, including drug fever and dermatitis, especially from local contact with streptomycin. Streptomycin is excreted by the kidney and its use is contra-indicated in anuric states.

The Tetracyclines

These comprise chlortetracycline (Aureomycin), oxytetracycline dihydrate (Terramycin) and tetracycline hydrochloride (Achromycin). They have a similar bacteriostatic range against a wide variety of organisms. Lately their value has become less because of the increase in bacterial resistance, particularly of *Staph. pyogenes*. They all share the disadvantage that gastro-intestinal complications are not uncommon.

INDICATIONS FOR TETRACYCLINE THERAPY

As the Drug of Choice

1. Rickettsial infections (typhus, Rocky Mountain spotted fever, Q fever, scrub typhus, tick-bite fever) which are rare in children.
2. Psittacosis, ornithosis, lymphogranuloma venereum.
3. Pertussis (if used in the early stages).
4. Severe staphylococcal infections—pneumonia, septicæmia, etc. (where the organism is known to be sensitive).
5. Inclusion conjunctivitis and trachoma.
6. Brucellosis (with streptomycin).

As an Alternative Drug

7. Gonorrhœa caused by gonococci resistant to penicillin.
8. Pyogenic infections (streptococcal, pneumococcal, *H. influenzæ*, Friedländer, etc.), where the organism is known to be sensitive.

For Long-term Prophylaxis

9. Long-term prophylactic treatment in bronchiectasis and fibrocystic disease.

DOSAGE (*see* Table XXIX, p. 656)

TOXIC EFFECTS

Tetracyclines cause rapid changes in flora of the respiratory and alimentary tract. In such conditions glossitis and ulcerative stomatitis may occur, and monilia infections, sometimes becoming widespread, may be dangerous, especially in newborn infants. For this reason, vitamin B preparations should be given together with any tetracycline. Intensive treatment with nystatin (*see* p. 656) should also be given, both locally as a paint and in tablet form, if signs of monilial infection are present. Of the direct toxic effects of the drug, nausea and vomiting are common and diarrhœa may occur.

Chloramphenicol

The antibiotic range of this drug is somewhat wider than that of the tetracyclines, and strains of resistant organisms are less commonly encountered. Owing to the presence of a benzene ring, chloramphenicol is capable of damaging the bone-marrow. In children, a very small number of cases of agranulocytosis or aplastic anæmia have been reported, usually only after excessive dosage, prolonged use, or after repeated courses. For this reason chloramphenicol must be regarded as a somewhat dangerous antibiotic. However, a single course of chloramphenicol lasting not more than seven days and in a dosage not exceeding that advised on p. 655 has been found effective in severe infections, within the range of its bacteriostatic action. High dosage is especially toxic to premature infants to whom half the usual weight-for-weight dose should be given; methicillin now provides a safer alternative.

INDICATIONS FOR CHLORAMPHENICOL

As the Drug of Choice

1. Typhoid fever, paratyphoid A and paratyphoid B.
2. *Staph. pyogenes* infections where the organism is known (or is likely) to be resistant to all other antibiotics.

As an Alternative Drug

3. Urinary infections (sulphonamides remain the first choice for routine treatment).
4. Rickettsial infections (alternative to tetracyclines).
5. Psittacosis, lymphogranuloma venereum (alternative to tetracyclines).
6. Primary atypical pneumonia (alternative to tetracyclines).
7. *H. influenzæ* infections, particularly meningitis (in combination with other antibiotics and sulphonamides).
8. Other pyogenic infections (streptococcal, staphylococcal, pneumococcal, Friedländer, etc.).

Chloramphenicol is useful and safe in topical treatment.   It can be used in a cream for staphylococcal and streptococcal skin infections.   It may also be used in the form of aural drops as a topical agent in eye infections and in otitis media.

DOSAGE (*see* Table XXIX, p. 655)

TOXIC EFFECTS

In addition to marrow damage, and in premature infants, chloramphenicol has toxic effects similar to those of the tetracyclines (*see* p. 652).

Erythromycin

This antibiotic is effective against the Gram-positive organisms, particularly *Staph. pyogenes*, Group A streptococci, and pneumococci. Unfortunately erythromycin-resistant strains of *Staph. pyogenes* rapidly appear, and the more widely that this antibiotic is used, the sooner will its usefulness diminish.

INDICATIONS

Staph. pyogenes infections of major severity where the organism is known to be resistant to penicillin and other antibiotics.

DOSAGE (*see* Table XXIX, p. 655)

TOXIC EFFECTS

Erythromycin may sometimes cause diarrhœa and vomiting.   Leucopenia has occasionally been noted.

Oleandomycin

This antibiotic has properties similar to those described for erythromycin, including the rapid development of resistant strains of *Staph. pyogenes*. Its use, therefore, should be rigorously restricted to severe *Staph. pyogenes* infections where the organism is known to be resistant to other antibiotics but sensitive to oleandomycin.

DOSAGE (*see* Table XXIX, p. 656)

TOXIC EFFECTS

Due to its powerful effect on the bacterial flora of the intestinal tract, diarrhœa may develop during treatment.   Concomitant treatment with vitamin B preparations should be given to prevent this complication.

Spiramycin

The properties of this antibiotic are very similar to those of erythromycin. *Staph. pyogenes* known to be resistant to erythromycin is likely to be resistant also to spiramycin. Its use in clinical medicine is therefore limited to the very exceptional *Staph. pyogenes* infections of major severity, in which the particular infecting strain is known to be resistant to all other antibiotics, including erythromycin, but sensitive to spiramycin. This antibiotic is somewhat unreliable in its effect since its absorption from the bowel is very variable.

DOSAGE (*see* Table XXIX, p. 656)

Novobiocin

The range of organisms against which novobiocin is effective includes the Gram-positive cocci and particularly *Staph. pyogenes*. *H. influenzæ* and some strains of *B. proteus* are also sensitive. As with the other newer antibiotics, resistant strains of organisms rapidly develop. Its use should be carefully restricted to those infections known to be resistant to other antibiotics but with proven sensitivity to novobiocin.

DOSAGE (*see* Table XXIX, p. 655)

Vancomycin

Vancomycin is an effective bacteriocidal agent against *Staph. pyogenes* and some Gram-negative organisms. It is at present available only in an intravenous form. Its place in therapy has yet to be fully assessed.

Polymixin B

Polymixin has a place in the treatment of *Pseudomonas* infections; apart from this it can be used as an alternative drug in other infections by Gram-negative bacilli when there is bacterial sensitivity.

INDICATIONS FOR POLYMIXIN

As an Alternative Drug

1. *Ps. pyocyaneæ* infections (local or general treatment), although Colomycin is likely to be the first choice.

2. *H. influenzæ* infections (usually combined treatment with sulphonamides).

DOSAGE (*see* Table XXIX, p. 656)

TOXICITY

Polymixin may give rise to fever, malaise, and a generalized pruritus which rapidly disappear when treatment is stopped. Patients with abnormal renal function may deteriorate on treatment.

Colomycin

Colomycin has recently been introduced as an antibiotic with both bacteriocidal and bacteriostatic actions against Gram-negative bacilli. It appears to be especially valuable for *Pseudomonas* infections. *E. coli* infections resistant to other treatment provide a further indication for its use. For dosage, *see* Table XXIX, p. 655.

Neomycin

Although neomycin has a very wide range of bacteriocidal action its parenteral use is contra-indicated by its highly toxic effects which include nerve deafness and renal damage.

Its use is therefore limited to oral administration (since its poor absorption from the alimentary tract removes the dangers attendant upon its parenteral use) and to topical applications.   Within these limits it is a highly effective antibiotic being active against some of the dysenteric organisms and against many of the pathogenic strains of *E. coli*.   It is also used as a local application for nasal, conjunctival and skin infections, and infected burns where the nature and antibiotic sensitivities of the infecting organism are known to be appropriate.

Bacitracin

Like neomycin, the general use of bacitracin is contra-indicated by its toxic effects upon the kidneys.   It has a wide range of antibacterial action and has a very useful place in the treatment of skin infections due to *Staph. pyogenes*.   In desperate cases its systemic use, with the attendant dangers of renal damage, may be necessary, as for example in *Staph. pyogenes* septicæmia.   In such circumstances a very high fluid intake and urine output must be assured.

Nystatin

Nystatin is an antifungal antibiotic, being effective against yeasts and fungi. Its principal use is to combat *Candida albicans* infections, which tend to become extensive in severely ill patients already under treatment with a broad-spectrum antibiotic.   It is available both for local use and as a general preparation given by mouth.   It is always advisable to give an extended course of treatment since, in severely ill patients on antibiotic treatment, monilial infection may extend far down the œsophagus or into the bronchial tree, where monilia may persist after the signs of oral infection have subsided.

DOSAGE (*see* Table XXIX, p. 656)

TOXIC EFFECTS

Nausea and diarrhœa may sometimes occur, but are seldom of a severe nature.

TABLE XXIX

DOSAGE OF ANTIBIOTICS

Antibiotic	Route	Total Daily Requirement (to be divided into individual doses)	Interval between Doses
Bacitracin (for contra-indications, *see* above)	Intramuscular Topical	500 units/Kg./body-wt. 500 units per G. ointment	6 hours
Chloramphenicol (dose for premature infants, *see* p. 652)	Oral Intramuscular Intravenous	40mg./Kg./body-wt. 40mg./Kg./body-wt. 40mg./Kg./body-wt.	6 hours 6 hours 6 hours
Colomycin	Oral Intramuscular Intravenous Intrathecal	100,000 units/Kg./body-wt 50,000 units/Kg./body-wt. 25,000/Kg./body-wt. 10,000–20,000 units	6–8 hours 6–12 hours slow infusion daily
Erythromycin	Oral Intravenous Intramuscular	20mg./Kg./body-wt. 20mg./Kg./body-wt. 20mg./Kg./body-wt.	6 hours 6 hours 6 hours
Neomycin	Oral	40–80mg./Kg./body-wt.	6 hours
Novobiocin	Oral	20mg./Kg./body-wt.	12 hours

TABLE XXIX (*continued*)

DOSAGE OF ANTIBIOTICS

Antibiotic	*Route*	*Total Daily Requirement* (to be divided into individual doses)	*Interval between Doses*
Nystatin	Oral	50,000 units/Kg./body-wt.	6 hours
	Topical	100,000 units per G.	
Oleandomycin	Oral	25–40 mg./Kg./body-wt.	6 hours
Penicillins			
Benzylpenicillin	Intramuscular	300,000–600,000 units	
(Penicillin G)	or intravenous	(under 15 Kg. body-wt.)	8 hours
		600,000–1,500,000 units	
		(over 15 Kg. body-wt.)	
	Intrathecal	5,000–10,000 units	
Procaine penicillin G	Intramuscular	150,000–300,000 units	daily
Benzathine penicillin	Oral or	300,000–600,000 units	6 hours
(as Penidural	intramuscular	(under 15 Kg. body-wt.)	orally,
combined with		600,000–1,200,000 units	daily if
benzyl penicillin)		(over 15 Kg. body-wt.)	intra-muscular
Penidural all-purpose	Intramuscular	1·2 mega units	weekly
Phenoxymethyl	Oral	250–500 mg.	6 hours
penicillin		(under 8 Kg. body-wt.)	
(Penicillin V)		500–1,000 mg.	
		(8–15 Kg. body-wt.)	
		1,000–2,000 mg.	
		(over 15 Kg. body-wt.)	
Propicillin	Oral	250–750 mg.	6 hours
(Brocillin, Ultrapen)			
Ampicillin	Oral	50–150 mg./Kg./body-wt.	6 hours
(Penbritin)			
Phenethicillin	Oral	250–750 mg.	6 hours
(Broxil)			
Methicillin	Intramuscular	100 mg./Kg./body-wt.	4–6 hours
(Celbenin)			
Cloxacillin	Oral	500–1000 mg.	6 hours
(Orbenin)	Intramuscular	250–500 mg.	6 hours
Polymixin B	Oral (intestinal infections only)	200,000 units/Kg./body-wt.	4 hours
	Intramuscular	50,000 units/Kg./body-wt.	6 hours
	Intrathecal	10,000 units	
Spiramycin	Oral	20 mg./Kg./body-wt.	6 hours
Streptomycin	Intramuscular	25–40 mg./Kg./body-wt.	12 hours
	Intrathecal	25–50 mg.	
Tetracycline	Oral	20 mg./Kg./body-wt.	8 hours
(Chlortetracycline)	Intramuscular		
(Oxytetracycline)	(not recommended for		
(Tetracycline)	prolonged use)	20 mg./Kg./body-wt.	
	Intravenous (usually initial dose only)	5–10 mg./Kg./body-wt.	single dose

Corticosteroid Therapy in Childhood

PHYSIOLOGY

THE adrenal cortex produces three main types of steroid hormone:

1. Mineralocorticoids (main example aldosterone)
2. Glucocorticoids (main example hydrocortisone)
3. Androgens.

The mineralocorticoids are concerned with the regulation of the water and electrolyte content of the body fluids. By their effect on renal tubular re-absorption, they tend to cause sodium retention and potassium excretion.

The actions of the glucocorticoids are threefold: (*a*) They have an anabolic effect on carbohydrate metabolism tending to increase the amounts of both liver glycogen and blood glucose. This is brought about by the diversion of amino-acids from protein metabolism towards carbohydrate synthesis (gluconeogenesis) leading indirectly to an increased nitrogen output. (*b*) The glucocorticoids are concerned with the maintenance of the arterial blood pressure. (*c*) They contain a factor which appears to reduce the tissue response to foreign substances, thus tending to suppress inflammatory reactions, allergic responses and antibody production.

The androgens are concerned with the development of the male secondary sex characteristics (virilism) but not directly with spermatogenesis.

In practice, there is considerable overlap in the effects of the individual compounds as between their mineralocorticoid, glucocorticoid and androgenic action. Thus hydrocortisone, though acting mainly as a glucocorticoid, when given in large amounts exerts both a mineralocorticoid and androgenic effect. Work on synthetic corticosteroids has been directed towards producing compounds which have a maximal " anti-inflammatory " action and a minimal sodium-retaining function. In addition, a preparation (spironolactone) has been isolated which is an inhibitor of the mineralocorticoid aldosterone.

The amount of hydrocortisone produced in the adrenal cortex is regulated by the anterior pituitary hormone ACTH. When the plasma level of hydrocortisone falls, there is a release of ACTH from the pituitary which stimulates hydrocortisone production. Conversely, when the plasma level of hydrocortisone is high, the level of ACTH output diminishes. Thus the effect of hydrocortisone or other corticosteroid therapy will be to reduce the ACTH output. If this is long continued, the lack of stimulus for endogenous hydrocortisone production will cause atrophy of the adrenal cortex.

INDICATIONS FOR CORTICOSTEROID THERAPY IN CHILDHOOD

REPLACEMENT THERAPY

Short-Term

In acute septicæmia, and particularly *septicæmic meningitis* (p. 402), acute adrenal hæmorrhage with destruction of the gland may occur (Waterhouse-

657

Friderichsen crisis) with symptoms of acute adrenal insufficiency. Emergency treatment with intravenous hydrocortisone, DOCA, fluids and electrolytes is essential.

In other overwhelming infections, such as acute broncholitis, a state of peripheral circulatory failure may occur. The effect of intravenous and intramuscular hydrocortisone may be dramatically helpful. It is a matter for conjecture as to how much of the benefit is the result of replacement therapy at a time when " adrenal exhaustion " has occurred or how much may be due to the relief of associated bronchospasm (see below) thus relieving a state of asphyxia.

Long-Term

Long-term replacement therapy is indicated in *Addison's disease* when the adrenal glands have atrophied or have been affected by tuberculosis or where *bilateral adrenalectomy* has been carried out. All of these are extremely rare in childhood.

Long-term corticosteroid therapy has revolutionised the treatement of the *adrenogenital syndrome* (p. 159). In this disorder there is a recessively inherited enzyme deficiency which interferes with the formation of hydrocortisone in the adrenal cortex. The resulting low-plasma level of hydrocortisone causes a greatly increased ACTH output and thus considerable hypertrophy of the adrenal cortex with an excessive production of androgens. Virilization occurs in both sexes with pseudo-hermaphroditism in females. The giving of exogenous hydrocortisone immediately inhibits the excessive ACTH production with subsequent reversal of the virilizing effect. This treatment, as with Addison's disease, has to be life-long. Some of these patients (*salt losers*) show considerable loss of sodium. In such cases replacement treatment with sodium chloride together with DOCA is required as well as regular treatment with hydrocortisone.

ANABOLIC EFFECT ON CARBOHYDRATE METABOLISM

In children with *idiopathic hypoglycæmia* (see p. 172) corticosteroids are effective treatment in the majority of patients. The dangerous effects of repeated hypoglycæmia may be averted by maintenance treatment with a very small dosage. In the majority of cases small children outgrow their hypoglycæmic tendency after the age of two or three years. Very rarely hypoglycæmia may be due to an islet-cell tumour of the pancreas; in such cases, and in others which have failed to respond to corticosteroids, consideration should be given to the need for partial pancreatectomy. Many patients will respond to this treatment even though no islet-cell tumour is found.

ANTI-INFLAMMATORY

Inflammation is the natural response of tissue to bacterial or other noxious stimuli. In certain diseases an excessive and harmful inflammatory reaction occurs which may cause as much, or even more, damage to the tissues as does the infection. It is in the attempt to reduce the extent of this excessive reaction that much of the corticosteroid therapy of the last decade has been undertaken. It was originally claimed that corticosteroids exerted a highly beneficial effect in the group of disorders which includes rheumatic carditis, rheumatoid arthritis, disseminated lupus erythematosis and peri-arteritis nodosa, in which infection may often appear to precipitate the illness, but in which the disease process persists long after the infection has cleared. A longer-term appraisal has failed to substantiate the *permanent* value of corticosteroid treatment in these diseases in almost every respect. There is no doubt that the disease processes can be modified by corticosteroids, with rapid relief from acute symptoms. The effect, however, is due to a suppression of symptoms, not to a cure of the disease process. Present evidence suggests that long-term treatment with corticosteroids has failed to reduce the incidence of permanent rheumatic endocarditis following acute rheumatism and that the long-term benefits in rheumatoid arthritis, disseminated lupus erythematosis and periarteritis are equally questionable. Corticosteroids, in short courses, would still appear to have a place in the short-term management of episodes of acute *rheumatic pancarditis* (*see* p. 309), enabling a patient to survive a severe crisis in the illness which might otherwise prove fatal. The same may well be true of the acute episodes of *pericarditis* which may complicate *rheumatoid arthritis* (*see* p. 317).

Corticosteroids, again in relatively short courses, may play a useful part in the treatment of *tuberculous meningitis* (p. 405) by reducing exudates and thus preventing the possible obstruction of the cerebrospinal fluid pathways. Similar effects may be achieved in the treatment of the severe *E. coli* meningitis of the newborn. Such treatment is not commenced until the underlying infection has been well controlled by chemotherapy.

SUPPRESSION OF ALLERGIC REACTIONS

ACTH and corticosteroids may be used in *emergency treatment* of severe allergic reactions and in status asthmaticus where there has been no response to adrenaline, aminophylline, etc.

Corticosteroids are used in the *maintenance therapy* of severe allergic states, but, because of the disadvantages of long-term treatment, this should be avoided whenever possible; for example, in asthma, corticosteroids should be used only when a child is progressing towards a state of irreversible pulmonary damage, because of persistent asthmatic attacks, and *when no other treatment will halt this progression.*

REDUCTION OF ANTIBODY PRODUCTION

Relatively short-term treatment (which in practice may mean approximately six weeks) with corticosteroids will usually produce a remission in cases of *acquired hæmolytic anæmia* (p. 338) and of *thrombocytopenic purpura* (p. 341).

Corticosteroids in high dosage will often produce a dramatic remission in children with *acute lymphatic leukæmia* (p. 347). The corticosteroid is followed up with an antimetabolite, such as 6-mercaptopurine. Unfortunately a remission of only some months or possibly a year or two is obtained and never a cure.

MISCELLANEOUS DISORDERS

Corticosteroids appear to have a useful place in the treatment of *nephrosis* (p. 370), both in bringing about a remission in an episode of nephrotic œdema with massive proteinuria, and also, in longer-term treatment, by reducing the number of relapses to which these patients are prone. Thus, high doses of corticosteroids are indicated for short-term treatment of the acute episodes, followed by a much smaller dosage for prolonged periods of two to three years. The action of corticosteroids in nephrosis seems to fall into the same nonspecific category as has been discussed in relation to their " anti-inflammatory " effect. In nephrosis, corticosteroids appear to prevent the gradual destruction of the nephrons that otherwise occurs in a proportion of the patients. By no means all patients are benefited by corticosteroids and a longer-term evaluation of their effect is still needed.

In ulcerative colitis (p. 203) corticosteroids may occasionally be required systemically to tide a patient over a severe episode of the disease. Their longer-term systemic use is seldom justified, although local treatment (with hydrocortisone sodium succinate retention enemata or prednisolone 21-phosphate) may need to be continued for some months.

LOCAL TREATMENT

The local application of one per cent. hydrocortisone ointment is an extremely valuable remedy in *infantile eczema* (p. 502). The local treatment of the skin however, is only one small part of the larger problem of the management of children with infantile eczema (p. 504). Stronger concentrations of hydrocortisone, up to 40 per cent., may be helpful in *psoriasis*.

The anti-inflammatory effect of corticosteroids is of particular value in ophthalmology. Thus, local treatment with hydrocortisone ophthalmic ointment (25 mg. per G.) or eye drops (one per cent.) is valuable in such conditions as *infective keratitis*, *iridocyclitis*, and *sympathetic ophthalmitis*.

DOSAGE

THE preparations available[1] and their relative potency by weight are:

	Relative Potency by Weight	*Salt Retaining Action*
Cortisone	1	Marked
Hydrocortisone	1·2	Marked
Prednisone	5	Slight
Prednisolone	5	Slight
Methyl prednisolone	6	None
Triamcinolone	6	None
Dexamethazone	35	Very slight
Betamethazone	35	Very slight

Hydrocortisone sodium succinate and prednisolone 21-phosphate may be used intravenously and cortisone acetate intramuscularly. There is no exact equivalent between ACTH and cortisone, etc. The strength of ACTH solutions is expressed in units. In practice, the daily dose of cortisone in milligrams is taken as corresponding roughly to the same number of units of ACTH. It will be appreciated from the relative potency by weight of the corticosteroid preparations listed above, that, for example, the equivalent dose of cortisone will be five times greater than that of prednisolone; similarly, the equivalent dose of dexamethazone will be seven times smaller than the equivalent dose of prednisone. Although weight-for-weight the potency of fludrocortisone is even greater, its salt-retaining action is very high.

SHORT-TERM TREATMENT

For *infants* requiring intensive treatment for a short period, an oral dosage of prednisone of 2·0 mg. per Kg. body-weight per day, given in two divided doses, is recommended. In acute illness, intravenous hydrocortisone sodium succinate may be given in doses of 1–2 mg. per Kg. body-weight, which may be

[1] Nabarro, J. D. N. (1961). In *Prescribers Journal 1*, No. 2.

repeated eight hourly; alternatively, a continuous infusion containing 0·1–0·2 mg. per Kg. body-weight per hour may be given.   In cases of acute adrenal hæmorrhage, twice or even three times this dose may be necessary, together with DOCA 5 mg. intramuscularly and intravenous fluid and salt replacement.

For a child of two years, an intensive course of oral prednisone should start with an initial daily dose of 20–30 mg.; at five years 30–40 mg. daily; at ten years 50–60 mg. daily.   Larger doses than these may be given in cases of urgency in severe illness.   The subsequent treatment depends upon the disease.   After four or five days, the dose is either *gradually reduced* to complete withdrawal or the patient is maintained on a much reduced dosage for a prolonged period.

LONG-TERM TREATMENT

The dangers of long-term corticosteroid therapy are so grave that it is advised that no practitioner should prescribe such treatment until he has sought a second opinion.

For long-term treatment, after an initial period of high dosage, prednisone may be continued in a dosage of 0·4–0·6 mg. per Kg. body-weight per day in infancy.   This is a relatively higher weight-for-weight ratio than that required in older children, who seldom need a maintenance dose of prednisone greater than 5 mg. or occasionally 10 mg. daily.

In infants with the adrenogenital syndrome who are also salt losers, maintenance treatment should include, in addition to cortisone, sodium chloride 3–6 G. daily and DOCA given initially in a daily intramuscular dosage of 2–5 mg., followed later by slow-acting implants or DOCA trimethyl acetate, 30 mg. crystules at monthly intervals.

Whenever prednisone is being given in high dosage, it is advisable to give also potassium chloride 0·5 G. with each dose to avoid hypokalæmia.

COMPLICATIONS OF CORTICOSTEROID THERAPY

THE dangers of prolonged corticosteroid therapy cannot be overemphasized. They already account for a number of deaths in children every year, many of which could have been avoided.   The ill-effects can be divided into those which occur whilst treatment is being continued and those which develop after withdrawal of the drug.

COMPLICATIONS WHILE ON TREATMENT

If corticosteroids are long continued at a relatively high dosage, the clinical picture of Cushing's syndrome (p. 150) will inevitably emerge—a moon face, striæ, obesity, hypertension and hirsutism.   Metabolic complications which may follow include hyperglycæmia and glycosuria, œdema, hypokalæmia, osteoporosis and a general failure of growth.   Due to the depressed inflammatory reaction, intercurrent infections may lack their usual symptoms and, with decreased antibody production, progress rapidly to septicæmia and even a fatal conclusion.   Peptic ulceration, going on to perforation or hæmorrhage, may occur.

COMPLICATIONS AFTER THE WITHDRAWAL OF TREATMENT

As has been already mentioned, the giving of exogenous corticosteroids depresses the output of ACTH and leads ultimately to adrenal cortical atrophy.

Even after a relatively short course of corticosteroids, however, withdrawal symptoms may occur if treatment is stopped suddenly rather than gradually reduced. These take the form of an Addisonian crisis with severe vomiting, hypotension, prostration and dehydration. Treatment consists in the immediate resumption of corticosteroid therapy and, in the most severe cases, the intensive programme already outlined for cases of acute adrenal hæmorrhage (pp. 657–658).

After more prolonged treatment with corticosteroids, the efficiency of the adrenal cortex may be atrophied permanently or may recover only after many years. Such an adrenal cortex is unable to respond to the stresses of intercurrent infections, trauma or surgical procedures—stresses to which the healthy adrenal greatly increases its secretory activities in response to increased ACTH production. The atrophied adrenal cortex is unable to respond in this way. Under such circumstances, an intercurrent illness or a surgical operation is likely to become complicated by the symptoms of acute adrenal insufficiency already described and which unchecked will lead to the death of the child.

Any patient, therefore, who has been given any corticosteroid treatment within the previous five years, or a prolonged course at any time in their lives should receive full doses of corticosteroids as a part of their preparation for operation. Treatment should subsequently be continued for an appropriate period afterwards. Likewise, any child who becomes ill less than two years after a course of corticosteroids is in an equally precarious position. There should be no hesitation in giving further corticosteroids on such occasions, especially if any symptoms such as vomiting or marked listlessness are present. *In the presence of vomiting the corticosteroid must be given intravenously or intramuscularly in full dosage.*

It is abundantly clear, therefore, that the parents of any child who has been given corticosteroids should be told of the treatment and preferably provided with a card which gives details of the dates and dosages. The parents should be told that because of the treatment some precautions are necessary and that they must always inform any doctor who sees their child of the details. During the first years after the withdrawal of corticosteroid therapy, they must be instructed to report immediately to their doctor any illness that the child may contract.

Dosages of Other Drugs in Childhood

To calculate the appropriate dosage of a drug for infants and children of different ages and weights is not always easy. Although some useful guides exist for this purpose, they have limitations because some drugs exert a relatively more pronounced effect in infancy and in the case of others the infant is relatively more tolerant. For example, the immature cerebral cortex of the infant is less sensitive to the action of caffeine, atropine and the barbiturates. On the other hand, drugs acting on the subcortical centres, such as the opium derivatives, should always be prescribed with extreme caution, and morphine is a dangerous drug.

FORMULÆ FOR CALCULATING DOSAGE

Under two years of age

Fried's Rule. Infant's dose $= \dfrac{\text{adult dose} \times \text{age in months}}{150}$

Over two years of age

Clark's Rule. Child's dose $= \dfrac{\text{adult dose} \times \text{weight in lb.}}{150}$

For various ages

Young's Rule. Child's dose $= \dfrac{\text{adult dose} \times \text{child's age}}{\text{child's age} + 12}$

For a particular patient, Clark's rule permits the calculation of dosages on a weight-for-weight basis proportionate to the standard adult dose. Under two years of age, however, modifications may be needed, since infants require relatively larger doses of antibiotics, antihistamines, antimalarials, barbiturates, corticosteroids, digitalis and sulphonamides, whilst smaller amounts of aminophylline and morphine are required by infants than might appear on a simple body-weight ratio.

TABLE XXX

DOSES IN INFANCY AND CHILDHOOD

(The amounts given are guides to individual doses, not twenty-four hour requirement, except where otherwise stated)

Drug	Birth	1 Year	5 Years	10 Years
Acetozolamide (Diamox)	—	—	125 mg.	250 mg.
Adrenaline	—	From 0·07–0·3 ml. (1–5 minims of a 1 in 1,000 solution subcutaneously)		
Aminophylline	3 mg./Kg. body-weight by mouth or I.M.I.; up to twice this dose by suppository.			
Amphetamine	—	—	2·5 mg.	5 mg.

Drug	*Birth*	1 *Year*	5 *Years*	10 *Years*
Antihistamines				
Diphenhydramine HCl (Benadryl)	1–1·5 mg. per Kg. body-weight			
Chlorpheniramine maleate (Piriton)	—	1 mg.	2 mg.	4 mg.
Mepyramine maleate (Anthisan)	—	—	$\frac{1}{2}$ adult dose	adult dose (25–100 mg.)
Promethazine HCl (Phenergan)	2·5 mg.	5 mg.	10 mg.	20 mg.
Aspirin	—	100–200 mg. ($1\frac{1}{2}$–3 grains)	150–300 mg. ($2\frac{1}{2}$–5 grains)	300–600 mg. (5–10 grains)
Atropine (by injection)	0·4 mg. ($\frac{1}{150}$ grain)	0·6 mg. ($\frac{1}{100}$ grain)	0·6 mg. ($\frac{1}{100}$ grain)	0·6 mg. ($\frac{1}{100}$ grain)
Atropine methonitrate (Eumydrin)	0·08–0·12 mg. ($\frac{1}{750}$–$\frac{1}{500}$ grain) to be increased as necessary			
Bromethol (B.P.) (Avertin) (basal narcotic dose)	0·1 ml. ($1\frac{1}{2}$ minims) per Kg. body-weight in $2\frac{1}{2}$% solution of distilled water per rectum			
Barbiturate group				
Amylobartitone (Amytal)	—	—	60 mg. (1 grain)	90 mg. ($1\frac{1}{2}$ grains)
Butobarbitone (Soneryl)	—	—	30 mg. ($\frac{1}{2}$ grain)	60 mg. (1 grains)
Methylphenobarbitone (Phemitone, Prominal)	—	15–30 mg. ($\frac{1}{4}$–$\frac{1}{2}$ grain)	30–60 mg. ($\frac{1}{2}$–1 grain)	30–90 mg. ($\frac{1}{2}$–$1\frac{1}{2}$ grains)
Pentobarbitone (Nembutal)	5 mg. ($\frac{1}{12}$ grain) per Kg. body-weight up to a maximum of 200 mg. (3 grains) (Obese children should not receive full dose)			
Phenobarbitone	7·5–15 mg. ($\frac{1}{8}$–$\frac{1}{4}$ grain)	15 mg. ($\frac{1}{4}$ grain)	15–30 mg. ($\frac{1}{4}$–$\frac{1}{2}$ grain)	15–30 mg. ($\frac{1}{4}$–$\frac{1}{2}$ grain)
Quinalbarbitone (Seconal)	5–7·5 mg. ($\frac{1}{12}$–$\frac{1}{8}$ grain) per Kg. body-weight up to a maximum of 200 mg. (3 grains) (Obese children should not receive full dose)			
Belladonna Tinct.	0·12 ml. (2 minims)	0·2 ml. (3 minims)	0·3 ml. (5 minims)	0·6 ml. (10 minims)
Bemegride	5 mg. ($\frac{1}{12}$ grain) per ml. (minim) for I. V. injection as indicated			
Bisacodyl	—	—	5 mg. ($\frac{1}{12}$ grain)	10 mg. ($\frac{1}{6}$ grain)
Carbimazole	—	—	—	5 mg.
Cascara Sagrada Elixir	—	—	2 ml. (30 minims)	4 ml. (60 minims)
Castor Oil	—	2–4 ml. ($\frac{1}{2}$–1 drachm)	4–8 ml. (1–2 drachms)	8–16 ml. (2–4 drachms)
Chenopodium, Oil of	—	—	0·12–0·3 ml. (2–5 minims)	0·3–0·6 ml. (5–10 minims)
Chloral Hydrate	30–60 mg. ($\frac{1}{2}$–1 grain) 4-hourly intervals	60–180 mg. (1–3 grains) 4-hourly intervals commencing with the smaller dose	180–540 mg. (3–9 grains)	600 mg. (10 grains)
Chloroquine Sulphate	—	50 mg.	100 mg.	200 mg.
Chlorothiazide	*See* p. 667			
Chlorpromazine (Largactil)	1 mg./Kg. body-weight up to 5 years		10–20 mg. ($\frac{1}{6}$–$\frac{1}{3}$ grain)	20–40 mg. ($\frac{1}{3}$–$\frac{3}{5}$ grain)
Codeine Phosphate	—	—	8 mg. ($\frac{1}{8}$ grain)	8·16 mg. ($\frac{1}{8}$–$\frac{1}{4}$ grain)
Cyancobalamin	50 micrograms by injection			
Digitalis	*See* p. 667			

Drug	Birth	1 Year	5 Years	10 Years
Ephedrine	—	8–15 mg. ($\frac{1}{8}$–$\frac{1}{4}$ grain)	15–30 mg. ($\frac{1}{4}$–$\frac{1}{2}$ grain)	30 mg. ($\frac{1}{2}$ grain)
Ethosuximide	—	—	250 mg.	500 mg.
Ferric Ammonium Citrate	100 mg. ($1\frac{1}{2}$ grains)	400 mg. (6 grains)	400 mg. (6 grains)	600 mg. (10 grains)
Ferrous Sulphate	60 mg. (1 grain)	90 mg. ($1\frac{1}{2}$ grains)	120 mg. (2 grains)	120 mg. (2 grains)
Folic Acid	—	5 mg.	10 mg.	10 mg.
Gentian Violet	—	10 mg. ($\frac{1}{6}$ grain)	20 mg. ($\frac{1}{3}$ grain)	30 mg. ($\frac{1}{2}$ grain)
Griseofulvin	—	—	0·5 G. (8 grains)	0·5 G. (8 grains)
Hexylresorcinol	—	—	0·5 G.	0·8 G.
Hydrochlorothiazide	—	—	12·5 mg. ($\frac{1}{5}$ grain)	25 mg. ($\frac{2}{5}$ grain)
Hydroxyzine Hydrochloride (Atarax)	—	—	10 mg.	10–20 mg.
Isoniazid	5–20 mg. per Kg. body-weight daily			
Isoprenaline Sulphate	—	—	10 mg. ($\frac{1}{6}$ grain) (used also as 1% spray)	20 mg. ($\frac{1}{3}$ grain)
Lobeline Hydrochloride	3 mg. ($\frac{1}{20}$ grain)	—	—	—
Mepacrine	(Antimalarial therapy, p. 610); Giardiasis, p. 633			
Mersalyl Injection	—	—	0·5 ml.	0·5 ml.
Methedrine	0·5–1·0 mg. ($\frac{1}{120}$–$\frac{1}{60}$ grain) as cerebral stimulant	—	—	—
Morphine	—	3 mg. ($\frac{1}{20}$ grain)	5 mg. ($\frac{1}{12}$ grain)	8 mg. ($\frac{1}{8}$ grain)
Nalorphine Hydrobromide	0·5–1 mg. ($\frac{1}{120}$–$\frac{1}{60}$ grain)	Thereafter 0·2 mg. ($\frac{1}{300}$ grain) per Kg. intravenously up to a maximum of 10 mg. ($\frac{1}{6}$ grain) per dose		
Nepenthe	—	0·12 ml. (2 minims)	0·3 ml. (5 minims)	0·6 ml. (10 minims)
Nikethamide Injection	$\frac{1}{4}$–$\frac{1}{2}$ ml. (4 minims)	1 ml. (15 minims)	2 ml. (30 minims)	2 ml. (30 minims)
Nitrofurantoin	5–8 mg. per Kg. body-weight per day (in four divided doses)			
Norethandrolone	—	—	2·5 mg.	5·0mg.
Opii Camphorata Tinct.	0·06 ml. (1 minim)	0·2 ml. (3 minims)	0·3 ml. (5 minims)	0·6 ml. (10 minims)
Para-aminosalicylate Sodium	—	4 G. (24-hour dose)	8 G. (24-hour dose)	12 G. (24-hour dose)
Paraffin Liquid Emulsion ⎫ Paraffin Liquid ⎭	—	2–4 ml. ($\frac{1}{2}$–1 drachm)	4–8 ml. (1–2 drachms)	4–12 ml. (1–3 drachms)
Paraldehyde	—	1 ml. (15 minims) (Oral)	2 ml. (30 minims) (Oral)	4 ml. (1 drachm) (Oral) Intramuscularly, 0·15 ml. (2$\frac{1}{2}$ minims) per Kg. body-weight Per rectum, 0·45–0·6 ml. (6–10 minims) per Kg. body-weight
Paramethadione	—	0·1 G.	0·3 G.	0·3 G.
Pethidine	—	—	12·5 mg.	25 mg.

Drug	Birth	1 Year	5 Years	10 Years
Phensuximide	—	—	—	250 mg.
Phenytoin Sodium (Epanutin)	—	—	50 mg. ($\frac{3}{4}$ grain)	100 mg. ($1\frac{1}{2}$ grains)
Piperazine Adipate ⎱ Piperazine Citrate ⎰	See p. 632			
Potassium Chloride	—	0·5 G. (8 grains)	0·5 G. (8 grains)	0·5 G. (8 grains)
Potassium Citrate	60 mg. (1 grain)	200 mg. (3 grains)	600 mg. (10 grains)	900 mg. (15 grains)
Potassium Iodide	—	—	120 mg. (2 grains)	200 mg. (3 grains)
Primidone (Mysoline)	—	—	125 mg.	250 mg.
Quinine	See p. 610			
Santonin	—	—	120 mg. (2 grains)	200 mg. (3 grains)
Senna, Syrup of	—	1 ml. (15 minims)	2 ml. (30 minims)	4 ml. (60 minims)
Sodium Bicarbonate	200 mg. (3 grains)	300 mg. (5 grains)	600 mg. (10 grains)	900 mg. (15 grains)
Sodium Salicylate	—	300 mg. (5 grains)	900 mg. (15 grains)	1,200 mg. (30 grains)
Stanolone	—	12·5 mg.	25 mg. (10-day course of treatment)	50 mg.
Stramonium, Tincture of	—	0·12 ml. (2 minims)	0·2 ml. (3 minims)	0·3 ml. (5 minims)
L-Thyroxin	—	0·025 mg.	0·05 mg.	0·05 mg.

0·05 mg. equivalent to $\frac{1}{2}$ grain thyroid

Vanillic acid diethylamide   0·1 ml. ($1\frac{1}{2}$ minims) of a 5% solution diluted to
(Vandid)   1·0 ml. (15 minims) intravenously for a newborn
                             infant.   Or one to two drops on to the tongue

For treatment of certain tropical disorders, see under the relevant section in Chapter 26; for treatment of parasitic infestations see also under specific infestations in Chapter 27.

DRUG COMPLICATIONS

No medication, when used incorrectly, is free of complications; some preparations cause untoward effects in susceptible individuals even when given in standard dosages.   It is not practicable here to describe fully the pharmacology and side-effects of all the substances mentioned (the more common complications of treatment have already been discussed under the descriptions of the relevant disorders).   The following comments cover only the commoner side-effects of standard dosages of the preparations listed in Table XXX; no mention is made of the effects of over-dosage (see p. 641).

Anabolic steroids are rarely indicated in childhood; two deaths from liver damage have followed the use of norethandrolone, and jaundice is not uncommon with all the oral preparations.   Virilizing effects may occur in females.   Prolonged use of tranquillizers, including chlorpromazine and hydroxyzine, may occasionally cause liver damage.   In addition to the potential ill-effects of sulphonamides and chloramphenicol, bone-marrow depression and particularly granulocytopenia may follow the use of carbimazole and paramethadione sufficiently often to warrant repeated checks on the peripheral white blood-cell count whilst these preparations are being administered.   Rashes may follow the use of many drugs (p. 515) and an inquiry as to the nature of any treatment should be the first question concerning any patient with an obscure rash. Other complications common to many drugs include nausea, malaise, vomiting, giddiness, and bowel upset. In some individuals, hæmatemesis follows the taking of aspirin. Tinnitus is a special complication of treatment with salicylates.

DOSAGE OF DIGITALIS

Weight-for-weight, infants require somewhat more digitalis than older children, and children somewhat more than adults. Differences in individual tolerance exist.

TABLE XXXI
MEAN DOSAGE FOR DIGITILIZATION

Under Two Years of Age		Total Dose per Kg. Body-weight	Over Two Years of Age		Total Dose per Kg. Body-weight
Digoxin	.. .. ..	0·08 mg.	Digoxin	.. ..	0·06 mg.
Lanatoside C	.. ..	0·06 mg.	Lanatoside C ..	..	0·04 mg.

The total digitalizing dose should be divided into 4 or 8 doses, which should be given 6-hourly over a period of 24–48 hours according to the degree of urgency.

Alternatively, the dose of digoxin can be calculated from a method based on the surface area of the child proportionate to the adult.[1] The following percentages of the full adult digitalizing dose of digoxin (2·0–3·0 mg.) are found to apply at the following body-weights:

Body-Weight			Percentage of Adult Dose of Digoxin
3·0 Kg. (6½ lb.)	..	.. ..	12%
4·5 Kg. (10 lb.)	..	.. ..	15%
9·0 Kg. (20 lb.)	..	.. ..	25%
11·5 Kg. (25 lb.)	..	.. ..	30%
13·5 Kg. (30 lb.)	..	.. ..	33%
22·5 Kg. (50 lb.)	..	.. ..	50%
40·5 Kg. (90 lb.)	..	.. ..	75%

Maintenance Dosage. For maintenance, one-sixth to one-quarter of the total digitalizing dose given as a single daily dose.

Toxicity. Vomiting is a warning symptom. Electrocardiographic changes appear early, particularly a shortening of the QT interval. Ectopic beats may occur. Coupled beats or pulsus bigeminus is a later sign.

DOSAGE OF CHLOROTHIAZIDE

Catzel[2] points out that the proportionate dosage based on the surface area, as given above for the dosage of digoxin, can be used in the calculation of the dose of chlorothiazide. The usual adult dose ranges from 0·5–2 G. daily.

[1] Butler, A. M., Richie, R. H. (1960). *New Eng. J. Med.*, **262**, 903.
Catzel P. (1962). " The Pædiatric Prescriber ." Oxford: Blackwell Scientific Publications,
[2] Catzel, P. (1962). *Lancet*, 2, 505.

TABLE XXXII

Approximate Equivalents of Doses in the Metric and Imperial Systems

Millilitres Grammes					Minims Grains	Milligrams					Grain
10	.	.	.	.	150	80	.	.	.	.	1·1/3
8	.	.	.	.	120	75	.	.	.	.	1·1/4
6	.	.	.	.	90	60	.	.	.	.	1
5	.	.	.	.	75	50	.	.	.	.	3/4
4	.	.	.	.	60	40	.	.	.	.	3/5
3	.	.	.	.	45	30	.	.	.	.	1/2
2·6	.	.	.	.	40	25	.	.	.	.	2/5
2	.	.	.	.	30	20	.	.	.	.	1/3
1·6	.	.	.	.	25	16	.	.	.	.	1/4
1·3	.	.	.	.	20	12	.	.	.	.	1/5
1	.	.	.	.	15	10	.	.	.	.	1/6
0·8	.	.	.	.	12	8	.	.	.	.	1/8
0·6	.	.	.	.	10	6	.	.	.	.	1/10
0·5	.	.	.	.	8	5	.	.	.	.	1/12
0·4	.	.	.	.	6	4	.	.	.	.	1/16
0·3	.	.	.	.	5	3	.	.	.	.	1/20
0·25	.	.	.	.	4	2·5	.	.	.	.	1/24
0·2	.	.	.	.	3	2	.	.	.	.	1/30
0·15	.	.	.	.	2½	1·5	.	.	.	.	1/40
0·12	.	.	.	.	2	1·2	.	.	.	.	1/50
0·1	.	.	.	.	1½	1	.	.	.	.	1/60

Other commonly accepted approximate equivalents include:

Weights		Fluids	
1 oz.	≏ 30 G.	1 oz.	≏ 30 ml.
1 lb.	≏ 0·45 Kg.	1 pint	≏ 560 ml.
1 Kg.	≏ 2·2 lb.	1 litre	≏ 35 oz.

When considering American measurements for fluid therapy and infant feeding, it is to be emphasised that the American pint is equal to 16 ounces, whilst the Imperial pint contains 20 ounces.

Electrolytes of the Body Fluids

Electrolytes may be defined as chemical compounds in solution which have undergone dissociation into their constituent ions. Therefore the electrolytes of the body fluids are in solution also and they exist for the most part in ionic, that is, electrically charged, form.

When, in order to help in clinical work, the concentrations of various ions in the plasma and other body fluids (chloride, bicarbonate, phosphate, sodium, potassium, etc.) were first estimated, it was customary to express the results in terms of weight per volume, usually in milligrams per cent., but in recent years it has become generally agreed that it is better to consider the different ions in terms of chemical equivalence, that is, chemical combining power, and to think in " milliequivalents per litre " instead of " milligrams per cent."

The *equivalent* or combining *weight* of any atom, radicle or molecule is its actual weight divided by its valence; one *equivalent* (Eq) is its atomic weight in grams divided by its valence. One *milliequivalent* (mEq) is one thousandth of an equivalent:

$$\frac{\text{atomic weight in milligrams}}{\text{valence}} = 1 \text{ milliequivalent (mEq)}$$

Equivalents and milliequivalents are units with which to measure the comparative weights of different elements, compounds and groups of ions, which are equivalent chemically in their combining power.

Thus, the cation sodium (Na^+) has an atomic weight of 23 and a valence of 1. The weight of 1 milliequivalent of sodium is arrived at as follows:

$$1 \text{ mEq of Na} = \frac{23 \text{ (in milligrams)}}{1 \text{ (valence)}} = 23 \text{ milligrams}$$

Similarly, the anion chlorine (Cl^-) has an atomic weight of 35 and a valence of 1 and the weight of 1 milliequivalent of this element is

$$1 \text{ mEq of Cl} = \frac{35 \text{ (in milligrams)}}{1 \text{ (valence)}} = 35 \text{ milligrams}$$

In other words, 23 milligrams of sodium and 35 milligrams of chlorine are chemically equivalent so that they balance each other in any solution and give electrochemical neutrality.

When the concentrations of electrolytes are expressed in milliequivalents per litre, the total amount of cation and anion in solution can be compared. For example, plasma contains approximately 155 milliequivalents of cation and an equal amount of anion. The well-known Gamble diagram illustrates this chemical balance.

Conversion

When the weight of a substance in solution is given in milligrams *per litre* the number of milliequivalents per litre can be calculated by the formula

$$\frac{\text{milligrams per litre} \times \text{valence}}{\text{atomic weight}} = \text{mEq/L}$$

But since the weight of the substance is more usually expressed in milligrams *per* 100 *millilitres*, while the number of milliequivalents is expressed *per litre*, the result will then have to be multiplied by the factor 10.

(1) Thus, to convert a value expressed as *milligrams per cent* into milliequivalents per litre, multiply by 10 and by the valence and divide by the atomic weight:

$$\frac{(mg./100 \; ml.) \times 10 \times valence}{atomic \; weight} = mEq/L$$

Example:—20 mg./100 ml. of K+ $= \dfrac{20 \times 10 \times 1}{39} = 5 \cdot 1$ mEq/L.

(2) To convert a value expressed as *milliequivalents per litre* into milligrams per cent., divide by 10 and by the valence and multiply by the atomic weight:

$$\frac{(mEq/L) \times atomic \; weight}{10 \times valence} = mg. \; per \; cent.$$

Example:—100 mEq/L of Cl $= \dfrac{100 \times 35}{10 \times 1} = 350$ mg. per cent.

(3) 1 mEq/L of NaCl represents 1 mEq of Na+ and 1 mEq of Cl−. When the chloride content of a solution is given as " milligrams per cent.", it may be expressed either " as chloride " or " as NaCl." The conversion of these values, being expressed in milligrams per cent., is as follows:—

580 mg. per cent. of chloride (as NaCl) $= \dfrac{580 \times 10 \times 1}{35 + 23} = 100$ mEq of Cl/L

350 mg. per cent. of chloride (as Cl) $= \dfrac{350 \times 10 \times 1}{35} = 100$ mEq of Cl/L

(4) Until recently it has been customary to express the bicarbonate content of the plasma in terms of the *carbon dioxide combining power* (*see* alkaline reserve, p. 671) given in volumes per cent. that is to say, the volumes of CO_2 bound as bicarbonate by 100 ml. of plasma. Since, however, 1 milliequivalent of any substance yields $22 \cdot 4$ ml. of gas at N.T.P., the CO_2 combining power of the plasma in volumes per cent. can be converted into milliequivalents.

Example:— 60 vols. per cent $CO_2 = \dfrac{60 \times 10}{22 \cdot 4} = 27$ mEq/L

Electrolyte Balance

It is well known that the electrochemical neutrality of the blood plasma depends on various processes which maintain its cations and anions in balance, each being approximately 155 mEq/L. Among the electrolytes of plasma, Na+ and Cl− are in highest concentration, yet quantitatively the total amount of the *non-electrolyte bodies*, such as glucose, amino-acids and urea, transported to and from the tissue cells in a given time, is greater than the total amount of *electrolyte* moved in the same time. But these non-electrolyte bodies require for their transport only the fluid medium of the extracellular compartment, whereas the electrolytes together form, with that fluid medium, the actual chemical framework upon which depends the physical properties of the extracellular fluid.

Acid–Base Balance

The extracellular fluid is concerned with the maintenance of hydrogen-ion concentration, and a remarkably efficient mechanism exists for retaining the *p*H of the blood plasma between $7 \cdot 3$ and $7 \cdot 5$, in spite of the ingestion of acid and basic substances and their formation by the tissues in considerable quantity. This mechanism is a continuous adjustment carried out by (1) compensatory alterations in the composition of the extracellular fluid, and (2) elimination of unwanted acid and basic ions by excretion in lungs and kidneys.

(1) The compensatory alterations in the extracellular fluid depend on the buffer systems which can soak up excess acid or excess alkali without the pH of the plasma being changed. The main buffer system is a rapid-acting one, namely, the bicarbonate-carbonic acid buffers. At pH 7·4 the following ratio obtains:

$$H.HCO_3 : B.HCO_3 = 1 : 20$$

When altered, important mechanisms exist for the rapid correction of this ratio. The phosphate buffers act more slowly because they depend on renal elimination of monosodium phosphate, a slower process than the elimination of CO_2 by the lungs. Other buffers exist in the form of plasma protein and hæmoglobin.

The amount of bicarbonate in the plasma, after all acid stronger than carbonic acid has been removed, is called the *alkaline reserve*. This measures the quantity of base available for the immediate neutralization of additional acid as this enters the plasma. A disturbance of acid-base balance is then reflected in an alteration in the alkaline reserve. The alkaline reserve is not, however, an indication of the total base in the plasma because a large amount of plasma sodium, being in balance with chloride, is not available for the neutralization of additional acid.

The alkaline reserve of the plasma is usually expressed as its *carbon dioxide combining power* in volumes CO_2 per cent. This value can be converted into milliequivalents (*see* p. 670).

(2) Both lungs and kidneys are concerned in the excretory side of acid-base regulation. The respiratory centre is sensitive to changes in pH and this, by regulating CO_2 elimination, adjusts alterations in the normal ratio already given above.

$$H.HCO_3 : B.HCO_3 = 1 : 20$$

" Fixed acids," such as sulphuric acid and phosphoric acid, which are produced by the breakdown of sulphur- and phosphorus-containing proteins, are neutralized by the buffer substances of the plasma; then the salts of these " fixed acids " are excreted by the kidneys. Excess sodium bicarbonate is also eliminated by the kidneys. The work of the phosphate buffers is completed by the excretion of monosodium phosphate in the urine.

A short book by Gamble[1] beautifully illuminates this subject and is recommended for further reading.

[1] Gamble, J. L. (1951). " The Companionship of Water and Electrolytes in the Organisation of Body Fluids." Lane Medical Lectures. London: Oxford University Press.

Normal Values for Height, Weight, Skull Circumference and Skeletal Maturation

HEIGHT AND WEIGHT

The charts on the following pages show the ranges of normal height and weight in childhood. They were prepared at the Institute of Child Health, Great Ormond Street, by Dr. J. M. Tanner and Mr. R. H. Whitehouse, who obtained the data for children aged 0–5 years from the Institute of Education, the Institute of Child Health, and the Child Study Centre of the University of London, and the Oxford Child Health Survey; the data for children aged 5–15 years was obtained from the London County Council Survey (1955). The children were measured without shoes for height and without clothes for weight. If a child is weighed with clothes, therefore, the appropriate adjustment should be made before the weight is charted.

In interpreting the findings, it is suggested that children outside the area of the tenth to nineteenth percentile range should be regarded with some suspicion, and those outside the third to ninety-seventh range as abnormal until proved otherwise.

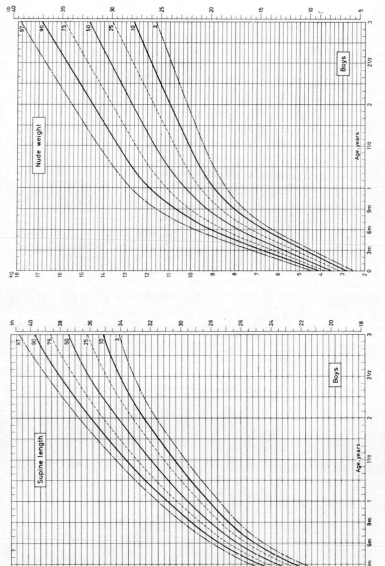

Boys 0–3 years: weight.

Boys 0–3 years: height.

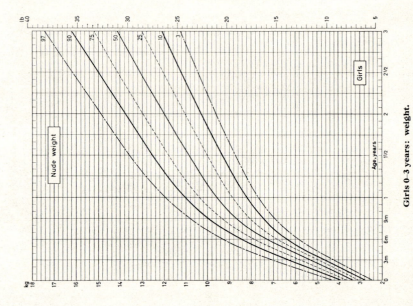

Girls 0-3 years: weight.

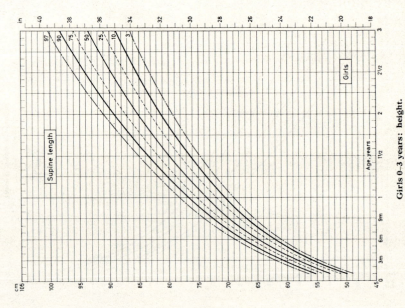

Girls 0-3 years: height.

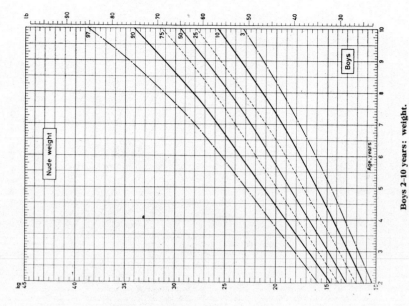

Boys 2-10 years: weight.

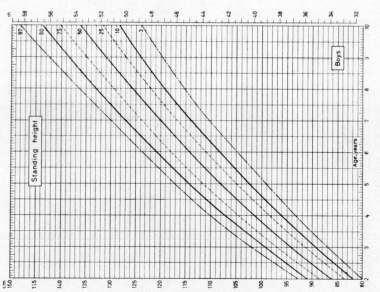

Boys 2-10 years: height.

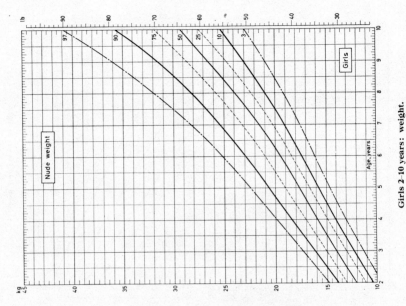

Girls 2–10 years: weight.

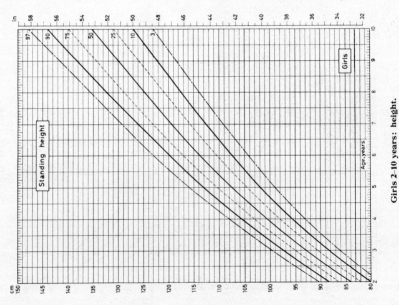

Girls 2–10 years: height.

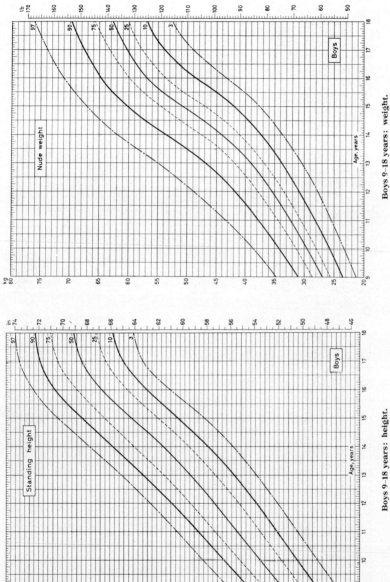

Boys 9–18 years: weight.

Boys 9–18 years: height.

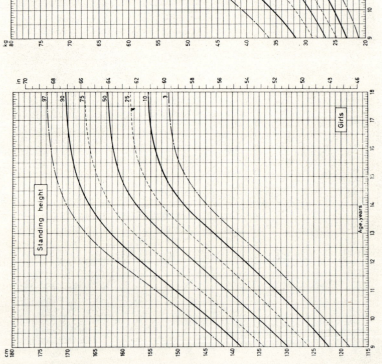

Girls 9–18 years: weight

Girls 9–18 years: height.

CHEST AND SKULL CIRCUMFERENCE

TABLE XXXIII

NORMAL VALUES FOR SKULL AND THORAX CIRCUMFERENCE
(the first figure refers to boys, the lower figure in brackets to girls)

Age	Chest Circumference (inches)	Head Circumference (inches)
At Birth	13·4	13·9 ($\pm$ ·5)
(Full Term)	(13·0)	(13·5)
6 months	16·5	17·0 ($\pm$ ·5)
	(16·1)	(16·6)
1 year	18·0	18·0 ($\pm$ ·5)
	(17·5)	(17·5)
1½ years	18·7	18·6 ($\pm$ ·5)
	(18·2)	(18·0)
2 years	19·3	19·2 ($\pm$ ·5)
	(18·8)	(18·6)
2½ years	19·8	19·5 ($\pm$ ·5)
	(19·3)	(19·0)
3 years	20·3	19·8 ($\pm$ ·5)
	(19·8)	(19·4)

OSSIFICATION DATA

THE development of the skeleton is marked by the appearance of the epiphyseal centres; there are considerable degrees of anatomical variability, as shown in the ossification table on the following pages. In order to estimate a child's skeletal age, an x-ray survey is made and the results are then compared with the data in the age columns.

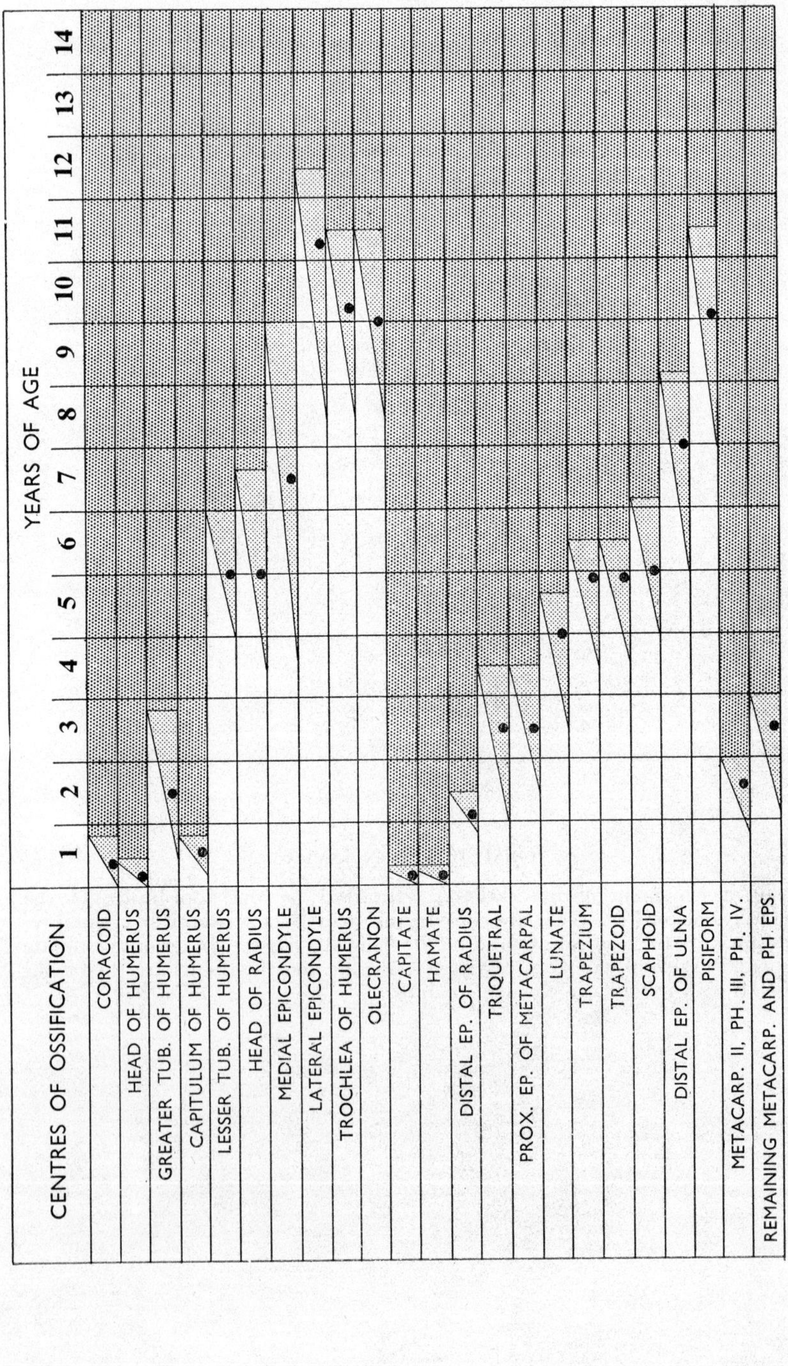
CENTRES OF OSSIFICATION
YEARS OF AGE
1
2
3
4
5
6
7
8
9
10
11
12
13
14
CORACOID
HEAD OF HUMERUS
GREATER TUB. OF HUMERUS
CAPITULUM OF HUMERUS
LESSER TUB. OF HUMERUS
HEAD OF RADIUS
MEDIAL EPICONDYLE
LATERAL EPICONDYLE
TROCHLEA OF HUMERUS
OLECRANON
CAPITATE
HAMATE
DISTAL EP. OF RADIUS
TRIQUETRAL
PROX. EP. OF METACARPAL
LUNATE
TRAPEZIUM
TRAPEZOID
SCAPHOID
DISTAL EP. OF ULNA
PISIFORM
METACARP. II, PH. III, PH. IV.
REMAINING METACARP. AND PH. EPS.

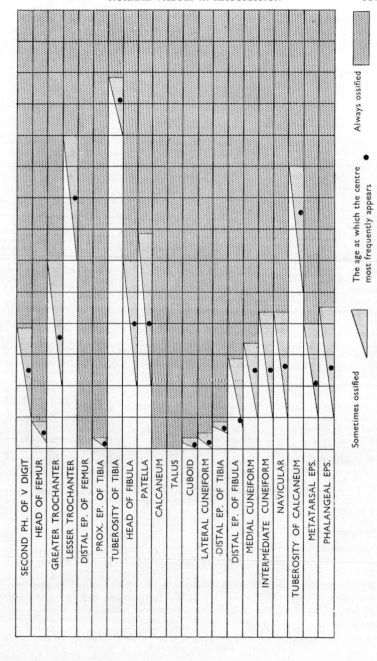

SECOND PH. OF V DIGIT
HEAD OF FEMUR
GREATER TROCHANTER
LESSER TROCHANTER
DISTAL EP. OF FEMUR
PROX. EP. OF TIBIA
TUBEROSITY OF TIBIA
HEAD OF FIBULA
PATELLA
CALCANEUM
TALUS
CUBOID
LATERAL CUNEIFORM
DISTAL EP. OF TIBIA
DISTAL EP. OF FIBULA
MEDIAL CUNEIFORM
INTERMEDIATE CUNEIFORM
NAVICULAR
TUBEROSITY OF CALCANEUM
METATARSAL EPS.
PHALANGEAL EPS.

Sometimes ossified

The age at which the centre
most frequently appears

Always ossified

Modified from Schmid and Halden (1949). Fortschr. Röntgenstr., 71, 6, 977.

Certain Special Diets

GLUTEN-FREE DIET[1]

FOR patients with cœliac disease (p. 143), a wheat and rye gluten-free diet can be constructed which is varied and interesting if full use is made of the wide range of foods allowed. It is particularly important to include generous amounts of milk and other dairy products such as butter and cheese.

FOODS ALLOWED IN A GLUTEN-FREE DIET

Almonds	Fish canned in brine, oil	Meat, fresh, all kinds
Bacon	or water	Milk, fresh
Bicarbonate of soda	Fruit, fresh, all kinds	Milk, tinned or dried
Bovril	Fruit juices and squashes	Olives
Boiled sweets (clear only)	Fruit tinned in syrup	Peels
Butter	Gelatin	Pickles, clear
Calves-foot jelly	Ginger	Prunes
Capers	Glucose	Raisins
Carraway seeds	*Gluten-free flour	Rice
Cheese	Herbs	Sago
Chicory	Honey	Salt
Cloves	Jam	Suet
Cocoa	Jam setters	Sugar
Coconut	Jelly (crystals, cubes, etc.)	Sultanas
Coffee	Junket (rennet)	Table waters
Colourings	Lard	Tapioca
Cooking-fat	Lemon juice	Tea
Cooking-oil	Lemonade (bottled) and	Treacle (golden syrup or
Cream, dairy or tinned	aerated waters	molasses)
Cream of tartar	Lentils	Vegetables, fresh or dried,
Dried fruits, all kinds	Lime juice	all kinds
Eggs	Margarine	Vegetables canned in brine
Essences	Marmalade	or water, all kinds
Fish, fresh, all kinds	Marmite	Vinegar
		Yeast, bakers'

* In the United Kingdom, gluten-free flour can be obtained; bread made from such flour is also available. Certain manufactured foods have been examined and found free of wheat or of gluten.

GLUTEN-FREE FLOUR

Gluten-free flour (that is, wheat flour from which all gluten has been removed) may be obtained in 7 lb. tins from Energen Foods Ltd., Birling Road, Ashford, Kent.

Bread made from gluten-free flour and yeast may be obtained by post from Birkett and Bostock Ltd., Dept. T.R.D., Coronation Bakery, Stockport, Cheshire. This firm also supplies wheat starch, gluten-free rusks, sweet

[1]Fletcher, R. F., McCririck, M. Y. (1958). Brit. med. J., 2,299.

biscuits, shortcake, and " Tendercake Dry-Mix ". The latter contains all the ingredients, except water, for gluten-free bread; instructions are enclosed. Local bakeries will sometimes bake gluten-free bread if there is a sufficient and regular demand, but most patients prefer to bake their own.

MANUFACTURED FOODS ALLOWED

Alfred Bird and Sons: Blancmange powder. Custard powder. Instant Postum. Instant Whip. Rice Toasties.

Brown and Polson Ltd.: Cornflour.

Cadbury Bros. Ltd.: All products at present except biscuits.

Cerebos Ltd. (Saxa): Bisto. Pepper. Spices.

Chocolate Tobler Ltd.: Toblerone and all assorted packs and bars.

Crosse and Blackwell Ltd.: Baked beans. Browning. Celery salt. Chef tomato ketchup. Fulcreem custard powder. Herring in tomato. Mayonnaise. Rennet essence. Salad cream. Sandwich spread. Sweet mango chutney. Sweet mixed pickles. Tomato ketchup.

Fray Bentos (Oxo) Ltd.: Beef: pressed, rolled and brisket. Chicken breasts in aspic. Corned beef. Crab. Cream of tomato soup. Lemco. Minced chicken. Ox tongues.

J. S. Fry and Sons Ltd.: All products at present except " Tiffin ".

H. J. Green and Co. Ltd.: Blancmange powder. Carmelle. Complete custard mix. Cornflour. Custard powder. Gravy salt. Lemonade powder.

H. J. Heinz and Co. Ltd.: Celery salt. Chutney. Gravy browning. Ideal sauce. Junior fruit dessert and pineapple. Mayonnaise. Pickle: Piccalilli, Ideal, Mixed, Royal. Potato salad. Salad cream. Sandwich spread. Soups: cream of asparagus, cream of celery, cream of green pea, cream of onion, cream of spinach, cream of tomato. Strained apples, apricots with rice, beetroot, carrots, rice pudding. Kipper spread. Chocolate pudding, cream cereal, egg custard with rice, green beans, peas, pineapples with rice. Tomato ketchup. Vegetable salad. Tomato juice. Worcestershire sauce.

H.P. Sauce Ltd.: H.P. baked beans. H.P. pickle. H.P. salad cream. H.P. tomato ketchup. H.P. tomato soup.

Keen Robinson and Co. Ltd.: Robinson's patent barley and patent groats. Ready-cooked groats and baby rice. Robsoup—chicken and bone and vegetable varieties. Three Bears oats.

James Keiller and Son Ltd.: All chocolate and sweet packs.

Kellogg and Co. Ltd.: Corn flakes. Rice Krispies. Sugar-frosted flakes. Sugar Ricicles.

Kraft Foods Ltd.: Processed cheeses, all varieties at present. Caramels. Mayonnaise. Miracle Whip. Salad cream. Salad dressing. Tomato chutney. Tomato ketchup.

J. Lyons and Co. Ltd.: Bev. Boiled sweets. Chico. Chocolate, all varieties. Custard powder. Meringues. Mousse, all flavours. Ready Brek. Strawberries in melba sauce.

Nestle Co. Ltd.: Chocolate—all varieties except Cracker Milk Bars, Crispette Biscuit Centres, and turkish delight chocolates. Lactogen. Milo chocolate food drink. Nesquik instant chocolate. Swiss Knight petit gruyére cheese.

Quaker Oats Ltd.: Oat Krunchies. Quaker one-minute oats.

Rowntree and Co. Ltd.: Aero. Beechnut chewing-gum. Elect cocoa. Fruit gums. Fruit pastilles. Milk Motoring chocolate. Polo fruits. Polo mints. Sunchoc.

A. R. Scott Ltd.: Scott's Porrage oats. Piper oatmeal. Scott's baby cereals: M.O.F., ready-cooked groats.

Smith's Potato Crisps Ltd.: Potato crisps.

A. Wander Ltd.: Vimaltol.

Ice Cream: J. Lyons and Co. Ltd.—all varieties except Wonder Ice Cake. Midland Counties Dairies Ltd. Tudor Dairies Ltd., Henley. T. Wall and Sons Ltd.—all varieties except Gaycakes.

LOW-PHENYLALANINE DIET

NATURAL PROTEIN

THE degree of restriction of dietary phenylalanine required to achieve and maintain a normal level of plasma phenylalanine varies in different patients, depending mainly upon the rate of growth and the age. Most patients require limitation of phenylalanine intake to between 10 and 30 mg./Kg./day, and in practice a diet containing 25 mg./Kg./day is started, and is varied slightly according to the resulting changes of plasma phenylalanine concentration. The calculated quantity of phenylalanine is provided in the form of natural foods, the exact amount and type of protein being selected from the food tables (*see* p. 686). Thus, an infant weighing 10 Kg. on 25 mg./Kg./day intake will require 250 mg. of phenylalanine, which can be selected from any of the foods listed. In young infants, milk or double cream will be chosen, but a more varied diet becomes important for older children. As the total quantity of natural protein which can be given is small and quite inadequate for nutritional needs, a supplement of phenylalanine/low-casein hydrolysate has to be given to provide adequate protein. The amounts of fat and carbohydrate included in these natural foodstuffs are also totally inadequate and have to be supplemented.

CALORIE REQUIREMENTS

The total calorie requirement depends upon the weight and age of the child (Table XXXIV). The calorie intakes suggested are 12 per cent. higher than those usually recommended for a normal diet, the additional quantity being necessary on account of the synthetic nature of the protein.

TABLE XXXIV

DAILY FOOD REQUIREMENTS

Age in Years	Calories (per Kg. Body-weight)	Protein* (G./Kg. Body-weight)	Fat† (G./Kg. Body-weight)	Carbohydrate‡ (G./Kg. Body-weight)
0–1	125	4·6	4·7	16·7
1–3	115	4·2	4·3	15·3
4–6	105	3·8	4·0	14·0
7–9	90	3·3	3·4	12·0
10–12	80	2·9	3·0	10·7
13–15	70	2·6	2·6	9·3
15–18	60	2·2	2·3	8·0

* 15% calorie intake.   † 35% calorie intake.   ‡ 50% calorie intake.

REQUIREMENTS OF PHENYLALANINE-LOW PROTEIN HYDROLYSATE

The main protein requirements are next calculated. These should amount to 15 per cent. of the total caloric intake (approximately 4 calories/G. protein) and are supplied as phenylalanine-low casein hydrolysate, the commercial preparations of which also include some carbohydrate, fat, vitamins, and mineral salts. For young infants up to 6 months, Minafen, a high-calorie phenylalanine-low artificial milk powder, can be prepared for use by the simple addition of an appropriate volume of water, and, apart from the essential natural protein requirements described above, together with extra vitamins and minerals, no further supplement is necessary, as this is a complete, balanced food preparation. Alternatively Lofenalac, which is also fortified with fat and carbohydrate, may be similarly used. In older children, more variety in the diet is highly desirable and Cymogran may be used to supplement the nitrogen requirements other than those supplied by natural protein. An equivalent of 40 G. of protein is supplied by every 100 G. of the preparation. Table XXXV gives the actual daily requirements of Cymogran per Kg. body-weight for each age, for two levels of phenylalanine intake.

TABLE XXXV

DAILY REQUIREMENTS OF CYMOGRAM, FAT, AND CARBOHYDRATE IN DIET

Age	Calories per Kg.	Cymogran (G./Kg.)	Fat (G./Kg.)	Carbohydrate (G./Kg.)
*Phenylalanine 25 mg./Kg. Body-Weight**				
1–3	115	14·0	3·0	10·0
4–6	105	11·5	2·5	9·5
7–9	90	9·5	2·3	8·2
10–12	80	8·5	2·0	7·3
13–15	70	7·2	1·8	6·4
15–17	60	5·9	1·6	5·6
Adult	45	4·0	1·3	4·4
Phenylalanine 10 mg./Kg. Body-Weight†				
1–3	115	14·0	3·0	9·0
4–6	105	12·5	2·5	8·5
7–9	90	10·7	2·3	7·0
10–12	80	9·5	2·0	6·3
13–15	70	8·0	1·8	5·1
15–17	60	7·0	1·6	4·5
Adult	45	5·0	1·3	3·5

* This diet allows 0·5 G. natural protein/Kg./day to supply phenylalanine needs.
† This diet allows 0·2 G. natural protein/Kg./day to supply phenylalanine needs.

CALCULATION OF ADDITIONAL CALORIES AND FAT

To achieve a balanced diet, 50 per cent. for the caloric requirements should be supplied as carbohydrate, 35 per cent. as fat, and 15 per cent. as protein (the relative proportions of Cymogran are 38 per cent., 20 per cent. and 40 per cent. respectively). Thus, after the protein needs and *some* of the calorie requirements in the older child have been supplied, *further* carbohydrate and fat are essential for normal weight gain and nutrition and also to maintain the effectiveness of the phenylalanine restriction, as an inadequate supply of calories, especially of carbohydrate, leads to negative nitrogen balance and elevation of the blood levels of phenylalanine. Gluten-free wheat starch, sugar, vegetable fat, and many of the low-protein foods may be used, and recipes have been developed for cakes, biscuits, sweets, vegetables, and fruit dishes to make the diet interesting. Table XXXIV gives the actual requirements for a given age and body-weight of the carbohydrate and fat which must be added to the Cymogran supplement to ensure adequate calories and a balanced diet.   These supplements do not include the fat and carbohydrate in the natural protein allowance, which will normally be insignificant.   Extra vitamins and minerals must be given in all low-phenylalanine diets.

QUANTITIES OF FOOD CONTAINING KNOWN AMOUNTS OF PHENYLALANINE

I. PHENYLALANINE = 200 mg.

Dairy Products

	grammes		grammes
Cheese, Cheddar	12	Milk, dried, skimmed	11
Egg, raw, boiled	31	Milk, dried, whole	14
Egg, fried	26	Trufood (reconstituted 1 part in 8 water)	222

II. PHENYLALANINE = 100 mg.

1. Dairy Products

Milk, double cream ..	107 ml.	Milk, dry, whole	7 G.
Milk, fresh	58 ml.	Trufood (1 part in 8) ..	111 G.
Milk, dry, skimmed ..	5 G.		

2. Meat

	grammes		grammes
Bacon, fried	13	Lamb chop, grilled	10
Beef, boiled	7	Lamb chop, fried	12
Beef, corned	10	Liver, ox, fried	6
Beef, roast, lean	8	Mutton, leg, boiled	10
Beef, steak, grilled	9	Mutton, leg, stewed	11
Beef, steak, fried	11	Mutton, leg, roast	11
Beef, steak, stewed	7	Pork, fresh, roast	10
Brain	16	Pork, salt, smoked	10
Chicken, boiled	9	Pork, chop, grilled	9
Chicken, roast	8	Rabbit, stewed	6
Duck, roast	11	Tongue, ox, boiled	13
Ham, boiled, lean	11	Turkey, roast	12
Heart, sheep, roast	7	Veal cutlet, fried	7
Kidney, stewed or fried	8	Veal, roast	7

3. Fish

	grammes		grammes
Cod, steamed	14	Lobster, boiled	16
Cod, fried	12	Mackerel, fried	13
Cod, grilled	9	Pollack, steamed	15
Crab, boiled	14	Pollack, fried	18
Haddock, steamed	11	Prawns, cooked	8
Haddock, fried	12	Salmon, fresh, steamed	8
Haddock, smoked, steamed ..	11	Salmon, tinned	13
Halibut, steamed	11	Sardines, tinned	12
Herrings, fried	11	Shrimps, cooked	11
Herrings, soused	10	Trout, steamed	10
Herring roe, fried	8	Turbot, steamed	27

4. *Cereals*

	grammes			grammes
All-bran	24	Grape-nuts	15
Baby cereal (Cow and Gate) ..	9	Groats (Robinson's)	12
Baby cereal, oats (Scott's) ..	19	Post Toasties	30
Baby cereal (Robinson's) ..	25	Robrex	12
Barley, peal, boiled	54	Shredded wheat	22
Cornflakes	30	Wheatflakes	20
Force	20		

5. *Bread, Biscuits, etc.*

	grammes		grammes
Bread, brown	24	Rice, raw	28
Bread, white	26	Sago	100
Ryvita	22	Tapioca	50
Vitawheat	24	Oatmeal	12

III. PHENYLALANINE = 20 mg.

1. *Fruit*

Apricot, fresh	66	Figs, dried, stewed	20
Apricot, dried, stewed	20	Gooseberries, raw	66
Apricot, tinned	80	Gooseberries, stewed	66
Banana	36	Grapes, black	66
Cherries, raw	66	Grapefruit	66
Blackberries, stewed	56	Grapes, white	66
Currants, black, stewed	66	Greengage, raw	50
Currants, red, stewed	50	Greengage, stewed	80
Currants, dried, stewed	23	Loganberries	36
Dates	20	Loganberries, tinned	66
Melon, cantaloup	40	Plums, raw	66
Melon, yellow	66	Plums, stewed	100
Nectarines	11	Prunes, stewed	44
Orange	45	Raisins, dried	36
Orange juice	66	Raspberries, raw	44
Peach, fresh	66	Raspberries, stewed	66
Peach, dried, stewed	33	Rhubarb, stewed	100
Peach, tinned	100	Strawberries, raw	66
Pear, tinned	100	Sultanas, dried	23
Pineapple, fresh	80		

2. *Vegetables*

Artichokes, boiled	28	Egg plant	56
Asparagus, boiled	16	Leeks, boiled	22
Beans, broad	14	Lettuce	36
Beans, French, boiled	76	Marrow, boiled	100
Beans, runner, boiled	76	Mushrooms, raw	16
Beetroot, boiled	58	Mushrooms, fried	14
Broccoli, boiled	14	Mustard and cress	25
Cabbage, raw	30	Onions, fried	52
Cabbage, boiled	83	Parsnips, raw	23
Carrots, raw	76	Parsnips, boiled	30
Carrots, boiled	35	Potatoes, raw	20
Cauliflower, boiled	38	Potatoes, boiled	28
Celery, raw	44	Potatoes, baked	17
Celery, boiled	66	Potatoes, roast	15

2. Vegetables—continued

	grammes		grammes
Potatoes, chipped 11		Sweet potatoes, boiled 36	
Pumpkin, raw 74		Tomatoes, raw 105	
Seakale, boiled 28		Tomatoes, fried 95	
Spring greens 23		Turnips, raw 50	
Swedes, raw 36		Turnips, boiled 56	
Swedes, boiled 44			

IV. PHENYLALANINE = 10 mg.

1. Fruit

Apple, raw 100		Loganberries, tinned 33	
Apple, baked 100		Melon, cantaloup 20	
Apricot, fresh 33		Melon, yellow 33	
Apricot, dried, stewed 10		Nectarines 22	
Apricot, tinned 40		Orange juice 22	
Banana 18		Oranges 33	
Blackberries, raw 15		Peach, fresh 33	
Blackberries, stewed 28		Peach, dried, stewed 16	
Cherries, raw 33		Peach, tinned 50	
Cherries, stewed 100		Pear, raw 66	
Currants, black, stewed 33		Pear, stewed 100	
Currants, red, stewed 25		Pear, tinned 50	
Currants, dried, stewed 11		Pineapple, fresh 40	
Damson, stewed 16		Pineapple, tinned 66	
Dates 10		Plums, raw 33	
Figs, dried, stewed 10		Plums, stewed 50	
Fruit salad, tinned 66		Prunes, stewed 22	
Gooseberries, raw 33		Raisins, dried 18	
Gooseberries, stewed 33		Raspberries, raw 22	
Grapes, black 33		Raspberries, stewed 33	
Grapes, white 33		Rhubarb, stewed 50	
Grapefruit 33		Strawberries, raw 33	
Greengage, raw 25		Sultanas, dried 11	
Greengage, stewed 40		Tangerines 22	
Loganberries 18			

2. Preserves

Blackcurrant puree 50		Jam—fruit with stones 50	
Cherries, glace 33		Marmalade 200	
Honey, comb 33		Mincemeat 33	
Honey in jars 50		Syrup, golden 33	
Jam—fruit with seeds 33		Treacle 16	

VITAMINS

Patients taking a low-phenylalanine diet require regular vitamin supplements. In the case of infants, some vitamins are contained in Minafen; Ketovite syrup (Paines & Byrne Ltd.) is designed to complete the vitamin requirement.

Ketovite Syrup, 5 ml., contains:

Vitamin A	2,500 units
Vitamin D	400 units
Choline chloride	150 mg.
Cyanocobalamin	12·5 microgrammes

Infants taking Minafen require 5 ml. daily. In addition, orange juice or other vitamin C to supply 50 mg. daily should be given.

For older children who may be taking Cymogran as their principal protein food, the additional vitamin needs are included in Ketovite tablets (Paines & Byrne Ltd.).

Ketovite tablets contain:

Aneurine hydrochloride	1·0 mg.
Riboflavin	1·0 mg.
Pyridoxine hydrochloride	0·33 mg.
Nicotinamide	3·3 mg.
Calcium pantothenate	1·16 mg.
Ascorbic acid	16·6 mg.
α-Tocopherol	5·0 mg.
Inositol	50·0 mg.
Biotin	0·17 mg.
Folic acid	0·25 mg.

Children on Cymogran should take three Ketovite tablets daily.

Legislation Concerning Children in the United Kingdom

EDUCATION

EDUCATION ACT 1944

THIS Act provides for the medical inspection, treatment and after-care of all children within compulsory school age: Sections 33 and 34 for the medical examination and placement of children requiring special forms of education on account of physical disability; Section 48 for medical inspection and free medical treatment; Section 49 for free milk and meals; Section 54 for compulsory cleansing of verminous or filthy children. Section 57, which made provision for the mentally subnormal child, is amended by the Mental Health Act 1959; this later Act makes more compassionate and comprehensive provision for the ascertainment, review and training of children of subnormal and severe subnormal mentality.

Special Education. In the United Kingdom, there are about 950 special schools which provide for physically and mentally handicapped children in the following categories: blind, partially-sighted, deaf, partially-deaf, delicate, educationally subnormal, epileptic, maladjusted, physically handicapped, and those with speech defects.

Child Guidance Clinics evaluate and treat children with emotional and behaviour problems. They are usually provided by the Local Education Authorities but in some cases come under the jurisdiction of Health Departments or, if in a hospital, the National Health Service. A clinic is staffed by a psychiatrist, a psychiatric social worker and an educational psychologist.

PROTECTION, CARE AND ADOPTION

NOTE

THE majority of children received into care are taken with the permission of the parents, thus by-passing the Courts; there having been no Court Order, the parents can at any time take their child back again. However, when there has been a Court Order, the child can be returned home only by a further Court Order. The Local Authority provides homes for such children or places them in voluntary homes or foster homes. The National Society for the Prevention of Cruelty to Children is a voluntary body which has no legal authority. This Society investigates reports of cruelty to children and, when there is sufficient evidence, can place a child in a " place of safety " without a Court Order, pending a hearing by the Magistrates' Court which decides the final disposition. Often a children's hospital is used as a " place of safety ".

CHILDREN AND YOUNG PERSONS ACT 1933

This Act provides for the care and protection of neglected or ill-treated children, and for those removed by the Courts from their parents. It makes the Local Authority responsible for the placement, with due regard to the age, aptitude and ability of the child.

An Amendment to this Act (1952) places a duty on the Local Authority to investigate information which it may receive suggesting that a child may be in need of care or protection, but it can refrain from making such investigation if not satisfied that it is necessary. This Act gives discretion to a Court to place a child in a Reception Centre for children or in a Remand Home.

CHILDREN ACT 1948

This Act, in making provision for children who suffer cruelty, neglect or loss of home life, overlaps with the Children and Young Persons Act 1933. The Children and Young Persons Act 1933 allows action to be taken through the Courts for the protection or care of a child, while the Children Act 1948 makes provision for a deprived child to be received into the care of the Local Authority; the latter is more passive, that is, it creates a favourable environment for a deprived child.

By virtue of these Acts, a doctor concerned for the well-being of his patient may bring the child to the Court, as in need of care or protection under the Children and Young Persons Act 1933, and request a Local Authority to investigate whether cruelty or neglect does in fact exist under the provision of the 1952 Amendment to this Act; he may advise the parents, because of their permanent or temporary incapacity to care for the child, to appeal under Section 1b of the Children Act 1948; or request the Local Authority to make a resolution on the child's behalf under Section 11b of this same Act.

This Act places a duty on the Local Authority to assume the care of a child where it appears to them that " (a) he has neither parent nor guardian or has been and remains abandoned by his parents or guardian, or is lost; or (b) that his parents or guardian are, for the time being or permanently, prevented by reason of mental or bodily disease or infirmity or other incapacity or any other circumstances, from providing for his proper accommodation, maintenance and upbringing; and (c) in either case, that the intervention of the Local Authority under this section is necessary in the interests of the welfare of the child ".

Having received a child into care, the Children Act 1948 empowers the Local Authority to make a resolution vesting the powers of the parent in the Children's Officer as follows: " Subject to the provisions of this Act, a Local Authority may resolve with respect to any child in their care in whose case it appears to them—

(a) that his parents are dead and that he has no guardian; or
(b) that his parent or guardian (hereinafter referred to as the person on whose account the resolution was passed) has abandoned him or suffers from some permanent disability rendering the said person incapable of caring for the child, or is of such habits or mode of life as to be unfit to have the care of the child,

that all the rights and powers which the deceased parents would have if they were still living, or, as the case may be, all the rights and powers of the person on whose account the resolution was passed, shall vest in the Local Authority ".

CHILDREN ACT AMENDMENT 1958

Part I of this Act makes provisions for child life protection which are in advance of those in the Public Health Acts of 1936. It places a duty on Local Authorities to ensure the well-being of foster-children, and defines the foster-child as "one placed with a person not related for a period longer than a month for payment or reward". The distinction between a foster-child, as defined above, and a " protected child ", i.e. one awaiting adoption, is clearly made. This Act also makes provision for the inspection of premises; it prohibits persons found unsuitable from having foster-children, and gives power to remove foster-children from such persons.

MENTAL HEALTH

MENTAL HEALTH ACT 1959

This Act repeals all previous Mental Deficiency Acts and the Mental Treatment Act, 1930. Its emphasis is on the community care of the mentally subnormal and the mentally ill.

Part I, Section 4, reclassifies mental deficiency as *subnormality* and *severe subnormality*, the old terms " idiot ", " imbecile ", and " feeble-minded " being thus superseded. Section V makes provision for the informal admission of patients to hospital and advises that there be less distinction made between the physically ill and the mentally ill, and less compulsion and formality in the admission and discharge of the mentally ill consistent with their own interests and those of the community.

Part II makes general provisions for Local Authority services. Section 6 groups the mentally ill with the physically ill for the purposes of the National Health Act, and makes provision for the " prevention of illness, care, and after-care of patients ". This is another advance towards the merging of mental and physical illness. Section 9 provides for a mentally subnormal or mentally ill child to be received into care for placement in a Reception Centre by a Children's Officer under the Children Act 1948. The section of the Education Act 1944, by which a child deemed ineducable (and therefore unable to be dealt with by the normal educational services) was supervised at home and only sometimes received at an Occupation Centre, is amended by the Mental Health Act 1959, which places a duty on the Local Authority to know of all such children, to provide medical inspection for them and to place them in Training Centres (formally known as Occupation Centres). Attendance at such a Training Centre is now compulsory in exactly the same way as education is compulsory. The penalties for failure on the part of the parents are the same, but the parent who can show evidence of comparable training in the home will be allowed to contract out if to do so is in the best interests of the child. The parent can appeal for review in the case of a child deemed " unsuitable for education ", whereas only the Institution where the child might be placed, or the Local Authority, could previously require this review.

INDEX

BIOCHEMICAL FINDINGS IN NORMAL CHILDREN

Continued from the front of the book.

Estimation	*Result*

DUODENAL JUICE

Amylase	500–1,500 Somogyi units/100 ml.
Lipase	Over 20 units/100 ml. (Anderson, 1942)
Trypsin	A dilution of 1 in 100 digests gelatin

SWEAT

Sodium	10–60 mEq/L.
Potassium	5–15 mEq/L.

FÆCES

Trypsin	Under 2 years of age, a 1 in 100 dilution of fresh stool usually digests gelatin
Fat	After 1 year of age, 95–98 per cent. of fat is absorbed (Van de Kamer, Huinink, and Weijers, 1949)

URINE

Creatinine clearance — Newborn infants and prematures: 40–65 cc./min./1·73 sq. m.
Children, boys: 98–150 cc./min./1·73 sq. m.
girls: 95–123 cc./min./1·73 sq. m.

Urea clearance

	Maximum clearance (ml./1·73 sq. m./minute)	Standard clearance (ml./1·73 sq. m./minute)	Clearance (ml./sq. m./minute)
Premature infants			15
Full-term infants			20
Children over 2 years	75	54	40

17-ketosteroids — 0–1 year: 0·25 ± 0·12 mg./24 hours (± S.D.)
1–5 years: 0·78 ± 0·46 mg./24 hours
6–10 years: 1·38 ± 0·74 mg./24 hours
11–17 years: 4·96 ± 2·06 mg./24 hours (Prout and Snaith 1958)

Total 17-hydroxycorticoids — There is a gradual rise during childhood with a sharp rise at puberty
Up to 10 years: 1·0–4·5 mg./24 hours
10–20 years: 4·5–19 mg./24 hours depending on age, sex and body build (Appleby, Gibson, Norymberski, and Stubbs, 1955)

CEREBRO-SPINAL FLUID

Pressure	50–150 mm. water
Sugar	70–85 mg./100 ml.
Chlorides	700–750 mg./100 ml.
Total protein	10–30 mg./100 ml.
Cells	Less than 5 lymphocytes per c.mm.

Details of blood chemistry are given at the front of the book.